Congenital Heart Disease in Adults

Cardiovascular Clinics Series

*Not Available

Congenital Heart Disease in Adults

William C. Roberts, M.D. | Editor

Chief, Pathology Branch
National Heart, Lung and Blood Institute
National Institutes of Health
Bethesda, Maryland

and

Clinical Professor of Pathology and Medicine (Cardiology)
Georgetown University
Washington, D.C.

CARDIOVASCULAR CLINICS

Albert N. Brest, M.D. | Editor-in-Chief

James C. Wilson Professor of Medicine
Director, Division of Cardiology
Jefferson Medical College
Philadelphia, Pennsylvania

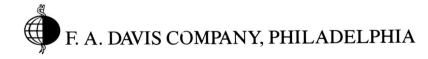 F. A. DAVIS COMPANY, PHILADELPHIA

Cardiovascular Clinics 10/1, Congenital Heart Disease in Adults

Copyright © 1979 by F. A. Davis Company
Second printing 1979
Third printing 1980
Fourth printing 1980
Fifth printing 1981
Sixth printing 1982

Printed in the United States of America

Library of Congress Cataloging in Publication Data
Main entry under title:

Congenital heart disease in adults.

  (Cardiovascular clinics ; 10/1)
  Includes bibliographical references and index.
  1. Heart—Abnormalities. I. Roberts, William
Clifford, 1932- II. Series. [DNLM: 1. Heart
defects, Congenital—In adulthood—Congresses. W1
CA77N v. 10 no. 1 / WG220 C754]
RC681.A1C27 vol. 10, no. 1 [RC687] 616.1'1008s
ISBN 0-8036-7419-8 [616.1'2'043] 78-21460

Preface

This is the first book, to my knowledge, to focus specifically on adults with major congenital malformations of the heart or great vessels. Primarily because of operative treatment, survival to adulthood of more and more infants and children with congenital cardiovascular anomalies affords adult cardiologists the opportunity to be involved with long-term follow-up of these patients.

Many questions regarding prognosis for adults with congenital cardiovascular anomalies treated definitively or incompletely in early life remain unanswered. How often will aortic isthmic coarctation resected in childhood restenose in adulthood? How many patients with aortic coarctation resected in childhood will need aortic valve replacement in adulthood because of stenotic or incompetent congenitally malformed aortic valves? Not all patients with tetralogy of Fallot "totally corrected" in early life are actually "totally corrected" in later life. How will the right ventricle function in later life when incised in childhood for closure of ventricular septal defect or partially excised for relief of outflow obstruction or when the stenotic pulmonic valve was partially excised? What will be the ultimate fate of the cleft and abnormally attached (by chordae tendineae to the left ventricular outflow tract) mitral valve in patients with atrioventricular canal who had the primum type atrial septal defect closed in childhood? Will the frequency of mitral valve prolapse in adult patients with fossa ovale type atrial septal defect be decreased by closure of the defect in childhood? These questions represent only a few of the many needing answers. The aim of this text is to present a better understanding of the problems and provide answers where possible.

The chapters dealing with specific congenital malformations generally are the result of the combined efforts of a pediatric cardiologist and an adult cardiologist. This approach by a combination of disciplines makes the presentation more comprehensive.

I thank the authors of the various chapters for providing superb information about adults with congenital cardiac disease and the F. A. Davis Company for their splendid cooperation and help.

William C. Roberts, M.D.
Guest Editor

Editor's Commentary

The broad clinical spectrum of congenital heart disease is manifested in full bloom in those patients who reach adulthood. The age range of individuals with congenital cardiac anomalies is steadily increasing by virtue of improved medical care in the young and by dint of palliative and corrective surgery. In recent years, too, we have come to better recognize certain congenital cardiac disorders which become manifest initially in adulthood. We have broadened our diagnostic and therapeutic approaches. We have a better understanding of natural evolution, including spontaneous (natural) "cures." This text explores comprehensively the natural and unnatural (i.e., changing postsurgical) history, clinical recognition and management of congenital heart disease in adults.

I am enormously grateful to Dr. William Roberts for his invaluable guidance in the formulation of this text and to the individual contributors for their truly outstanding contributions.

Albert N. Brest, M.D.
Editor-in-Chief

Contributors

Robert J. Adolph, M.D.
Professor of Medicine, Director, Cardiac Research Laboratories, University of Cincinnati, College of Medicine, Cincinnati, Ohio

Denton A. Cooley, M.D.
Clinical Professor of Surgery (Cardiovascular and Thoracic), University of Texas Medical School at Houston; Surgeon-In-Chief, Texas Heart Institute of St. Luke's Episcopal Hospital and Texas Children's Hospital, Houston, Texas

J. Michael Criley, M.D.
Professor of Medicine, University of California, Los Angeles; Chief, Division of Cardiology, Harbor General Hospital, Torrance, California

James E. Dalen, M.D.
Professor of Medicine, University of Massachusetts Medical School, Worcester, Massachusetts

Gordon K. Danielson, M.D.
Professor of Surgery, Mayo Medical School, Rochester, Minnesota

Lewis Dexter, M.D.
Professor Emeritus of Medicine, Harvard Medical School, Boston, Massachusetts

Jesse E. Edwards, M.D.
Director of Laboratories, United Hospitals-Miller Division, St. Paul, Minnesota

Larry P. Elliott, M.D.
Professor and Director, Division of Cardiac Radiology, University of Alabama Medical Center, Birmingham, Alabama

R. Curtis Ellison, M.D.
Senior Associate in Cardiology, Chief, Cardiology Department, Children's Hospital Medical Center, Boston, Massachusetts

Mary Allen Engle, M.D.
Professor of Pediatrics, Cornell University Medical College; Director of Pediatric Cardiology, The New York Hospital, New York, New York

Stephen E. Epstein, M.D.
Chief, Cardiology Branch, National Heart, Lung, and Blood Institute, National Institutes of Health, Bethesda, Maryland

Victor J. Ferrans, M.D., Ph.D.
Chief, Ultrastructure Section, Pathology Branch, National Heart, Lung and Blood Institute, National Institutes of Health, Bethesda, Maryland

William J. French, M.D.
Assistant Professor of Medicine, University of California, Los Angeles, School of Medicine; Co-Director, Cardiac Catheterization Laboratory, Harbor General Hospital, Torrance, California

William F. Friedman, M.D.
Professor of Pediatrics and Chief, Pediatric Cardiology, University of California, San Diego, School of Medicine, La Jolla, California

Gottlieb C. Friesinger, M.D.
Professor of Internal Medicine and Director, Division of Adult Cardiology, Vanderbilt University Medical Center, Nashville, Tennessee

Arthur Garson, Jr., M.D.
Fellow, Pediatric Cardiology, Baylor College of Medicine and, Texas Children's Hospital, Houston, Texas

Thomas P. Graham, Jr., M.D.
Professor of Pediatrics and Director, Pediatric Cardiology, Vanderbilt University Medical Center, Nashville, Tennessee

Charles I. Haffajee, M.D.
Assistant Professor of Medicine, University of Massachusetts Medical School, Worcester, Massachusetts

Wade T. Hamilton, M.D.
Clinical Fellow, Pediatrics, Harvard Medical School, Boston, Massachusetts

W. Proctor Harvey, M.D.
Professor of Medicine and Director, Division of Cardiology, Georgetown University Medical Center, Washington, D.C.

Joel Heger, M.D.
Fellow in Cardiology, University of California, Los Angeles School of Medicine, Harbor General Hospital Campus, Torrance, California

Walter L. Henry, M.D.
Senior Investigator, Cardiology Branch, National Heart, Lung and Blood Institute, National Institutes of Health, Bethesda, Maryland

J. O'Neal Humphries, M.D.
Robert Levy Professor of Cardiology, The Johns Hopkins University, School of Medicine, Baltimore, Maryland

Allen D. Johnson, M.D.
Assistant Professor of Medicine, University of California, San Diego School of Medicine, La Jolla, California

Michael Jones, M.D.
Senior Surgeon, Surgery Branch, National Heart, Lung and Blood Institute, National Institutes of Health, Bethesda, Maryland

Samuel Kaplan, M.D.
Professor of Pediatrics and Associate Professor of Medicine, University of Cincinnati College of Medicine; Director, Division of Pediatric Cardiology, Children's Hospital Medical Center, Cincinnati, Ohio

David T. Kelly, M.D.
Scandrett Professor of Cardiology and Director, Hallstrom Institute of Cardiology, University of Sydney, Camperdown, New South Wales, Australia

Langford Kidd, M.D.
Harriet Lane Home Professor of Pediatric Cardiology and Director, Division of Pediatric Cardiology, Johns Hopkins University, School of Medicine, Baltimore, Maryland

Susan Anderson Kline, M.D.
Clinical Associate Professor of Medicine, Cornell University Medical College; Director, Adult Cardiac Catheterization Laboratory, The New York Hospital, New York, New York

Barry J. Maron, M.D.
Senior Investigator, Cardiology Branch, National Heart, Lung and Blood Institute, National Institutes of Health, Bethesda, Maryland

Dwight C. McGoon, M.D.
Chief of Thoracic Surgery, Mayo Clinic, Rochester, Minnesota

Dan G. McNamara, M.D.
Professor of Pediatrics and Chief of Cardiology Section, Baylor College of Medicine and Texas Children's Hospital, Houston, Texas

Alexander S. Nadas, M.D.
Professor of Pediatrics, Harvard Medical School; Chief, Cardiology Department, Children's Hospital Medical Center, Boston, Massachusetts

Valerie Novak
Senior Medical Student, University of California, San Diego School of Medicine, La Jolla, California

Joseph K. Perloff, M.D.
Professor of Medicine and Pediatrics, University of California, Los Angeles School of Medicine, Los Angeles, California

William C. Roberts, M.D.
Chief, Pathology Branch, National Heart, Lung and Blood Institute, National Institutes of Health, Bethesda, Maryland; Clinical Professor of Pathology and Medicine (Cardiology), Georgetown University, Washington, D.C.

Laurence J. Sloss, M.D.
Instructor in Medicine and Pediatrics, Harvard Medical School; Director, Heart Station, Peter Bent Brigham Hospital, Boston, Massachusetts

Renu Virmani, M.D.
Staff Fellow, Pathology Branch, National Heart, Lung and Blood Institute, National Institutes of Health, Bethesda, Maryland

Contents

Classification of Congenital Heart Disease in the Adult*

Jesse E. Edwards, M.D.

The adult studied for congenital heart disease symptoms may not have been previously suspected of having such a condition. The following classification of congenital heart disease in the adult deviates from standard classifications. It is, rather, an approach through dominant clinical states that may be shared with various forms of acquired heart disease. The groupings presented here will hopefully aid the clinician in considering particular types of congenital heart disease as he evaluates the patient with a particular clinical pattern. With this end in view, a classification of congenital heart disease in the adult is presented (Table 1).

Table 1. Classification of congenital heart disease in the adult.

1. Acyanotic types
    a. Prominence of pulmonary arteries
        (1) Presence of pulmonary venous obstruction
        (2) Absence of pulmonary venous obstruction
    b. Left ventricular outflow obstruction
    c. Hypertension
    d. Aortic regurgitation
        (1) Regurgitation through valve
        (2) Left-to-right shunts originating in aorta
2. Cyanotic types
    a. Presence of right ventricular hypertrophy
    b. Absence of right ventricular hypertrophy

ACYANOTIC TYPES

The acyanotic types of congenital heart disease observed in adults include states in which the dominant picture is (1) prominence of the pulmonary arteries as seen in roentgenograms, (2) signs of left ventricular outflow obstruction, (3) systemic hypertension, and (4) pulse characteristics in common with aortic regurgitation.

Prominence of the major pulmonary arteries occurs either without or with pulmonary venous obstruction. Without pulmonary venous obstruction, the common causes of prominence of the pulmonary arteries are (1) poststenotic or idiopathic dilatation of the pulmonary trunk, and (2) left-to-right shunts, particularly those occurring at defects between the cardiac chambers or great arteries. These conditions are usually associated

*This study was supported by Public Health Service Research Grant 5 RO1 HL05694 from the National Heart, Lung and Blood Institute, and by the Saint Paul Foundation, St. Paul, Minnesota.

1

with normal pulmonary arterial "wedge" pressures, although in some conditions the pulmonary arterial pressure may be elevated. With pulmonary venous obstruction, both the pulmonary arterial and pulmonary arterial "wedge" pressures are elevated.

Prominence of Pulmonary Arteries without Pulmonary Venous Obstruction

Prominence of the pulmonary arteries without pulmonary venous obstruction may be a manifestation of (1) poststenotic or idiopathic dilatation of the pulmonary trunk, (2) shunts resulting from septal defects or (3) communications between the great arteries.

Poststenotic Dilatation of the Pulmonary Trunk

Poststenotic dilatation of the pulmonary trunk is a classic feature of congenital pulmonary valvular stenosis with intact ventricular septum.[1] The basic abnormality is the dome-shaped stenosis of the pulmonary valve (Fig. 1). The valvular tissue fails to form distinct commissures and takes the configuration of a truncated cone. As a result, the effective orifice of the valve may be only a few millimeters in diameter, while the diameter of the pulmonary trunk is many times wider than the effective orifice. The branches of the pulmonary trunk usually are not involved in dilatation. The marked elevation of right ventricular pressure incident to the obstructed valve is accompanied by corresponding concentric hypertrophy of the right ventricular wall. This condition may lead to secondary muscular infundibular stenosis. If the foramen ovale is anatomically sealed, no shunt is possible; if it is potentially patent, a right-to-left shunt may occur. The latter aspect of pulmonary valvular stenosis with intact septum will be covered in the section dealing with cyanotic types.

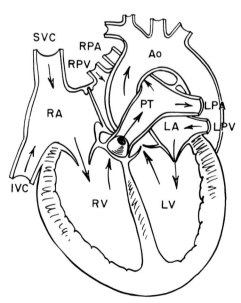

Figure 1. Pulmonary valvular stenosis with intact ventricular septum and poststenotic dilatation of pulmonary trunk.

2

Idiopathic Dilatation of the Pulmonary Trunk

Idiopathic dilatation of the pulmonary trunk is characterized by asymptomatic dilatation of the pulmonary trunk in the absence of the usual causes of pulmonary arterial widening. The peripheral pulmonary arteries are normal. The condition appears to be a manifestation of cystic medial necrosis of the vessel and may be viewed as a variant of arachnodactyly (Marfan's syndrome).[2] The diagnosis is made by excluding other conditions that cause enlargement of the pulmonary trunk, particularly pulmonary valvular stenosis[3] and pulmonary parenchymal disease.

Septal Defects

Septal defects, including patent ductus arteriosus and aorticopulmonary window, are causes of prominence of the major pulmonary arteries. Atrial septal defect is the most common cause in the adult. In contrast to the two previously cited conditions, the peripheral pulmonary arteries are also dilated.

ATRIAL SEPTAL DEFECT. The anatomic locations of atrial septal defects vary. The *ostium secundum* type is most common and is located at the fossa ovalis[4] (Fig. 2a). Probably the next most common is the *sinus venosus* type (Fig. 2b), which lies superior to the fossa ovalis. This defect is near the entrance of the superior vena cava and may be overhung by that vessel. It is part of a developmental complex that includes anomalous termination of right pulmonary veins either into the terminal part of the superior vena cava or the nearby right atrium. Consistently, the vein of the upper lobe of the right lung is involved and, in some instances, the entire venous drainage of the right lung may terminate anomalously in the manner described.

A third type of atrial septal defect, *ostium primum,* is that involving the lowermost part of the atrial septum. This defect characteristically is associated with deficiency of the ventricular septum and clefts in the atrioventricular valves—a complex known as *persistent common atrioventricular canal* or *endocardial cushion defect* (Fig. 2c). Clefts in both the mitral and tricuspid valves and interventricular communication are common here. This combination usually leads to death in infancy; the exception occurs when the condition includes a large interventricular communication, and the tetralogy of Fallot is associated. The pulmonary stenosis of the associated tetralogy protects from the effects of the large interventricular communication and allows survival into adulthood.[5]

When the endocardial cushion defect is not associated with an interventricular communication, survival into adulthood is common since the heart shows an ostium primum atrial septal defect and a cleft only in the mitral valve. Such patients have been known to survive to the eighth decade.[6]

The least common of the atrial septal defects is that which lies in the *posteroinferior angle of the atrial septum* at the usual position of the right atrial ostium of the coronary sinus (Fig. 2d). Such defects, which in some cases are confluent with an ostium primum type of defect, are part of a developmental complex which includes absence of the coronary sinus and termination of a persistent left superior vena cava in the left atrium.[7]

Regardless of specific anatomic type, atrial septal defects are for many years associated with a large left-to-right shunt and normal pulmonary arterial pressure. As a consequence of the shunt, there is enlargement—without hypertrophy—of the right atrium and ventricle. The entire pulmonary vascular bed is wider than normal.

Complicating obstructive pulmonary vascular disease does not usually develop until the third or fourth decade. The resulting pulmonary hypertension is responsible for right ventricular hypertrophy, and the latter may underlie the appearance of a right-to-left shunt (Fig. 3).

ANOMALOUS CONNECTION OF PULMONARY VEINS. Anomalous connection of pulmo-

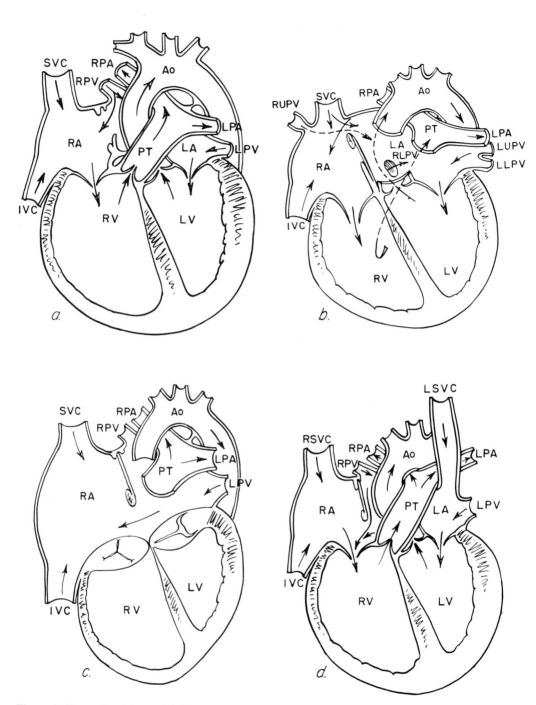

Figure 2. Types of atrial septal defect with sole or dominant left-to-right shunt. a. Fossa ovalis type with left-to-right shunt. b. Sinus venosus type. Anomalous pulmonary venous connection from the right lung is a component. c. Defect involving the lowermost part of the atrial septum with cleft mitral valve, known as ostium primum defect with cleft mitral valve. d. Developmental complex of atrial septal defect in the posterior-inferior angle of the atrial septum, absence of the coronary sinus, and union of the left superior vena cava with the left atrium.

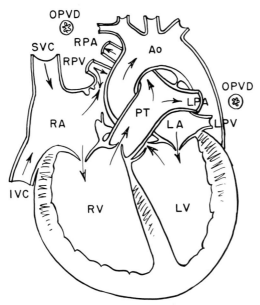

Figure 3. Atrial septal defect with right-to-left shunt. Right ventricular hypertrophy is present and is the underlying basis for the right-to-left shunt.

nary veins, total or partial, either into a systemic vein or into the right atrium, may be observed in the adult and yields states which are functionally akin to atrial septal defect.[8,9] In the total form, an interatrial communication is universally present, while in patients with partial anomalous connection the atrial septum may be intact or have an opening. For individuals to reach adulthood there can be no element of pulmonary venous obstruction which would tend to cause death at an early age. Since pulmonary venous obstruction is usually not observed in adult patients with anomalous pulmonary venous connection, the characteristic sites of anomalous pulmonary venous termination seen in the adult are supradiaphragmatic in position and include the left innominate vein (Fig. 4), the coronary sinus, or the superior vena cava. Less common sites include the left superior vena cava and, uncommonly, the azygos vein.[10] A patient may show termination of the right pulmonary veins into the inferior vena cava in close relationship with the diaphragm, but this is rare as an isolated entity. Some such terminations may be part of the scimitar syndrome.[11] In addition to anomalous termination of right pulmonary veins into the inferior vena cava, this syndrome may include other anomalies, such as right pulmonary arterial supply from the descending thoracic or abdominal aorta, bronchial abnormalities, dextrocardia, and sequestration of the right lung.[11,12]

Post-tricuspid shunts may occur at the level of the ventricular septum or between the pulmonary arteries. At the ventricular septum, the anomaly is most commonly that of a ventricular septal defect (VSD). The so-called left ventricular—right atrial communication is uncommon.

Ventricular Septal Defect. VSDs may be considered from an anatomic or from a functional point of view. It is beyond the scope of this presentation to enter into a detailed consideration of the various anatomic types and locations of VSDs. This subject has been covered in existing reports.[13,14] From a functional point of view, VSD may be classified into two types, the small VSD and the large VSD, with recognized gradations from one to the other. Defects which are of about the same diameter as the aortic valvular orifice function as *large VSDs*,[15] while those smaller than the orifice function as *small VSDs*.

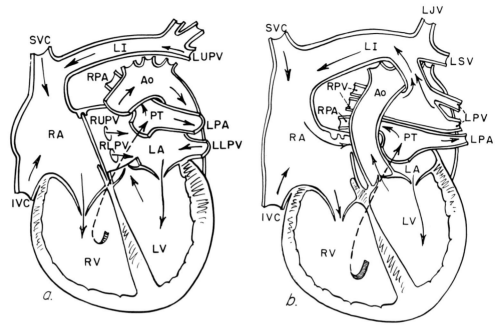

Figure 4. Anomalous connection of pulmonary veins to the left innominate vein (LI). a. The partial type. b. The total type.

The small VSD (Fig. 5a) has the characteristics of an obstructed opening between the two ventricles and, as such, prevents transmission of left ventricular pressure into the right ventricle. Characteristically, the pressure in the latter chamber and in the pulmonary arterial system is normal. Right ventricular hypertrophy is absent and the associated left-to-right shunt is of limited volume. Thus, the demands upon circulatory dynamics are minimal and allow subjects to reach adult life. The one significant potential problem with small VSD is the patient's susceptibility to bacterial endocarditis arising from the traumatic effects of the jet-like stream constituting the left-to-right shunt.

A large VSD (Fig. 5b) is an unobstructed opening between the ventricles. As such, it allows equalization of pressures between the ventricles, with the systemic and pulmonary arterial systolic pressures being equal to each other and to the ventricular systolic pressures. Thus, pulmonary hypertension is a component of the hemodynamic state in large VSD. A left-to-right shunt is the early characteristic feature, and this may be lethal in infancy. Those patients who survive infancy are subject to ultimate development of obstructive pulmonary vascular disease and its associated right-to-left shunt. This complicated state is usually reached by adolescence, leaving relatively few surviving adult patients. The majority of patients that do reach adult life with a large VSD harbor obstructive pulmonary vascular disease. In this state, patients are subject to intensification of the right-to-left shunt whenever the systemic arterial pressure falls for any reason (Fig. 6). Childbirth represents a major challenge and is peculiarly responsible for catastrophic intensified hypoxia associated with a fall in systemic pressure.

It is to be emphasized that the right-to-left shunt commonly present in adult subjects with large VSD is the result of complicating obstructive pulmonary vascular disease, rather than the result of details in relationship between the aorta and the right ventricle.[16]

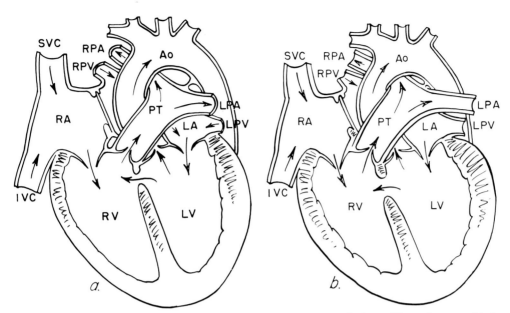

Figure 5. Two functional types of VSD. a. The small type. The right ventricular wall is not hypertrophied and the shunt is limited in extent. b. Large type. The defect is an unobstructed communication. Right ventricular hypertrophy and pulmonary hypertension are associated. Phase of left-to-right shunt is shown.

Functionally similar to VSD are anomalies which carry specific anatomic designations, such as single ventricle without pulmonary stenosis (Fig. 7a), certain forms of double outlet right ventricle (Fig. 7b), and persistent truncus arteriosus (Fig. 7c). As these states are distinctly less common than VSD and carry the same chance of death by adolescence, it is uncommon to observe adults with these conditions, but brief mention of each is justified at this point.

Single ventricle, as the name implies, represents absence of the ventricular septum, and the outflow portion is usually subdivided into subaortic and subpulmonary

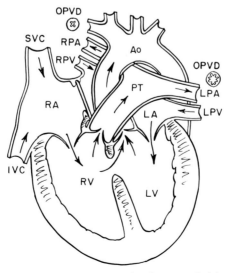

Figure 6. Large VSD with obstructive pulmonary vascular disease and right-to-left shunt.

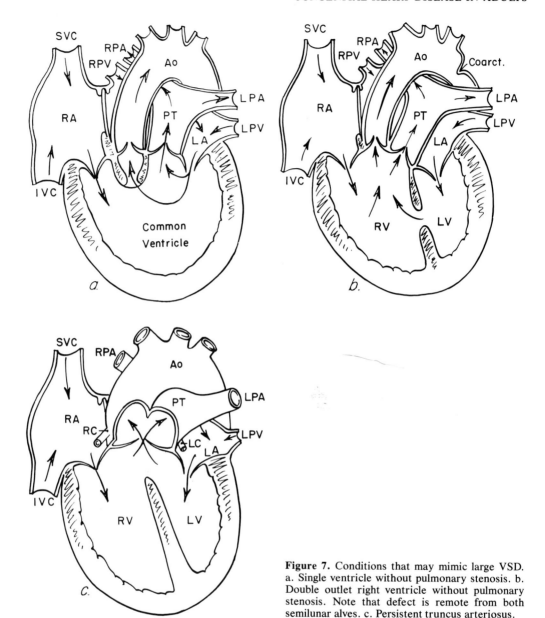

Figure 7. Conditions that may mimic large VSD. a. Single ventricle without pulmonary stenosis. b. Double outlet right ventricle without pulmonary stenosis. Note that defect is remote from both semilunar alves. c. Persistent truncus arteriosus.

portions.[17-20] Pulmonary or subpulmonary stenosis may be present, and tend to place the case into a different functional category than that under discussion (acyanotic type). When pulmonary stenosis is absent, the dynamics are like those in large VSD. Usually, the great vessels do not exhibit normal relationships; the ascending aorta arises anteriorly with respect to the origin of the pulmonary trunk. In classic examples of single ventricle both atrioventricular valves are present. The tricuspid valve is not usually atretic, and only rarely is the mitral valve atretic, since most patients with either tricuspid or mitral atresia succumb long before adulthood.

Double outlet right ventricle occurs when both great arterial vessels originate from the right ventricle and the only outlet for the left ventricle is a VSD. There is variation with regard to the relationship between the position of the VSD and the origins of the great vessels.[21] Also, pulmonary stenosis may be present or absent. Those cases of double outlet right ventricle with hemodynamics like large VSD usually exhibit no pulmonary stenosis and a close relationship between the VSD and the aortic origin.[22]

Persistent truncus arteriosus is characterized by biventricular origin of a single arterial vessel above a VSD. From the single vessel arise (1) the coronary arteries, (2) the aorta, and (3) the pulmonary arterial system. Until obstructive pulmonary vascular lesions appear there is a strong tendency for the left ventricular output to be directed to the aorta and for the right ventricular output to flow toward the pulmonary arterial system. Survival into adulthood is rare, and when it does occur obstructive pulmonary vascular disease with a dominant right-to-left shunt is usually manifest.[23]

A variant of classical VSD is the type of defect that lies in that part of the ventricular septum interposed between the left ventricle and right atrium (Fig. 8), the condition known as *left ventricular–right atrial communication*. This leads to a clinical picture which is like that of a small VSD, except that the left-to-right shunt is into the right atrium rather than into the right ventricle.[24]

Communications Between the Great Arteries

PATENT DUCTUS ARTERIOSUS. Of the communications between the great arteries, patent ductus arteriosus (PDA) is the more common and classic example. The patent channel, the PDA, runs between the proximal part of the left pulmonary artery, below, and the inferior aspect of the aorta, just beyond the level of origin of the left subclavian artery, above. Just as there are two functional types of VSDs, so are there two types of PDAs. The small VSD is comparable to the typical PDA (Fig. 9a), in which the channel is narrow enough to allow a difference in pressure between the aorta and the pulmonary arterial system. The large VSD is comparable to the wide or hypertensive PDA (Fig. 9b).

Classic PDA is characterized by normal or near-normal pulmonary arterial pressure. The shunt is entirely left-to-right. Of the cardiac chambers, only the left-sided ones

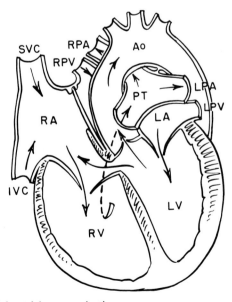

Figure 8. Left ventricular–right atrial communication.

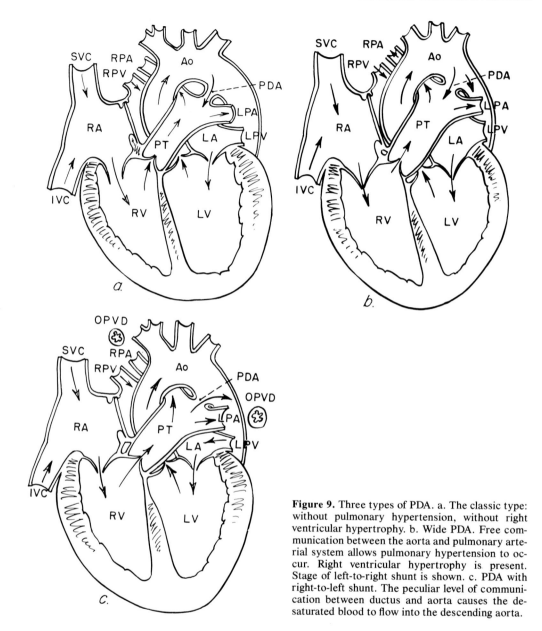

Figure 9. Three types of PDA. a. The classic type: without pulmonary hypertension, without right ventricular hypertrophy. b. Wide PDA. Free communication between the aorta and pulmonary arterial system allows pulmonary hypertension to occur. Right ventricular hypertrophy is present. Stage of left-to-right shunt is shown. c. PDA with right-to-left shunt. The peculiar level of communication between ductus and aorta causes the desaturated blood to flow into the descending aorta.

carry the shunted blood. Left ventricular dilatation and, at times hypertrophy, are characteristic features. Just as the effects of small VSD are well tolerated, so are those of classic PDA. The chief danger to the adult with this condition is bacterial infection of the pulmonary arterial system at the site of impact of the jet-like stream constituting the left-to-right shunt. This may lead to mycotic saccular pulmonary arterial aneurysm.[25] In rare instances, the ductus may become thrombosed and lead to systemic embolism.[26] Also rare is the possibility of aneurysmal formation of the classic ductus. This lesion often involves the aortic end of the ductus and so may be confused with an aortic aneurysm.

The wide or hypertensive ductus which is not treated is often lethal in early life. Some individuals do reach adulthood with this condition, at which point hypertensive pulmonary vascular disease is usually present and an associated right-to-left shunt exists (Fig. 9c). This stage has been referred to as "reversing patent ductus." Because of the anatomic site of entry of the ductus into the aorta, the desaturated blood entering the aorta is carried principally to the lower part of the body, so that the lower part may be cyanotic while the head and arms are not (differential cyanosis). In some instances, some of the right-to-left shunt is driven into the left subclavian artery, resulting in cyanosis of the left upper extremity associated with a normal-colored right upper extremity.

Coarctation of the aorta has been noted occasionally in adults with PDA.[27]

AORTICOPULMONARY SEPTAL DEFECT. The less common type of congenital communication between the great arteries is the aorticopulmonary septal defect or aorticopulmonary window.[28] This is a simple communication between the adjacent portions of the ascending aorta and the pulmonary trunk (Fig. 10a). In the latter vessel, the opening is peculiarly close to the origin of the right pulmonary artery. The fundamental hemodynamics of aorticopulmonary septal defect are like those in hypertensive PDA, except that the entire aorta will receive a right-to-left shunt (Fig. 10b). There may be a tendency for streaming, so that differential cyanosis, though not expected, may occur in aorticopulmonary septal defect. Rarely, a dissecting aneurysm may begin at the abnormal communication and yield a state wherein a large cavity receives the origins of the aorta and pulmonary trunk and gives rise to three branches: the distal ascending aorta, and the right and left pulmonary arteries. Since congenital aorticopulmonary septal defect is particularly uncommon in adults, its differential diagnosis must include an aortic aneurysm that has penetrated into the pulmonary artery.

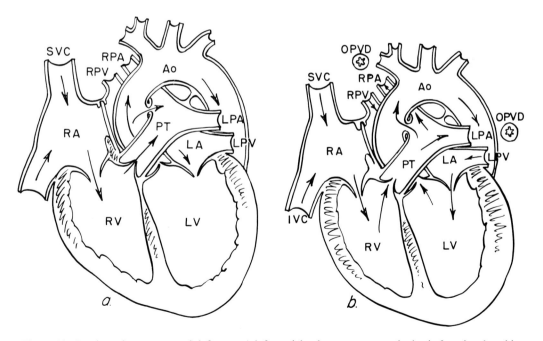

Figure 10. Aorticopulmonary septal defect. a. A left-to-right shunt represents the basic functional problem. b. With obstructive pulmonary vascular disease, a right-to-left shunt may occur as in VSD or wide PDA.

Prominence of Pulmonary Arteries
with Pulmonary Venous Obstruction

Congenital anomalies that are responsible for pulmonary venous obstruction are either stenotic or are represented by mitral regurgitation. The conditions are numerous. Most cause profound symptoms and death in infancy, so that only a small number of adult patients are represented.

The obstructive conditions that may be seen in adults include cor triatriatum, the Shone syndrome, and constrictive endocardial fibroelastosis. Mitral regurgitation on a congenital basis may also occur but is uncommon.

Cor triatriatum is a condition wherein the left atrium is subdivided by a perforated membrane into upper and lower segments.[29] The upper segment (accessory left atrium) receives the pulmonary veins (Fig. 11). It is separated by a perforated membrane from the lower chamber (the true left atrium). The latter chamber communicates with the left atrial appendage and leads through a normal mitral valve into the left ventricle. The basis for pulmonary venous obstruction is the narrowness of the perforation in the membrane between the two left atrial chambers. Resection of the membrane results in normal cardiac function.

In 1963, Shone and associates[30] reported a developmental complex which has come to be known as the Shone syndrome. In its full state, this consists of four obstructive anomalies: (1) a supravalvular ring of the left atrium, (2) a parachute mitral valve, (3) subaortic stenosis, and (4) coarctation of the aorta (Fig. 12). In some patients, only two or three of these conditions are present and the anomalies are not always functionally significant. The supravalvular ring is characterized by a fibrous encirclement at the inlet of the mitral valve. In this position, in contrast to cor triatriatum, the obstructive lesion lies downstream from the left atrial appendage. The parachute mitral valve is characterized by only one papillary muscle, and the chordae of both mitral leaflets insert into

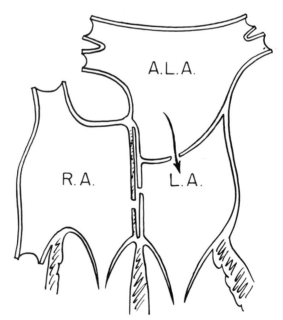

Figure 11. Cor triatriatum. The pulmonary veins lead into an accessory left atrial chamber (A. L. A.). This chamber communicates through a perforated diaphragm with the true left atrium (L.A.). The narrow state of the opening between the accessory and true left atria accounts for obstruction of blood flow from the lungs.

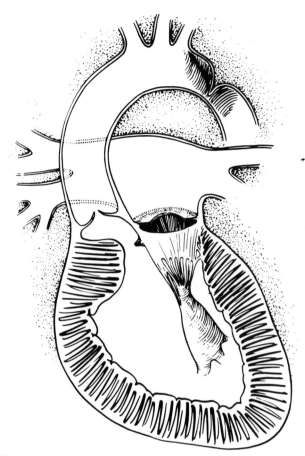

Figure 12. Shone syndrome characterized by four obstructive lesions in the left side of the circulation. These are supravalvular ring of left atrium, parachute mitral valve, subaortic stenosis, and coarctation of aorta. (Reproduced with permission of the American Heart Association, Inc.)

it. Flow from the left atrium must pass through interchordal spaces to reach the left ventricle and, if these are narrow, mitral stenosis occurs. We have observed an adult patient with a stenotic mitral valve that appeared to be a variant of the classic parachute valve.[31]

Constrictive endocardial fibroelastosis is characterized by a normal-sized or somewhat smaller than normal left ventricle, of which the endocardium is grossly thickened by collagenous and elastic tissue. This tissue appears to exert a constricting effect upon the left ventricle, resulting in restriction of diastolic excursion. This rare condition may have a familial tendency.[32] Constrictive endocardial fibroelastosis should be distinguished from the restrictive types of cardiac myopathy, which are functionally similar.

Congenital *mitral regurgitation* may take the form of an intrinsic anomaly of the mitral valve or it may be secondary to an anomaly extrinsic to the mitral valve, with the latter occurring more often. If classic prolapse of the mitral valve is considered a congenital anomaly, it is then the most common type of mitral regurgitation of congenital origin in the adult. Detailed considerations of this entity and its complications have been covered elsewhere.[33]

Other forms of intrinsic mitral valvular anomalies that cause mitral regurgitation in the adult are uncommon to rare.[34,35] One such defect is characterized by a cleft in the

13

anterior mitral leaflet associated with a persistent ostium primum. The defect and the cleft valve together may be considered as the partial form of persistent common atrioventricular canal or endocardial cushion defect. It is to be remembered, however, that the mitral valve will not always be incompetent in such cases. An uncommon variant takes the form of a simple cleft in the anterior mitral leaflet, but with the cardiac septa intact.

Other forms of intrinsic valvular abnormalities that lead to mitral regurgitation include ectopic lower insertion of chordae and double orifice of the mitral valve. To be included under intrinsic valvular anomalies causing "mitral insufficiency" are the changes in the left atrioventricular valve (the anatomic tricuspid valve) that are associated with corrected transposition of the great vessels. This condition is characterized by inversion of the ventricles and atrioventricular valves, and transposition and inversion (l-transposition) of the great vessels. However different from the normal heart, the anatomic arrangements in corrected transposition allow a normal route for the flow of blood. Were it not for associated anomalies, corrected transposition would not disturb the circulation. The common forms of associated conditions, either alone or in combination, are pulmonary stenosis, VSD, and anomalies of the left atrioventricular valve; the latter causes insufficiency of the valve. The anomaly of the left atrioventricular valve may take the form of Ebstein-like deformity[36] or show dysplastic changes of the chordae tendineae.

Mitral regurgitation on a congenital basis commonly results from anomalies originating in some structure other than the mitral valve.[37] Included in these are the dilated type of endocardial fibroelastosis, aortic stenosis, and origin of the left coronary artery from the pulmonary trunk. These conditions are usually lethal in childhood or infancy, but an occasional patient lives to adult life. Congenital aortic valvular stenosis causing mitral regurgitation in an 18-year-old boy has been reported,[38] as has anomalous origin of the left pulmonary artery from the pulmonary trunk causing mitral regurgitation in a 26-year-old woman.[39] The frequent occurrence of mitral regurgitation in the hypertrophic muscular type of subaortic stenosis is commonly recognized.

Left Ventricular Outflow Obstruction

A congenital basis for left ventricular outflow obstruction in the adult may take the form of (1) obstruction at the aortic valve (aortic valvular stenosis), the subaortic portion of the left ventricle (subaortic stenosis) or in the ascending aorta (supravalvular aortic stenosis),[40] or (2) systemic hypertension, usually associated with coarctation of the aorta. The latter condition will be considered in another section.

Aortic Valvular Stenosis

In the adult, aortic valvular stenosis caused by congenital disease takes two forms: intrinsic stenosis and calcification of congenitally bicuspid aortic valve.

The dominant structural type of congenitally intrinsic aortic valvular stenosis is that of a modified dome, or unicuspid, unicommissural aortic stenosis.[41] This condition usually is severe, causing death in infancy or childhood with few exceptions. There is a tendency toward calcification of the valve so that the usual example of congenital aortic stenosis in the adult is associated with severe calcification of the valve. Adults with this deformity may exhibit a mild degree of intrinsic stenosis. Prior to calcification, incompetence of the valve is prevented by a flutter valve action of the pliable dome forming the valve. As calcification develops, the flutter action is lost, incompetence appears, and stenosis increases to the point of being significant (Fig. 13).

The congenital bicuspid valve may be associated with mild and unnoticed stenosis.

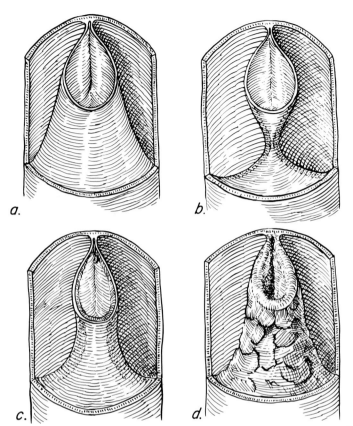

Figure 13. a. Congenital unicuspid aortic valvular stenosis. b. In the uncomplicated state, the valve may close during ventricular diastole by a flutter valve action. c. and d. Ultimately, calcification appears which may accentuate the stenosis.

This valve, while subject to intrinsic incompetence and to infective endocarditis, is most likely to become calcified and stenotic. The present-day view is that most calcific aortic stenosis occurs in congenitally bicuspid valves.[40,42] In such cases, mitral valvular disease is not usually present and aortic regurgitation is absent or inconsequential.

Subaortic Stenosis

Subaortic stenosis may be either of the primary or the secondary type. The primary type may be one of three varieties: (1) asymmetrical septal hypertrophy, (2) membranous type, and (3) tunnel type.[43]

Asymmetrical septal hypertrophy, also known as hypertrophic muscular subaortic stenosis, is a primary disease of the myocardium. It is characterized by localized hypertrophy of the base of the ventricular septum in the part which forms the outflow tract of the left ventricle. While hypertrophy of the left ventricle may occur generally, the greatest degree of change occurs typically in the septal wall of the outflow tract. Current observations suggest that the basis for the left ventricular outflow obstruction is failure of the anterior mitral leaflet to move away from the ventricular septum during ventricular systole (Fig. 14). This abnormality causes left ventricular outflow obstruction and mitral regurgitation simultaneously.[44]

The *membranous type* of subaortic stenosis is characterized by a fibrous ring which

15

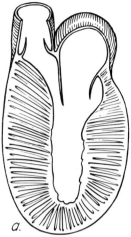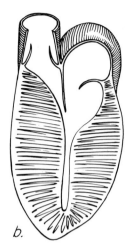

Figure 14. Hypertrophic muscular subaortic stenosis. a. Diastolic phase. There is prominence of the ventricular wall, especially in the outflow tract. b. Systolic phase. The posterior mitral leaflet moves in a normal position, but the anterior leaflet flutters in a relatively open state against the hypertrophied ventricular septum, causing subaortic stenosis and mitral insufficiency.

encircles the left ventricular outflow tract and causes it to be narrow.[40] As the encircling ring attaches partly to the anterior leaflet of the mitral valve, mitral regurgitation may occur. Resection of the ring may cause injury to the mitral valve.

In contrast to muscular hypertrophic subaortic stenosis, the membranous type is usually associated with traumatic jet lesions on the contact surfaces of the aortic leaflets. The traumatic effect is probably the underlying basis for the not uncommon complication of aortic valvular infective endocarditis in the membranous type.

The *tunnel type* of subaortic stenosis is characterized by a relatively long and narrow left ventricular outflow tract.[43] Although endocardial fibrous thickening may occur in the wall of the narrow channel, the basic condition is to be distinguished from the membranous type. Hypoplasia of the aortic anulus may be associated.

There are many secondary types of subaortic stenosis, each usually representing a different malformation of the mitral valve.[45] Included in these are accessory masses of tissue involving the ventricular aspect of the anterior mitral leaflet and anomalous attachment of the center of the anterior mitral leaflet to the ventricular septum. Such anomalous attachment may be of the leaflet itself but is more commonly caused by the presence of aberrant chordae which interpose between the leaflet and the ventricular septum.

Supravalvular Aortic Stenosis

Stenosis of the ascending aorta is commonly called supravalvular aortic stenosis. Three types have been described: (1) hourglass, (2) hypoplastic, and (3) membranous[46] (Fig. 15).

The hypoplastic type is not likely to be seen in adults, since its degree of obstruction is so severe. The entire ascending aorta may be narrow, and major and diffuse stenosis of the pulmonary trunk is not uncommon. The membranous type is least common and is represented by a fibrous encirclement of the ascending aorta. The hourglass type is the variation most likely to be seen in adults. The shape of the ascending aorta leads to the designation for this type. Coronary arterial abnormalities include hypertrophy of the medial layers, and premature atherosclerosis[47] and narrowing of the ostia.[48] In some

16

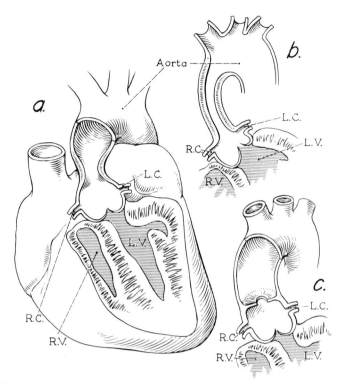

Figure 15. Supravalvular aortic stenosis of three types. a. Hourglass. b. Hypoplastic. c. Membranous.

cases the coronary ostia may be involved either directly by the aortic lesion or indirectly through abnormal attachment of aortic cusps to the aortic wall.[49] Stenosis of branches of the aortic arch[50] and of the pulmonary arteries is commonly observed.[51] Infective aortitis may occur at the stenotic segment of the aorta.

Hypertension

In the adult, congenital systemic hypertension is most commonly caused by coarctation of the aorta. Fibromuscular hyperplasia of a renal artery and polycystic kidneys are also causes, but these conditions are beyond the scope of this presentation.

Coarctation of the aorta is a localized narrowing which most often occurs between the arch and the descending portion of the vessel (Fig. 16). The anomaly is characterized externally by an indentation of the superior aspect of the aorta at the site of involvement. Internally, the external indentation creates a curtain-like fold of tissue which projects into the lumen from the superior, anterior, and posterior aspects of the aorta; the inferior wall is uninvolved. The orientation of the curtain causes the aortic lumen to be narrow and eccentric, so that along the inferior wall of the aorta the lumen is usually only a few millimeters wide. The basic structure of the curtain is localized thickening of the media.[52] There may be secondary intimal thickening on top of this basic lesion, which, in time, contributes slightly to the narrowness of the lumen.

Secondary changes include poststenotic dilatation of the aorta, and a localized jet lesion which may form in the upper descending aorta at the site of impact of the jet-like stream flowing through the narrow aortic segment. Left ventricular hypertrophy is a response to the hypertension.

The adult with coarctation usually has a well developed collateral system which

17

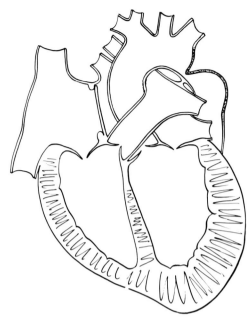

Figure 16. Coarctation of the aorta represented by focal indentation in the superior aspect of the aorta which causes the aortic lumen to be eccentric and narrow.

causes blood to flow from the upper compartment to the lower (Fig. 17). Two basic subdivisions of the collateral system are evident, the anterior and the posterior,[53] and both begin in the subclavian artery. The carotid arterial system does not play a material role in the collateral function.

The anterior segment of the system is concerned primarily with delivery of blood to the lower extremities. It begins in the subclavian artery and proceeds through the internal mammary arteries. In the upper anterior abdominal wall these vessels join the superior epigastric arteries. Flow is then carried into the inferior epigastric arteries which arise from the external iliac arteries and carry blood in a retrograde direction into the ileofemoral system of arteries. Thus, the lower extremities are supplied by blood that bypasses the lower thoracic and abdominal segments of the aorta.

The posterior segment of the collateral system is concerned with carrying blood into the descending and abdominal aorta for supply of the abdominal viscera. This segment also originates in the subclavian arteries and mainly employs those branches which supply the parascapular aspect of the thoracic wall. From such branches, blood flows through the posterior portion of the intercostal arteries and into the descending thoracic aorta. The characteristic notching of ribs observed in coarctation is secondary to the dilatation and tortuosity of those segments of the intercostal arteries that participate in the collateral system. The anterior spinal artery may contribute to the posterior system of collaterals since this vessel runs continuously past the level of the aortic obstruction. It receives blood from branches of the subclavian arteries and delivers it through intercostal and lumbar arteries to the distal aorta.

In exceptional cases of coarctation there is a significant difference in systolic pressures between the two upper extremities. If pressure is higher in the right arm than in the left there may be either narrowing of the ostium of the left subclavian artery, or coarctation lying proximal to the left subclavian artery in the segment between the origin of this vessel and that of the left common carotid artery. A lower pressure in the right arm may be a manifestation of either isolated stenosis of the origin of the right

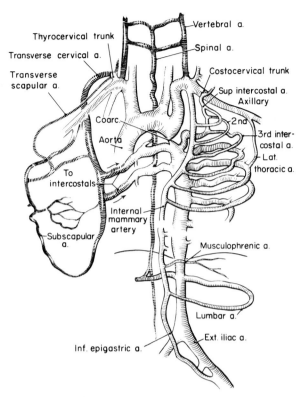

Figure 17. Collateral circulation in coarctation of the aorta. The right side shows the anterior system in which the internal mammary artery leads to flow which ultimately is carried into the lower extremities. The left side shows the posterior system and scapular vessels through which blood is carried via intercostal arteries into the lower aortic segment to supply the abdominal viscera.

subclavian artery or an aberrant right subclavian artery which arises distal to the coarctation.

Complications involving the congenital bicuspid valve are found in about 50 percent of patients with coarctation of the aorta. Infective endocarditis, intrinsic aortic regurgitation, and calcific aortic stenosis may appear even after the coarctation has been treated surgically.

Other complications of coarctation may be classified as cardiac, aortic, and those of the central nervous system.[54]

Aside from complications occurring in the congenital bicuspid valve, the main cardiac complication is left ventricular failure resulting from systemic hypertension. The aortic complications are those of dissecting or saccular-type aneurysm formations.[55] Dissecting aneurysm occurs more often in the proximal aorta. There are two main types of saccular aneurysms. The first type involves the descending aorta, where infective aortitis may begin at the site of a jet lesion.[56] The other type of saccular aneurysm results from a laceration of the aorta, as in dissecting aneurysm, but does not involve intramural dissection of blood. External rupture of the aorta may complicate either dissecting or saccular aneurysm and the resulting hemorrhage enters the pericardial or a pleural (usually left) cavity.

It is the author's view that pseudocoarctation, or "kinked aorta," is anatomic coarctation with little or no obstruction.[57]

19

Aortic Regurgitation

Congenital disease may cause aortic regurgitation or hemodynamic states resembling this condition, such as a shunt from the aorta into another vessel or a cardiac chamber.[58] Regurgitation through the aortic valve on a congenital basis may result either from malformation of the aortic valve or the aortic wall. Isolated congenital aortic regurgitation usually is a manifestation of a congenital bicuspid aortic valve in which the conjoined cusp is excessively long. This accounts for prolapse of this cusp so that during ventricular diastole its free edge comes to lie well below the free edge of the second cusp. The result is faulty closure of the valve and regurgitation.

In some cases of VSD, particularly the supracristal type, the root of the aorta is inadequately supported. This results in a "tipping" of the aorta with consequent malalignment of the cusps, and regurgitation through the valve ensues.

Congenital weakness of the aortic wall is usually the result of extensive cystic medial necrosis. Some subjects harboring such aortae manifest the body physique of arachnodactyly (Marfan's syndrome). The aortic regurgitation is probably compounded of aortic dilatation and coexisting mucinous change ("floppiness") of the aortic valve.[59]

Hemodynamics like those of aortic regurgitation may result from a congenital anomaly that allows a shunt from the aorta into another vessel or a cardiac chamber. One such condition is congenital aneurysm of an aortic sinus (Valsalva). Two of the sinuses are particularly susceptible: the posterior (noncoronary) and the right. The basic lesion appears to be a weakness in support of the aortic root at its aortic valvular anular attachment.[60] This allows avulsion of the aortic origin from the anulus with the result that the structure lying against the involved part of the aorta is called upon to support aortic pressure. An aneurysm results, and if this ruptures a shunt is established.

Those congenital aneurysms involving the posterior aortic sinus involve the right atrial aspect of the atrial septum.[61] Rupture leads to a communication between the aorta and right atrium (Fig. 18a). In cases of congenital aneurysm of the posterior aortic sinus, VSD usually is not associated. This is in contrast to congenital aortic sinus aneurysm involving the right aortic sinus. Such aneurysms present in the outflow tract of the right ventricle and are typically associated with a subjacent VSD (Fig. 18b).

PDA and aorticopulmonary septal defect have been covered in another section, but are mentioned here because they involve a large left-to-right shunt. Either of these communications may yield a high pulse pressure and thus may be confused with aortic regurgitation.

Congenital communications of a coronary artery either with a cardiac chamber (Fig. 19a) or the pulmonary trunk (Fig. 19b) may be associated with a run-off from the aorta large enough to cause a high systemic pulse pressure.

CYANOTIC TYPES

In adults, cyanosis from congenital heart disease is commonly the result of acquired pulmonary vascular disease and resulting right-to-left shunt in various conditions that, in early life, are manifested by left-to-right shunts. The principal conditions are atrial septal defect, PDA, and large VSDs. Less common conditions are those in which a right-to-left shunt occurs in the basic hemodynamics of certain anatomic states. Many anatomic forms of cyanotic congenital heart disease have yielded exceptional cases that survive into adulthood; there also are certain specific types in which such survival is not exceptional. The latter group includes the tetralogy of Fallot and its functional variants, pulmonary stenosis with intact ventricular septum, Ebstein's anomaly of the tricuspid valve, and pulmonary arteriovenous fistula. The presence or absence of right ventricular hypertrophy is an important point in differential diagnosis.

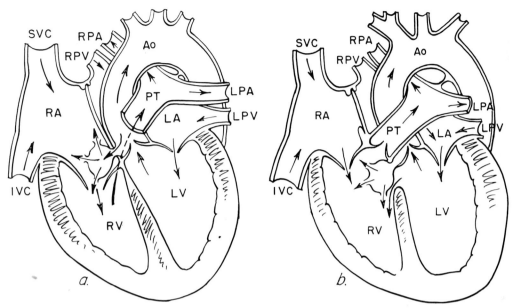

Figure 18. Ruptured aortic sinus aneurysm. a. Aneurysm of the posterior aortic sinus leads into the right atrium. The ventricular septum is intact. b. Aneurysm of the posterior aortic sinus leads from the aorta into the outflow tract of the right ventricle. VSD, commonly associated with this type of congenital aortic sinus aneurysm, is shown also.

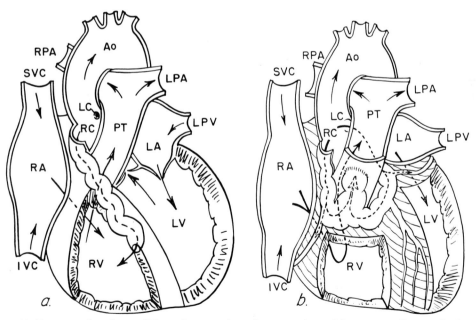

Figure 19. Two examples of run-off from the aorta through coronary arterial system. a. Communication of a coronary artery with a cardiac chamber (the right ventricle, in this instance). b. Accessory coronary artery originating in the pulmonary trunk and making collateral communications with each of the two normally located coronary arteries. Through the collateral system, a shunt has developed whereby aortic blood is carried into the pulmonary trunk.

The potential danger of cerebral abscess is a peculiarity of persistent right-to-left shunt in the absence of intracardiac infection. About ten percent of adult patients with a chronic right-to-left shunt develop this complication.[62]

Presence of Right Ventricular Hypertrophy

Congenital right-to-left shunt in adults may be categorized on the basis of whether right ventricular hypertrophy is present or absent. The tetralogy of Fallot and pulmonary stenosis with intact ventricular septum constitute the main conditions in the adult which present right ventricular hypertrophy.

Tetralogy of Fallot

This well-known entity is characterized by pulmonary stenosis and biventricular origin of the aorta above a VSD (Fig. 20a). The pulmonary stenosis is usually most marked in the outflow tract of the right ventricle. Complications in the adult include cerebral abscess, congestive heart failure (particularly in cases with a mild degree of pulmonary stenosis),[63] hypoxic spells (especially in association with systemic hypotension), and infective endocarditis. The latter may originate at the tricuspid or pulmonary valves, but is usually found at the stenotic right ventricular infundibulum.

Anatomic states which differ from the tetralogy of Fallot, but which have common functional features and may allow survival into adulthood, include single ventricle with pulmonary stenosis, double outlet right ventricle with pulmonary stenosis, and solitary arterial trunk.[64] With solitary aortic trunk the aorta is the only great vessel, and pulmonary blood flow is facilitated by either bronchial arteries or true pulmonary arteries with ductal origins in the aorta.

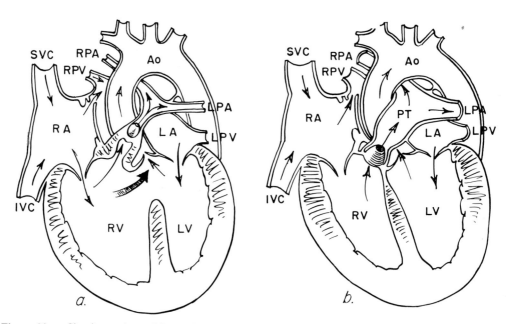

Figure 20. a. Classic tetralogy of Fallot. b. Pulmonary stenosis with intact ventricular septum and right-to-left shunt through a patent foramen ovale.

Pulmonary Stenosis with Intact Ventricular Septum

This condition is characterized by an intact ventricular septum and a deformed pulmonary valve that has the shape of a truncated cone ("dome" stenosis). The basis for a right-to-left shunt is flow across a patent foramen ovale or, less commonly, through a true atrial septal defect (Fig. 20b). If the atrial septum is sealed, no shunt occurs and cyanosis is absent. Right ventricular systolic hypertension and concentric, often marked right ventricular hypertrophy are classic findings. The hypertrophy may underlie acquired right ventricular infundibular stenosis, as the muscle bundles of the right ventricular outflow tract participate in the hypertrophy. As with the tetralogy of Fallot, infective endocarditis is an important potential complication.

Absence of Right Ventricular Hypertrophy

The two most common cyanotic conditions without right ventricular hypertrophy seen in adults are Ebstein's malformation of the tricuspid valve and pulmonary arteriovenous fistula.

Ebstein's Anomaly of Tricuspid Valve

In this uncommon condition the tricuspid valve is highly malformed and there is downward displacement of valvular elements which usually involves the septal and posterior leaflets. The basal attachments of the involved leaflets adhere to the right ventricular wall some distance below the true anulus of the valve. Additional abnormalities include features which have been termed dysplasia (Fig. 21a). These include broad attachment of the downwardly displaced leaflets to the right ventricular wall and

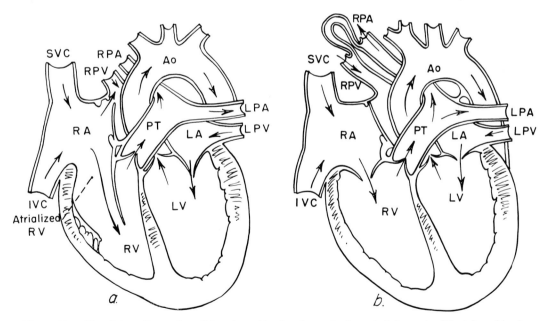

Figure 21. a. Ebstein's malformation of the tricuspid valve. Low attachment of elements of the tricuspid valve functions in such a way that part of the right ventricle is common with the right atrium. The effective right ventricular cavity is reduced in size. b. Arteriovenous fistula. Shown is one communication between a pulmonary artery and a pulmonary vein through which desaturated blood is carried from the pulmonary arterial system into the systemic circulation.

poorly developed papillary muscles and chordae, so that the free edges of the involved leaflets are attached directly to the apical part of the right ventricular free wall. The anterior leaflet is not usually involved and thus supplies the sole flap-like valve function.

In this condition part of the right ventricle lies above the tricuspid valve and, together with the right atrium, contributes to the receiving chamber. At the same time, the effective right ventricular chamber is reduced in volume. During ventricular systole, the large anterior leaflet bulges, as an aneurysm, toward the right atrium, reducing the effectiveness of right ventricular contraction. The malformed valve may be stenotic or incompetent, but is usually neither. The reduced right ventricular chamber prevents a full forward flow, and right atrial blood is, in part, shunted into the left atrium. The shunt typically occurs through either a patent foramen ovale or an atrial septal defect. The major symptoms relate to poor cardiac output, right-to-left shunting, and a strong tendency for arrhythmias.[65]

Pulmonary Arteriovenous Fistula

Though not a cardiac anomaly, pulmonary arteriovenous fistula may be confused with congenital heart disease, especially when sufficient right-to-left shunting occurs to be responsible for evident cyanosis. This condition has a familial tendency and may be part of a systemic vascular anomalous condition known as the Rendu-Osler-Weber syndrome.[66] The fistulous condition has various forms, ranging from a solitary lesion to a highly complex multiple fistulous state (Fig. 21b). Infection of the fistula is not often encountered.

REFERENCES

1. Dow, J. W., Levine, H. D., Elkin, M., et al.: *Studies of congenital heart disease. IV. Uncomplicated pulmonic stenosis.* Circulation 1:267, 1950.

2. Tung, H.-L., and Liebow, A. A.: *Marfan's syndrome. Observations at necropsy: With special reference to medionecrosis of the great vessels.* Lab. Invest. 1:382, 1952.

3. Greene, D. G., Baldwin, E. F., Baldwin, J. S., et al.: *Pure congenital pulmonary stenosis and idiopathic congenital dilatation of the pulmonary artery.* Am. J. Med. 6:24, 1949.

4. Bedford, D. E.: *The anatomical types of atrial septal defect. Their incidence and clinical diagnosis.* Am. J. Cardiol. 6:568, 1960.

5. Tandon, R., Moller, J. H., and Edwards, J. E.: *Tetralogy of Fallot associated with persistent common atrioventricular canal (endocardial cushion defect).* Br. Heart J. 36:197, 1974.

6. Tandon, R., Moller, J. H. and Edwards, J. E.: *Unusual longevity in persistent common atrioventricular canal.* Circulation 50:619, 1974.

7. Raghib, G., Ruttenberg, H. D., Anderson, R. C., et al.: *Termination of left superior vena cava in left atrium, atrial septal defect, and absence of coronary sinus. A developmental complex.* Circulation 31:906, 1965.

8. Swan, H. J. C., Burchell, H. B., and Wood, E. H.: *Differential diagnosis at cardiac catheterization of anomalous pulmonary venous drainage related to atrial septal defects or abnormal venous connections.* Proc. Mayo Clin. 28:452, 1953.

9. Burchell, H. B.: *Total anomalous pulmonary venous drainage: Clinical and physiological patterns.* Proc. Mayo Clin. 31:161, 1956.

10. Burroughs, J. T., and Edwards, J. E.: *Total anomalous pulmonary venous connection.* Am. Heart J. 59:913, 1960.

11. Frye, R. L., Marshall, H. W., Kincaid, O. W., et al.: *Anomalous pulmonary venous drainage of the right lung into the inferior vena cava.* Br. Heart J. 24:696, 1962.

12. Halasz, N. A., Halloran, K. H., and Liebow, A. A.: *Bronchial and arterial anomalies with drainage of the right lung into the inferior vena cava.* Circulation 14:826, 1956.

13. Becu, L. M., Fontana, R. S., DuShane, J. W., et al.: *Anatomic and pathologic studies in ventricular septal defect.* Circulation 14:349, 1956.

14. Goor, D. A., Lillehei, C. W., Rees, R., et al.: *Isolated ventricular septal defect. Development basis for various types and presentation of classification.* Chest 58:468, 1970.

15. SELZER, A.: *Defect of the ventricular septum: Summary of 12 cases and review of the literature.* Arch. Intern. Med. 84:798, 1949.

16. EDWARDS, J. E.: *The Lewis A. Conner Memorial Lecture. Functional pathology of the pulmonary vascular tree in congenital cardiac disease.* Circulation 15:164, 1957.

17. VAN PRAAGH, R., ONGLEY, P. A., AND SWAN, H. J. C.: *Anatomic types of single or common ventricle in man. Morphologic and geometric aspects of 60 necropsied cases.* Am. J. Cardiol. 13:367, 1964.

18. ANSELMI, G., ARMAS, S. M., DE LA CRUZ, M. V., ET AL.: *Diagnosis and classification of single ventricle. Report on seventeen cases with an anatomoembryologic discussion.* Am. J. Cardiol. 21:813, 1968.

19. LEV, M., LIBERTHSON, R. R., KIRKPATRICK, J. R., ET AL.: *Single (primitive) ventricle.* Circulation 39:577, 1969.

20. MARIN-GARCIA, J., TANDON, R., MOLLER, J. H., ET AL.: *Single ventricle with transposition.* Circulation 49:994, 1974.

21. ZAMORA, R., MOLLER, J. H., AND EDWARDS, J. E.: *Double-outlet right ventricle. Anatomic types and associated anomalies.* Chest 68:672, 1975.

22. SRIDAROMONT, S., FELDT, R. H., RITTER, D. G., ET AL.: *Double outlet right ventricle: Hemodynamic and anatomic correlations.* Am. J. Cardiol. 38:85, 1976.

23. CARTER, J. B., BLIEDEN, L. C., AND EDWARDS, J. E.: *Persistent truncus arteriosus. Report of survival to age of 52 years.* Minn. Med. 56:280, 1973.

24. ELLIOTT, L. P., GEDGAUDAS, R., LEVY, M. J., ET AL.: *The roentgenologic findings in left ventricular-right atrial communication.* AJR 93:304, 1965.

25. DETERLING, R. A., JR., AND CLAGETT, O. T.: *Aneurysm of the pulmonary artery: Review of the literature and report of a case.* Am. Heart J. 34:471, 1947.

26. JAGER, B. V., AND WOLLENMAN, O. J., JR.: *An anatomical study of the closure of the ductus arteriosus.* Am. J. Pathol. 18:595, 1942.

27. EDWARDS, J. E., DOUGLAS, J. M., BURCHELL, H. B., ET AL.: *Pathology of the intrapulmonary arteries and arterioles in coarctation of the aorta associated with patent ductus arteriosus.* Am. Heart J. 38:205, 1949.

28. NEUFELD, H. N., LESTER, R. G., ADAMS, P., JR., ET AL.: *Aorticopulmonary septal defect.* Am. J. Cardiol. 9:12, 1962.

29. VAN PRAAGH, R., AND CORSINI, I.: *Cor triatriatum: Pathologic anatomy and a consideration of morphogenesis based on 13 postmortem cases and a study of normal development of the pulmonary vein and atrial septum in 83 human embryos.* Am. Heart J. 78:379, 1969.

30. SHONE, J. D., SELLERS, R. D., ANDERSON, R. C., ET AL.: *The developmental complex of "parachute mitral valve," supravalvular ring of left atrium, subaortic stenosis, and coarctation of aorta.* Am. J. Cardiol. 11:714, 1963.

31. DA SILVA, C. L., AND EDWARDS, J. E.: *Parachute mitral valve in an adult.* Arq. Bras. Cardiol. 26:149, 1973.

32. MOLLER, J. H., FISCH, R. O., FROM, A. H. L., ET AL.: *Endocardial fibroelastosis occurring in a mother and son.* Pediatrics 38:918, 1966.

33. GUTHRIE, R. B., AND EDWARDS, J. E.: *Pathology of the myxomatous mitral valve. Nature, secondary changes and complications.* Minn. Med. 59:637, 1976.

34. EDWARDS, J. E., AND BURCHELL, H. B.: *Pathologic anatomy of mitral insufficiency.* Proc. Mayo Clin. 33:497, 1958.

35. LEVY, M. J., AND EDWARDS, J. E.: *Anatomy of mitral insufficiency.* Prog. Cardiovasc. Dis. 5:119, 1962.

36. EDWARDS, J. E.: *Differential diagnosis of mitral stenosis. A clinicopathologic review of simulating conditions.* Lab. Invest. 3:89, 1954.

37. DAVACHI, F., MOLLER, J. H., AND EDWARDS, J. E.: *Diseases of the mitral valve in infancy. An anatomic analysis of 55 cases.* Circulation 43:565, 1971.

38. EDWARDS, J. E.: *An Atlas of Acquired Diseases of the Heart and Great Vessels.* Vol. I, *Diseases of the Valves and Pericardium.* W. B. Saunders, Philadelphia, 1961. p. 94.

39. USMAN, A., FERNANDEZ, B., URICCHIO, F. J., ET AL.: *Aberrant origin of left coronary artery combined with mitral regurgitation in an adult.* Am. J. Cardiol. 8:130, 1961.

40. ROBERTS, W. C.: *Valvular, subvalvular, and supravalvular aortic stenosis: morphologic features.* Cardiovasc. Clin. 5(1):98, 1973.

41. EDWARDS, J. E.: *Pathologic aspects of cardiac valvular insufficiencies.* Arch. Surg. 77:634, 1958.

42. EDWARDS, J. E.: *The congenital bicuspid aortic valve.* Circulation 23:485, 1961.

43. MARON, B. J., Redwood, D. R., Roberts, W. C., ET AL.: *Tunnel subaortic stenosis. Left ventricular outflow tract obstruction produced by fibromuscular tubular narrowing.* Circulation 54:404, 1976.

44. WIGLE, E. D., HEIMBECKER, R. O., AND GUNTON, R. W.: *Idiopathic ventricular septal hypertrophy causing muscular subaortic stenosis.* Circulation 26:325, 1962.

45. SELLERS, R. D., LILLEHEI, C. W., AND EDWARDS, J. E.: *Subaortic stenosis caused by anomalies of the atrioventricular valves.* J. Thorac. Cardiovasc. Surg. 48:289, 1964.

46. PETERSON, T. A., TODD, D. B., AND EDWARDS, J. E.: *Supravalvular aortic stenosis.* J. Thorac. Cardiovasc. Surg. 50:734, 1965.

47. PEROU, M. L.: *Congenital supravalvular aortic stenosis: A morphological study with attempt at classification.* Arch. Pathol. 71:453, 1961.

48. WOOLEY, C. F., HOSIER, D. M., BOOTH, R. W., ET AL.: *Supravalvular aortic stenosis: Clinical experiences with four patients including familial occurrence.* Am. J. Med. 31:717, 1961.

49. KREEL, I., REISS, R., STRAUSS, L., ET AL.: *Supravalvular stenosis of the aorta.* Ann. Surg. 149:519, 1959.

50. TAYLOR, R. R., AND POLLOCK, B. E.: *Coarctation of the aorta in three members of a family.* Am. Heart J. 45:470, 1953.

51. BOURASSA, M. G., AND CAMPEAU, L.: *Combined supravalvular aortic and pulmonic stenosis.* Circulation 28:572, 1963.

52. EDWARDS, J. E., CHRISTENSEN, N. A., CLAGETT, O. T., ET AL.: *Pathologic considerations in coarctation of the aorta.* Proc. Mayo Clin. 23:324, 1948.

53. EDWARDS, J. E., CLAGETT, O. T., DRAKE, R. L., ET AL.: *The collateral circulation in coarctation of the aorta.* Proc. Mayo Clin. 23:333, 1948.

54. REIFENSTEIN, G. H., LEVINE, S. A., AND GROSS, R. E.: *Coarctation of the aorta. A review of 104 autopsied cases of the "adult type," 2 years of age or older.* Am. Heart J. 33:146, 1947.

55. EDWARDS, J. E.: *Aneurysms of the thoracic aorta complicating coarctation.* Circulation 48:195, 1973.

56. CLAGETT, O. T., KIRKLIN, J. W., AND EDWARDS, J. E.: *Anatomic variations and pathologic changes in coarctation of the aorta. A study of 124 cases.* Surg. Gynecol. Obstet. 98:103, 1954.

57. SMYTH, P. T., AND EDWARDS, J. E.: *Pseudocoarctation, kinking or buckling of the aorta.* Circulation 46:1027, 1972.

58. EDWARDS, J. E.: *Lesions causing or simulating aortic insufficiency.* Cardiovasc. Clin. 5(1):128, 1973.

59. READ, R. C., THAL, A. P., AND WENDT, V. E.: *Symptomatic valvular myxomatous transformation (the floppy valve syndrome). A possible forme fruste of the Marfan syndrome.* Circulation 32:897, 1965.

60. EDWARDS, J. E., AND BURCHELL, H. B.: *The pathological anatomy of deficiencies between the aortic root and the heart, including aortic sinus aneurysms.* Thorax 12:125, 1957.

61. SAKAKIBARA, S., AND KONNO, S.: *Congenital aneurysm of the sinus of Valsalva. Anatomy and classification.* Am. Heart J. 63:405, 1962.

62. SANCETTA, S. M., AND ZIMMERMAN, H. A.: *Congenital heart disease with septal defects in which paradoxical brain abscess causes death. A review of the literature and report of two cases.* Circulation 1:593, 1950.

63. HIGGINS, C. B., AND MULDER, D. G.: *Tetralogy of Fallot in the adult.* Am. J. Cardiol. 29:837, 1972.

64. RAO, B. N. S., AND EDWARDS, J. E.: *Conditions simulating the tetralogy of Fallot.* Circulation 49:173, 1974.

65. BIALOSTOZKY, D., HORWITZ, S., AND ESPINO-VELA, J.: *Ebstein's malformation of the tricuspid valve. A review of 65 cases.* Am. J. Cardiol. 29:826, 1972.

66. DINES, D. E., ARMS, R. A., BERNATZ, P. E., ET AL.: *Pulmonary arteriovenous fistulas.* Proc. Mayo Clin. 49:460, 1974.

Postpediatric Congenital Heart Disease: Natural Survival Patterns

Joseph K. Perloff, M.D.

In any large series of geriatric necropsies . . . atrial septal defect is always well represented; where's the maladie de Roger? Assuming it does provide immortality, it must either close spontaneously in middle life or have long since run its mortal course.[1]

Congenital is derived from the Latin "con," meaning together, and "genitus," meaning born, but the simple implication that congenital heart disease merely means "present at birth" requires qualification. The ductus in a premature infant may remain widely patent for months, finally closing spontaneously, leaving the baby with a normal heart. A ventricular septal defect that delivers a large left-to-right shunt in infancy may gradually develop progressive infundibular pulmonic stenosis, presenting years later with the physiologic and clinical picture of cyanotic Fallot's tetralogy. A congenital bicuspid aortic valve that is functionally normal at birth may take two, three, or more decades to stiffen, calcify, and present as overt aortic stenosis. Accordingly, congenital heart diseases should not be viewed narrowly as static anatomic defects, but instead as a dynamic group of anomalies that originate in utero and change anatomically and functionally during the course of their natural histories. A given defect may exist in harmony with the fetal circulation, but is confronted with dramatic circulatory changes at birth that alter this harmony to widely varying degrees. The physiologic adaptations of the *normal* heart to the events at birth are remarkable enough; it is no surprise that *congenital* defects of the heart or circulation will variably interact with, or be modified by, adaptations to extrauterine life. The principle to be extracted is clear. The anatomy and physiology of the heart and circulation in congenital heart disease change with the passage of time from the fetus, to the dramatic changes at birth, to further changes in the infant, child, adolescent, and adult survivor. Some of these changes result in neonatal death; others express themselves gradually, over weeks, months, years, or decades. A satisfactory comprehension of the clinical manifestations of congenital heart disease requires that these patterns be understood.

Postpediatric survival occurs as a result of natural selection or operative intervention. Palliative or corrective surgery is now possible in almost all—even the most complex—anomalies, so that survival patterns have been significantly affected.[2] We are therefore confronted with a changing population of patients with congenital cardiac malformations, a population that requires an understanding of the basic disorders as well as their surgical modifications. Operation may not only increase life span in patients with anomalies that have a natural tendency to adult survival, but may also permit increasing numbers of patients with disorders previously fatal in infancy or early childhood to reach adult life. The following discussion deals with naturally occurring adult survival in congenital heart disease, i.e., anomalies which have not been operated upon. Such malformations are classified as follows: (1) *common* congenital cardiac defects in which adult survival is *expected*, (2) *uncommon* congenital cardiac defects in which adult survival is *expected*, (3) *common* congenital cardiac defects in which adult survival is *exceptional*, and (4) *uncommon* congenital cardiac defects in which adult survival is *exceptional*. It should be remembered, however, that as time goes on, more and more postpediatric patients with congenital cardiac defects will have had surgery. This is only as it should be.

COMMON CARDIAC DEFECTS WITH EXPECTED ADULT SURVIVAL

For the purpose of this essay, the largest and most important group of defects are the *common* malformations in which adult survival is *expected* (Table 1).

Bicuspid Aortic Valve

The incidence of congenital bicuspid aortic valve—functionally normal, stenotic, or incompetent—may approach 2 percent of the population.[3,4] If this estimate is correct, it means that the bicuspid aortic valve is the commonest congenital malformation of the heart or great vessels;[3,4] it also means, paradoxical though it may seem, that the commonest congenital cardiac defect is most prevalent in adults. The natural history of a bicuspid aortic valve varies. Such a valve may be functionally normal at birth and may continue to function normally throughout life, presenting as an incidental necropsy finding in late adulthood. The greatest tendency is for the functionally normal bicuspid aortic valve to become thickened, fibrotic, calcified, and stenotic during early or middle adulthood.[3] Osler called attention to the peculiar susceptibility of the bicuspid aortic valve to infective endocarditis,[3] which may convert a physiologically benign lesion into the catastrophic mechanical fault of acute severe aortic regurgitation.[5] Less commonly, one or both cusps progressively evert or prolapse, causing aortic regurgitation which may become severe.[6] Unicommissural unicuspid aortic valves may exhibit a similar natural history but this is less common.[7] It follows that the most frequent cause of anatomically isolated valvular aortic stenosis presenting from the third to the sixth decade results from thickening, fibrosis, and calcification of a congenital bicuspid valve that was functionally normal or nearly so at birth.

Coarctation of the Aorta

Coarctation of the aortic isthmus is most likely to produce significant symptoms in early infancy or between ages 20 and 30.[8] The majority of unoperated patients live to adulthood, but only a minority reach age 40.[8] The longest known survival was reported in 1828 in Reynaud's account of a 92-year-old man.[8]

Table 1. Common congenital cardiac defects in which adult survival is expected

Functionally normal bicuspid aortic valve
Valvular aortic stenosis and/or regurgitation
Coarctation of the aorta
Valvular pulmonic stenosis
Atrial septal defect (ostium secundum)
Patent ductus arteriosus
Ventricular septal defect with pulmonic stenosis

Coarctation can present as congestive heart failure in adults previously devoid of significant cardiac symptoms.[9] Three other major complications occur, namely, rupture of the aorta or dissecting aneurysm (most often in the third or fourth decade), infective endocarditis (highest incidence in the second to fifth decades), and cerebral hemorrhage which is usually caused by rupture of an aneurysm of the circle of Willis (generally in the second or third decade).[8] Coarctation of the aorta is readily recognized early in life since diagnosis requires only routine palpation of the brachial and femoral arterial pulses for initial suspicion. The malformation is included in this discussion principally to call attention to the coexistence of congenital bicuspid aortic valve (upwards of 25 percent) which poses inherent problems whether or not the coarctation is corrected[2,10] (Fig. 1). The most common site of infective endocarditis is not on the coarctation itself, but on the peculiarly susceptible bicuspid aortic valve.[8]

Valvular Pulmonic Stenosis

Isolated valvular pulmonic stenosis is a relatively common congenital cardiac defect that often permits adult survival. In one study of anatomically proven valvular pulmonic stenosis, seven patients survived to age 50 and three of these were between 70 and 75

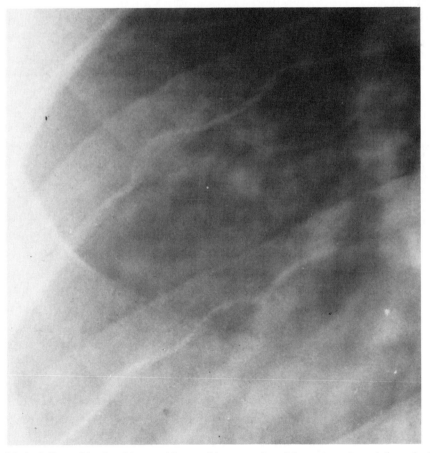

Figure 1. Marked rib notching in a 54-year-old man with coarctation of the aorta and coexisting valvular aortic stenosis caused by a congenital bicuspid valve. (Courtesy of Dr. Miles Schwartz, New York, N.Y.)

29

years old.[11] I have seen six such patients between the ages of 42 and 48 (Fig. 2), and one of Wood's patients was aged 67.[12] Additional examples of survival into the sixth, seventh, and eighth decades have been recorded; one patient lived to age 78.[8]

The adaptive response of the right ventricle to valvular obstruction differs appreciably from patient to patient. Subjective complaints tend to increase with age, although equivalent degrees of stenosis may handicap one patient in childhood and leave another relatively unaffected in the fourth decade.[8] Mild pulmonic stenosis causes no symptoms, but an appreciable number of patients with moderate to severe obstruction are also virtually asymptomatic.[8] One group of patients with right ventricular pressures of 50 to 100 mm. Hg included a New England long-distance swimmer, a female athlete, a British hockey captain, and a long-distance runner.[12] These favorable reports should not obscure the fact that asymptomatic persons may deteriorate rapidly, although one patient with right ventricular pressure exceeding 200 mm. Hg had recurrent ascites for seven years before death at age 60.[8]

Atrial Septal Defect

Ostium secundum atrial septal defect is one of the commonest forms of congenital heart disease found in adults.[13,14] Symptoms are often absent or unnoticed for decades and physical signs may be disarmingly subtle. The relatively soft pulmonic midsystolic murmur can be easily overlooked in children and mistaken for an innocent murmur in both children and young adults. Although life expectancy is shortened in patients with atrial septal defects, adult survival is the rule and many live to advanced ages[8] (Fig. 3). Atrial septal defects beyond age 70 are not rare, and the malformation has occasionally been seen in patients in their 80s or 90s. Since the natural history spans the childbearing age and since the majority of patients with an atrial septal defect are female, pregnancy is anticipated and is usually well tolerated. Complications generally arise after the third or fourth decade and practically all who survive to the sixth decade are

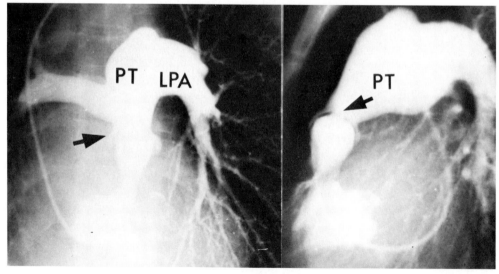

Figure 2. Angiocardiograms with contrast material injected into the right ventricle of a 47-year-old woman with severe valvular pulmonic stenosis (gradient, 106 mm. Hg). In the posteroanterior projection the dilatation of the pulmonary trunk (PT) is not especially evident, but the left branch (LPA) is conspicuously dilated. Arrow points to the level of the stenotic valve. In the lateral projection the dome-shaped stenotic pulmonary valve (arrow) is well seen, and poststenotic dilatation of the pulmonary trunk is readily apparent.

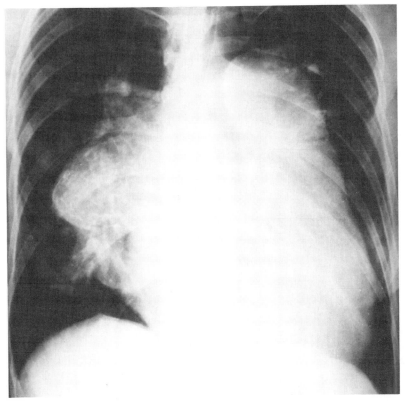

Figure 3. X-ray of a 64-year-old mildly cyanotic woman with a pulmonary hypertensive ostium secundum atrial septal defect and persistent small left-to-right shunt. The pulmonary trunk and its right branch are aneurysmal, and the wall of the right branch contains calcium. (With permission, W.B. Saunders Co.)

symptomatic, although there are notable exceptions.[15] Older patients deteriorate from (1) a decrease in left ventricular compliance which augments the left-to-right shunt in the presence of normal or increased pulmonary arterial pressure, and (2) the advent of atrial arrhythmias—fibrillation, flutter, or occasionally paroxysmal supraventricular tachycardia.

An uncomplicated ostium secundum atrial septal defect in the young is among the most easily diagnosed congenital malformations of the heart, but this same defect may be among the most difficult to recognize in some adults. Despite sophisticated clinical assessment, an adult with an ostium secundum atrial septal defect is occasionally considered to have acquired heart disease. The error stems from a number of ambiguities, some of which are avoidable or understandable (Table 2). This catalog of misleading clinical features is impressive, but confrontation with all or most of them at once is rare. Even when the entire clinical picture is considered, the correct diagnosis may remain in doubt, although enough clues generally emerge to provide the background for an intelligently planned laboratory investigation.

Patent Ductus Arteriosus

This anomaly predominates in females, with a sex ratio of 2 or 3 to 1; female preponderance is even greater in older patients[8] (Fig. 4). Congestive heart failure and infective endarteritis are the commonest natural causes of death related to the ductus itself.[8]

31

Table 2. Secundum atrial septal defect—diagnostic ambiguities in adults

1. Coexisting acquired disease
   a. Coronary artery disease
   b. Systemic hypertension
   c. Inverted left precordial T waves
   d. Atrial arrythmias
2. Mitral stenosis
   a. Dyspnea, orthopnea
   b. Atrial fibrillation
   c. Increased V wave in jugular venous pulse
   d. Right ventricular impulse
   e. Loud S_1
   f. P_2 mistaken for opening snap
   g. Mid-diastolic murmur
   h. X-ray—vascular lungs, dilated right ventricle and pulminary trunk, dilated left atrium
3. Mitral regurgitation
   a. Atrial fibrillation
   b. Apical holosystolic murmur
   c. Wide splitting of S_2
   d. Short middiastolic murmur
   e. Third heart sound

After the first year of life, most children with a ductus arteriosus are asymptomatic. At the beginning of the second decade, the risk of infective endarteritis is believed to exceed the risk of congestive heart failure.[16] Beginning with the third decade (occasionally earlier), cardiac failure develops in an increasing number of patients with large shunts,[16] while those with small communications remain asymptomatic. One woman led an active life as a school teacher and died at age 85 because of gastrointestinal bleeding without ever experiencing heart failure.[17] A number of other reports have called attention to survival beyond age 60, and one patient died at age 90.[8] The ductus arteriosus normally closes spontaneously in early neonatal life. However, *delayed* spontaneous closure sometimes occurs, especially in premature infants and sometimes in older children, but rarely in adults.[18] Campbell described an impressive case of a 45-year-old man who had the continuous murmur of patent ductus arteriosus between the ages of 12 and 17 years.[16] Many years later, only a faint continuous murmur was heard. At age 44, the patient was accepted for life insurance because the murmur had vanished. Such a case exemplified disappearance of the ductus murmur because of late spontaneous closure, not because of abolition of the left-to-right shunt by increased pulmonary vascular resistance.[18] Patent ductus with pulmonary hypertension and reversed shunt is uncommon, but adult survival (second or third decade) is often encountered. The typical continuous murmur is not present since the left-to-right shunt is abolished. In addition, cyanosis is easily overlooked since reversed flow through the ductus results in selective cyanosis of the feet which may not be properly examined.

Ventricular Septal Defect with Pulmonic Stenosis

Isolated ventricular septal defects—irrespective of size—are seldom seen in adults. However, the coexistence of pulmonic stenosis favorably influences the natural history of a large ventricular septal defect and often permits adult survival[8,19] (Fig. 5). In such patients, the early history may be dominated by the ventricular septal defect itself; the acquisition (or early presence) of obstruction to right ventricular outflow curtails excessive pulmonary blood flow and thus relieves volume overload of the left ventricle.

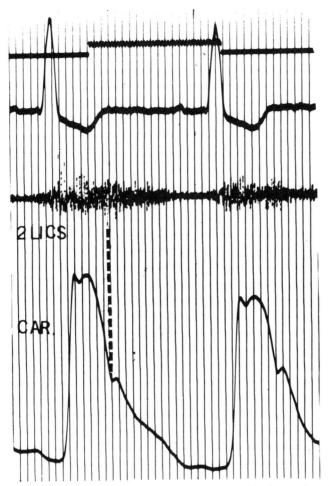

Figure 4. Phonocardiogram of an 84-year-old woman with angiographically confirmed patent ductus arteriosus. Phonocardiogram shows typical continuous murmur. 2 LICS = second left intercostal space; CAR = carotid artery. (Courtesy of Dr. Lucia Gomez, Washington, D.C.)

Symptoms related to the large left-to-right shunt diminish, physical development improves, and adult survival is not only possible but likely. This is especially true when the ideal balance is achieved, i.e., pulmonary blood flow is sufficiently curtailed to relieve the left ventricle but still adequate for oxygenation.[8]

The combination of a large ventricular septal defect with pulmonic stenosis and a balanced or small left-to-right shunt has been called "acyanotic Fallot's tetralogy." Physiologically, a large ventricular septal defect with pulmonic stenosis and reversed shunt is *cyanotic* Fallot's tetralogy. After age 4, the majority of cyanotic children with congenital heart disease have this anomaly.[22] The malformation is also present in the largest number of cyanotic adults with congenital heart disease.[21-24] Fallot recognized this tendency when he wrote, "We have seen from our observations that cyanosis, especially in the adult, is a result of a small number of cardiac malformations well determined . . . One of these cardiac malformations is much more frequent than others . . .", namely, the tetralogy of which he wrote.[8]

33

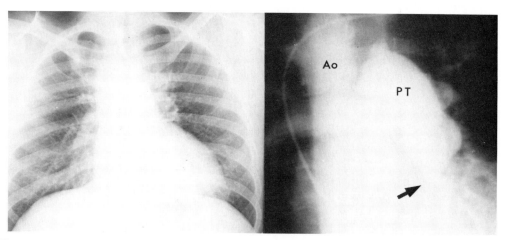

Figure 5. X-ray and angiocardiogram from a 57-year-old man with a large ventricular septal defect and infundibular pulmonic stenosis (arrow). The degree of stenosis was virtually ideal in regulating pulmonary blood flow. The lung vascularity is normal (arterial oxygen saturation 94 percent). Note the right aortic arch (Ao). PT = pulmonary trunk.

UNCOMMON CARDIAC DEFECTS WITH EXPECTED ADULT SURVIVAL

Let us now turn to uncommon defects with expected adult survival (Table 3). These anomalies vary in incidence from uncommon to rare, but when present, postpediatric survival is the rule.

Situs Inversus (Mirror Image Dextrocardia)

This cardiac malposition generally occurs in hearts that are otherwise normal, and is likely to be discovered accidentally during routine physical examination or on chest x-ray[8] (Fig. 6). Patients with uncomplicated situs inversus have normal life spans and hence fall into age groups susceptible to acquired cardiac disorders (Fig. 6). Symptoms related to the acquired diseases may lead to the discovery of the previously unsuspected cardiac malposition. However, the malposition will not be missed if gastric tympany, hepatic dullness, and cardiac dullness are identified by simple percussion, and if the right and left designations on frontal chest x-rays are routinely identified. In the

Table 3. Uncommon congenital cardiac defects in which adult survival is expected

Situs inversus (mirror image dextrocardia)
Dextroversion of the heart
Congenital complete heart block
Congenitally corrected transposition of the great arteries
Idiopathic dilatation of the pulmonary trunk
Congenital pulmonary valve regurgitation
Ebstein's anomaly of the tricuspid valve
Primary pulmonary hypertension
Congenital pulmonary arteriovenous fistula
Lutembacher's syndrome
Common atrium
Coronary arteriovenous fistula
Congenital aneurysm of a sinus of Valsalva
Vena cava to left atrial connection

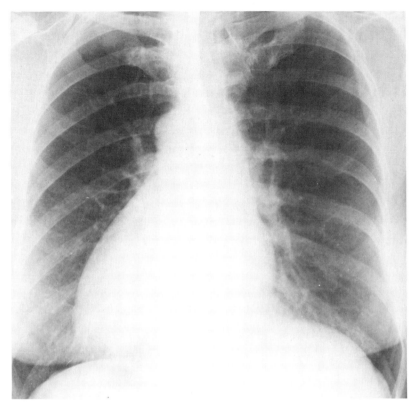

Figure 6. X-ray showing mirror image dextrocardia in a 65-year-old man who had right precordial and retrosternal anginal pain. Congenital heart disease was not present.

electrocardiogram, the standard leads resemble tracings taken with reverse placement of right and left arm leads; aVR and aVL are the reverse of normal. Inspection of the precordial leads avoids the error of considering incorrect limb lead placement, since left thoracic leads show progressively diminishing QRS amplitudes.

Dextroversion of the Heart

This positional anomaly is characterized by situs solitus (thoracic and abdominal viscera in normal position) with the cardiac apex in the *right* chest (right thoracic heart). Gastric tympany is on the left; hepatic dullness is on the right; the chest film shows the stomach normally located, with the aorta descending on the left, but the cardiac apex is on the right. Coexisting congenital malformations are almost invariable; some of these, such as isolated left-to-right shunts at the atrial level or ventricular septal defect with pulmonic stenosis, permit adult survival.[8]

Congenital Complete Heart Block

Congenital complete atrioventricular block has probably been recognized since the turn of the century.[8] As a rule, the disorder is accidentally discovered because of inappropriately slow heart rates in otherwise healthy asymptomatic children or young adults.[8] Confirmation of the diagnosis requires nothing more than a standard scalar electrocardiogram. The P-wave (atrial activity) and the QRS complex (ventricular activ-

35

ity) are completely independent. The ventricular rate—though slower than the atrial rate—is rapid relative to other forms of complete heart block since the depolarization focus is above the bifurcation of the His bundle. Accordingly, the QRS complex generally has a normal or near normal configuration.

One reported patient with congenital complete heart block was a hockey player and other patients have included Air Force officers, a 56-year-old woman who worked on a farm for 20 years and walked two miles daily to her job, and a 38-year-old man who had won several boxing matches in his youth.[8] Although postpediatric survival in patients with uncomplicated congenital complete heart block is the rule, the unqualified air of optimism that previously prevailed cannot be justified.[25,26]

Congenitally Corrected Transposition of the Great Arteries

In this anomaly, the anatomic left ventricle and mitral valve are found in the right heart interposed between a normal right atrium and the pulmonary trunk; an anatomic right ventricle and tricuspid valve are found in the left heart interposed between the normal left atrium and aorta.[8] Since the pulmonary trunk arises from an anatomic left ventricle and since the aorta originates from an anatomic right ventricle (ventricular–great artery discordance), the term "transposition of the great arteries" is appropriate. However, since right atrial blood finds its way into the pulmonary trunk (albeit via a mitral valve and anatomic left ventricle) and since left atrial blood finds its way into the aorta (albeit via a tricuspid valve and anatomic right ventricle), the transposition is physiologically "corrected." The anatomic derangement itself causes little or no functional disturbance in early life,[2] but only a small portion of patients with congenitally corrected transposition have hearts with no coexisting defects. The most common associated anomalies are: (1) large ventricular septal defect, (2) Ebstein-like malformations of the left atrioventricular (tricuspid) valve, and (3) disturbances in atrioventricular conduction. Adult survival is expected in patients with no coexisting defects or with minimal defects (normal or slightly prolonged atrioventricular conduction or mild incompetence of the left A-V valve). Survivals to the fourth through early eighth decades have been reported.[2] On the other hand, spontaneous failure of the systemic ventricle in uncomplicated congenitally corrected transposition of the great arteries has been described in the adult, indicating limited durability of an anatomic right ventricle as a systemic pump.[27]

Idiopathic Dilatation of the Pulmonary Trunk

This uncommon malformation is characterized by congenital dilatation of the pulmonary trunk and occasional dilatation of its main branches with no discernible anatomic or physiologic cause.[8] The anomaly is usually suspected because of an enlarged pulmonary trunk on routine chest x-ray or because of auscultatory detection of a pulmonic ejection sound and a soft short pulmonic systolic murmur.[8] It is important to distinguish idiopathic dilatation of the pulmonary trunk from mild valvular pulmonic stenosis with poststenotic dilatation and from atrial septal defect.

Congenital Pulmonary Valve Regurgitation

The first clinical diagnosis of this anomaly was made in an asymptomatic 24-year-old medical student.[28] The lesion initially comes to attention because of a murmur or because of a dilated pulmonary arterial trunk on chest x-ray.[8] Children, adolescents, and young adults are typically asymptomatic when the defect is discovered, and generally tolerate the malformation through middle age, and, occasionally, into the sixth, seventh, or eighth decade. Congenital absence of the pulmonary valve has been reported in a 73-year-old man.[29] It is worth emphasizing that the murmur of congenital pulmonary valve regurgitation is medium- to low-pitched; crescendo-decrescendo in configuration; delayed in onset after the second heart sound; and short in duration, ending well before the subsequent first heart sound. Low diastolic pressure in the pulmonary trunk generates a low rate of regurgitant flow and a correspondingly low-pitched murmur.[8] This condition contrasts sharply with pulmonary hypertensive pulmonary regurgitation in which high velocities of regurgitant flow exist throughout diastole, so that the accompanying murmur is high frequency, decrescendo, and often holodiastolic.[30]

Ebstein's Anomaly

The basic anatomic fault in Ebstein's anomaly is displacement of fused, malformed tricuspid valvular tissue into the right ventricular cavity.[8] The portion of right ventricle underlying the adherent valve is thin and functions as a receiving chamber analogous to the right atrium. Abnormal function of the right heart in Ebstein's anomaly is related to three derangements: (1) the malformed tricuspid valve, (2) the "atrialized" portion of right ventricle, and (3) the reduced capacity of the pumping portion of the right ventricle.[8] Ebstein's anomaly is compatible with a relatively long and active life; the majority of patients survive into the second, third, or fourth decade[31] (Fig. 7). As a rule, the later the onset of cyanosis, the longer the survival; recurrent paroxysms of rapid heart action tend to counter this trend. Nevertheless, about 5 percent of patients live beyond age 50.[31] Survival into the seventh and eighth decades has been reported, and one patient died two months before age 80.[32] Another patient, a 79-year-old woman, died of noncardiac causes despite rather marked deformity of the tricuspid valve.[33] Ebstein's anomaly was discovered at necropsy in a 75-year-old man who had been a lumberjack during his youth; he apparently had been asymptomatic until his 50s, during which he was once obliged to outrun an irate female bear.[34]

Primary Pulmonary Hypertension

This disorder is characterized by increased pulmonary arteriolar resistance with no apparent cause.[30] The disease is typically found in young women but ranges from infancy to the eighth decade, with the highest incidence occurring between 12 and 40 years of age.[8,30] Longevity is related to the severity of pulmonary vascular obstruction (and pulmonary hypertension): the higher the pressure, the graver the outlook. The disorder often progresses rapidly in younger patients, and death within four or five years after the onset of symptoms is common.[8] Those with milder disease may survive for 10 to 20 years after clinical recognition.[8] The presence of dyspnea, weakness, fatigue, syncope, and chest pain in an otherwise healthy acyanotic woman without a cardiac murmur suggests primary pulmonary hypertension on the basis of the history alone.[8]

Pulmonary Arteriovenous Fistula

The fistulas can be solitary or multiple, unilateral or bilateral, minute or large; most of them involve the lower lobes or right middle lobe (Fig. 8). The arterial supply is usually from one or more abnormally enlarged, tortuous branches of the pulmonary artery, and the fistula almost always drains through anatomically recognizable dilated pulmonary veins.[8] Physiologic consequences of pulmonary arteriovenous fistulas depend chiefly upon the amount of unoxygenated blood delivered through the communication. The essence of the disturbance is the right-to-left shunt. An interesting aspect

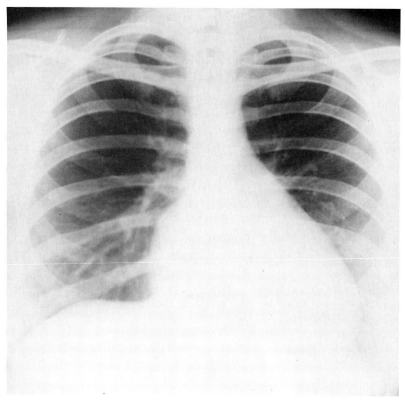

Figure 7. X-ray from a 23-year-old woman with Ebstein's anomaly. She was acyanotic and asymptomatic except for recurrent bouts of paroxysmal rapid heart action, which occurred despite the absence of pre-excitation. The lung fields (middle and outer thirds) are relatively clear. The ascending aorta and main pulmonary artery are small, resulting in a narrow vascular pedicle. There is a prominent right atrial convexity along the lower right cardiac border. The left upper border of the heart is straight because of enlargement of the right ventricular outflow tract. (With permission, W.B. Saunders Co.)

of the disorder is its association with Rendu-Osler-Weber disease (hereditary hemorrhagic telangiectasia). Most pulmonary arteriovenous fistulas are not recognized until adult life. Asymptomatic fistulas come to light because of the accidental discovery of abnormal shadows in the chest x-rays (Fig. 8) or the detection of cyanosis or telangiectasia.[8]

Lutembacher's Syndrome

Lutembacher's syndrome is a congenital atrial septal defect upon which acquired mitral stenosis is imposed.[8] In an atrial septal defect of any given size, the more severe the mitral stenosis, the larger the left-to-right shunt. On the other hand, the interatrial communication constitutes an exit for the left atrial blood. If the defect is large enough, the left atrium decompresses and the gradient across the stenotic mitral valve diminishes, vanishes altogether, or appears only during exercise.[35] Lutembacher's syndrome has a predilection for females, which is understandable because both atrial septal defects and rheumatic mitral stenosis are more prevalent in this sex.[8] When a large atrial septal defect decompresses the left atrium in mitral stenosis, the symptoms

38

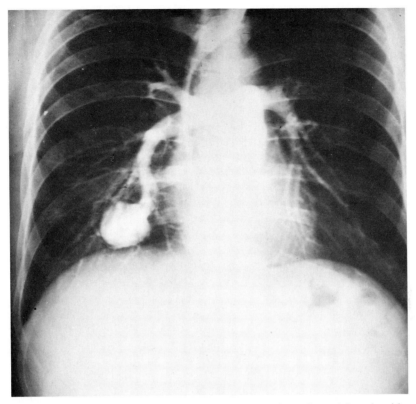

Figure 8. Angiocardiogram (following pulmonary arterial dye injection) of an adult male with a congenital pulmonary arteriovenous fistula of the right lower lobe. The circumscribed fistula is shown with its vascular connections to the right hilus. (With permission, W.B. Saunders Co.)

of mitral valve obstruction are attenuated but replaced by fatigue from low cardiac output. The ameliorating effect of an atrial septal defect was pointed out in early descriptions. Lutembacher's original patient was a 61-year-old woman who had undergone seven pregnancies, and an earlier patient reported in the German literature (and referred to by Lutembacher) was a 74-year-old woman who had experienced 11 pregnancies.[8] Survival to advanced age has been reconfirmed in an 81-year-old woman who lived a normal life with no symptoms related to her disease until age 75.[36]

Common Atrium

In this relatively rare form of interatrial communication, the septum is virtually or completely absent.[8,37,38] There are two atrial appendages and two identifiable atrial chambers but without septal partition. The physiologic consequences are akin to those of a large atrial septal defect.[8,37,38] However, varying degrees of venoarterial mixing are more likely, and systemic arterial oxygen unsaturation exists despite persistence of the left-to-right shunt.[8] Symptoms resemble those of large atrial septal defect but are generally earlier in onset and more marked. Nevertheless, some patients appear relatively well even in late childhood or early adolescence, and one patient lived to age 53.[8] Common atrium often accompanies the Ellis-Van Creveld syndrome (dwarfism with polydactyly and ectodermal dysplasia).[8]

Coronary Arteriovenous Fistula

Both coronary arteries arise from appropriate aortic sinuses, but a fistulous branch of one communicates directly with a cardiac chamber or vessel (Fig. 9). Most fistulas enter the right atrium, coronary sinus, or right ventricle.[8,39] The coronary artery that forms the fistula (right coronary is involved more often than left) is characteristically dilated, elongated, and tortuous. Physiologic disturbances caused by the coronary arteriovenous fistula relate to: (1) the amount of blood flowing through the communication, i.e., the magnitude of the left-to-right shunt; (2) the chamber or vessel into which the fistula drains; and (3) myocardial ischemia believed to result from fistulous bypass (coronary steal). Adult longevity is the rule,[8,39] although life expectancy is not normal. Nevertheless, survivals to ages 64, 75, 76, 84 and 85 have been recorded.[8] It is wise to consider the diagnosis whenever an acyanotic patient exhibits a precordial continuous

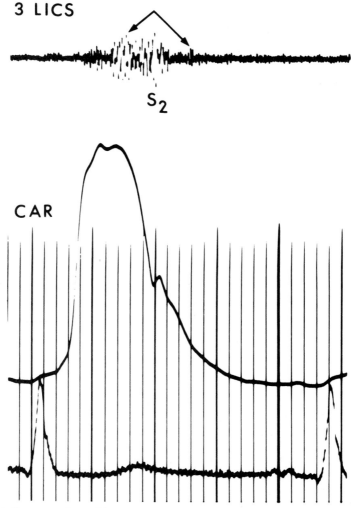

Figure 9. Phonocardiogram and carotid pulse tracing of a 47-year-old man with a coronary arteriovenous fistula between the right coronary artery and the right ventricle. The continuous murmur was maximal in the third left intercostal space (3 LICS) and louder in systole (arrows). CAR = carotid. (With permission, W.B. Saunders Co.)

murmur in an atypical site (Fig. 9). The location of the murmur is determined by the chamber or vessel that receives the communication and not by the coronary artery that gives rise to it.[39]

Aneurysm of a Sinus of Valsalva

The typical aneurysm begins as a blind pouch or diverticulum originating from a localized site in one aortic sinus.[8] The entire sinus is not dilated; instead, the aneurysm protrudes as a finger-like or nipple-like projection.[8] The common form of congenital aortic sinus aneurysm is found in the right or noncoronary sinus and is apt to perforate into the right ventricle or right atrium. The developmental fault—but not the aneurysm itself—is present or is likely to be present at birth. The physiologic consequences attending rupture depend upon: (1) the amount of blood shunted through the abnormal communication, (2) the rapidity with which the perforation develops, and (3) the chamber that receives the shunt. Ruptured aneurysms of a sinus Valsalva are found predominantly in males, with a sex ratio as high as 4:1. Most ruptures develop in patients well beyond puberty but before age 30,[8] so that the disorder is typically seen in young adult males. Perforations rarely occur in infancy and childhood, and equally rarely as late as the seventh decade.[8] Death ordinarily follows within a year after rupture if the defect is not corrected, but longer survival can occur. One patient lived 30 years, and another report described a ruptured aortic sinus aneurysm in a 65-year-old man who died 10 years later of carcinoma.[40] Gradual development of a small perforation may go unnoticed until a continuous murmur is detected. An acute, large rupture is dramatically heralded by sudden, severe, retrosternal or upper abdominal pain accompanied by marked dyspnea. Acute symptoms generally last for hours or days and may partially subside, leaving the patient comparatively improved. After a variable latent period, congestive heart failure reappears and usually progresses relentlessly.[8]

Connection of Vena Cava to Left Atrium

Uncomplicated isolated connection of superior or inferior vena cava to the left atrium is a very rare congenital malformation.[8,41] The average age of such patients is about 21 years, with a range of 2 to 37 years.[8] Cardiac symptoms may be minimal or absent; the anomaly is usually suspected because of cyanosis that dates from birth or early childhood. One man with this defect did heavy manual labor and had no difficulty during periods of rigorous training while in the Armed Services.[41] Clinical suspicion depends upon the combination of cyanosis with a dominant left ventricle.

COMMON CARDIAC DEFECTS WITH UNEXPECTED ADULT SURVIVAL

Let us finally turn to those congenital cardiac defects—first the common (Table 4) and then the uncommon—in which postpediatric survival is exceptional.

Table 4. Common congenital cardiac defects in which adult survival is exceptional

Ventricular septal defect
Ventricular septal defect with aortic regurgitation
Endocardial cushion defects
Tricuspid atresia
Complete transposition of the great arteries

Ventricular Septal Defect

In 1879 Henri Roger wrote, "Among the congenital defects of the heart compatible with life and perhaps a long one, one of the most frequent which I have encountered . . . is the communication between the two ventricles because of failure of occlusion of the interventricular septum in its upper portion."[8] In actual fact, uncomplicated isolated ventricular septal defect is relatively common, but *not* in adults.

Three regulatory mechanisms affect the volume and direction of the interventricular shunt in infants born with large ventricular septal defect:[8] (1) the pattern taken by the pulmonary resistance, (2) the tendency of the defect to decrease in size, and (3) the development of obstruction to right ventricular outflow (previously discussed as ventricular septal defect with pulmonic stenosis). When the defect is small, longevity should be normal or nearly so. However, even small ventricular septal defects are seldom seen in adults,[42] although patients in the sixth decade (Fig. 10) and one at age 79 have been reported.[43] Relatively few adults are seen with ventricular septal defects, not because of fatality, but probably because the communication has spontaneously closed or diminished to the point where it is clinically unrecognizable.[18,42,43,44] In the presence of a large ventricular septal defect, mortality is highest in early childhood; in those who succumb, the large left-to-right shunt is not adequately regulated and death results from congestive heart failure. Conversely, a decrease in volume overload of the left heart with clinical improvement may be the result of any of the three previously cited regula-

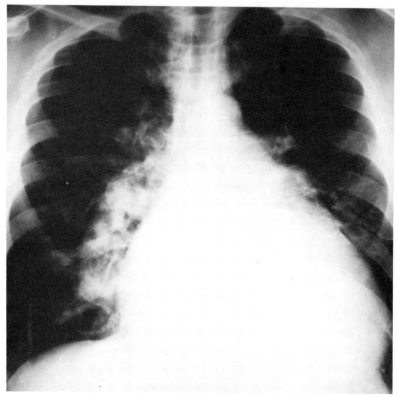

Figure 10. X-ray of an acyanotic 51-year-old man who had a large ventricular septal defect with prominent pulmonary trunk and central branches and a conspicuous right atrial silhouette to the right of the vertebral column. The left ventricle occupies the apex. A 2.8:1 left-to-right shunt and pulmonary hypertension were present. (Courtesy of Dr. Andrew G. Morrow, Bethesda, Md.; with permission, W.B. Saunders Co.)

tory mechanisms. A rise in pulmonary vascular resistance is the least desirable of the three; volume overload of the left heart is relieved, but if pulmonary resistance progresses, the left-to-right shunt is reversed and cyanosis appears, rendering the patient hypoxemic and inoperable. The term "Eisenmenger's complex" is then applied. Wood's summary of Eisenmenger's original account[45] is appropriate: "Eisenmenger's patient was a powerfully built man of 32 who gave a history of cyanosis and moderate breathlessness since infancy. He managed well enough . . . until January 1894 when dyspnea increased and edema set in. . . . he improved with rest and digitalis, but collapsed and died more or less suddenly . . . following a large hemoptysis." At necropsy a defect, 2 by 2.5 cm., was found in the membranous septum.

Aortic regurgitation may be a part of the natural course of ventricular septal defect.[8] The regurgitation typically develops insidiously between ages 3 and 8 years. Occasionally, the defect decreases in size while the aortic regurgitation progresses. Such patients may present as examples of pure or nearly pure aortic regurgitation with postpediatric survival.

Endocardial Cushion Defect

Longevity is greatest with partial endocardial cushion defect, especially when an isolated ostium primum exists with a competent mitral valve.[8] Under these circumstances, the longevity patterns are similar to ordinary ostium secundum atrial septal defect. However, the electrocardiogram is likely to distinguish the two conditions since an endocardial cushion defect usually displays counterclockwise depolarization, left axis deviation and splintering of the S waves in leads 2, 3, and aVF, together with the rSr' right precordial pattern of ostium secundum atrial septal defect.[8,46] When an ostium primum defect exists with mitral regurgitation, longevity depends upon the degree of valvular incompetence. If the physiologic derangement is comparatively mild to moderate, survival through childhood occurs with little or no cardiac failure, and symptoms may be delayed for one or two decades. Patients come to attention during this period because of the mitral regurgitant murmur. When the defect in the atrial septum is absent or small in the presence of a cleft and incompetent mitral valve, the history resembles pure mitral regurgitation. The early onset of the murmur helps identify the disorder as congenital, but when such history is not available, a mistaken diagnosis of acquired mitral regurgitation is often made.

Tricuspid Atresia

In tricuspid atresia, right atrial blood exits exclusively via the atrial septum into the left atrium and left ventricle. The important anatomic variations beyond the mitral valve consist of: (1) the presence or absence of transposition of the great arteries, (2) the presence or absence of pulmonic stenosis, and (3) the condition of the ventricular septum. These variations are the chief determinants of pulmonary blood flow and pressure; longevity varies accordingly. Life expectancy is best when the degree of pulmonic stenosis permits adequate but not excessive pulmonary blood flow and prevents pulmonary vascular disease.[8,43] When the great arteries are not transposed, subpulmonic obstruction takes the form of a small, slitlike ventricular septal defect, and most such patients die in the first year of life. Nevertheless, sporadic survivals to the second through the fifth decades have been recorded;[8] one exceptional patient lived to age 57.[47] When the great arteries are transposed, appropriate degrees of pulmonic stenosis occasionally permit survival into the second, third, or fourth decade; one patient died at 56.[43] When tricuspid atresia exists without pulmonic stenosis, pulmonary vascular resistance per se seldom accomplishes satisfactory regulation of blood flow to the lungs, and survival is limited.[8] Longevity beyond infancy is exceptional; one such patient with normally related great arteries and no pulmonic stenosis lived to age 45,[48] and another with transposed great arteries and no pulmonic stenosis lived to age 18.[8] The occasional long-term survivor with tricuspid atresia is therefore likely to have coexisting pulmonic stenosis with favorable regulation of pulmonary blood flow.

Complete Transposition of the Great Arteries

The right atrium communicates with the anatomic right ventricle that gives rise to the aorta (ventricular–aortic discordance), while the left atrium communicates with the anatomic left ventricle that gives rise to the pulmonary trunk (ventricular–pulmonary artery discordance).[8] Survival requires a means of exchange between the pulmonary and systemic circulations. Most unoperated patients with complete transposition die in the first year of life, often within the first six months. Sporadic examples of unusual longevity have been recorded with survival into the second, third, or fourth decade;[8] one patient came to necropsy at age 56.[49]

UNCOMMON CARDIAC DEFECTS WITH EXCEPTIONAL ADULT SURVIVAL

Uncommon congenital cardiac defects with exceptional adult survival are listed in Table 5.

Subvalvular Aortic Stenosis

The morphologic bases of congenital subvalvular aortic stenosis in hearts with ventricular–great artery concordance are many and varied. Nevertheless, there are two relatively common varieties of discrete subvalvular obstruction: (1) the localized fibromembranous type, and (2) the tunnel, tubular, or fibromuscular type.[4,50] The distinction is important since the natural histories differ.

Fibromembranous subaortic stenosis is characterized by a relatively localized, thin, crescent-shaped fibrous membrane located 2 cm. or less from the aortic valve.[4] Except for the membrane, the outflow tract is not narrow and the aortic ring is normal in size. The aortic valve is equipped with three cusps which are frequently malformed and thickened on their ventricular surfaces, resulting in aortic regurgitation.[4]

"Tunnel" subaortic stenosis is represented by a relatively long, diffuse, narrow fibromuscular channel.[50] The aortic ring tends to be abnormally small (hypoplastic). Aortic cusps show fibrous thickening analogous to that in the localized fibromembranous obstruction. It has been proposed that discrete subaortic stenosis includes a morphologic spectrum encompassing mild localized membranous deformity at one end, and severe tunnel obstruction at the other.[50] The spectrum has been further broadened to include at least some patients with asymmetric septal hypertrophy.[50]

Table 5. Uncommon congenital cardiac defects in which adult survival is exceptional

Discrete subvalvular or supravalvular aortic stenosis
Anomalous origin of the left coronary artery from the pulmonary trunk
Cor triatriatum
Total anomalous pulmonary venous connection
Right ventricular origin of both great arteries
Truncus arteriosus
Single ventricle

Discrete subaortic stenosis of the tunnel, tubular, or fibromuscular variety is characteristically severe and is seldom seen beyond childhood.[50] The localized fibromembranous variety is more variable in severity at its onset but is also seldom seen in adults.[8,51] Just why fibromembranous subaortic stenosis has a relatively high incidence in the young but is virtually nonexistent in middle-aged adults is a question that has received little attention.[51] Inherent severity, progression in severity, and perhaps later development of fibromuscular (tunnel) and/or asymmetric septal hypertrophy may conspire to shorten the life span and thus account for the difference in prevalence of fibromembranous subaortic stenosis between children and adults.

Supravalvular Aortic Stenosis

This form of obstruction to left ventricular outflow is usually the result of a localized, segmental, hourglass narrowing located immediately above the aortic sinuses.[4] Supravalvular obstruction can also be caused by a fibrous diaphragm or by a uniform tubular narrowing of the entire ascending aorta that begins above the origins of the coronary arteries.[8] Hourglass supravalvular aortic stenosis commonly coexists with branch stenosis of the pulmonary arteries.[8] There is a significant tendency for familial recurrence in some forms. The presence of mental retardation is presumptive evidence that aortic stenosis is supravalvular, especially if there is a history of infantile hypercalcemia;[8] stenosis of the pulmonary artery and its branches almost invariably coexists. Afflicted individuals resemble each other as strikingly as do subjects with Down's syndrome; the chin is small (hypoplastic mandible), the mouth large, the lips patulous, the nose blunt and upturned, the eyes wide-set with occasional internal strabismus, the forehead broad, the cheeks baggy, the teeth malformed, and the bite abnormal (malocclusion). This variety of supravalvular aortic stenosis is nonfamilial. There is another variety that can be sporadic *or* familial with normal facial appearance. Supravalvular aortic stenosis is seldom found in adults, probably because of its inherent severity as well as the deleterious effect of the obstruction on coronary arterial circulation.[8]

Anomalous Origin of the Left Coronary Artery from the Pulmonary Trunk

In this malformation, the right coronary artery arises normally from the aorta, while the left coronary artery arises from the pulmonary trunk. The natural history of anomalous origin of the left coronary artery from the pulmonary trunk is a continuum from death in infancy to asymptomatic adult survival, with many gradations in between.[8] About 15 to 20 percent of patients are believed to reach adulthood.[52] Interestingly, one of the first known cases of this anomaly was that of a 60-year-old woman.[53] However, the majority die within the first year of life.[8] Occasionally, an infant with serious cardiac failure improves, only to die suddenly during a relatively asymptomatic childhood or adolescence. At other times the anomaly is discovered in an asymptomatic child with a murmur but little or no history of cardiac disease. Adults may present with mitral regurgitation (papillary muscle dysfunction), with or without symptoms. In some instances the disorder is not suspected until a previously healthy adult develops cardiac failure or angina or dies suddenly.[8] One patient, a 33-year-old woman, had been operated on for suspected patent ductus arteriosus (mistaken interpretation of a continuous murmur related to intercoronary anastomoses).[8] She had no cardiac symptoms until adulthood, when onset of atrial fibrillation provoked chest pain. The electrocardiogram exhibited only digitalis effects. She had undergone five pregnancies and carried three to term with no cardiac complications. It should be emphasized, however, that sudden death is a constant threat, and few patients survive beyond age 30.

Cor Triatriatum

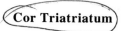

This anomaly is represented by a left atrium that is partitioned into proximal and distal compartments; the latter communicates with the mitral valve and contains the left atrial appendage and usually the fossa ovalis.[8] The fibrous or fibromuscular diaphragm that partitions the left atrium has one or more openings, the size of which determines the degree of obstruction. Functional consequences of cor triatiatum are analogous to mitral stenosis. Clinical manifestations depend upon the degree of obstruction, which can range from insignificant to complete absence of a connection between upper and lower atrial compartments. Cor triatriatum usually is manifest in infants or young children, but symptoms occasionally await adolescence or adulthood.[54] Patients with mild obstruction may be entirely asymptomatic, as typified by a 70-year-old man in whom anatomic evidence of cor triatriatum was an incidental finding at necropsy.[55] Conversely, symptomatic and radiologic evidence of pulmonary venous congestion together with a small left atrium, no enlargement of the left atrial appendage (which is located in the distal or low pressure compartment), and no murmur of mitral stenosis should arouse suspicion of cor triatriatum.[8]

Total Anomalous Pulmonary Venous Connection

All venous blood from both lungs enters the right atrium directly or through one of its tributary veins.[8] The anomalously connecting pulmonary veins emerge individually from the lungs and enter either the right atrium or, as is more often the case, unite in the mediastinum to form a confluence. A separate vascular channel connects this confluence of veins to a systemic vein that lies either within the thorax or within the abdomen. Blood from this systemic vein ultimately finds its way to the right atrium, so that the circuit from pulmonary veins to right atrium is complete.[56] Total anomalous pulmonary venous connection should be suspected in patients, especially males, who have clinical signs of an atrial septal defect with large left-to-right shunt and cyanosis, particularly when the cyanosis dates from infancy or childhood. The diagnosis is most apparent in patients with the characteristic radiographic appearance of the "figure of 8" or "snowman."[8] The silhouette occurs when the confluence of four pulmonary veins gives rise to a left vertical vein that bulges to the left before joining a left innominate vein. This innominate vein crosses the midline and connects with a large bulging right superior vena cava. Life expectancy is best when there is a large coexisting atrial septal defect that allows the systemic bed to receive the mixture of pulmonary and systemic venous blood from the right atrium. When the pulmonary resistance is low or relatively low, pulmonary blood flow is substantially increased, oxygenation is good, and cyanosis is slight. A patient in this category occasionally reaches adulthood with comparatively little disability, although symptoms usually occur earlier.[8] Such patients resemble those with isolated atrial septal defects except for accompanying mild cyanosis. Survival has occurred into the second, third, and early fourth decades. In one case surgical correction was successfully accomplished at age 49.[8]

Right Ventricular Origin of Both Great Arteries

This malformation is characterized by normal origin of the pulmonary trunk but an aorta that arises entirely from the right ventricle.[56] A ventricular septal defect provides the left ventricle with its only outlet. Pulmonic stenosis may or may not coexist; the ventricular septal defect can either be below the crista (infracristal or subaortic) or above the crista (supracristal or subpulmonic). Right ventricular origin of both great arteries with an infracristal ventricular septal defect and no pulmonic stenosis closely resembles an ordinary large ventricular septal defect with left-to-right shunt and pulmonary hypertension.[8] As with ordinary ventricular septal defect, few of these patients reach adulthood, although favorable regulation of pulmonary blood flow has allowed sporadic survival in the postpediatric period. One such patient underwent successful surgical correction at age 53 (Fig. 11).

When pulmonic stenosis exists with right ventricular origin of both great arteries, the physiology of the circulation closely resembles ventricular septal defect with pulmonic stenosis. The history may be similar to cyanotic Fallot's tetralogy and include the practice of squatting. Right ventricular origin of both the great arteries with a supracristal ventricular septal defect and no pulmonic stenosis has been called the Taussig-Bing anomaly.[8] Occasionally, pulmonary vascular resistance delicately regulates pulmonary blood flow so that longevity improves; these patients are rare, but may live into the second, third, or even fourth decade. One such patient died at age 40.[57]

Truncus Arteriosus

In this anomaly, a single great artery leaves the base of the heart via a single semilunar valve.[56] The truncus is situated above a ventricular septal defect, receives blood from both ventricles, and gives rise to the coronary arteries and the pulmonary and systemic circulations.[56] The physiologic consequences of truncus arteriosis depend

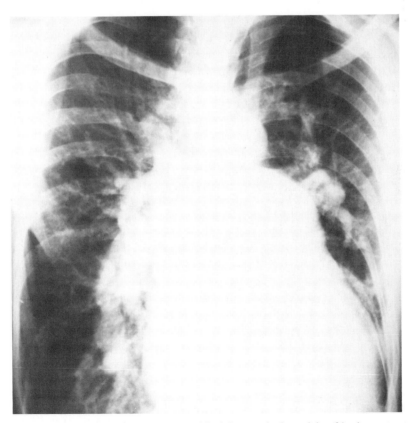

Figure 11. X-ray of an acyanotic 53-year-old man with right ventricular origin of both great arteries and a large infracristal ventricular septal defect. The pulmonary trunk and its right branch are markedly dilated. (Courtesy of Dr. Andrew G. Morrow, Bethesda, Md.; with permission, W.B. Saunders Co.)

chiefly upon the presence and size of the pulmonary arteries and the resistance to flow through the lungs.[8] Longevity is improved if the vessels that spring from the truncus are moderately obstructed; this permits adequate but not excessive pulmonary blood flow and prevents pulmonary vascular disease. A few patients with favorably regulated pulmonary circulations have survived into the third or fourth decades and one patient died at age 43.[8]

Single Ventricle

In this condition there are two atria but only one morphologic ventricular chamber that receives both the mitral and tricuspid valves. The usual type of single ventricle is a morphologic left ventricle with a small outlet chamber that represents the infundibular portion of the otherwise absent right ventricle. The great arteries are almost always transposed so that the pulmonary trunk springs from the single left ventricle while the aorta arises from the outlet chamber (infundibulum). Pulmonic stenosis may or may not coexist. Survival depends largely upon a favorable balance between the resistance to flow into the pulmonary bed and the resistance into the aorta. An appropriate degree of pulmonic stenosis occasionally regulates pulmonary flow so that it is sufficient for oxygenation but not hemodynamically excessive. Survival into adolescence or early adulthood is then possible (Fig. 12), and occasionally longevity extends into the third, fourth, or even fifth decades. One such patient lived to age 56.[8]

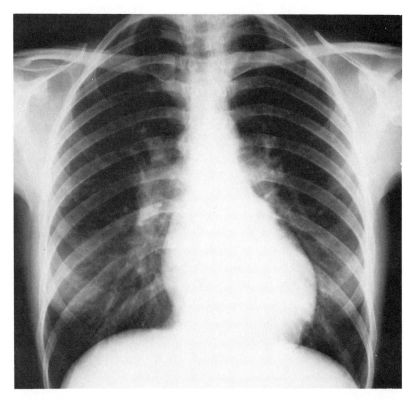

Figure 12. X-ray of a 30-year-old cyanotic woman with a single ventricle and pulmonary stenosis. The heart size is virtually normal. The distinctive feature is the vascular pedicle, which is narrow because the anterior aorta courses vertically upward and the pulmonary trunk is posterior and medial. The patient was married at age 15 and had had two successful pregnancies. (Courtesy of Dr. Stephen Epstein, Bethesda, Md.; with permission, W.B. Saunders Co.)

SUMMARY

Congenital cardiac anomalies in which postpediatric survival occurs because of natural selection rather than surgical intervention may be classified as follows: (1) common defects in which adult survival is expected, (2) uncommon defects in which adult survival is expected, (3) common defects in which adult survival is exceptional, and (4) uncommon defects in which adult survival is exceptional.

The age range of patients with congenital heart disease is steadily increasing because of palliative and corrective surgery. Physicians who care for this new population of patients with congenital cardiac disorders must understand the natural survival patterns before they can understand the effects of operative intervention.

REFERENCES

1. WOOD, P.: *Forward,* in Bedford, P.D., and Caird, F. L.: *Valvular Diseases of the Heart in Old Age.* Little, Brown & Co., Boston, 1960.
2. PERLOFF, J. K.: *Pediatric congenital cardiac becomes a post-operative adult: The changing population of congenital heart disease.* Circulation 47:606, 1973.
3. ROBERTS, W. C.: *The congenitally bicuspid aortic valve.* Am. J. Cardiol. 26:72, 1970.
4. ROBERTS, W. C.: *Valvular, subvalvular, and supravalvular aortic stenosis: Morphologic features.* Cardiovas. Clin. 5(1):97, 1973.
5. MORGANROTH, J. PERLOFF, J. K., ZELDIS, S. M., ET AL.: *Acute severe aortic regurgitation— pathophysiology, clinical recognition and management.* Ann. Intern. Med. 87:223, 1977.
6. CARTER, J. B., SETHI, S., LEE, G. B., ET AL.: *Prolapse of semilunar cusps as causes of aortic insufficiency.* Circulation 43:922, 1971.
7. FALCONE, M. W., ROBERTS, W. C., MORROW, A. G., ET AL.: *Congenital aortic stenosis resulting from a unicommissural valve.* Circulation 44:272, 1971.
8. PERLOFF, J. K.: *The Clinical Recognition of Congenital Heart Disease,* ed. 2. W. B. Saunders Company, Philadelphia, 1978.
9. CAMPBELL, M., AND BAYLES, J. H.: *Course and prognosis of coarctation of the aorta.* Br. Heart J. 18:475, 1956.
10. TAWES, R. L., BERRY, C. L., AND ABERDEEN, E.: *Congenital biscuspid aortic valves associated with coarctation of the aorta in children.* Br. Heart J. 31:127, 1969.
11. GREENE, D. G., BALDWIN, E. D., BALDWIN, J. S., ET AL.: *Pure congenital pulmonary stenosis and idiopathic dilatation of the pulmonary artery.* Am. J. Med. 6:24, 1949.
12. WOOD, P.: *Diseases of the Heart and Circulation,* ed. 2., J. B. Lippincott Company, Philadelphia, 1956.
13. CAMPBELL, M.: *Natural history of atrial septal defect.* Br. Heart J. 32:820, 1970.
14. COOLEY, D. A., HALLMAN, G. L., AND HAMMAN, A. S., *Congenital cardiovascular anomalies in adults.* Am. J. Cardiol. 17:303, 1966.
15. GAULT, J. H., MORROW, A. G., GAY, W. A., ET AL.: *Atrial septal defect in patients over age 40 years.* Circulation 37:261, 1968.
16. CAMPBELL, M.: *Natural history of patent ductus arteriosus.* Br. Heart J. 30:4, 1968.
17. BAIN, C. W. C.: *Longevity in patent ductus arteriosus.* Br. Heart J. 19:574, 1957.
18. PERLOFF, J. K.: *Therapeutics of nature—the invisible sutures of spontaneous closure.* Am. Heart J. 82:581, 1971.
19. SHEPHARD, R. L., GLANCY, D. L., JAFFE, R. B., ET AL.: *Acquired subvalvular right ventricular outflow obstruction in patients with ventricular septal defect.* Am. J. Med. 53:446, 1972.
20. ELLIOTT, L. P., AND SCHIEBLER, G. L.: *X-ray Diagnosis of Congenital Heart Disease.* Charles C Thomas, Springfield, Ill., 1968.
21. MARQUIS, R. M.: *Longevity and the early history of tetralogy of Fallot.* Br. Med. J. 1:819, 1956.
22. WHITE, P. D., AND SPRAGUE, H. B.: *Tetralogy of Fallot: Report of a case in a noted musician who lived to his 60th year.* JAMA 92:787, 1929.
23. MEINDOK, H.: *Longevity in the tetralogy of Fallot.* Thorax 19:12, 1964.
24. BAIN, G. O.: *Tetralogy of Fallot; survival to seventieth year.* Arch. Pathol. 58:176, 1954.
25. CAMPBELL, M., AND EMMANUEL, R.: *Six cases of congenital complete heart block followed for 34–40 years.* Br. Heart J. 29:577, 1967.

26. McHenry, M. M.: *Factors influencing longevity in adults with congenital complete heart block.* Am. J. Cardiol. 29:416, 1972.

27. Nagle, J. P., Cheitlin, M. D., and McCarty, R. J.: *Corrected transposition of the great vessels without associated anomalies: Report of a case with congestive failure at age 45 years.* Chest 60:367, 1971.

28. Kedzi, P., Priest, W. S., and Smith, J. M.: *Pulmonic regurgitation.* Q. Bull. Northwestern U. Med. School 29:368, 1955.

29. Pouget, J. M., Kelly, C. E., and Pilz, C. G.: *Congenital absence of the pulmonic valve. Report of a case in a 73-year-old man.* Am. J. Cardiol. 19:732, 1967.

30. Perloff, J. K., and Szidon, P.: *Pulmonary hypertension,* in Willerson, J. T., and Sanders, C.: *Practice, Theory and Science of Clinical Cardiology.* Grune and Stratton, New York, 1977.

31. Genton, E., and Blount, S. G.: *The spectrum of Ebstein's anomaly.* Am. Heart J. 73:395, 1967.

32. Makous, N., and VanderVeer, J. B.: *Ebstein's anomaly and life expectancy.* Am. J. Cardiol. 18:100, 1966.

33. Adams, J. C. L., and Hudson, R.: *Case of Ebstein's anomaly surviving to age 79.* Br. Heart J. 18:129, 1956.

34. Harris, R. H. D.: *Ebstein's anomaly, discovered in a seventy-five-year-old subject in the dissecting laboratory.* Can. Med. Assoc. J. 83:653, 1960.

35. Goldfarb, B., and Wang, Y.: *Mitral stenosis and left to right shunt at atrial level.* Am. J. Cardiol. 17:319, 1966.

36. Rosenthal, L.: *Atrial septal defect with mitral stenosis (Lutembacher's syndrome) in a woman of 81.* Br. Med. J. 2:1351, 1956.

37. Munoz-Armas, S., Gorrin, J. R. D., Anselmi, G., et al.: *Single atrium. Embryologic, anatomic, electrocardiographic and other diagnostic features.* Am. J. Cardiol. 21:639, 1968.

38. Hung, J., Ritter, D. G., Feldt, R. H., et al.: *Electrocardiographic and angiographic features of common atrium.* Chest 63:970, 1973.

39. Sakakibara, S., Yokoyama, M., Takao, A., et al.: *Coronary arteriovenous fistula.* Am. Heart J. 72:307, 1966.

40. Sorenson, E. W., and Kolsaker, L.: *Ruptured aneurysm of sinus of Valsalva.* Acta Med. Scand. 172:369, 1962.

41. Meadows, W. R., Bergstrand, I., and Sharp, J. T.: *Isolated anomalous connection of a great vein to the left atrium.* Circulation 24:669, 1961.

42. Walker, W. J., Garcia-Gonzalez, E., Hall, R. J., et al.: *Interventricular septal defect: Analysis of 415 catheterized cases, 90 with serial hemodynamic studies.* Circulation 31:54, 1965.

43. Fontana, R. S., and Edwards, J. E.: *Congenital Cardiac Disease.* W. B. Saunders Company, Philadelphia, 1962.

44. Hoffman, J. I. E.: *Natural history of congenital heart disease.* Circulation 37:97, 1968.

45. Wood, P.: *The Eisenmenger syndrome or pulmonary hypertension with reversed central shunt.* Br. Med. J. 2:701, 1958.

46. Feldt, R. H.: *Atrioventricular Canal Defects.* W. B. Saunders Company, Philadelphia, 1976.

47. Jordan, J. C., and Sanders, C. A.: *Tricuspid atresia with prolonged survival. A report of two cases with a review of the world literature.* Am. J. Cardiol. 18:112, 1966.

48. Guller, B., Titus, J. L., and DuShane, J. W.: *Electrocardiographic diagnosis of malformations associated with tricuspid atresia: correlation with morphologic features.* Am. Heart J. 78:180, 1969.

49. Kato, K.: *Congenital transposition of the vessels; clinical and pathological study.* Am. J. Dis. Child. 39:363, 1930.

50. Maron, B. J., Redwood, D. R., Roberts, W. C., et al.: *Tunnel subaortic stenosis—left ventricular outflow tract obstruction produced by fibromuscular tubular narrowing.* Circulation 54:404, 1976.

51. Greenspan, A. M., Morganroth, J., and Perloff, J. K.: *Discrete subaortic stenosis—survival patterns in the adult.* Cardiology, in press.

52. Wesselhoeft, H., Fawcett, J. B., and Johnson, A. L.: *Anomalous origin of the left coronary artery from the pulmonary trunk.* Circulation 38:403, 1968.

53. Abbott, M. E.: *Congenital cardiac disease,* in Osler, W.: *Modern Medicine.* Philadelphia, Lea & Febiger, 1908.

54. McGuire, L. B., Nolan, T. B., Reeve, R., et al.: *Cor triatriatum as a problem of adult heart disease.* Circulation 31:263, 1965.

55. Leoffler, E.: *Unusual malformation of left atrium.* Arch. Pathol. 48:371, 1949.

56. Edwards, J. E., Carey, L. S., Neufeld, H. N., et al.: *Congenital Heart Disease.* W. B. Saunders Company, Philadelphia, 1965.

57. PERLOFF, J. K., URSCHELL, C. W., ROBERTS, W. C., ET AL.: *Aneurysmal dilatation of the coronary arteries in cyanotic congenital cardiac disease.* Am. J. Med. 45:802, 1968.
58. MACARTNEY, F. J., PARTRIDGE, J. B., SCOTT, O., ET AL.: *Common or single ventricle.* Circulation 53:543, 1976.
59. ANDERSON, R. H., DECKER, A. E., WILKINSON, J. L., ET AL.: *Morphogenesis of univentricular hearts.* Br. Heart J., 38:558, 1976.

Auscultatory Features
of Congenital Heart Disease*

W. Proctor Harvey, M.D.

The first suspicion of congenital heart disease is often afforded by the detection of a precordial murmur; less commonly, the electrocardiogram or x-ray provides the first clue, while at other times unexplained hypertension or polycythemia and/or cyanosis suggest a congenital anomaly. The echocardiogram has proved to be a useful tool for confirming or supporting the diagnosis. This chapter, however, places special emphasis on the auscultatory features of congenital heart disease. My discussion will dwell on the congenital heart lesions in the adult that the practicing physician is most likely to encounter.

Although auscultation alone may at times make a specific diagnosis, it must be appreciated that it is only one very important aspect of the physical examination and it is most informative when combined with the other findings from the total evaluation of the patient.

ATRIAL SEPTAL DEFECT

Uncomplicated atrial septal defect (ostium secundum)[1,2,8] (Fig. 1) can be accurately diagnosed on clinical grounds. Of particular importance is the presence of a systolic murmur together with wide splitting of the second heart sound heard over the pulmonic area and/or third intercostal space along the left sternal border (Fig. 2). The murmur generally averages grade 3 (grading on the basis of 1 to 6). It is short and occurs in early- to mid-systole. Although the systolic murmur generally is best heard over the pulmonic area, occasionally it is more prominent at the third or fourth left intercostal spaces. It is not usually loud enough to be associated with a palpable thrill, but it can be grade 4 or even louder and then a thrill may be palpated. The absence of a systolic murmur with uncomplicated atrial septal defect is rare.†

---

*Supported in part by the Special Cardiac Research, Public Health Grants, Benjamin May Memorial Fund, and the Metropolitan Heart Guild.

†I often made the statement that I had never seen a patient with this type of atrial septal defect who did not have a systolic murmur, even though it might be faint (grade 1 or grade 2). Because of this, I was shown a patient at Walter Reed Army Hospital during a conference; the other typical findings of atrial septal defect were present, but no murmur was detected at that time. The patient had just come from the cardiac catheterization laboratory where an ostium secundum septal defect was documented. Then, because of the absence of murmur, I suggested that the patient be presented at our own weekly conference in order to show an exception to the rule. At the weekly conference, however, a systolic murmur was heard. It is likely that in the immediate postcardiac catheterization period changes in hemodynamic state with some decrease in blood pressure and cardiac output were responsible for the decrease in the intensity and the resulting absence of the murmur.

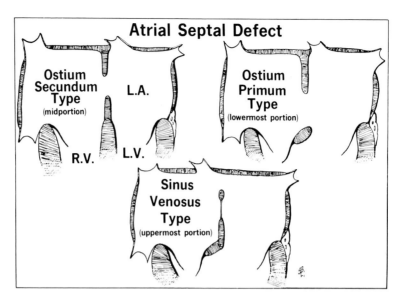

Figure 1. Artist's drawing of three types of atrial septal defect. The ostium secundum is the most common type.

The other finding typical of atrial septal defect is wide splitting of the second heart sound heard over the pulmonic area or along the left sternal border (Figs. 2 and 3). This represents an important auscultatory finding in patients with atrial septal defect.[1-3,8] The second component of the widely split sound is primarily caused by delayed closure of the pulmonic valve. The so-called "fixed" splitting of the second heart sound was emphasized by Leatham some years ago.[2] Some patients, however, have wide splitting that increases further on inspiration. In fact, by listening carefully, some increase in the degree of splitting coincident with inspiration will be detected in over one third of patients with atrial septal defect. Another important auscultatory truism is that of the unusual patient with an uncomplicated ostium secundum atrial septal defect whose second sound becomes single with expiration. It does occur but it is not likely. Following closure of the defect, the splitting of the second heart sound may become more normal, although it is not unusual to find persistent wide splitting. The intensity of the pulmonic component of the second heart sound varies; when accentuated it suggests pulmonary hypertension.

The simple combination of the systolic murmur plus wide splitting of the second heart sound over the pulmonic area or along the left sternal border affords an immediate clue to atrial septal defect. By putting together the other aspects of the total cardiovascular evaluation this diagnosis can be made with a high degree of accuracy. In fact, the diagnosis of atrial septal defect can be one of the easiest in cardiology; uncommonly, it is one of the most difficult.

Since the predominant shunt is from left to right through the defect in the atrial septum, cyanosis is absent except in complicated cases where associated defects or pulmonary hypertension are present. Blood flow is increased through the right atrium, right ventricle, pulmonary artery, and lungs, with little of the burden placed on the left ventricle. Therefore, the right atrium is enlarged, often greatly, and there is concomitant enlargement of the right ventricle and the pulmonary artery and its branches. The lungs are plethoric, but the left atrium is usually not enlarged. Thus, right atrial and right ventricular enlargement in the absence of an increase in size of the left atrium on

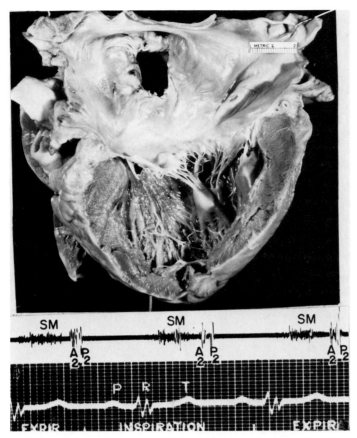

Figure 2. Ostium secundum atrial septal defect. Note systolic murmur (SM) in early to mid-systole and wide splitting of the second heart sound (A_2, P_2) which widens slightly on inspiration.

barium swallow, plus enlargement of the pulmonary trunk and increased vascularity of the lung fields, produce the characteristic roentgenologic picture. The electrocardiogram aids in diagnosis of a great majority of patients by showing right ventricular conduction delay with incomplete or complete right bundle branch block, or right ventricular hypertrophy. These electrocardiographic findings are particularly reflected in lead V_1. The presence of right ventricular hypertrophy should raise the suspicion of associated pulmonary hypertension or associated defects, such as pulmonic stenosis or ventricular septal defect.

The systolic murmur of atrial septal defect may mimic an innocent systolic murmur which also is frequently heard over the same areas (Fig. 4). However, the presence of wide splitting of S_2, which does not become single with expiration, serves as an immediate differential point, as would the presence of an ejection sound, which would not be heard with an innocent murmur.[4] The other clinical findings readily make the diagnosis, but all too often an atrial septal defect has been overlooked because the murmur has been misinterpreted as an innocent murmur. Diastolic murmurs also may be present in some patients and are of two types. The first, an early blowing diastolic murmur consistent with pulmonic regurgitation, may be heard along the left sternal border. It is most audible when the diaphragm of the stethoscope is used. This murmur is not a common finding in atrial septal defect and is more likely to occur with the advent of

55

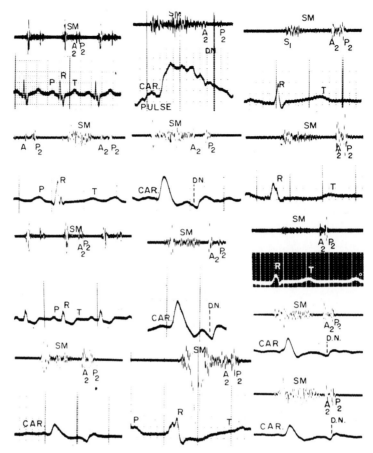

Figure 3. Wide splitting of second sound and pulmonic systolic murmur in 13 patients with atrial septal defect.

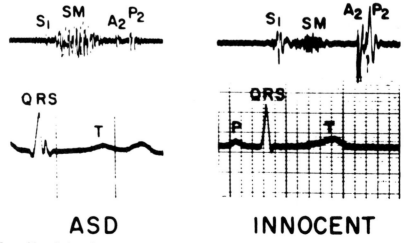

Figure 4. Note wide splitting of second sound (A_2, P_2) and systolic murmur (SM) with atrial septal defect. The innocent murmur does not have the "fixed" wide splitting of the second sound.

pulmonary hypertension, the so-called Eisenmenger type of atrial septal defect (to be discussed subsequently). The second type is found at the mitral or tricuspid area. A diastolic rumble may be present and is usually heard in a well localized spot along the lower left sternal border[5] (Fig. 5); it is generally best detected with the bell of the stethoscope. With inspiration, the murmur can increase in intensity. This rumble is attributed to increased blood flow across the tricuspid valve, resulting from the shunting of blood from left to right atrium. It is likely that the shunt across the atrial septal defect is large since the rumble is usually not heard with a small shunt. A holosystolic murmur due to mitral regurgitation is sometimes present at the apex; it occurs with an ostium secundum defect but is more frequently heard with an ostium primum defect.

Ostium Primum Defect

The auscultatory findings encountered with the ostium primum defect may be the same as those with the secundum defect, and often the first and only clue to this disorder is the finding of left axis deviation on the elctrocardiogram. Right ventricular hypertrophy is more common with the ostium primum defect, as is a holosystolic murmur along the lower left sternal border, indicating tricuspid and/or mitral valve regurgitation.[6,7,8]

Atrial Septal Defect with Pulmonary Hypertension

Physical findings vary in these patients, depending on the degree of pulmonary hypertension. The second sound becomes less widely split and louder, and is often easily palpated (Fig. 6). The systolic murmur over the pulmonic area is still present and, in addition, an early blowing diastolic murmur of pulmonic regurgitation is sometimes

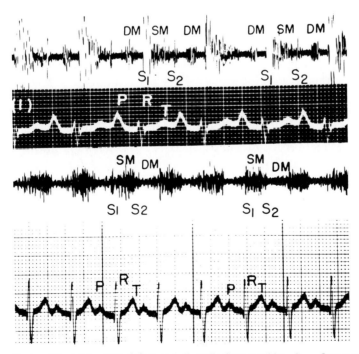

Figure 5. Two patients with atrial septal defect and diastolic flow rumbles. S_1 = first sound, S_2 = second sound, SM = systolic murmur, DM = diastolic murmur.

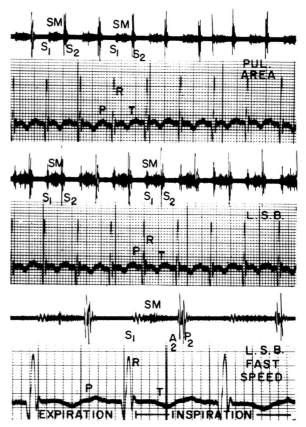

Figure 6. Atrial septal defect with pulmonary hypertension. Note systolic murmur (SM) and closely split second sound (S_2) over pulmonic area and left sternal border (LSB). The closely split second sound (A_2, P_2) widens slightly on inspiration (bottom tracing).

heard along the left sternal border. This murmur is of a high frequency type similar to that of aortic regurgitation, which also is best heard with the diaphragm of the stethoscope pushed firmly against the chest wall. A diastolic rumble can also be heard along the lower left sternal border in some patients. An interesting and worthwhile point concerning the Eisenmenger type of atrial septal defect is that the splitting, even though it becomes narrower, is generally wide enough to identify both the aortic and pulmonic components if one listens carefully. This is in contradistinction to the Eisenmenger type of ventricular septal defect in which the second heart sound becomes very closely split, as it does at times also in the patient with patent ductus arteriosus and pulmonary hypertension. In such instances, the splitting may widen slightly with inspiration, though to a lesser degree than with the atrial septal Eisenmenger defect.

Mitral Valve Prolapse Associated with Atrial Septal Defect

Prolapse of the mitral valve is common in patients with atrial septal defect. The finding of a click or clicks in systole, or a click plus a systolic murmur— either holosystolic or mid to late systolic—should raise the possibility of mitral valve prolapse. Thus, this combination of lesions can be suspected when the usual features of the atrial septal defect are found over the pulmonic area and the third interspace along the left sternal border, and when the auscultatory findings of the click/murmur syndrome are heard along the lower left sternal border and apex.

Another auscultatory feature of atrial septal defect is the finding of a louder tricuspid (second) component of the first sound than mitral (first) component.[1,2,9] Normally the opposite exists. This finding is frequent enough to provide additional evidence for suspecting atrial septal defect.

A clue to atrial septal defect with a large shunt is the finding of a murmur heard peripherally (over the back, axillae, right and left sides of the chest, anteriorly as well as posteriorly). Initially, one may think this murmur is caused by associated pulmonary branch stenosis. It has been determined, however, that flow across the large pulmonary vessels accounts for most of these peripheral murmurs.[10] Of course, peripheral arterial branch stenosis can also coexist with atrial septal defect.

When pulmonary hypertension is present, a holosystolic murmur of tricuspid regurgitation may appear and become progressively more prominent with increasing degrees of pulmonary hypertension; the pulmonary hypertensive Graham-Steell murmur may also be heard then. Both filling sounds, i.e., atrial (S_4) and ventricular diastolic (S_3) gallops, are likely to be present with progression of pulmonary hypertension. Another important auscultatory finding is a pulmonary ejection sound which is more likely to be encountered with pulmonary hypertension than in the uncomplicated ostium secundum septal defect.

Thus, the following signs represent clinical bedside features of pulmonary hypertension: a loud, closely split second heart sound (easily palpable) which widens slightly on inspiration; an atrial sound (S_4) in presystole and sometimes a ventricular gallop (S_3); a pulmonary ejection sound; a mid systolic murmur over the pulmonic area; a holosystolic murmur of tricuspid regurgitation; and a high frequency, early blowing diastolic murmur of pulmonic valve regurgitation (Graham-Steell type).

It is important not to confuse the wide splitting of the second heart sound due to aortic and pulmonic valve closures with an extra sound, such as the opening snap of mitral stenosis, a pericardial knock sound, a normal third heart sound, or a ventricular diastolic gallop. As mentioned, there may be a diastolic flow rumble associated with larger defects, which is heard along the lower left sternal border and is occasionally loudest at the apex, especially if more advanced degrees of right ventricular hypertrophy are present. Because of these findings there may be confusion with the rumble of mitral stenosis. The murmur of tricuspid regurgitation occurs when the heart dilates; it is characteristically holosystolic and increases in intensity with inspiration. The pulmonary systolic ejection sound is infrequently heard in patients with atrial septal defect without pulmonary hypertension; however, it is the rule with mild to moderate degrees of pulmonic stenosis and it is also commonly detected in patients with idiopathic dilatation of the pulmonary artery. It is important to differentiate the pulmonary ejection sound from the loud second component of the first heart sound.

PULMONIC STENOSIS

Uncomplicated pulmonic stenosis generally presents characteristic features that enable the diagnosis to be made with a high degree of accuracy.[1,11-15] It is first suspected when a systolic murmur is heard at the pulmonary area (Fig. 7). The murmur is harsh and rough—similar to the sound one makes when clearing the throat—has its maximum peak around mid systole or shortly thereafter and thereby produces a "diamond or kite-shaped" murmur, and from auscultation alone can simulate the murmur of aortic stenosis. It is generally best heard in the second left intercostal space and is frequently widely transmitted over the precordium. It may also be well heard in the first left intercostal space and occasionally is loudest over the third left intercostal space. The

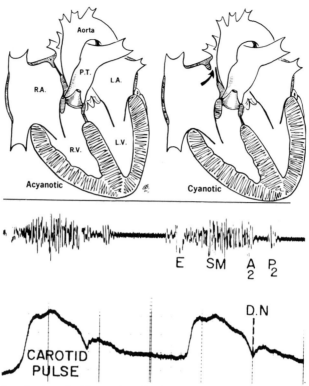

E SM A₂ P₂

D.N

CAROTID PULSE

Figure 7. Valvular pulmonic stenosis. Note pulmonic ejection sound (E) and diamond-shaped systolic murmur (SM) extending to aortic valve closure (A₂). The pulmonic valve closure (P₂) is delayed, producing wide splitting of the second heart sound. The artist's drawing shows the mechanism of cyanosis resulting from the shunting of blood through a patent foramen ovale.

murmur of subvalvular or infundibular stenosis is generally heard lower—at the third or fourth left intercostal spaces—than the valvular type, which is loudest over the pulmonary area. If the murmur is grade 4 a palpable thrill is frequently present, the direction of which is toward the left side of the neck and shoulder, in contrast to the thrill of aortic stenosis, which is directed toward the right side of the neck and shoulder. When the murmur is loud it is often heard well in the back and is frequently heard better in the left upper back than in the right. A diastolic murmur of pulmonic regurgitation is unusual, but it can occur.

The typical loud murmur of pulmonic stenosis usually presents no diagnostic problem. In general, the loudness of the murmur tends to correlate with the degree of stenosis. Fainter murmurs, which usually signify a milder degree of stenosis, are occasionally difficult to inerpret. The possibility of an innocent murmur may arise, but an important differential point is the presence of an ejection sound, typically present with pulmonic stenosis, but not heard with an innocent murmur.[4] Also, with milder degrees of pulmonic stenosis, the second heart sound is widely split (Fig. 8), as in atrial septal defect; hence, it may be difficult, at times, to differentiate between atrial septal defect and mild pulmonic stenosis. However, an ejection sound is much more likely in a patient with mild pulmonic stenosis than it is in a patient with atrial septal defect. Also, right ventricular hypertrophy on the electrocardiogram is more common with mild pulmonic stenosis. With moderate or severe stenosis, the systolic murmur over the pulmonary area lengthens to envelop or obscure the aortic component of the second sound (Figs. 9–11). The pulmonic valve closure, because of the stenosis, is delayed and becomes

60

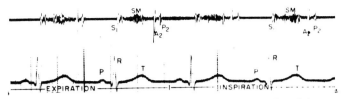

Figure 8. Mild pulmonic stenosis. As with atrial septal defect, the wide splitting of the second sound does not become single with expiration.

fainter. In some patients, particularly in those with more severe stenosis, it is necessary to listen carefully to detect the delayed pulmonic component after the ending of the murmur. Actually, the second sound is widely split, but the first component (aortic valve closure) is "covered up" by the prolonged murmur. By listening along the lower left sternal border, the wide splitting may be identified; in some patients it widens even further with inspiration. It is probable that the degree of splitting increases with more severe grades of stenosis. On the other hand, if wide splitting of the second heart sound is easily identified over the pulmonic area, the diagnosis of moderate or severe stenosis is unlikely, since the aortic component is generally obscured in such cases.

An early systolic sound, the ejection sound, is commonly heard over the pulmonary area; it moves closer to the first heart sound with increasing grades of stenosis and the murmur becomes louder and longer, with the aortic closure sound obscured and the pulmonic closure more delayed and fainter. Also, with increasing stenosis an atrial sound (S_4) is more likely to be heard, and in some patients a murmur in presystole is present. This presystolic murmur may be the result of low frequency vibrations accompanying and following the atrial sound; it could also be related to atrial contraction producing increased blood flow across the obstructed pulmonic valve. The pulmonic ejection sound is a characteristic finding of valvular (but not subvalvular) stenosis; it characteristically decreases with inspiration and sometimes even disappears, but it is easily heard with expiration. The ejection sound occurring shortly after the first heart sound coincides with the "doming" or "checking" (deceleration) of the stenotic pulmonic valve in systole. An interesting explanation of the behavior of the ejection sound with respiration is that with expiration, pressure in the pulmonary artery slightly exceeds the end-diastolic pressure in the right ventricle. Therefore, with each systole the right ventricle moves the stenotic valve forward, producing the ejection sound. During inspiration, however, right ventricular end-diastolic pressure slightly exceeds that in the pulmonary artery and the pulmonic valve may have already moved to its "domed" position; thus, with right ventricular systole there is very little additional movement of the pulmonic valve to produce the ejection sound.[13]

Isolated pulmonic stenosis in most patients is valvular in origin. However, in some

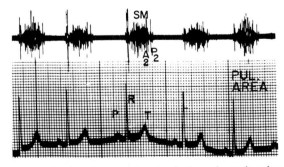

Figure 9. The systolic murmur of pulmonic stenosis extends through aortic valve closure (A_2).

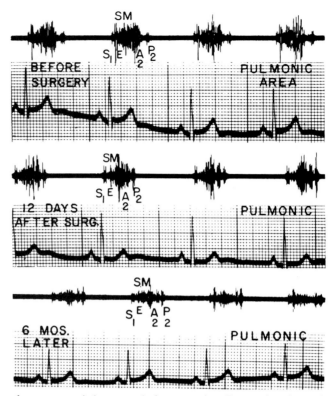

Figure 10. Valvular pulmonic stenosis before and after operation. Top tracing shows the typical "diamond-shaped" or "kite-shaped" systolic murmur (SM) of pulmonic stenosis, tending to mask aortic valve closure (A_2). The ejection sound (E) and the systolic murmur decreased in intensity following operation.

patients with infundibular pulmonic stenosis significant delay of pulmonic valve closure may also be encountered. The murmur of valvular pulmonic stenosis is more likely to be heard higher over the pulmonic area than the murmur of infundibular stenosis. For that reason, the palpable thrill is also higher. Both the murmur and thrill may be maximal at the third interspace along the left sternal border with infundibular stenosis; less commonly, they can be located another interspace lower.

Cyanosis is absent in uncomplicated, isolated pulmonic stenosis; if it is present one would immediately suspect an associated anomaly, the most common one being an atrial or ventricular septal defect. X-ray and fluoroscopic examinations show clear lung fields, especially in the periphery. The pulmonary trunk is often enlarged with valvular stenosis. The electrocardiogram characteristically shows right axis deviation and right ventricular hypertrophy.

Although the murmur of pulmonic stenosis is similar in quality to that of aortic stenosis, there should be no confusion between the two. With pulmonic stenosis the murmur is heard over the pulmonic area and is accompanied by a palpable thrill that radiates toward the left side of the neck or shoulder. With aortic stenosis the murmur and palpable thrill are commonly most prominent at the aortic area or third interspace along the left sternal border with the thrill directed toward the right side of the neck and shoulder. Right ventricular hypertrophy is present with pulmonic stenosis, as evidenced by the x-ray examination and electrocardiogram; left ventricular hypertrophy accompanies aortic stenosis. A left ventricular precordial impulse is present with aortic

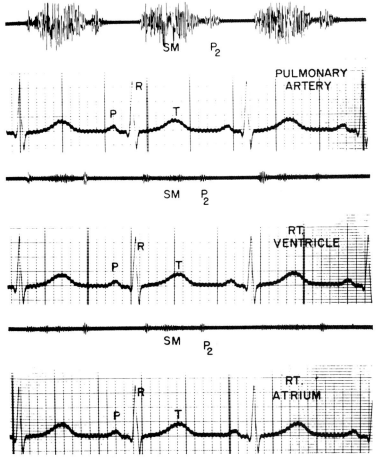

Figure 11. Intracardiac phonocardiogram of pulmonic stenosis. The systolic murmur (SM) is clearly loudest in the pulmonary artery (top tracing), as compared with the right ventricle and right atrium.

stenosis, whereas a right ventricular impulse is encountered with pulmonic stenosis. The second heart sound is diminished over the pulmonary area in pulmonic stenosis, while the same sound is normal or accentuated in aortic stenosis (except with the advanced, heavily calcified immobile valves). All of these findings, in addition to others from the total cardiovascular evaluation, should assist in differentiating these lesions.

After valvulotomy for pulmonic stenosis the systolic murmur usually persists, although it is decreased in intensity. At times there is little change in the murmur in the immediate postoperative period. With the passage of time, however, the murmur may decrease (Fig. 10). After successful valvulotomy, the pulmonic component of the second sound may become less delayed and the splitting closer; it may subsequently be normal.

Intracardiac phonocardiograms demonstrate the site of maximum intensity of the murmur of pulmonic stenosis. As shown in Fig. 11, the murmur is loudest in the pulmonary artery just beyond the valve. Figure 12 illustrates the decrease in intensity of the murmur from within the pulmonary artery to the external chest wall; comparable tracings were recorded at the same volume, and it is apparent that a considerable dampening of the murmur takes place by the time one listens with the stethoscope.

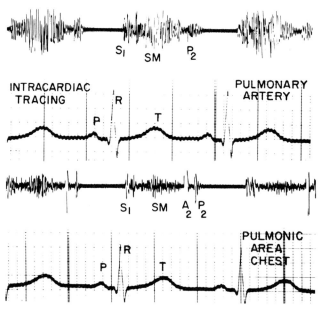

Figure 12. Pulmonic stenosis. Note the striking increase in the systolic murmur (SM) recorded in the pulmonary artery, as compared to the pulmonic chest wall area.

PULMONARY ARTERIAL BRANCH STENOSIS

Peripheral pulmonary arterial stenosis or branch stenosis is one of the most frequent cardiovascular complications occurring in children of mothers who had rubella during pregnancy. Stark, sobering statistics point out the tragic complications of maternal rubella infection in Fowler's report of Kaplan's experiences at Children's Hospital in Cincinnati.[16] Thirty children whose mothers had rubella during the first trimester of pregnancy were studied. All babies had the rubella virus and pulmonary branch stenosis; four also had pulmonic stenosis. Twenty-two had patent ductus arteriosus and five had coarctation of the aorta. Septal defects were not encountered. Most patients had deafness and cataracts and some exhibited mental retardation.

The clue to detection of this condition is the presence of murmurs heard over the periphery of the lungs. One should listen routinely and carefully for any murmurs outside of the usual cardiac areas, including the left and right anterior chest, axillary lines, upper and lower back, the interscapular area, and over the spine. The peripheral murmurs of pulmonary arterial branch stenosis are generally systolic, grade 2 or 3 in intensity, fairly long, and crescendo-decrescendo with a maximum intensity around mid systole; they are rarely continuous. The loudness of the murmurs usually is about the same in the front of the chest as over the axilla and back, and they may increase in intensity during inspiration. The second heart sound is usually of average intensity and splits normally; occasionally, it is widely split. A pulmonary ejection sound is generally absent. Chest x-ray usually shows little or no dilatation of the pulmonary artery segment.

AORTIC STENOSIS

Aortic stenosis can be of several types: valvular, supravalvular, and subvalvular.[1,15-19] Valvular aortic stenosis is congenital in origin more often than realized; in fact, as emphasized by Roberts, isolated aortic stenosis in an adult below the age of 65 is congenital in the great majority of cases. This concept contrasts sharply with the prevailing beliefs held several decades ago when a rheumatic etiology was considered the more likely cause. Roberts stresses further that the congenitally bicuspid aortic valve probably represents one of the most common of all congenital heart anomalies.

It is now known that a patient can have an ejection sound as the only clinical manifestation of aortic stenosis. This sound may be heard in young people without any symptoms or other findings of aortic stenosis, but it is often overlooked. Even more likely is the presence of a short systolic murmur in early to mid systole, which is mistaken for an innocent murmur. The presence of an aortic ejection sound (Fig. 13) should afford an immediate clue that the murmur is not innocent. Subsequently, the same patient may have a louder, longer systolic murmur and an aortic diastolic murmur may also be heard; in some, the ejection sound is encountered with an isolated murmur of aortic regurgitation. More commonly, however, a systolic murmur is present in association with a faint, high frequency, aortic diastolic murmur.

An isolated systolic murmur is often not recognized as being caused by aortic stenosis until a patient is in his thirties or forties; there may then be a progressive increase in the intensity and duration of the murmur, and around the age of 50 or older, symptoms related to the aortic stenosis become manifest. Calcium is frequently found in the valve at that time. This course often represents the natural history of a congenitally bicuspid valve; in others, however, the lesion does not progress, remains asymptomatic, and can be a surprise finding at necropsy. Thus, the natural history can be quite variable.

In general, the findings observed with congenital aortic stenosis are similar to those of acquired stenosis. A loud, harsh systolic murmur best heard over the aortic region is usually present (Figs. 13,14). It begins a few hundredths of a second after the first sound, peaks about mid-systole, and ends before the aortic component of the second sound. A palpable systolic thrill may accompany the murmur. Usually, the murmur ranges in intensity from grade 3 to grade 6. Sometimes it is best heard along the left sternal border, and in early infancy or childhood this may lead to the misdiagnosis of atrial septal defect, pulmonic stenosis, or innocent murmur. When the murmur is best heard at the base or the left sternal border, an important point for differential diagnosis is the direction of the palpable thrill. The thrill of pulmonic stenosis radiates toward the left shoulder and left side of the neck, whereas that of aortic stenosis is transmitted toward the right shoulder and right side of the neck. The murmur of aortic stenosis also is usually heard at the apex and neck, and, if it is loud enough, over the back. In some patients, a thrill or "shudder" can be palpated over both carotid arteries or in the suprasternal notch. As a rule, the degree of aortic stenosis is reflected by the loudness of the murmur; but this relationship can be quite variable. For example, in a patient who has low cardiac output associated with congestive heart failure, a murmur which formerly was known to be of grade 5 intensity can be reduced to an insignificant grade of 1 or 2.

When there is no calcium in the valve of a patient with congenital aortic stenosis, the aortic closure of the second sound is easily heard and may even be accentuated. It is rarely absent. With more severe grades of stenosis, aortic closure may be delayed so that it occurs paradoxically after pulmonic valve closure (Fig. 15). (Paradoxical splitting of the second sound is more common in idiopathic hypertrophic cardiomyopathy than with valvular aortic stenosis).

An important auscultatory finding is a systolic ejection sound heard at the apex, left sternal border, aortic area, and over the carotid arteries (Fig. 13); often it is best heard at the apex where it may be mistaken for the first heart sound or for a split first sound. In contrast to the ejection sound of pulmonic valvular stenosis, there is no respiratory variation.

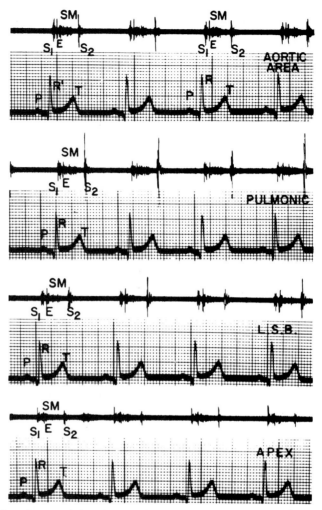

Figure 13. Congenital aortic stenosis in a 24-year-old man. In addition to the systolic murmur (SM), which was best heard over the aortic area, an early systolic ejection sound (E) was heard over all areas. Note the normal to slightly accentuated second sound (S_2).

The characteristic murmur of aortic stenosis is diamond-shaped, with a harsh quality similar to the sound one makes when clearing the throat. In elderly patients with emphysema or other forms of chronic pulmonary disease, the murmur sometimes has a high frequency musical quality often better appreciated at the apex; in such patients the murmur might not be heard as well over the aortic area, although a systolic murmur of a harsher quality is commonly audible over the supraclavicular areas and the carotid arteries. Since bone is one of the best conducting media, listening with the stethoscope over the clavicles may also identify a more characteristic, louder murmur. The murmur of aortic stenosis is generally heard equally well on both sides of the neck, and it is also well heard over the suprasternal notch. Absence of the ejection sound of congenital aortic stenosis indicates that the valve is no longer mobile because of increased scarring and calcium deposition. The probable cause of progression of the stenosis is "wear and tear," which occurs more commonly with a bicuspid than with a tricuspid valve.

The diagnosis of congenital aortic stenosis is usually established by the following

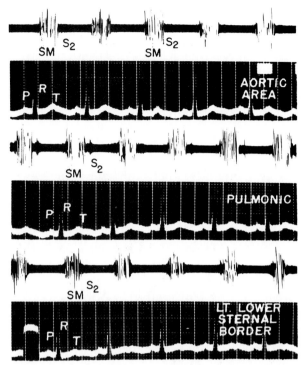

Figure 14. Congenital aortic stenosis. The harsh aortic systolic murmur (SM) was transmitted widely over the precordium. Clinically, the second sound (S_2) was louder than recorded.

findings: a history of a murmur detected in early infancy or childhood in the absence of a history of rheumatic fever; a loud, harsh, aortic systolic murmur indicating an isolated lesion, with a palpable thrill which is directed rightward; an aortic ejection sound; a normal or even slightly accentuated aortic component of the second heart sound; electrocardiographic evidence of left ventricular hypertrophy; and x-ray evidence of left ventricular hypertrophy without pulmonary artery enlargement.

VENTRICULAR SEPTAL DEFECT

The clinical features of ventricular septal defect depend on several factors, including size, location, and the presence or absence of pulmonary hypertension.[1,20,21] The most important factor appears to be the size of the defect. The presence of associated congenital defects causes the clinical picture to vary considerably. The small, uncomplicated defect is not uncommon in infants and children, but is infrequently encountered in adults. This obviously means that a large number of the small defects have closed by the time the patient reaches adulthood. The diagnosis of ventricular septal defect is statistically unlikely in a patient between 40 and 60 years old whose main clinical finding is a systolic murmur; more likely diagnoses in such a patient would be mitral valve regurgitation, aortic stenosis, or pulmonic stenosis.

On auscultation, the usual finding is a moderately loud or very loud holosystolic murmur. It is typically crescendo-decrescendo, peaking around mid-systole and best heard along the lower left sternal border rather than at the apex (Figs. 16 and 17). Sometimes, however, it is best heard over the third left interspace (Fig. 18), or, uncommonly, over the pulmonic area (Fig. 19). The extent of its transmission will depend on its intensity; and if the murmur is loud enough, it can be widely transmitted over the

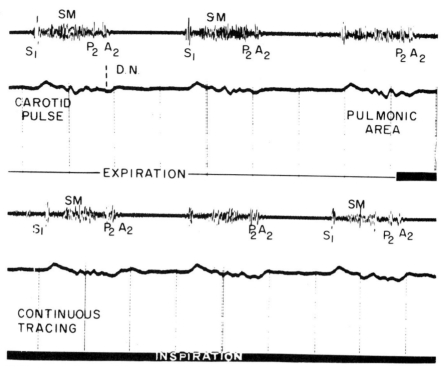

Figure 15. Severe aortic stenosis in a 43-year-old woman. Note the paradoxical splitting of the second sound (P_2A_2): wide with expiration and close with inspiration.

precordium or heard over the back. Furthermore, it may closely simulate the murmur of mitral regurgitation or aortic stenosis. Helpful in differential diagnosis is the knowledge that a murmur was present shortly after birth or heard in the first few years of life, or that it appeared after an attack of rheumatic fever.

An unexplained, moderately loud holosystolic murmur (averaging about grade 4) heard along the lower left sternal border in a young patient suggests ventricular septal defect. The murmur is often harsh, though not to the degree of aortic or pulmonic stenosis murmurs. An important additional finding is a palpable thrill along the lower left sternal border. Remember that when palpating thrills, the palm of the hand should be used rather than the tips of the fingers. Gentle stroking with the fingers of the opposite hand—starting with the tips of the fingers and them moving over the entire palmar surface of the hand—will quickly reveal that the palm at the junction of the fingers is generally more sensitive. Both hands should be tried since one hand may be more sensitive than the other. The presence of a thrill affords an immediate clue to the diagnosis of ventricular septal defect. The thrill is usually specifically located along the lower left sternal border; this area also marks the site of maximum intensity of the murmur, which radiates outward in various directions like spokes of a wheel from its hub. The detection of a palpable thrill generally means that the murmur is at least of grade 4 intensity.

The finding of a holosystolic (pansystolic) murmur generally connotes three important conditions: mitral regurgitation, tricuspid regurgitation, or ventricular septal defect. This knowledge is helpful in differentiating the murmur from that of aortic or pulmonic stenosis, which can be confusing. The stenotic murmurs, as already mentioned, tend to have a harsh quality (similar to clearing the throat), are not holosystolic, and end before the second heart sound; they are diamond- or kite-shaped, and both aortic and pul-

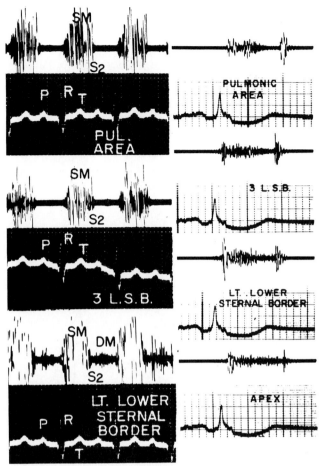

Figure 16. Two patients with ventricular septal defect. The crescendo-decrescendo systolic murmurs (SM) were best heard at the lower left sternal border. A diastolic flow rumble murmur (DM) was heard in the patient on the left.

monic stenosis are more likely to be associated with an ejection sound (which is not encountered with ventricular septal defect in the absence of pulmonary hypertension).

The small ventricular septal defect, or one that is spontaneously closing, may produce a very short murmur in early to mid-systole (Fig. 20). This type of murmur can be confused with an innocent murmur. However, the history will be helpful because the patient with the closing ventricular septal defect might have had a known systolic murmur since birth or infancy; the murmur then gradually decreases in intensity and shortens in duration, and may ultimately disappear with closure of the defect. Sometimes the small closed or nearly closed defect has a sound in early systole called the "wind sock" sound, a term derived from an airport device which indicates wind direction. A ventricular septal defect which is closing or closed can be demonstrated on angiogram to abruptly protrude, like a wind sock, into the right ventricle during the early part of systole, thereby producing this sound.

As a rule, it is not difficult to differentiate an innocent from a significant murmur. This is accomplished by combining all of the findings from the total cardiovascular evaluation. The murmur of uncomplicated ventricular septal defect is typically holosystolic as compared with an innocent murmur which is short, occurring in early to mid-systole.

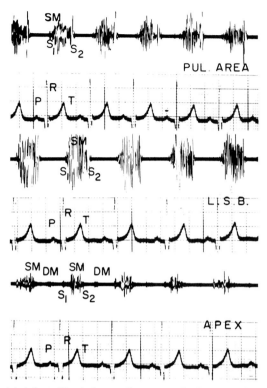

Figure 17. Ventricular septal defect. The holosystolic crescendo-decrescendo murmur was loudest at the lower left sternal border (LSB) but was also well heard over the pulmonic area.

The presence of a palpable thrill would be another point against an innocent murmur, but consistent with ventricular septal defect. Furthermore, there may be electrocardiographic or x-ray abnormalities that fit with ventricular septal defect, but such findings would not be present with an innocent murmur. The second heart sound over the pulmonic area is split, sometimes widely, with ventricular septal defect, although generally not as widely as with atrial septal defect. The splitting usually increases with inspiration. However, as with mitral regurgitation, the second heart sound usually does not become single with expiration; there is apt to be early closure of the aortic component of the second heart sound and this is one of the factors which produces the wider splitting.

Ventricular septal defects with large shunts result in increased blood flow to the right ventricle, pulmonary artery, lungs, left atrium, and left ventricle. These various cardiac chambers enlarge accordingly. Pulmonary vascular resistance and right-sided pressures also may increase and additional abnormalities then become evident. The electrocardiogram may show right and left ventricular hypertrophy. Careful auscultation at the apex or lower left sternal border may reveal a diastolic rumble, presumably caused by increased flow across the mitral valve (Figs. 16 and 17). The pulmonic component of the second heart sound accentuates as a result of the increase in pulmonary artery pressure. The second heart sound becomes more closely split but still widens slightly with inspiration. The x-ray findings vary. With a small defect there may be no apparent abnormality or only slight pulmonary artery segment enlargement. With larger defects, cardiomegaly is present with associated enlargement of the left atrium, right ventricle, and pulmonary artery. The electrocardiogram can be normal with small uncomplicated

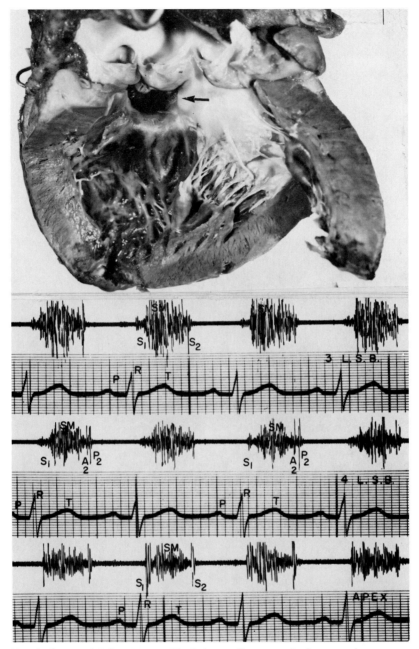

Figure 18. Ventricular septal defect (arrow). The holosystolic crescendo-decrescendo murmur was transmitted widely but was loudest at the third interspace along the left sternal border (3LSB).

defects, but with larger defects, right and/or left ventricular hypertrophy and conduction defects—such as right bundle branch block or first degree heart block—may be encountered.

With increasing pulmonary hypertension, the auscultatory findings of ventricular septal defect are altered strikingly. The murmur is quite variable; it may be heard in

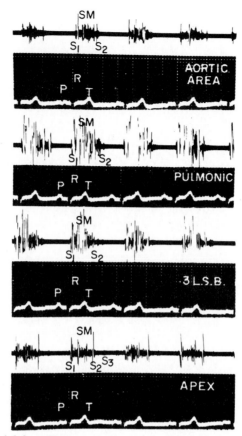

Figure 19. Ventricular septal defect. The pansystolic murmur (SM) was loudest over the pulmonic area but was well transmitted over the entire precordium. At the apex, first (S_1), second (S_2), and third (S_3) heart sounds were audible.

early systole or may extend from early to mid-systole; at times, it is holosystolic and can peak in the latter part of systole. Other important auscultatory findings include a pulmonary ejection sound which may vary with respiration, becoming fainter on inspiration and louder with expiration (similar to the behavior of the pulmonary ejection sound in valvular pulmonic stenosis), but there may also be little or no respiratory variation. The second heart sound becomes loud, closely split, and at times appears to be single (Figs. 21 and 22); however, careful auscultation will usually detect a very close

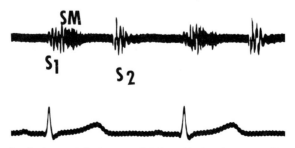

Figure 20. Spontaneously closing ventricular septal defect. Early, short systolic murmur (SM) was heard along the left sternal border.

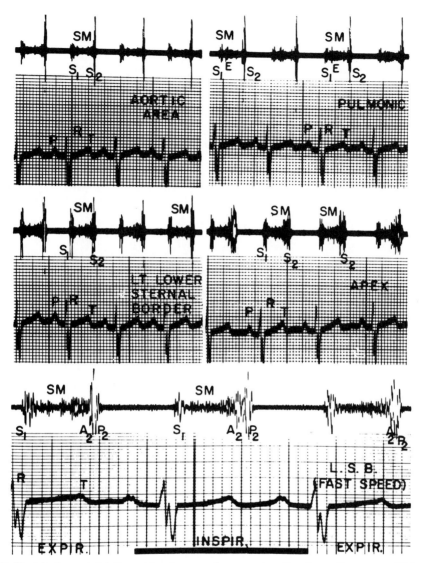

Figure 21. Ventricular septal defect with pulmonary hypertension. Loud systolic murmur (SM) was prominent along the left lower sternal border. The second sound (S₂) was accentuated and closely split. The closely split second sound (A₂P₂) became wider with inspiration. Systolic ejection sound (E) was heard over the pulmonic area.

splitting that increases slightly with inspiration. The pulmonic valve closure of the second heart sound can be felt easily on palpation. The pulmonary hypertensive ventricular septal defect may be accompanied by a murmur of Graham Steell type. This is a high frequency, early, blowing diastolic murmur heard best with the diaphragm of the stethoscope pressed firmly along the left sternal border. The development of significant pulmonary hypertension increases right ventricular pressure and thereby reduces the left-to-right shunt, which in turn decreases the murmur. Thus, the systolic murmur from such a defect is sometimes barely audible and may even disappear. With increasing pressures on the right side of the heart a right-sided (S₄) gallop may be evident and with the onset of congestive heart failure a ventricular diastolic gallop develops.

73

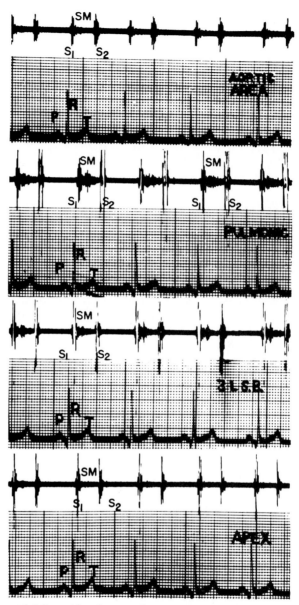

Figure 22. Ventricular septal defect with pulmonary hypertension and approximately balanced pressures in both ventricles. Systolic murmur (SM) was loudest over the pulmonic area and third interspace along the left sternal border. Second heart sound (S₂) was markedly accentuated, and closely split (second and third tracings).

Supracristal ventricular septal defects generally have a murmur that is crescendo-decrescendo, peaks around mid-systole, and is heard over the pulmonic area or first intercostal space. It may radiate to the left supraclavicular area and may be well heard over the left clavicle, since bone is an excellent transmitter of sound. This disorder may be misdiagnosed as valvular pulmonic stenosis.

Ventricular Septal Defect and Aortic Regurgitation

A ventricular septal defect may be located in such a way that aortic regurgitation develops (Fig. 23). This often represents a source of much diagnostic confusion. Patent ductus arteriosus has often been erroneously diagnosed, and some patients have been subjected to ill-advised operations. Some years ago a patient was referred to our hospital for operation for patent ductus. A cardiac catheterization had been performed at the referring hospital and revealed findings consistent with patent ductus arteriosus, i.e., an increase in oxygen content in the pulmonary artery. At operation, however, no ductus was found. Another cardiac catheterization after surgery again showed the increase in oxygen content in the pulmonary artery. However, on review of the phonocardiogram in this particular patient, it was noted that the typical *envelopment* of the second heart sound by the "continuous" murmur was not present. A comparison of the typical murmurs of patent ductus arteriosus and of ventricular septal defect associated with aortic regurgitation is shown in Fig. 23. In our patient with ventricular septal defect and aortic regurgitation, the actual peak intensity of the murmur was in mid-systole, and the murmur decreased before the second heart sound, as compared with the "enveloping" of the second heart sound with the classic murmur of patent ductus. Since that time we have paid more attention to the auscultatory findings and have found other patients in whom ventricular septal defect with associated aortic regurgitation simulated patent ductus. The proper diagnosis can generally be made from the total cardiovascular evaluation. The important diagnostic features of VSD with aortic regurgitation are: x-ray findings of an enlarged pulmonary trunk; electrocardiographic evidence of both right and left ventricular hypertrophy; a murmur which peaks in mid-systole rather than "enveloping" the second heart sound; and, an additional point, a murmur which can be

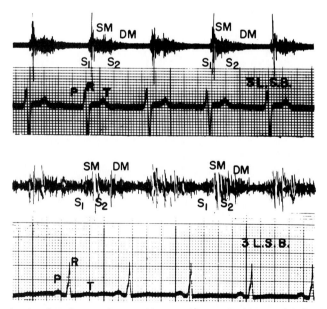

Figure 23. Upper tracing is taken from a 30-year-old man with ventricular septal defect and deformed aortic valve which resulted in aortic regurgitation. Atrial septal defect was also proved at necropsy. Both systolic (SM) and diastolic (DM) murmurs were heard over the precordium. Some observers erroneously diagnosed patent ductus. However, note that the systolic murmur peaked in mid systole and did not envelop the second sound (S_2). Lower tracing is taken from a 20-year-old man with typical continuous murmur (SM,DM) of patent ductus. The murmur enveloped the second sound (S_2).

75

best heard in the third and fourth interspace along the left sternal border rather than over the pulmonic area as with the usual patent ductus arteriosus.

PATENT DUCTUS ARTERIOSUS

Patent ductus arteriosus is now encountered less commonly in the adult than it was several decades ago.[1] This is because the murmur is detected earlier, generally during infancy and childhood, and operation is performed before adulthood. In the uncomplicated patient with patent ductus, there are usually few or no abnormalities other than the characteristic auscultatory findings. There is no cyanosis or digital clubbing, and many patients have no cardiac enlargement. There may be no significant electrocardiographic abnormalities, and most patients are asymptomatic. A few have stunted bodily development. The pulse pressure is characteristically increased, with a lowered diastolic pressure comparable with levels obtained in patients with aortic regurgitation. X-ray findings are often helpful, but not always diagnostic.

The murmur of patent ductus is commonly described as machinery-like and continuous in character, and usually it is best heard in the second left interspace (pulmonic area). Occasionally, it is as loud or louder in the third left interspace. It generally increases in intensity in the latter part of systole, "envelops" the second heart sound, and then continues throughout most or all of diastole (Figs. 24 and 25). The murmur is typically loudest in systole, while the diastolic component is usually greatest in early diastole and less prominent toward the end of diastole; occasionally, however, the murmur is louder in diastole than systole. When the murmur is very loud, as it often is, it can be heard all over the chest and back. Although the characteristic murmur is continuous, it may have a "to-and-fro" quality with distinct systolic and diastolic components, thereby simulating acquired aortic valve disease, but this is uncommon. With a large ductus a diastolic rumble may be heard at the apex, and occasionally the latter is confused with mitral stenosis. This rumble is due to rapid ventricular filling with increased blood flow shunted to the left side of the heart across the mitral valve. The effect of respiration on the continuous murmur is variable; in some cases the murmur increases with inspiration, while in others it decreases (Fig. 26). The continuous mur-

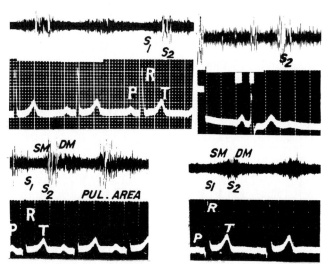

Figure 24. Tracings from four patients with patent ductus arteriosus showing typical machinery-type murmur (SM,DM) enveloping the second heart sound (S₂).

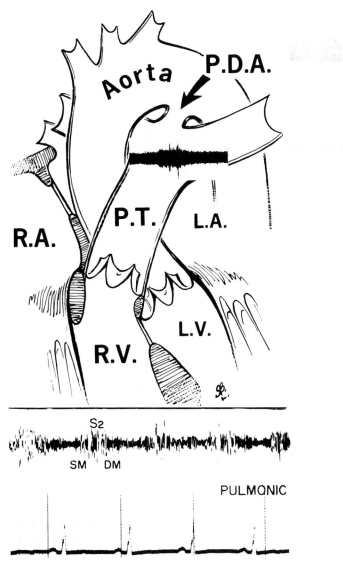

Figure 25. Patent ductus arteriosus. The continuous murmur (SM,DM) envelops the second heart sound (S_2). RA=right atrium, RV=right ventricle, PT=pulmonary trunk, LA=left atrium, LV=left ventricle.

mur is often heard clearly. In some cases, however, the murmur is inconspicuous or faint and of high frequency; as a rule such characteristics are more likely to be associated with a small ductus. The very loud murmurs often have low frequencies and may be associated with intermittent sounds throughout systole and diastole called "eddy" sounds. These findings are more typical of large ducti.

Worthy of re-emphasis is the fact that the most important auscultatory finding in the diagnosis of patent ductus is a continuous murmur that *envelops* the second heart sound. When the second sound is not enveloped, always consider the possibility of another lesion simulating patent ductus or of an associated defect. Remember, "all that is continuous is not patent ductus." In fact, there are about 30 causes of so-called continuous murmurs. When an associated congenital defect is present with patent

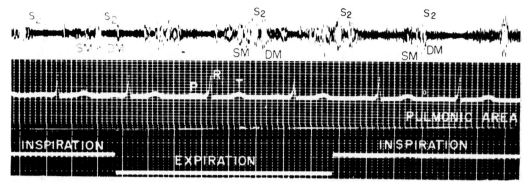

Figure 26. Patent ductus arteriosus. The continuous murmur decreases with inspiration.

ductus arteriosus, the classical machinery-like murmur may be changed when combined with the auscultatory features of the associated lesions.

It is important to listen carefully with both the bell and diaphragm of the stethoscope. Sometimes the continuous murmur is best heard with the diaphragm; at other times it is better heard with the bell (applying light pressure). A personal clinical impression is that there is a correlation between the size of the ductus and the sound frequencies of the murmur. A small ductus is more likely to have higher frequencies which are best heard with the diaphragm (applying firm pressure). The lower frequencies, associated with "eddy" sounds and louder murmurs, are more common with larger ducti and are heard best with the bell. However, there appears to be no absolute correlation between the size of the ductus and the intensity of the murmur.

During the first years of life the signs may be atypical and difficult to interpret. The characteristic machinery-like murmur is not heard at birth, and only the systolic component of the murmur is audible. The diastolic component may not appear for many months and sometimes does not appear for two or three years. For this reason, one should not rule out patent ductus on the basis of the absence of the continuous murmur until the first few years of life have passed. This delay is ordinarily not clinically significant, although in some cases recognition and surgery may be needed even in the first weeks or months of life. After closure the continuous murmur disappears (Fig. 27), but in many cases a slight pulmonic systolic murmur persists. This may be the result of either dilatation of the pulmonary artery that persists for weeks, months, or years, or blood being ejected from the right ventricle.

Patent Ductus Associated with Pulmonary Hypertension

It is probable that the great majority of patients with patent ductus have the characteristic machinery-type murmur. If this murmur is not heard in the adult or in the child after the first several years of life, the possibility of patent ductus is unlikely. The development of associated pulmonary hypertension, however, can greatly alter the typical murmur. Depending upon the degree of pulmonary hypertension, there may be no murmur or the murmur may be only systolic; occasionally the murmur is "to-and-fro" type, and only uncommonly is it diastolic. A high-pitched, blowing diastolic murmur suggests pulmonic regurgitation (Graham Steell murmur). In such instances, the murmur characteristically follows a loud, closely split, often palpable pulmonic closure of the second heart sound. A systolic murmur or a diastolic rumble, or both, may be heard at the apex. In some patients, a continuous murmur is intermittent, and its presence and disappearance suggests fluctuation of the level of pulmonary hypertension. Cyanosis may be absent or marked, depending on the degree of reversal of flow

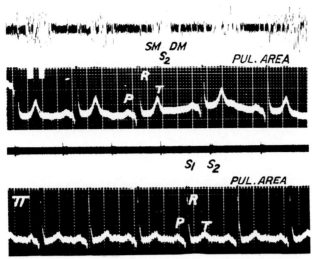

Figure 27. Tracings from a 24-year-old man with patent ductus arteriosus. Before operation (upper tracing) the loud machinery-type murmur was best heard over the pulmonic area. The murmur accentuates in late systole and envelops the second sound. Two weeks following operation (lower tracing) the murmur was no longer heard.

through the patent ductus. Sometimes cyanosis is limited to the legs or may be greater in the arms. This discrepancy, together with the absence of the typical machinery-type murmur, may be a first clue to this complication.

In the uncomplicated patent ductus, heart sounds are of little diagnostic importance. As a rule, the continuous murmur envelops and obscures the second sound over the pulmonary area. In patients with a less intense murmur the second sound may be of normal intensity or accentuated and normally split. In some instances, the splitting is noted to be paradoxical—it becomes narrow with inspiration and wider with expiration. When this occurs, it is generally associated with a large ductus. The second heart sound can usually be heard best by listening along the mid left sternal edge. A third heart sound may be heard at the apex and would indicate increased rate and volume of filling of the left ventricle. Left ventricular enlargement may be noted on palpation, particularly with a large ductus.

With the development of pulmonary hypertension, the second heart sound characteristically becomes accentuated and more closely split (Figs. 28 and 29). In fact, since patients who have pulmonary hypertension with reversal of flow may have atypical murmurs of patent ductus, the diagnosis might be first suspected upon detection of a loud, accentuated, closely split second sound over the pulmonary area together with an ejection sound (Figs. 28–30). The added presence of cyanosis, especially a greater degree of cyanosis of the toes than the fingers, is further evidence of patent ductus with pulmonary hypertension. To determine this difference the patient should be asked to perform an exercise which might accentuate the cyanosis of the toes. A pulmonary ejection sound is commonly heard in the presence of pulmonary hypertension. This sound may vary with respiration and become less intense with inspiration, but there may also be little respiratory variation.

The electrocardiogram is normal in the uncomplicated ductus. With development of pulmonary hypertension, however, right ventricular hypertrophy is evident. Fluoroscopic and x-ray examinations in the patient with uncomplicated ductus may show varying enlargement of the pulmonary trunk and its branches; the peripheral vascular markings also vary from normal to increased. As a rule the heart size is normal;

79

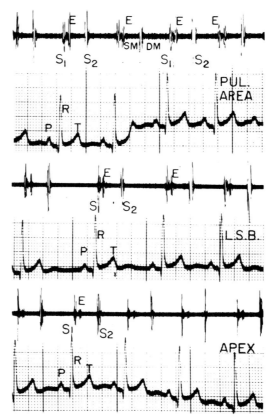

Figure 28. Tracings from a 28-year-old woman with patent ductus arteriosus, pulmonary hypertension, and reversal of shunt. Instead of the typical continuous murmur, faint systolic (SM) and diastolic (DM) murmurs were heard. The second sound (S_2) over the pulmonic area was very loud and closely split. A prominent ejection sound (E) was loudest over the pulmonic area, but widely transmitted over the entire precordium.

occasionally it is enlarged. The pulmonary trunk and its branches may show further enlargement in association with pulmonary hypertension; in such instances the peripheral lung fields generally become less vascular, increasing enlargement of the right ventricle is noted, and a right ventricular atrial (S_4) gallop is usually present. With cardiac decompensation, a right-sided ventricular diastolic (S_3) gallop is generally heard.

TETRALOGY OF FALLOT

The basic defects of this condition are pulmonic stenosis and ventricular septal defect; the clinical manifestations, as well as auscultatory findings, are dependent on the severity of each.[1,23,24] Although tetralogy of Fallot encompasses a wide spectrum of findings, the classic patient has severe pulmonic stenosis and a large ventricular septal defect. In the typical cyanotic patient with this disorder a systolic murmur, grade 3 to 4, is usually present (Fig. 31). As a rule the murmur is best heard over the third left interspace, but it may be heard equally well over the pulmonic area and at the fourth interspace along the left sternal border. The origin of the murmur is believed to be the pulmonic stenosis.

A palpable systolic thrill over the pulmonic area or the third left interspace is a clue

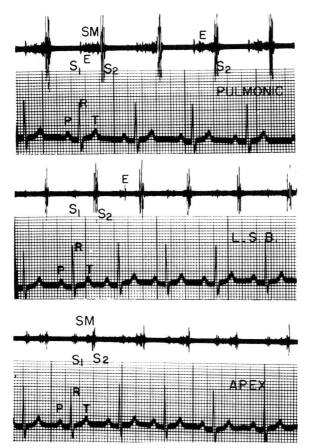

Figure 29. Patent ductus arteriosus with pulmonary hypertension and reversal of shunt. Systolic murmur (SM), closely split second sound (S₂), and ejection sound (E) were best heard over the pulmonic area. There was no diastolic murmur.

that the murmur is at least grade 4, and also that the pulmonic valve is significantly stenotic. Pulmonic ejection sounds are unusual because the stenosis is generally infundibular and the pulmonary trunk is seldom dilated. A pulmonic ejection sound indicates valvular stenosis. The incidence of aortic ejection sounds varies with the degree of right ventricular outflow obstruction. The more severe the obstruction, the more likely an aortic ejection sound. The latter is generally heard best along the upper right sternal border; if it is loud it may also be heard along the left sternal border and toward the apex. The aortic component of the second heart sound is usually well heard and is of moderate or even accentuated intensity (Fig. 31). The pulmonic valve closure is faint and rarely heard with classic tetralogy of Fallot (Fig. 32); thus, a prominent splitting of the second sound would be a point against its diagnosis. Also, a diastolic murmur is not encountered. The first heart sound at the apex is generally not remarkable, but in some patients an early systolic ejection sound is heard; this may be misinterpreted as a splitting of the first heart sound.

When a large ventricular septal defect is associated with mild pulmonic stenosis, the auscultatory signs are similar to those of uncomplicated ventricular septal defect. A wide splitting of the second sound suggests associated pulmonic stenosis, but occasionally this can occur as a result of the ventricular septal defect. The electrocardiographic

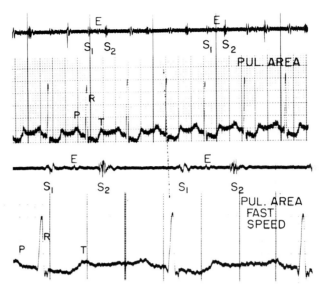

Figure 30. Tracings from a 30-year-old woman with patent ductus arteriosus, pulmonary hypertension, and balanced shunt. There were no significant murmurs. An ejection sound (E) was noted in mid-systole and was best heard over the pulmonic area.

findings in such cases are consistent with isolated ventricular septal defect. The x-ray may show an enlarged heart with increased vascularity of the lung fields.

When severe pulmonic stenosis and a small ventricular septal defect are present, the auscultatory features are those of pulmonic stenosis. The murmur is generally well heard over the pulmonic area or third left interspace. Sometimes the murmur is loudest even lower, over the fourth interspace along the left sternal border. In the latter instances the diagnosis of subvalvular stenosis is likely. The electrocardiogram reveals right ventricular hypertrophy, and the chest x-ray may show an enlarged pulmonary trunk with normal or decreased vascular markings.

The extreme type of tetralogy (pseudotruncus) consists of pulmonic atresia and a large ventricular septal defect. Such patients usually present with cyanosis, and continuous murmurs are heard over the anterior chest and back as a result of blood flow through collateral vessels (Fig. 33). A continuous murmur over the pulmonic area may simulate that of patent ductus; it differs in that it is generally well heard over the entire chest.

Still another combination in the spectrum of defects is slight pulmonic stenosis and small to medium-size ventricular septal defect. These patients have few symptoms and no cyanosis. On auscultation, a loud systolic murmur is usually heard and a thrill is palpated along the left sternal border. The second heart sound varies in intensity; it may be normally split or wide. Fluoroscopy shows normal or slightly increased vascularity of the lung fields. The pulmonary trunk may be enlarged and the heart size may be normal or slightly increased.

COARCTATION OF THE AORTA

The diagnosis of coarctation is generally suspected on the basis of two abnormal findings: hypertension in the arms and systolic murmurs at the base of the heart.[1] In coarctation the systolic blood pressure is elevated in the arms but not in the legs, whereas normally the pressure is greater in the legs. Palpation over the back and chest may reveal pulsating intercostal arteries, which are not present normally. X-ray exami-

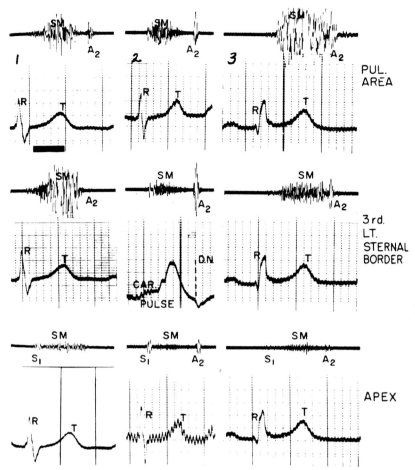

Figure 31. Tracings from three patients with pulmonic stenosis and ventricular septal defect. The systolic murmurs were best heard over the pulmonic area or left sternal border. The aortic component of the second sound (A₂) was well heard in each.

nation of the chest may show notching of the lower ridges of the ribs—an important confirmatory finding along with absence of an aortic knob on the left.

A systolic murmur, usually grade 2 or 3, is heard over the pulmonic and/or aortic areas. In itself this finding would be of little value since basal systolic murmurs are quite common in a variety of heart diseases and even in patients without organic heart disease. What is helpful is that the systolic murmur is also audible in the interscapular region or over some of the arterial pulsations in the back. It is particularly characteristic of coarctation that the systolic murmur can be clearly heard in the back, even when anteriorly it is only slight or moderate in intensity (Fig. 34). The reason for this is that the site of origin of the murmur is about as far from the front as it is from the back of the thoracic cage. The systolic murmur heard over the back may also originate from the enlarged, tortuous, intercostal arteries that are frequently present. A systolic murmur, generally one grade louder than that over the base of the heart or back, is almost always heard over the supraclavicular fossae. Presumably, this latter murmur is also produced by the engorged collaterals. The systolic murmur over the back accentuates late in systole, apparently the result of a lag between systole of the heart and the resultant flow of blood through the collaterals around the coarcted segment.

83

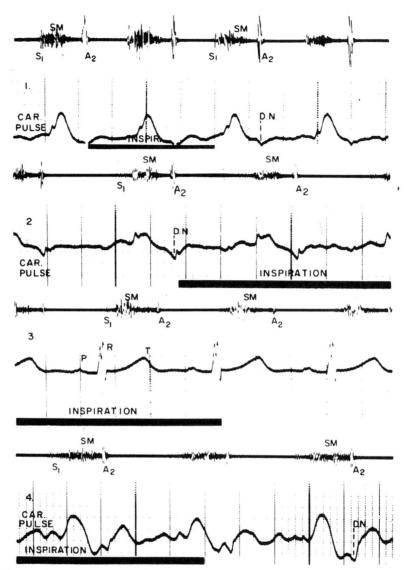

Figure 32. Tracings from four patients with pulmonic stenosis and ventricular septal defect. The systolic murmurs occupy the initial two thirds of systole so that aortic closure sounds (A$_2$) are not masked. Pulmonic valve closure was not heard in any instance. With inspiration, splitting of the second sound was not noted in any patient.

Associated defects should be also considered when additional murmurs are heard over the precordium. A bicuspid aortic valve is the most common associated defect. An early blowing high-pitched diastolic murmur, heard over the aortic area and/or along the lower left sternal border, is consistent with the diagnosis of aortic regurgitation from incompetent bicuspid aortic valve (Figs. 35 and 36). An early systolic ejection sound is another important clue to the presence of a bicuspid valve. Severe aortic regurgitation may occasionally be produced by an incompetent bicuspid valve. The presence of coarctation may be overlooked in such cases because the femoral arteries are often easily palpated and may even be accentuated in amplitude. However, one clinical pearl

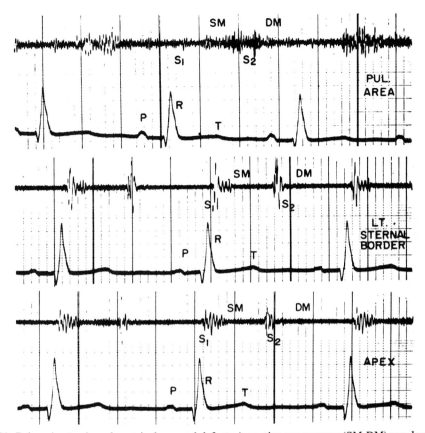

Figure 33. Pulmonic atresia and ventricular septal defect. A continuous murmur (SM,DM) was loudest over the pulmonic area.

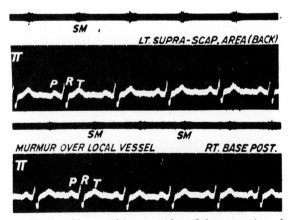

Figure 34. Tracings from a 22-year-old man with coarctation of the aorta. A grade 2 systolic murmur (SM) was heard in the left posterior cervical triangle (upper tracing). At the right base of the chest posteriorly, definite collateral pulsations of the intercostal arteries were felt and a grade 2 systolic murmur (SM) was heard over the vessel (lower tracing).

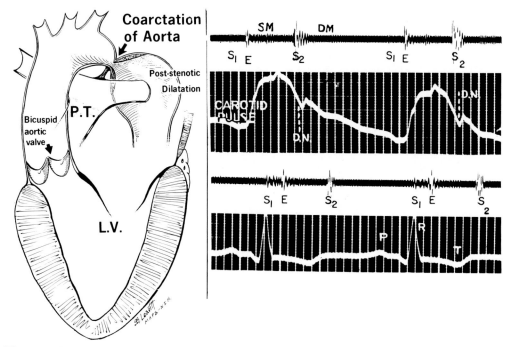

Figure 35. Drawing shows coarctation of the aorta and associated bicuspid aortic valve. Tracings are from a 20-year-old man with coarctation of the aorta and bicuspid aortic valve. Over the aortic area (upper tracing), a systolic ejection sound (E), systolic murmur (SM), and early diastolic murmur (DM) were present. At the apex (lower tracing), a prominent ejection sound (E) and faint systolic murmur (SM) were heard.

is to simultaneously feel both the femoral and the radial arteries; the finding of more prominent pulsations in the radials than in the femorals can be an immediate clue to the diagnosis of combined aortic regurgitation and coarctation of the aorta.

With aortic coarctation the first heart sound is generally normal. However, an early systolic ejection sound is frequently heard over the aortic and mitral areas, and also over the carotid arteries (Figs. 35 and 37); this is sometimes mistaken for the first heart sound or a splitting of the first heart sound. A bicuspid aortic valve is likely when this ejection sound is present. The bicuspid aortic valve may present as only an aortic ejection sound, but if aortic stenosis is present, there is an accompanying systolic

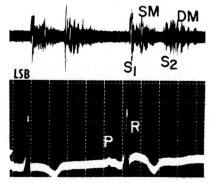

Figure 36. Tracing from a 31-year-old woman with coarctation of the aorta and severe aortic regurgitation. Systolic murmur (SM) and prominent, blowing, early diastolic murmur (DM) were heard.

86

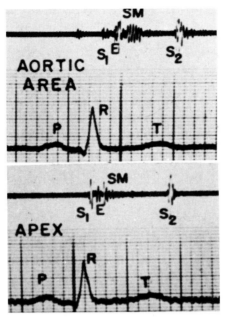

Figure 37. Coarctation of aorta. A systolic murmur and an ejection sound were present over the aortic area and apex. The ejection sound suggested an accompanying bicuspid aortic valve.

murmur which varies in intensity depending on the severity of the stenosis. As mentioned, aortic regurgitation of varying severity is also not uncommon with bicuspid aortic valve. Thus the spectrum of findings associated with the bicuspid valve includes an ejection sound, a systolic murmur at the apex and base, or an aortic diastolic murmur, and these may be encountered alone or in combinations.

In a case of suspected coarctation of the aorta, the presence of (1) a systolic murmur heard over the abdomen anteriorly and posteriorly, (2) palpable lower intercostal arteries, and (3) rib notching involving only the lower ribs, are clues that the coarctation may be located in the abdominal aorta instead of the thoracic. Abdominal aortic coarctation is more common in females, whereas thoracic coarctation is much more common in males.

CONGENITAL PULMONIC REGURGITATION

Although this lesion is uncommon, it is worth discussing; if one is aware of its characteristic features, it will not be overlooked or confused with other conditions.[1,25] Pulmonic regurgitation may result from various congenital abnormalities of the pulmonic valve. It is generally well tolerated and the patients usually are asymptomatic; such patients are usually referred for the evaluation of a low-frequency rumbling diastolic murmur detected along the left sternal border. The murmur is usually grade 1 to 3 in intensity and often increases in intensity with normal inspiration (Fig. 38). There is often a brief interval following the second heart sound to the beginning of the short low-frequency murmur, although in some patients the diastolic murmur is high-frequency in character and begins immediately after pulmonic valve closure. The murmur of congenital pulmonic regurgitation should not be confused with that of aortic regurgitation, in the latter condition, signs of left ventricular enlargement are typically present, the aortic murmur is not affected by respiration, and the peripheral arterial pulsations are hyperkinetic.

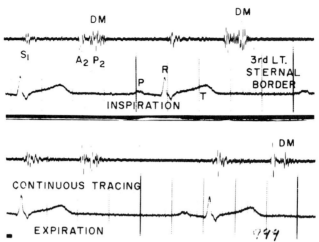

Figure 38. Congenital pulmonic regurgitation. An early diastolic murmur was heard at a distinct interval after aortic valve closure and increased on inspiration.

The patient with the Graham Steell diastolic murmur of pulmonary hypertension is also easily differentiated. Signs of right ventricular enlargement are present along with a palpable closure of the second sound related to the loud pulmonic valve closure. The decrescendo murmur follows immediately after the closure of the pulmonic valve and is high-frequency in character, similar to that of aortic regurgitation (Fig. 39). An ejection sound occurring in the early part of systole is a frequent finding; in some patients the sound may decrease with inspiration. In addition, patients with pulmonary hypertension are generally symptomatic and their x-ray and ECG findings provide further clues useful in the differentiation.

Congenital pulmonic regurgitation also may be associated with idiopathic dilatation

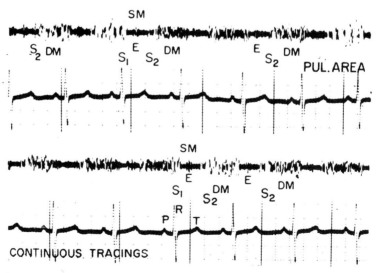

Figure 39. Tracing from a 31-year-old woman with patent ductus arteriosus and severe pulmonary hypertension with reversal of shunt. A very loud diastolic murmur (DM) was heard together with a softer systolic murmur (SM) and an ejection sound (E). The murmurs in no way resembled the typical continuous murmur of patent ductus.

of the pulmonary artery, a combination which is generally well tolerated by the patient. After operation for tetralogy of Fallot, a patient may also show signs of pulmonic regurgitation; the murmur may increase with inspiration and even be loud enough to be associated with a palpable thrill.

ACKNOWLEDGMENTS

Appreciation is expressed for the secretarial assistance of Miss Sharon Federation and Miss Jonnie Morrow.

Illustrations in this manuscript are used with permission of the author and publisher of *Clinical Auscultation of the Heart* (2nd ed.), W. Proctor Harvey and W. B. Saunders Company, respectively. The artist's drawings and the necropsy specimens used in some of the composite figures are supplied through the courtesy of Dr. William C. Roberts.

REFERENCES

1. LEVINE, S. A., AND HARVEY, W. P.: *Clinical Auscultation of the Heart,* ed. 2. W. B. Saunders Company, Philadelphia, 1959.
2. LEATHAM, A., AND GRAY, I.: *Auscultatory and phonocardiographic signs of atrial septal defect.* Br. Heart J. 18:193, 1956.
3. LEATHAM, A.: *Auscultation of the Heart and Phonocardiography,* ed. 2. Churchill, Livingstone, Edinburgh, 1975, p. 93.
4. HARVEY, A. P.: *Innocent vs. significant murmurs.* Curr. Probl. Cardiol. 1(8), 1976.
5. WENNEVOLD, A.: *The diastolic murmur of atrial defects as detected by intracardiac phonocardiography.* Circulation 34:132, 1966.
6. PRYOR, R., WOODWARK, M., AND BLOUNT, S. G., JR.: *Electrocardiographic changes in atrial septal defect: Ostium secundum defect vs. ostium primum (endocardial cushion defect).* Am. Heart J. 68:689, 1959.
7. DuSHANE, J. W., WEIDMAN, W. H., BRANDENBURG, R. O., ET AL.: *Differentiation of interatrial communications by clinical methods: ostium secundum, ostium primum, common atrium, and total anomalous pulmonary venous connection.* Circulation 21:363, 1960.
8. DE LEON, A. C., JR.: *Atrial septal defect in the adult.* Curr. Probl. Cardiol. 1(9), 1976.
9. SCHRIRE, W., AND VOGELPOEL, L.: *Atrial septal defect.* Am. Heart J. 68:263, 1964.
10. PERLOFF, J. K., CAULFIELD, W. H., AND DE LEON, A. C.: *Peripheral pulmonary artery murmur of atrial septal defect.* Br. Heart J. 29:411, 1967.
11. LEATHAM, A., AND WEITZMAN, D.: *Auscultatory and phonocardiographic signs of pulmonary stenosis.* Br. Heart J. 19:303, 1957.
12. GAMBOA, R., HUGENHOLTZ, P. G., AND NADAS, A. S.: *Accuracy of phonocardiogram in assessing severity of aortic and pulmonic stenosis.* Circulation 30:35, 1964.
13. HULTGREN, H. N., REEVER, R., COHN, K., ET AL.: *The ejection click of valvular pulmonic stenosis.* Circulation 40:631, 1969.
14. VOGELPOEL, L., AND SCHRIRE, W.: *Auscultatory and phonocardiographic assessment of pulmonary stenosis with intact septum.* Circulation 22:55, 1960.
15. SHAH, P. M., AND ROBERTS, D. L.: *Diagnosis and treatment of aortic valve stenosis.* Curr. Probl. Cardiol. 2(6): 1977.
16. FOWLER, N. O.: *Cardiac Diagnosis and Treatment,* ed. 2. Harper and Row, Hagerstown, Maryland, 1976, p. 344.
17. HANCOCK, E. W.: *Origin of the ejection sound in aortic stenosis.* Clin. Res. 13:209, 1965.
18. HANCOCK, E. W.: *Origin of the ejection sound in aortic stenosis.* Am. J. Med. 40:569, 1966.
19. SHAVER, J. A., GRIFF, F. W., AND LEONARD, J. U.: *Ejection sounds of left-sided origin.* In *Physiologic Principles of Heart Sounds and Murmurs.* American Heart Assoc. Monograph 46, 1975, p. 27.
20. LEATHAM, A., AND SEGAL, B.: *Auscultatory and phonocardiographic signs of ventricular septal defect with left to right shunt.* Circulation 25:318, 1962.
21. LEATHAM, A. AND SEGAL, B.: *The spectrum of ventricular septal defect.* In *Physiologic Principles of Heart Sounds and Murmurs.* American Heart Assoc. Monograph 46, 1975, p. 135.

22. LEATHAM, op. cit., p. 102.

23. MCCORD, M. C., VAN ELK, J., AND BLOUNT, S. G., JR.: *Tetralogy of Fallot: clinical and hemodynamic spectrum of combined pulmonary stenosis and ventricular septal defect*. Circulation 16:736, 1957.

24. MARTIN, C. E., SHAVER, J. A., ET AL.: *Ejection sounds of right-sided origin*. In *Physiologic Principles of Heart Sounds and Murmurs*. American Heart Assoc. Monograph 46, 1975, p. 35.

25. CRISCITIELLO, M. G., AND HARVEY, W. P.: *Clinical recognition and congenital pulmonary valve insufficiency*. Am. J. Cardiol. 28:765, 1971.

Radiologic Differentiation
of the Common Congenital Malformations
of the Heart and Great Vessels

Larry P. Elliott, M.D.

To properly interpret the thoracic roentgenogram in patients with congenital heart disease, the physician must develop an *approach*. The proposed diagnostic approach is based upon a strict set of priorities and encompasses four major facets. The first is *technical analysis*. The second, analysis of the *extracardiac structures,* involves an evaluation of other thoracic structures such as ribs (looking for signs of a previous operation)[1] and vertebrae, and evaluation of abdominal structures such as the liver, spleen, and stomach. The third and most important facet, the hemodynamic or *physiologic aspect,* necessitates a detailed analysis of the pulmonary vasculature and lung parenchyma before analyzing any cardiac structure.[2] The fourth facet is specific stepwise analysis of the *anatomic structures* forming the heart and great arteries (e.g., position of aortic arch and size of left atrium).

A fundamental rule of any approach is that the physiologic interpretation always takes precedence over interpretation of the cardiovascular anatomy. In other words, *abnormalities of the atria, ventricles, and great arteries only make sense if the pulmonary vasculature is properly interpreted*. The first three steps are always the same, regardless of the type of heart disease. Variations in approach occur in the fourth step, analysis of cardiovascular anatomy.

ROENTGENOLOGIC TECHNIQUES FOR CARDIAC EVALUATION

Any adult patient suspected of heart disease should have at least a posteroanterior (PA) and lateral view with an esophagram. Barium in the esophagus is indispensable for determining the presence of an aberrant right or left subclavian artery, left atrial enlargement, and lesions mimicking angina pectoris such as a hiatal hernia, systemic collateral arteries, etc. Ideally, the patient should have a cardiac series which includes right anterior oblique (RAO) and left anterior oblique (LAO) views as well.

It is my opinion that *cardiac fluoroscopy* should only be performed in adults in whom there is the likelihood of a *calcium-producing lesion* (i.e., aortic and mitral valves, coronary arteries, tumors, etc.). I have rarely found it useful in detecting abnormal pulsations of the ventricles and aorta, and it is worthless in determining increased pulmonary arterial pulsations among patients with left-to-right shunts. By the time the fluoroscopic findings are positive, the plain film findings are obvious.

TECHNICAL ANALYSIS

Technical analysis involves first an evaluation of the PA chest film with regard to alignment. Is the patient rotated? Even minor degrees of rotation will accentuate normal structures so that they appear abnormal. Second, the technical quality of the film should then be ascertained. Is the film overexposed, resulting in vascular markings that are not apparent, or is it too light, risking overinterpretation of the vascularity? Is the diaphragm too high, suggesting pseudocardiomegaly, nonexistent shunts or infiltrates in the lung?

EXTRACARDIAC STRUCTURES

The first step in this phase is to recognize those roentgen signs which indicate that the patient has had a palliative or corrective operation.[1,2] Previous surgery can distort familiar landmarks. A careful examination of the bony thorax and soft tissues can determine whether there has been prior surgery. This is translated radiologically as evidence of thoracotomy on the right side, left side, sternum, or any combination thereof.

The next step in the extracardiac phase of interpretation is to determine the relative position of upper abdominal structures, especially the contour of the *liver,* the presence of the *spleen,* and the position of the *stomach.* Figure 1 shows two adults with malposition of the stomach (visceral heterotaxy). Their cardiac and visceral relationships are virtually pathognomonic of polysplenia with absent hepatic segment of the inferior vena cava, regardless of the presence or absence of congenital heart disease.

The third step, which is not specifically extracardiac, should determine the positions of the *transverse aortic arch, aberrant subclavian artery, pulmonary trunk,* and *eparterial bronchus.* Several questions should be answered.

Does the aortic arch course to the left or right side of the trachea? In patients with cyanotic heart disease it is important to determine whether or not the patient has a right aortic arch (Fig. 2). If so, is there an anomalous left subclavian artery (Fig. 2B)? In patients with a left aortic arch, examine the upper barium column for signs of an anomalous right subclavian artery. This is important if catheterization is to be performed from the right brachial artery.

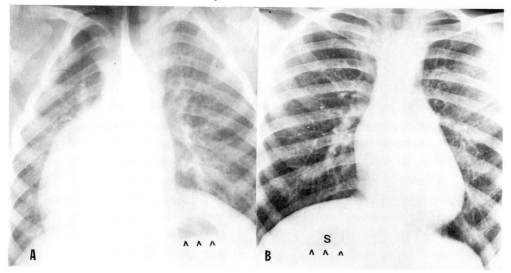

Figure 1. Two cases of polysplenia syndrome with absent hepatic segment of the inferior vena cava. A, The thoracic contents appear to be in the mirror-image normal position (situs inversus), yet the stomach (carets) is left-sided. B, The thoracic contents appear in normal position (situs solitus), yet the stomach (carets-S) is right-sided. Both thoraco-abdominal situations are termed visceral heterotaxia and almost invariably indicate these splenic and venous anomalies.

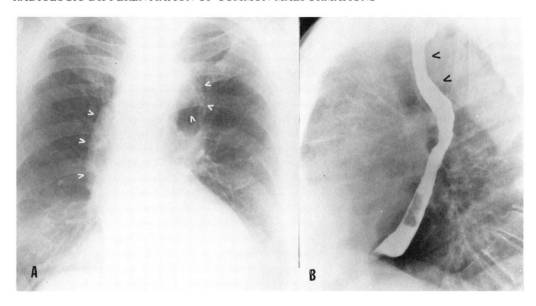

Figure 2. A, Right aortic arch with aberrant left subclavian artery. This elderly male was referred because of a right- and left-sided mediastinal mass (carets). In reality, the patient is normal and has a right aortic arch and an aberrant left subclavian artery. The so-called mass to the right of the spine is the tortuous descending thoracic aorta and the upper left mediastinal mass is the aortic diverticulum from which the left subclavian artery arises. B, The carets point out diffuse posterior indentation on the esophagus by the aortic diverticulum from which the left subclavian artery arises.

Determine the presence of a pulmonary trunk density (Fig. 3). Whether it is normal-sized or enlarged *its presence,* by inference, virtually rules out (1) those forms of transposition of the great arteries which are termed admixture lesions, and (2) corrected transposition of the great arteries.[3]

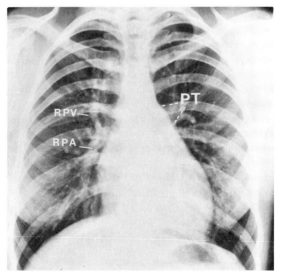

Figure 3. Normal pulmonary vascularity. This PA chest film shows the normal right and left hila and distribution of the pulmonary arteries and veins. The right upper lobe pulmonary veins (RPV) and right lower pulmonary artery (RPA) form the right hilar Y turned on its side (>—). This is a young adult who shows a normal pulmonary trunk (PT).

PHYSIOLOGIC ASPECT

The most important factor in the physiologic interpretation of any heart lesion is the radiographic appearance of the pulmonary vessels and lung parenchyma.[2] Initially, there are three possible findings regarding vasculature: it may appear normal, prominent, or diminished (Table 1).

The only approach to the various cardiac defects via the x-ray is a proper analysis of pulmonary vascularity. Our roentgen approach allows us to place lesions within certain *major* categories before identifying a specific lesion. At times, the x-ray allows us to delineate only a major disease grouping (e.g., a shunt lesion) and nothing more; at other times, the x-ray may be specific for a given entity (e.g., coarctation of the aorta).

The following major disease groups include nearly all forms of heart disease: (1) shunt lesions, which are characterized by an abnormal communication between the systemic and pulmonary circulations; (2) primary disease processes at or proximal to the mitral valve; (3) left ventricular stress problems; (4) right ventricular stress problems; and (5) combinations of these four disorders.

Normal Pulmonary Vascularity

Interpretation of the pulmonary vascular markings is often difficult, particularly when they border on the normal. The criteria for normal vascularity change with age. For example, vascular markings which appear normal in the neonate may actually be increased while markings which appear mildly increased in young adults are probably normal.

Analysis of pulmonary vascularity begins at the hilum. In the PA view, the vast majority of the middle and lower aspects of the right and left hilar densities are formed by the right and left main pulmonary arteries, respectively (Fig. 3). In young adults, the left hilar density is difficult to evaluate in the PA view, owing to superimposition of the pulmonary trunk; it is best evaluated in the LAO and lateral views. In middle-aged and elderly adults, the left hilum is apparent, owing to the absence of pulmonary trunk density. Absence of a pulmonary trunk density creates a concave mid-left heart border. This results in a cardiac shape termed left ventricular configuration (LVC).

The upper portion of the hilar densities (particularly the right hilum) are formed by the upper lobe pulmonary veins and the pulmonary artery (Fig. 3). In the normal person, the right hilum often assumes the shape of a Y turned on its side (Y). The vascular structures which form both hila are discrete and sharply marginated. The cartilaginous bronchi form only a small component of the normal hila. Often an individual bronchus can be seen on end as a thin, discrete, radiodense ring.

The intrapulmonary arteries extend in a tree-like manner from the hilum to the lung, producing a distinct radiographic pattern termed the *vascular markings* or *intrapulmonary vessels* (Figs. 3 and 4A). Although distribution of the vascular markings throughout the lung is uniform, one of the most important concepts for the reader to understand is that the intrapulmonary vessels coursing in the lower lobes are relatively large. One of the early signs of pulmonary venous hypertension may simply be a slight decrease in the size of the lower lobe pulmonary arteries and veins.

Peripheral pulmonary veins play some part in producing a normal vascular pattern (Fig. 4B). The proximal pulmonary veins play a significant role in producing the vascular markings in the bases, as well as forming the upper outer limbs of the pulmonary vessels in the upper lobes.

The pulmonary arteriogram is important in showing the relatively large size of the pulmonary arteries in the bases and the relative distribution of flow (Fig. 4). The upper portion of the right lower pulmonary artery can usually be measured on PA films. A

Table 1. Physiologic aspects of pulmonary vascularity with corresponding anatomic structures

Types of Vascularity	Physiologic Conclusion	Anatomic Analysis	Key Anatomic Structures
1. Prominent			
a. Shunt	Shunt lesions	Levels → Atrial, Ventricular, Great vessel	Left atrium; Aortic arch; Right upper pulmonary vein; Left atrial appendage and/or PT; △Triangle-shaped heart / LVC
b. PVH (postcapillary hypertension)	Conditions beyond capillaries causing obstruction to pulmonary flow	Disease process at or proximal to MV; Left ventricular stress	Aortic valve (Ca^{++}) = A.S.; Ascending aorta; Aortic arch = CoA
c. Precapillary hypertension	Disease process causing severe hyperresistance in capillaries or arteries	End-stage shunt; Lung disease; Occlusion of arteries	
d. Systemic collaterals	Pulmonary valve atresia and VSD		
2. Normal	Normal patient; Obstructive lesions; Small shunt	Sides → Left side, Right side	LVC, ascending aorta, arch; Pulmonary trunk, left pulmonary artery; Size of aorta, right atrium and heart
		Levels → Associated VSD (or single ventricle), Intact ventricular septum, Asplenia	Liver, spleen, eparterial bronchus
3. Diminished	Obstruction at or below pulmonary valve	Levels	

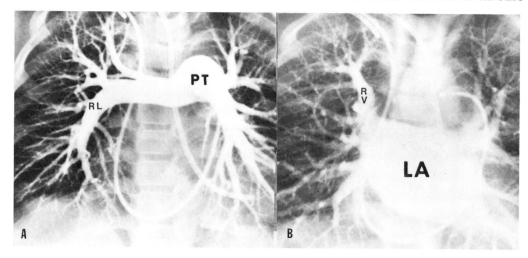

Figure 4. Normal pulmonary arteries and veins. A, The arterial phase shows the pulmonary trunk (PT), right and left pulmonary arteries with dichotomous branching into the periphery of the lung. The right lower pulmonary artery (RL) is one artery that is measurable on a PA chest film. The arteries run in a somewhat vertical manner, particularly in the bases. B, The pulmonary veins in the bases course in a more horizontal fashion than the arteries. The upper pulmonary veins form the outer limb of the vascular structures seen in the PA chest film. The right upper pulmonary vein (RV) forms the upper limb of the right hilar Y. LA = left atrium.

measurement over 17 mm. is highly suggestive of increased flow.[4] Note that the velocity of flow is uniform throughout the entire lung; contrast material reaches the periphery of the lung in the upper lobes in the same instant it reaches the midlobe and lower lobe regions. This concept is important in understanding the mechanism of changes seen in shunts and in pulmonary venous hypertension.

Prominent Pulmonary Vascularity

Prominent pulmonary vascularity can be subdivided into four major categories: (1) shunt lesions, (2) pulmonary venous hypertension (postcapillary hypertension), (3) precapillary hypertension, and (4) systemic collateral arteries (see Table 1).

Shunt Lesions

Uniform prominence of the hilar and intrapulmonary arteries and veins is the hallmark of the shunt, regardless of the location of the defect. Although the pulmonary trunk is often enlarged, there is no correlation between the size of the pulmonary trunk and the size of the shunt. Moreover, shunts at any level may not reveal a prominent pulmonary trunk. Changes in the pulmonary arteries and veins (pulmonary vessels) reflect the increased pulmonary blood flow and/or pressure which occur in conjunction with these abnormal communications (Figs. 5 and 6). When increased vascularity is in question, analysis of the hilar and intrapulmonary vessels in the lateral and oblique views will often provide the answer. With a significant shunt, the hilar and proximal pulmonary vessels appear abnormally large and dense in the lateral view (Fig. 5B). With the large shunts, regardless of site, vascularity is unequivocally abnormal, whereas in most small shunts the vasculature is normal. In moderate-sized shunts vascularity may be difficult to interpret, ranging from normal to overtly increased. A right lower pulmonary artery over 14 mm. would suggest increased flow, while one measuring 17 mm. or more is highly indicative of increased flow.[4]

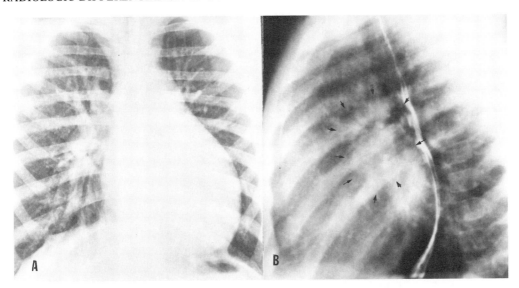

Figure 5. Shunt vascularity. In the PA view (A), shunt vascularity is simply indicated by a prominence of the pulmonary vessels. Shunt vessels in adults usually maintain a well delineated discrete margin, an important point distinguishing them from the vessels in PVH. The vessels can often be seen as prominent, well-defined structures below the diaphragm, particularly on the right side. In the lateral view (B) (different case), the right pulmonary artery on end becomes so large that it presents as a mass-like effect (arrows). There is a moderate degree of left atrial enlargement shown by the deviation of the barium-filled esophagus.

The presence of shunt vascularity usually indicates congenital heart disease. Occasionally, the vessels of patients with high flow syndromes or increased metabolic demands such as *anemia, pregnancy, thyrotoxicosis,* or *A-V fistulas* will mimic a shunt lesion. The *teenager* and *well-conditioned athlete* may also exhibit prominent vascularity.

In those patients with signs of a shunt lesion, and in whom it is determined there is a normal hematocrit and no clinical evidence of desaturation (cyanosis), the functional interpretation of left-to-right (L–R) shunt can be made. Now the observer is ready to utilize certain anatomic structures—notably, the *left atrium, transverse aortic arch,* and *right upper pulmonary vein.* These will be discussed in the anatomic phase of analysis.

Pulmonary Venous Hypertension

The type and severity of the vascular changes reflected in the chest film depend directly on the degree of pulmonary venous hypertension (PVH). In the roentgenogram, the physiologic and anatomic responses of the pulmonary vasculature to PVH are manifested by (1) redistribution of blood flow to the upper lobes and a corresponding decrease of blood flow to the lower lobes, and (2) edema around the bronchi, pulmonary vessels, and interlobular septa and in the air spaces.

Once again, pulmonary arteriography is important in showing the mechanism of changes depicted on the plain chest films (Fig. 7). The redistribution phenomenon is reflected as a decrease in size of the arteries and veins in the lower lobes (Fig. 7, A and B). The concomitant decrease in the velocity of blood flow to the lower lobes as compared to the upper lobes is shown by the capillary phase appearing in the upper lobes before it appears in the lower lobes, and by the upper lobe pulmonary veins filling before the lower lobe veins (Fig. 7, B and C). Another characteristic of PVH is a distinct tendency for the upper lobe pulmonary veins to show relatively more dilatation than their companion arteries. The plain film signs are as follows.

97

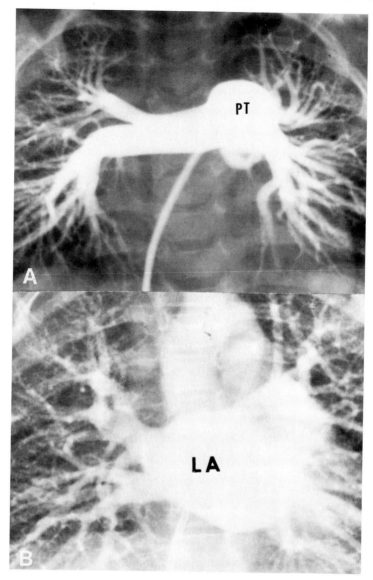

Figure 6. Pulmonary arteriogram with shunt vascularity. A, The pulmonary trunk (PT) and central pulmonary arteries are simply increased in size from the normal. This is a reflection of increased flow through the arterial system. In the venous phase B, the pulmonary veins are also enlarged as a reflection of the increased flow. The percentage of shunt must be at least 40 percent before definitive plain film signs are apparent. LA = left atrium.

HILAR VESSELS. One of the earliest signs of PVH is seen in the right hilum as loss of the normal hilar angle or ✕. This is caused by dilatation of the right upper lobe vein, interstitial and perivascular edema, or both (Figs. 8 and 9A).

In patients with moderate or severe PVH the hila become dense and prominent and are thus similar to the hila of a shunt. But unlike those of a shunt, the hila in PVH appear ill-defined or fuzzy, often creating the appearance of an indistinct "blob" (Figs. 8 and 9B). Moreover, the bronchi which are seen on end reveal indistinct margins with thick, dense cuffs of edema around their periphery (Fig. 8A).

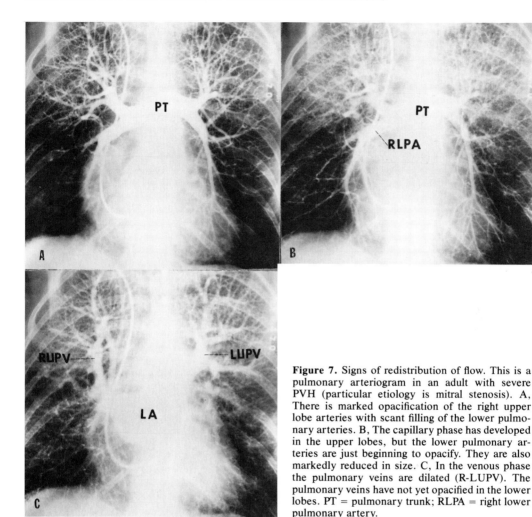

Figure 7. Signs of redistribution of flow. This is a pulmonary arteriogram in an adult with severe PVH (particular etiology is mitral stenosis). A, There is marked opacification of the right upper lobe arteries with scant filling of the lower pulmonary arteries. B, The capillary phase has developed in the upper lobes, but the lower pulmonary arteries are just beginning to opacify. They are also markedly reduced in size. C, In the venous phase the pulmonary veins are dilated (R-LUPV). The pulmonary veins have not yet opacified in the lower lobes. PT = pulmonary trunk; RLPA = right lower pulmonary artery.

INTRAPULMONARY VESSELS. The hallmark of PVH is a relative decrease in the size of the lower lobe vessels and a concomitant increase in size of the upper lobe veins (Figs. 8 and 9A). With moderate to severe PVH the lower lobe vessels are difficult to identify (Fig. 8). The upper lobe vessels are not only prominent but reveal well delineated, tapering margins.

In the lung bases perivascular edema results in a "veiling" phenomenon in which the bases appear to show a hazy veil in front of the vessels (Fig. 8B). This is best evaluated on the right side for obvious reasons.

If the mean pulmonary venous pressure (or pulmonary arterial wedge pressure) exceeds the oncotic pressure (usually 20 to 25 mm. Hg), the lymphatic channels of the interlobular septa in the bases of the lung become prominent (Fig. 9B). These are reflected radiologically as thin, dense, horizontal streaks, often termed *Kerley B-lines*.

Air space edema indicates severe PVH and occurs when the mean left atrial pressure is 25 mm. Hg or more (Fig. 9A). It has a homogenous appearance and is evanescent.

Once the observer has determined that he is dealing with some degree of PVH, he must next define the level of obstruction. Roentgenologically, all causes of PVH can be separated into two major categories: (1) a primary disease process at or proximal to the

99

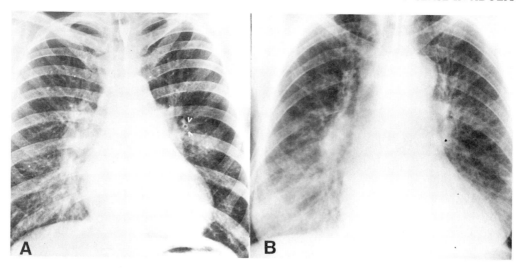

Figure 8. Plain film signs of pulmonary venous hypertension. A, Redistribution of flow is indicated by dilated upper lobe veins, reduction in size of the lower lobe vessels, a hazy reticulation in the right lung base owing to perivascular edema, peribronchial edema (carets), a hazy, ill-defined but prominent hilum, and an overall reticulation to the lung fields. (Compare this right hilum with the one in Fig. 5A). B, The findings are relatively the same. The "veiling" and reticulation and perivascular edema is even greater in the right base. There are interstitial Kerley B-lines in the left base. In A, the pulmonary trunk is dilated; when combined with severe PVH this indicates a mechanical obstruction at or proximal to the mitral valve. This patient has mitral stenosis and the atrial appendage has been amputated. In B, the PVH is secondary to left ventricular decompensation, indicated by the concave left heart border which invariably implicates the left ventricle as the offending site of PVH.

mitral valve (this includes all mechanical obstructive lesions at or proximal to the mitral valve and also rheumatic mitral valve incompetence), and (2) some condition stressing the left ventricle to the point that the end-diastolic pressure is elevated. The mechanisms of approach beyond this point will be dealt with in the anatomic phase of analysis.

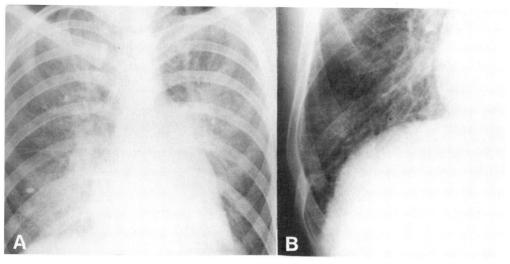

Figure 9. Pulmonary venous hypertension. A, The PVH is severe, with interstitial edema throughout most of the lung fields and *air space edema* in the right base. B, A closeup view of the right base shows the horizontal streaks or interstitial Kerley B-lines.

Precapillary Hypertension

This roentgen pattern indicates a severe degree of hypertension on the precapillary side of the pulmonary vascular bed (Fig. 10). The pulmonary artery and right ventricular pressures are usually equal to or greater than systemic arterial pressure.

A common etiology among adult patients with congenital heart disease is that of a large shunt lesion anywhere within the heart or great vessels. The roentgen findings in practically all shunt lesions in the hyperresistant or Eisenmenger stage are so similar that separate roentgen descriptions for each entity are unrewarding. Two conditions, patent ductus arteriosus (PDA) and total anomalous pulmonary venous connection (TAPVC), may show characteristic x-ray features. The PDA may show calcium in the wall of the ductus or aneurysmal dilatation of the ductus itself (Fig. 10B).

The fundamental roentgen findings are those involving the hilar and central pulmonary arteries (Fig. 10). As with L-R shunt lesions, the size of the pulmonary trunk per se plays no role in diagnosis. A prominent pulmonary trunk is common, but the diagnosis of precapillary hypertension does not depend upon its presence; it depends, instead on prominent, well-defined central pulmonary arteries together with a diminution and/or distortion in the size and course of the intrapulmonary arteries. In adults, calcium may be present in the pulmonary trunk and in the proximal pulmonary arteries (Fig. 10A). This almost invariably indicates (1) a longstanding chronic hypertensive state and (2) pulmonary artery pressures equal to or greater than systemic pressures.

The large hilar arteries together with the distinct decrease in size of the intrapulmonary arteries will often result in the "pruned-tree" appearance of the lung field (Fig. 10). The cardiovascular silhouette is usually normal or only slightly enlarged, but the right ventricle and right atrium appear prominent.

It must be stated that hyperresistant type pulmonary vascularity in some patients may appear to be essentially *normal*. We have witnessed this in several older children and young adults with large ventricular septal defect (VSD) and hyperresistance.

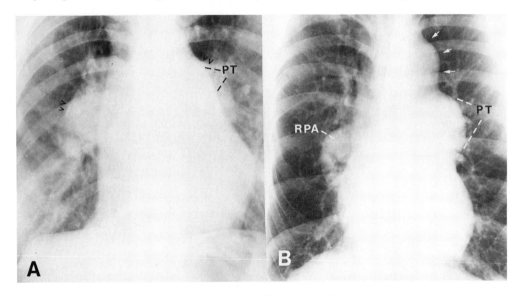

Figure 10. Precapillary hypertension. In both (A) VSD and (B) PDA the pulmonary trunk is exceedingly prominent (PT). The central pulmonary arteries are also prominent and the vessels beyond the central arteries are diminished and distorted. A, There is calcification in the wall of the right pulmonary artery and left pulmonary artery (carets). B, The arrows show a prominent vascular density which represents the dilated ductus infundibulum (outer wall of the ductus). Both patients were mildly cyanotic.

Systemic Collateral Arteries

Uncommonly, the pulmonary vasculature appears slightly prominent and/or reticulated owing to an increase in flow through systemic collateral arteries. This occurs almost invariably in patients with atresia of the pulmonary valve, VSD, and a single aortic trunk. The so-called end-stage tetralogy of Fallot, or pseudotruncus, is by far the most common lesion showing this pattern. Other lesions characterized by a *single aortic trunk*, pulmonary atresia, and VSD may show identical x-ray findings.

Making the distinction between prominent pulmonary arteries and systemic collateral arteries is usually not difficult. In the latter instance the vessel pattern, although prominent, is disorganized and has a more stringy or reticulated appearance (Fig. 11). More important, the hila are not large and are disorganized or even inapparent in the lateral view (Fig. 11B). The arteries seem most prominent over the area of the main stem bronchi (Fig. 11A). Clinically, these patients are cyanotic by the time they reach adulthood, with digital clubbing and elevated hematocrits.

Decreased Pulmonary Vascularity

Decreased pulmonary vascularity indicates severe obstruction to the flow of blood from the ventricle out of which the pulmonary artery arises. This may be a right, left, or single (primitive) ventricle. The chest film cannot identify the site of origin of the pulmonary valve. The obstruction itself is usually at the pulmonary valve or just below, in the infundibulum, or at both sites. Severe obstruction of flow at the inflow portion of the right ventricle (anomalous muscle bundle) or above the pulmonary valve is uncommon to rare.

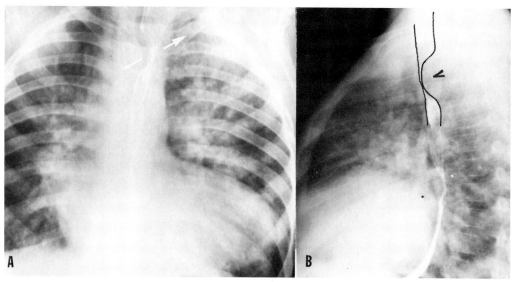

Figure 11. Systemic collateral vascularity. This is an adult with end-stage tetralogy (pseudotruncus arteriosus). A, The overall vascular picture appears prominent, yet there are no well-defined central arteries. The prominence is not uniform and is centered around the major bronchi and the left upper lobe. There is a right aortic arch (deviation of the trachea to the left) with an aberrant left subclavian artery. Right arch occurs in 50 percent of pseudotruncus cases. B, The lateral view shows prominence of the vessels throughout the lung but there are no well-defined hilar vessels (compare with Fig. 5B). The arrow in (A) and the caret in (B) point out the compression by the aortic diverticulum in the retroesophageal position from which the aberrant left subclavian artery arises.

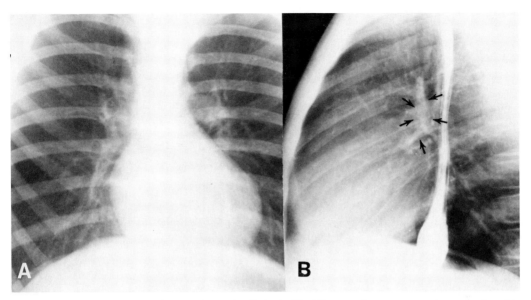

Figure 12. Diminished vascularity (tetralogy of Fallot). A, The hilar vessels are apparent but are reduced in size; the right lower pulmonary artery is particularly small and is the easiest to evaluate. The lungs often appear to be overexposed or hyperlucent with this condition. B, The lateral view shows a small or hypoplastic right hilum (arrows).

When the obstruction is severe enough to result in diminished pulmonary flow, the hilar and intrapulmonary vessels appear small (Fig. 12). The hilar vessels appear reduced in size and are also less dense than normal.

In adults, the lungs may have an emphysema-like appearance (Fig. 12A).

ANATOMIC STRUCTURES

Once a physiologic interpretation of pulmonary vascularity is achieved, the anatomy of the atria, ventricles, and great arteries assumes greater meaning.

Prominent Vascularity

There are four basic types of prominent vascularity. The presence of shunt vascularity or systemic collaterals almost invariably indicates a congenital cardiovascular lesion. Pulmonary venous hypertension and precapillary hypertension are seen in both congenital and acquired diseases. Lesions showing PVH at or proximal to the mitral valve are usually acquired, with rheumatic endocarditis of the mitral valve being the most common.

Acyanotic Lesions with Shunt Vascularity

There are four acyanotic lesions that comprise approximately 90 percent of the shunts encountered, regardless of age: (1) VSD, (2) PDA, (3) atrial septal defect (ASD), and (4) some form of endocardial cushion defect. *In adults, ASD is the lesion encountered at least 80 to 90 percent of the time.* If an adult female presents with shunt, the chances are greater than 90 percent that the patient has ASD. This is because the other forms of shunt lesions have usually undergone operative repair in childhood, and because ASD occurs in a female:male ratio of 4:1.

103

Left-to-right shunts are traditionally analyzed based upon the *level* of the shunt, i.e., the atrial level, the ventricular level, and the great artery level.

The pulmonary vascularity does not indicate the site of the shunt; it simply indicates its magnitude. Moreover, small defects or communications at any level do not show abnormal vascularity. The shunt must be at least 40 percent before the vascularity shows clear-cut changes. In infants and children the level of the shunt is best determined by the presence or absence of left atrial enlargement. When the shunt is at the "atrial level," there is no left atrial enlargement because through most of the cardiac cycle the left atrium can discharge the excess blood into the right atrium as well as into the left ventricle during diastole. When the atrial septum is intact and the shunt is of sufficient magnitude, the body of the left atrium enlarges (Fig. 5B); the left atrial appendage enlarges only rarely. [6]

Although there is an increase in blood flow through the left atrium in all shunts below the AV valves, most adults with such lesions do not show left atrial enlargement. When they are small, VSD and PDA show no plain film abnormalities at all. In adults, the moderate- and large-sized VSD and PDA show left atrial enlargement in a very small percentage of cases; here the atrial enlargement is usually secondary to intrinsic disease of the mitral valve, since adults with ASD often have prolapsing mitral valve as well.[7] Left atrial enlargement may also be generated by mitral or common AV valve incompetence that occurs in the persistent AV canal group of lesions. These are most commonly a partial or complete form of AV canal.

After the left atrium is analyzed, the transverse aortic arch region should be examined for evidence of a ductus infundibulum (Fig. 13A). The ductus infundibulum will sometimes produce a convex density just below the transverse arch, and this is the only reliable indication of a PDA.

In those few patients that reach adulthood with PDA, the ductus is small and the chest film, including the transverse arch, is normal. Those adult patients with PDA and an abnormal chest film almost invariably present with high resistance vascularity (precapillary hypertension). This is because the high resistance was present in infancy and a murmur was never apparent. As discussed previously, the outer wall of the ductus may calcify or become aneurysmally dilated (Fig. 10B).

The third step in analysis is an evaluation of the right upper hilum. In patients with a sinus venosus–type ASD there is a high incidence (at least 90 percent) of partial anomalous pulmonary venous connection of the right upper pulmonary vein to the superior vena cava. This vein can often be seen coursing in a more horizontal manner than the normal right upper pulmonary vein (Fig. 13B).

Since any adult with a L-R shunt (with or without left atrial enlargement) is diagnosed as having ASD until proven otherwise, a few additional points about ASD should be mentioned.

1. The dilated pulmonary trunk and/or infundibulum may fuse together and mimic the leftward ascending aorta in corrected transposition (Fig. 13C).

2. Middle-aged and elderly adults with ASD may show signs of right ventricular failure—dilated azygous vein and a dilated right atrium and ventricle.

3. Although the pulmonary vascularity in the adult with ASD may appear as precapillary hypertension, the flow is often predominantly left-to-right (Fig. 13D). In other words, the x-ray may be misleading in this regard.

Cyanotic Lesions with Shunt Vascularity

Within this category complete transposition of the great arteries is by far the most common condition among infants. Unless a palliative or corrective operation has been performed, these patients usually expire in their first year. However, there are other

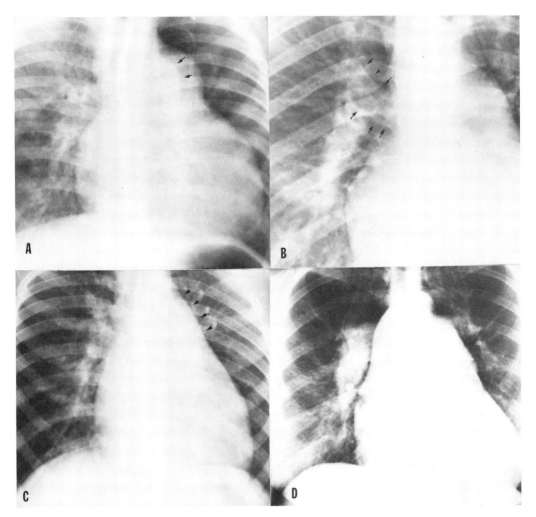

Figure 13. Left-to-right shunt lesions. A, PDA. The arrows indicate the outer wall of the ductus infundibulum which is seen through the dilated pulmonary trunk. B, ASD, sinus venosus type. The right upper lobe pulmonary vein (arrows) courses in a horizontal manner towards the superior vena cava. The normal vein shows a more vertical course. This is highly suggestive of partial anomalous pulmonary venous connection of the right upper lobe to the superior vena cava which by inference suggests a sinus venosus type ASD. C, ASD, ostium secundum type. The left upper mediastinum shows a linear density (arrows) which mimics *l*-transposed ascending aorta, but is actually the pulmonary trunk. This is a common sign in ASD, especially when the ascending aorta and transverse aortic arch are inapparent, as they often are. D, ASD in an elderly adult. The vascularity shows the criteria for precapillary hypertension of Eisenmenger physiology; however, this patient showed a predominant L-R shunt lesion at catheterization.

admixture lesions that may present with identical or similar x-ray findings because the physiology of the anomalies is similar. *In adults,* single ventricle with transposition is the most common defect presenting with cyanosis and shunt vascularity (Fig. 14). Persistent truncus arteriosus is the second most common cause (Fig. 15A), and is distinguished from the rest by a high incidence of right aortic arch and skeletal anomalies.

Among patients with cyanotic heart disease and shunt vascularity, the left atrium plays a minor role in analysis. It may be enlarged in any of these admixture lesions as

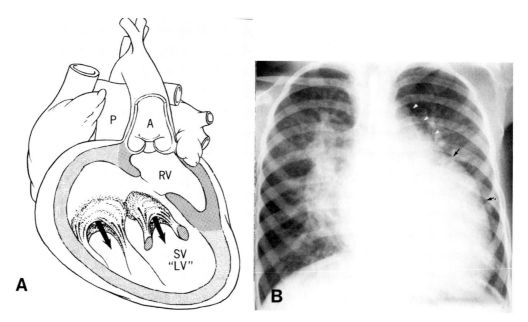

Figure 14. Single ventricle with inversion of the rudimentary right ventricle and transposition of the great arteries. A, A schematic representation shows both atrioventricular valves empty into the single (primitive) ventricle (SV). The rudimentary right ventricle (RV), or outlet chamber, is located along the left shoulder of the heart. The ventricular septum, because of its high insertion along the left heart border, allows the rudimentary RV to form a characteristic bulge. The ascending aorta (A) usually arises with a convexity to the left (*l*-transposition). B, The black arrows indicate the limits of the rudimentary RV and the ascending aorta is marked by the white arrowheads. In addition, there is evidence of profuse shunt vascularity. With SV the right hilum characteristically has a waterfall appearance.

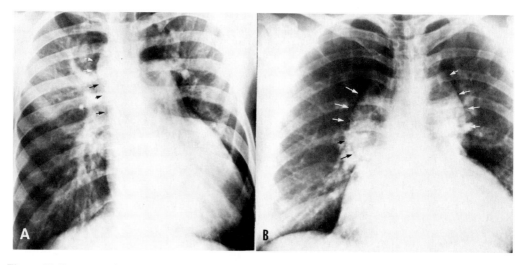

Figure 15. Two cyanotic heart lesions with shunt vascularity. A, Two x-ray features which should support persistent truncus arteriosus as the initial diagnosis in an adult patient with cyanosis. These are (1) shunt vascularity, and (2) a *right aortic arch* (arrows). B, This adult female shows the classic "figure of 8" or "snowman's" cardiac configuration seen in TAPVC to the innominate vein. The arrows at left point out the vertical vein; the arrows at right, the dilated superior vena cava.

long as the atrial septum is intact. The presence of an enlarged left atrium simply rules out TAPVC and common atrium. TAPVC is rare in adults but may present with the characteristic "figure of 8" cardiovascular silhouette (Fig. 15B).

The one cyanotic condition which presents with shunt vascularity and virtually pathognomonic chest film signs is single (or primitive) ventricle with an inverted infundibulum (or outlet chamber) located along the left shoulder of the heart and *l*-transposition (Fig. 14A.) The left heart border is characteristic. The ascending aorta forms the upper left mediastinal density, and the rudimentary right ventricle forms a discrete bulge along the upper left heart border (Fig. 14B).

Pulmonary Venous Hypertension

The causes of PVH may be categorized on the basis of the obstruction's relation to the mitral valve. These include (1) a primary disease process at or proximal to the mitral valve (Figs. 8A, 9A, and 16A), and (2) left ventricular stress problems (Figs. 8B and 16B). The appearance or type of PVH is related to severity and duration of the disease process, not to any particular lesion.

PRIMARY DISEASE PROCESSES AT OR PROXIMAL TO THE MITRAL VALVE. This category includes both mechanical obstructive lesions at or proximal to the mitral valve and primary mitral valve incompetence. The vast majority of obstructive lesions occur at the mitral valve and are *rheumatic* in origin. Other obstructive lesions, such as left atrial tumors, cor triatriatum, and stenosis of the individual pulmonary veins, are rare. The roentgen hallmark of a mechanical obstructive lesion is *severe PVH* and a *prominent pulmonary trunk* (Fig. 8A).

When mitral valve incompetence occurs as an isolated lesion and results in PVH, it is usually rheumatic in origin (Fig. 16A). Congenital mitral valve incompetence most often occurs as an isolated lesion in the form of a prolapsing mitral valve, or in association with a shunt lesion such as an endocardial cushion defect. In the former, the vascularity is usually *normal;* in the latter, the *shunt* vascularity dominates the roentgen picture.

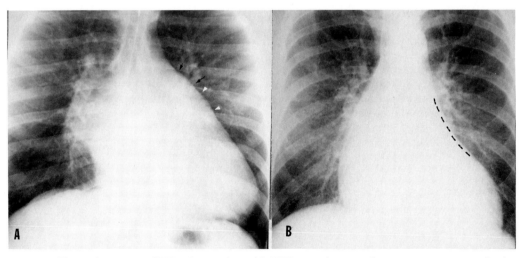

Figure 16. Two major causes of PVH. A, A patient with PVH secondary to a disease process at or proximal to the mitral valve. With PVH, this assumption is based upon the filled-in left heart border. Pulmonary trunk is indicated by black arrows; left atrial appendage by white arrowheads. This adult has rheumatic mitral valve insufficiency. B, The PVH is secondary to left ventricular decompensation. This assumption is valid when the heart shows a left ventricular configuration, characterized by an overt concavity (broken line) of the mid-left heart border.

Other primary forms of mitral incompetence are uncommon and are usually noticed in childhood.

Secondary forms of mitral valve incompetence are usually part of a more complex process affecting the left ventricle. For instance, mitral valve incompetence secondary to an infarcted papillary muscle, torn chordae tendineae, and left ventricular dilatation almost invariably presents within the framework of the stressed left ventricle.

In adults, rheumatic endocarditis of the mitral valve may result primarily in stenosis or incompetence, but almost invariably produces PVH. Therefore, PVH of some degree is the primary roentgen sign in the diagnosis of rheumatic heart disease. A secondary sign is the shape of the heart: in primary disease processes at or proximal to the mitral valve it almost always assumes a triangular shape which is accentuated by a filled-in or convex left heart border (Figs. 8A and 9A). The latter is usually formed by a normal-sized or dilated pulmonary trunk and dilated left atrial appendage. We feel that a dilated left atrial appendage is nearly pathognomonic of rheumatic endocarditis of the mitral valve.[6] When the pulmonary trunk and left atrial appendage (LAA) are apparent, this is termed a *mitral configuration*. This type of cardiac silhouette may be normal in size or enlarged. Congenital heart lesions which cause PVH at or proximal to the mitral valve are rare.

LEFT VENTRICULAR STRESS. When the left ventricle is placed under stress for any reason, the heart exhibits what is termed a *left ventricular configuration* (LVC), a shape that is entirely different from the one found in those patients with primary disease processes at or proximal to the mitral valve (Fig. 16B). It should be remembered that this is a normal configuration in most adults as long as the left ventricle is normal in size.

The primary feature of LVC is an overt concavity of the mid-left heart border in the PA view (Figs. 8B and 16B). The apex is usually rounded and the aorta (both the ascending and transverse arches) may be normal, prominent, or inapparent. There is often enlargement of the *body* of the left atrium; however, LAA and pulmonary trunk prominence are not present.

In summary, patients with a primary disease process at the mitral valve have a heart that is triangular in shape or a left heart border filled in by a prominent pulmonary trunk, LAA, or both. On the other hand, PVH and LVC indicate that some disease entity is stressing the left ventricle. This is true regardless of whether the LV is normal in size or enlarged. Enlargement of the body of the left atrium plays no role in differentiation between primary mitral valve disease and left ventricular stress, since it may occur in both major groups. But the enlarged LAA and prominent pulmonary trunk are fundamental indications of primary disease processes at the mitral valve; these diseases are usually acquired and will not be dealt with further.

APPROACH TO PATIENTS WITH PVH DETERMINED ON THE BASIS OF A STRESSED LEFT VENTRICLE (Table 2). Diseases which result in LVC can be divided into five general categories: (1) *pressure overload* in which there is obstruction to the flow of blood leaving the left ventricle; (2) *volume overload* in which an excess amount of blood returns to the left ventricle, the prime example being aortic valve incompetence; (3) *disorders of contraction and/or relaxation* of the left ventricle (i.e., cardiomyopathy); (4) *coronary ischemia,* regardless of cause; and (5) *any combination* of diseases in these four categories, e.g., coarctation of the aorta with aortic valve incompetence.

In patients with PVH and LVC, there is overall enlargement of the heart (see Table 2), although occasionally a patient will present with severe PVH and normal-sized left ventricle. These patients usually have had a sudden and severe myocardial infarction, acute renal shutdown, or fluid overload.[8] Regardless of the heart size, the observer can predict with confidence that the left ventricle has failed. Toxic, neurologic, and allergic causes must also be ruled out.

Table 2. Roentgenologic approach to left ventricular stress

Normal Vascularity		Pulmonary Venous Hypertension	
Normal-sized LVC	*Enlarged LVC*	*Normal-sized LVC*	*Enlarged LVC*
1. Normal	1. Aortic valve in-competence	1. Acute myocardial in-farction	Any of the afore-mentioned conditions in left ventricular failure
2. Obstructive lesions	a. Intrinsic aortic valve disease	2. Acute renal shut-down	
a. Systemic hyper-tension	b. Condition as-cending aorta	3. Fuid overload	
b. Coarctation of aorta	(1) Cystic medial necrosis	4. Toxic, neurologic, etc.	
c. Aortic valve stenosis	(3) Chronic dis-section		
d. Postoperative coarctation	2. Cardiomyopathy		
e. Discrete sub-aortic stenosis	3. ASH		
f. IHSS	4. Athletic heart		
3. Coronary ischemia			

The *first step* of the LV stress analysis is to rule out *calcific aortic valve stenosis,* a lesion that is extremely common and almost invariably congenital.[9] In adults, always examine the aortic valve region for calcium in the lateral and RAO views (Fig. 17). The aortic valve is obscured by the spine in the PA view and by the lower right pulmonary artery in the LAO view. When in doubt, *fluoroscope the patient.*

The *second step* is to analyze the left ventricular border in the PA and other views for irregularities and/or calcium that would suggest an aneurysm or areas of dyskinesis. An

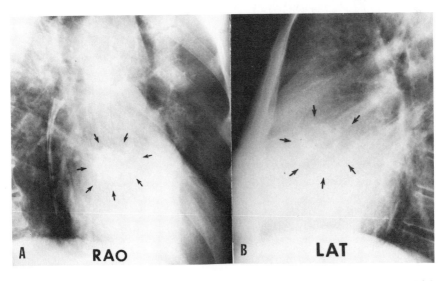

Figure 17. Left ventricular stress secondary to congenital calcific aortic valve stenosis. A, Right anterior oblique (RAO) view. B, Lateral view. In both views, the arrows surround the calcified aortic valve.

unusual convex bulge along the entire left heart border in the PA view suggests asymmetrical septal hypertrophy.

The *third step* is to analyze the ascending aorta for prominence and calcium deposits. Congenital lesions which may be reflected in this area are aortic valve stenosis producing poststenotic dilatation of the ascending aorta and cystic medial necrosis resulting in an extremely prominent aorta.

The *fourth step* is analysis of the transverse aortic arch (Fig. 18) and descending thoracic aorta. The premier sign of coarctation of the aorta is a disruption or distortion in the contour of the normal curvilinear density formed by the transverse arch or aortic knob (Fig. 18).

With regard to the diagnosis of specific lesions stressing the left ventricle, the remainder of the examination will yield little information. In fact, if the LV stress analysis outlined here proves negative, the lesion is usually one involving primarily the heart muscle, such as a cardiomyopathy or hypertrophic subaortic stenosis.

Precapillary Hypertension

The anatomic findings yield few clues to possible etiologies. Calcium in the wall or aneurysmal dilatation of the ductus infundibulum (Fig. 10B) indicate a patent ductus arteriosus as the offending lesion, and TAPVC to the innominate vein may show the "figure of 8" cardiac configuration. When there is high vascular resistance the vertical vein may be less apparent.

Systemic Collateral Arteries

As mentioned previously, patients with this condition almost invariably have pulmonary atresia with a large VSD, and these lesions are collectively known as single aortic

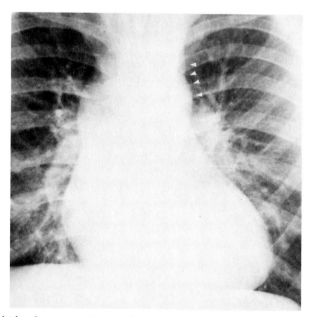

Figure 18. Left ventricular decompensation owing to coarctation of the aorta. This patient shows signs of PVH. Left ventricular decompensation causing PVH is based on the enlarged left ventricular configuration. The prominent ascending aorta could fit many lesions. The key roentgen finding is the distorted transverse aortic arch (arrowheads).

trunk. The end-stage tetralogy, or pseudotruncus, is the most common cause. The arteries themselves may produce small indentations in the posterior wall of the barium-filled esophagus. The heart usually shows an upturned apex, and a normally formed pulmonary trunk is absent. There is a high incidence (50 percent) of right aortic arch in pseudotruncus arteriosus (Fig. 11).

Normal Vascularity

In the presence of *normal vascularity,* the patient may be normal; he may also have a small to moderate sized shunt, obstructive lesions, or some other form of mild heart disease.

In the patient with normal vascularity and normal-sized heart, the *left atrium, pulmonary trunk,* and *aorta* are then analyzed. If these structures are normal, the chances of the x-rays yielding any other pertinent information from a cardiac viewpoint are minimal.

Obstructive Lesions

Obstructive lesions confronting the right ventricle almost invariably show either an abnormally prominent pulmonary trunk and/or left pulmonary artery, while left-sided obstructions usually show a prominent ascending aorta or calcified aortic valve. Both great arteries are extremely sensitive and will respond to mild nonobstructive or anatomic valve deformities by dilatation. Regardless of which side is confronted, the vascularity remains *normal* as long as the ventricle proximal to the obstruction maintains compensation. Right-sided obstructive lesions at or proximal to the pulmonary valve result in right ventricular failure, right atrial and azygous vein enlargement, and, in severe cases, show decreased vascularity. Obstructive lesions of the left ventricle causing left ventricular decompensation show PVH of varying degrees.

OBSTRUCTIVE LESIONS CONFRONTING THE RIGHT VENTRICLE. Significant obstructive lesions beyond the pulmonary trunk such as pulmonary hypertension from various causes (including reversal of shunt) are suspected on the basis of the pattern of precapillary hypertension.

Pulmonary valve stenosis is a common lesion. In the mild-to-moderate cases, its only means of x-ray presentation may be an enlarged pulmonary trunk and/or left pulmonary artery (Fig. 19). The key roentgen finding is unilateral prominence of the left hilum, regardless of the presence (Fig. 19A) or absence (Fig. 19B) of a prominent pulmonary trunk. However, idiopathic dilatation of the pulmonary trunk cannot be distinguished from pulmonary stenosis on plain films. In some adults, the pulmonary trunk may assume a near vertical course and mimic an *l*-transposed ascending aorta (Fig. 19C).

Left Ventricular Stress

We have discussed left ventricular stress problems that present with PVH. In those patients in whom the left ventricle has maintained its compensatory state, the vascularity will remain normal. Patients with *normal vascularity* can be divided into two major groups: those with a normal-sized LVC and those with an enlarged LVC (Table 3).

NORMAL VASCULARITY AND NORMAL-SIZED LVC. The vast majority of patients in this category are normal. The LVC is actually a normal contour in nearly all adults, even though in young children it should be considered abnormal until proven otherwise. Among older children and young adults LVC is often normal, but should be viewed with suspicion.

Of the five major categories of disease processes stressing the left ventricle, the most common lesions with normal vascularity and LVC are the obstructive lesions.

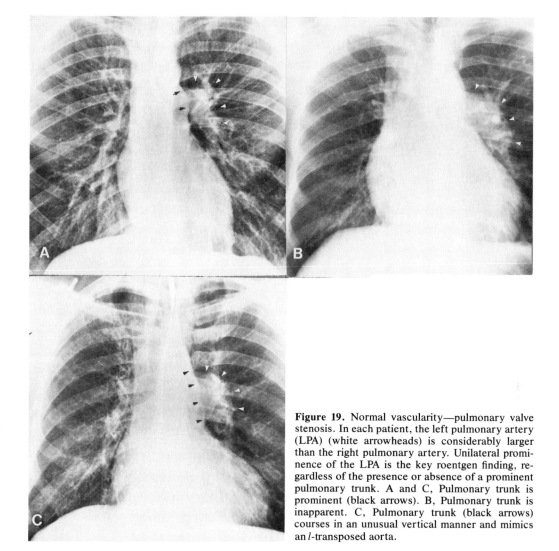

Figure 19. Normal vascularity—pulmonary valve stenosis. In each patient, the left pulmonary artery (LPA) (white arrowheads) is considerably larger than the right pulmonary artery. Unilateral prominence of the LPA is the key roentgen finding, regardless of the presence or absence of a prominent pulmonary trunk. A and C, Pulmonary trunk is prominent (black arrows). B, Pulmonary trunk is inapparent. C, Pulmonary trunk (black arrows) courses in an unusual vertical manner and mimics an *l*-transposed aorta.

Obstructing the blood from the left ventricle at any site (e.g., systemic hypertension or aortic valve stenosis) results in left ventricular hypertrophy. This pathologic term implies an increase in muscle mass and a small left ventricular cavity. Radiologically, left ventricular hypertrophy should be suspected when the left heart border shows an unusual convexity even if there is no overt cardiac enlargement.

Table 2 provides a radiologic classification which includes most diseases affecting primarily the left ventricle. The format for their analysis is the same as for LVC and PVH.

From a strict radiologic viewpoint, the obstructive lesions which are most easily diagnosed are the congenital disorders, *aortic valve stenosis* and *coarctation of the aorta*.

Aortic Valve Stenosis. It has been well documented that most cases of isolated aortic valve disease (stenosis and/or insufficiency) occur on a congenital basis.[9] The most reliable indication of a congenitally malformed valve is the presence of calcium in the valve itself, but this sign is not found in children and young adults. In my experience, calcified aortic valve is a rare finding in patients under age 30. Unless a lateral chest film

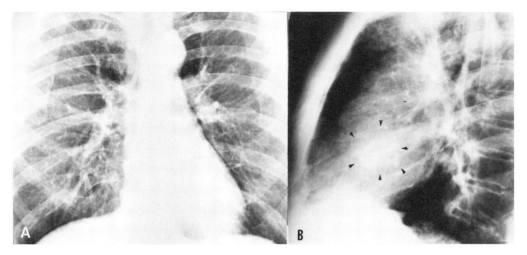

Figure 20. Normal vascularity—normal LVC configuration—calcific aortic stenosis. A, The PA chest film appears normal. B, The lateral film, however, shows dense calcification of the aortic valve (arrows). The calcified aortic valve lies over the calcified spine in the PA view, and is therefore obscured.

is obtained, most cases of calcific aortic stenosis will be missed, at least radiographically (Fig. 20).

Coarctation of the Aorta. The localized or juxtaductal type is the most common and the x-ray signs are nearly always diagnostic. The *sine qua non* of coarctation is an abnormal or disfigured transverse aortic arch region (Figs. 18 and 21). The clear, uninterrupted curvilinear configuration of the aortic knob seen in aortic valve stenosis or systemic hypertension is absent. Rib notching is present in over 50 percent of the adult patients (Fig. 21A). An earlier sign is a sclerotic reaction and density involving the lower rib margin (Fig. 21A).

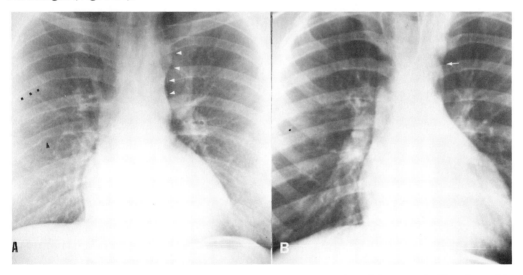

Figure 21. Normal vascularity—left ventricular configuration—coarctation of the aorta. A, There is notching of a mid-right posterior rib (black arrowhead) and an increased density to the lower margin of the ribs on the right side (squares). The *sine qua non* of coarctation lies in the distorted transverse aortic arch and upper descending thoracic aorta region (white arrowheads). B, The distortion of the transverse aortic arch is of a more classic variety (arrow), sometimes termed the "figure of 3" deformity.

Many adult patients with coarctation of the aorta (CoA) who underwent surgical repair in childhood will confront the cardiologist with calcific aortic valve stenosis or aortic valve incompetence. This is because of the high associated incidence of *aortic valve deformity* with CoA. In my personal angiographic experience the incidence is at least 70 percent.

Some adults will present with mild or nonobstructive forms of CoA with x-ray evidence of a disfigured aortic arch. When the transverse aortic arch eventually undergoes the normal changes of advanced age (tortuosity, etc.), the area of mild CoA becomes more apparent (Fig. 22A). This phenomenon has inappropriately been termed pseudocoarctation. There is nothing false about this situation, since these patients have (1) a bona fide CoA, which is simply nonobstructive, and (2) are as prone to a high incidence of aortic valve deformity (bicuspid aortic valve, etc.) and its complications as the hemodynamically significant CoA (Fig. 22B).

Discrete Subvalvular Aortic Stenosis. The changes on plain film may be identical to aortic valve stenosis. The diagnosis can be made only with left ventriculography. In approximately 50 percent of patients with this condition the ascending aorta appears prominent.

Systemic Hypertension. This is not an x-ray diagnosis. The ascending aorta may be prominent and the descending aorta, tortuous. A prominent aorta, however, does *not* indicate a dilated aorta (a common misconception). A dilated aorta can be detected only by delineating both aortic walls, either by aortography or calcium deposits in the posterior wall.

Asymmetrical Septal Hypertrophy. At least two thirds of these patients have a normal-sized LVC. The hallmark is an unusually convex left heart border with a normal-sized ascending aorta. There may be left atrial enlargement (body) secondary to mitral valve incompetence.

NORMAL VASCULARITY AND ENLARGED LVC. Radiographically, aortic valve incompetence (AI) should be suspected in the presence of an enlarged LVC and normal

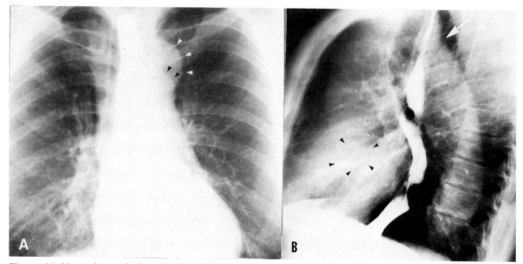

Figure 22. Normal vascularity—LVC—mild coarctation of the aorta (pseudocoarctation). A, Roentgen findings are normal except for the double density and distortion of the transverse aortic arch region. The white arrowheads indicate what appears to be an aneurysm of the aorta. The pulses were normal in the lower extremities. B, The lateral view shows a mild coarctation of the aorta. The posterior indentation can be seen clearly (white arrow). More importantly, these patients have the same tendency to also develop calcific aortic valve disease (black arrowheads) as those with hemodynamically significant CoA.

114

vascularity. When the other major causes of left ventricular stress result in overt left ventricular enlargement (obstructive lesions, coronary ischemia, etc.), signs of PVH are usually obvious.

Precise radiographic diagnosis of AI can be made only by aortic root aortography. Significant AI may be reflected at fluoroscopy by increased pulsations of the entire thoracic aorta. However, *auscultation is far more sensitive than fluoroscopy in detecting AI.*

In evaluating a patient with AI, the observer must determine whether the disease process is the result of *intrinsic aortic valve disease* or a disease process *affecting only the media of the wall of the ascending aorta,* or *both.*

Intrinsic Aortic Valve Incompetence. Pure aortic valve incompetence from intrinsic valvular disease usually results in only mild prominence of the ascending aorta (Fig. 23A). The most common cause of valvular AI is a congenital bicuspid valve, often associated with infective endocarditis. An uncommon cause is rheumatic endocarditis of the aortic valve.

Aortic valve incompetence of rheumatic origin is usually associated with significant mitral valve disease. To the radiologist this usually presents within the framework of PVH and a triangle-shaped or mitral configuration heart, not a LVC. Left ventricular dilatation, infarction, and papillary muscle dysfunction are the usual causes of mitral valve incompetence in patients with congenital aortic valve disease.

Extrinsic Aortic Valve Incompetence. Pronounced dilatation or calcification of the ascending aorta in a patient with AI usually indicates that the AI is secondary to a disease process involving the media of the aortic wall.

Cystic medial necrosis of the ascending aorta (CMN-AA) occurs in two groups of young patients: those with the Marfan syndrome, and those with so-called idiopathic CMN-AA who are otherwise normal.

In patients with the Marfan syndrome and signs of AI, diagnosis of CMN-AA on the plain film is relatively simple. In patients with normal body habitus and CMN-AA, the

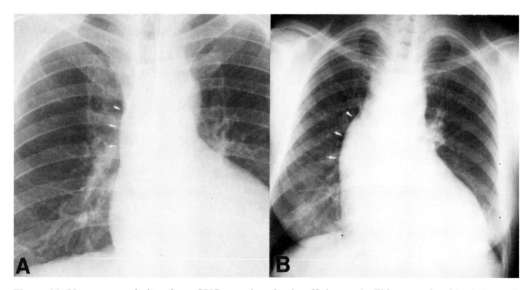

Figure 23. Normal vascularity—large LVC—aortic valve insufficiency. A, This example of *intrinsic aortic valve insufficiency* (AI) is based on the fact that the ascending aorta shows only mild prominence (arrows). The descending thoracic aorta is usually tortuous in AI. B, The ascending aorta is extremely prominent (arrows). This suggests that the AI in this patient is secondary to a condition of the ascending aorta. This degree of dilatation in an adult with AI strongly suggests cystic medial necrosis of the ascending aorta.

115

radiographic appearance is still consistent. In both cases, the ascending aorta is exceedingly prominent (Figure 23B). CMN-AA has been described in Ehlers-Danlos syndrome and osteogenesis imperfecta. In patients with these syndromes and AI, the diagnosis of CMN-AA can be made confidently.

Diminished Vascularity

Once severe pulmonary stenosis or atresia had been determined by the appearance of the pulmonary vascularity (Figs. 12 and 24), such patients can be divided into two major subdivisions[5] (Table 3): (1) those associated with VSD (or single ventricle) with the R-L shunt occurring from the ventricles (or ventricle) into the aorta (ventricular level), and (2) those with an intact ventricular septum with the R-L shunt occurring from the right atrium into the left atrium (atrial level). Most adult patients with severe pulmonary stenosis or atresia with VSD have tetralogy of Fallot. Since this is the most common

Table 3. Roentgenologic approach to cyanotic heart disease

Prominent Vascularity	*Decreased Vascularity or Systemic Collateral (severe pulmonary stenosis or atresia)*
A. Shunt vascularity	A. Associated large ventricular septal defect (or single ventricle)

1. Single ventricle with transposition
     a. Noninversion
     b. Inversion
	1. Tetralogy of Fallot

	2. Tricuspid atresia and pulmonary stenosis (or atresia), with or without transposition
2. Persistent truncus arteriosus	

3. Tricuspid atresia
     a. Normally related great vessels
     b. Transposition
	3. Single ventricle with inversion or non-inversion plus pulmonary stenosis (or atresia)

4. Total anomalous pulmonary venous connection above diaphragm	4. Complete transposition plus ventricular septal defect plus pulmonary stenosis (or atresia)
5. Double outlet right ventricle	5. Corrected transposition plus ventricular septal defect plus pulmonary stenosis (or atresia)
6. Common atrium	
B. Shunt vascularity with pulmonary trunk 1. Type I truncus	6. Double outlet right ventricle plus pulmonary stenosis (or atresia)
	7. Pulmonary atresia with hypoplastic right ventricle
2. Tricuspid atresia with normally related great vessels	
	8. Asplenia syndrome
3. Total anomalous pulmonary venous connection to coronary sinus, right atrium	B. Decreased vascularity with intact ventricular septum 1. Pulmonary stenosis or atresia
4. Double outlet right ventricle	2. Ebstein's anomaly

entity within the first category, it is considered the prototype. However, virtually any of the aforementioned admixture lesions with VSD and shunt vascularity (e.g., complete transposition, single ventricle, etc.; see Table 3), may have superimposed severe pulmonary stenosis or atresia. Thus, these patients usually present with roentgen findings similar or identical to those encountered in tetralogy of Fallot.

Roentgenologic findings indicating VSD (or single ventricle) in association with severe pulmonary stenosis (or atresia) are (1) prominent aorta with a left arch or a right aortic arch, (2) normal-sized right atrium, and (3) normal-sized heart or *mild* cardiomegaly (Fig. 24A). These anatomic findings indicate that the R-L shunt is at the ventricular level. With a large VSD (or a single ventricle), there is no tricuspid valve incompetence, and thus no stimulus to right atrial enlargement. The embryologic background in these conditions invariably decrees a *large aorta* and/or *a right arch*. In patients with normal arrangement of the ventricles, the convexity of the ascending portion of the aorta is usually to the right (Fig. 24A). In those with ventricular inversion, the convexity is usually to the left and results in a left superior mediastinal density of varying size.

Ninety percent of the adult patients who present with such findings will have tetralogy of Fallot. Far less common is corrected transposition with VSD and pulmonary stenosis followed by tricuspid atresia and single ventricle.

Patients with *severe pulmonary stenosis* and an *intact ventricular septum* represent the prototype of conditions having a R-L shunt at the atrial level. The major x-ray findings are virtually opposite to those just mentioned and consist of (1) an inapparent aorta (right arch is rare), and (2) moderate-to-severe cardiomegaly secondary to right atrial and/or right ventricular dilatation (Fig. 24B). The dilatation is caused by massive tricuspid valve incompetence of varying degrees which is usually a part of the disease process. The differential diagnosis of conditions associated with these radiologic circumstances is not as voluminous as those listed with the prototype conditions, complete transposition and tetralogy of Fallot (Table 3). Severe pulmonary stenosis and Ebstein's anomaly comprise over 90 percent of the conditions that will be encountered in adults. Tricuspid atresia appears in all categories. Other entities of a *rare* nature to be considered are (1) pericardial effusion, (2) tricuspid stenosis, (3) giant right atrium, and (4) Uhl's anomaly of the right heart.

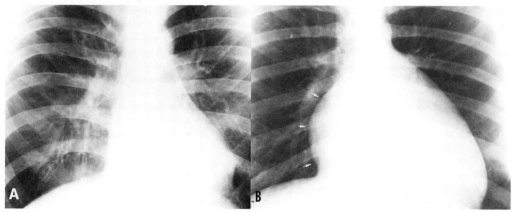

Figure 24. Diminished vascularity with R-L shunt at ventricular and atrial levels. A, In the presence of decreased vascularity the indications for a R-L shunt at the ventricular level are (1) the normal-size right atrium, (2) normal-size heart, and (3) slightly prominent aorta. More than 90 percent of the adult patients will have a tetralogy of Fallot. B, The findings indicating a R-L shunt at the atrial level are (1) prominent right atrium (arrows), (2) generalized cardiomegaly, and (3) an inapparent or normal-size aorta. Most adults who present with these findings will have either severe pulmonary stenosis or Ebstein's malformation of the tricuspid valve.

117

REFERENCES

1. CURRY, G. C., VICTORICA, B. E., AND ELLIOTT, L. P.: *Radiologic changes following repair and palliation of right-to-left and admixture shunts*. Radiol. Clin. North Am. 9:177, 1971.

2. ELLIOTT, L. P.: *A Roentgenologic Approach to Heart Disease*. MEDCOM, Inc. New York, N.Y. 1974.

3. TONKIN, I. L., KELLEY, J. M., BREAM, P. R., ET AL.: *The frontal chest film as a method of suspecting transposition complexes*. Circulation 53:1016, 1976.

4. ABRAMS, H. L.: *Radiologic aspects of increased pulmonary artery pressure and flow: preliminary observations*. Stanford Medical Bull. 14:97, 1956.

5. ELLIOTT, L. P., AND SCHIEBLER, G. L.: *A roentgenologic-electrocardiographic approach to cyanotic forms of heart disease*. Pediatr. Clin. North Am. 18:1133, 1971.

6. KELLEY, M. J., ELLIOTT, L. P., SCHULMAN, S. T., ET AL.: *The significance of the dilated left atrial appendage in rheumatic heart disease*. Circulation 54:146, 1976.

7. VICTORICA, B. E., ELLIOTT, L. P., AND GESSNER, I. H.: *Ostium secundum atrial septal defect associated with balloon mitral valve in children*. Am. J. Cardiol. 33:668, 1974.

8. HARLE, T. S., KOUNTOUPIS, J. T., BOONE, M. L. M., ET AL.: *Pulmonary edema without cardiomegaly*. Am. J. Roentgenol. 103:555, 1968.

9. ROBERTS, W. D.: *Anatomically isolated aortic valve disease: the case against its being rheumatic etiology*. Am. J. Med. 49:151, 1970.

Electrocardiographic Features of Congenital Heart Disease in the Adult

R. Curtis Ellison, M.D., and Laurence J. Sloss, M.D.

In the adult with congenital heart disease, the electrocardiogram often provides a valuable clue to the presence and nature of the cardiac lesion. Occasionally, abnormalities of P wave morphology, the sequence of ventricular depolarization, or patterns of marked hypertrophy or hypoplasia may point to a specific congenital cardiac diagnosis. More often, the electrocardiogram reflects only the hemodynamic consequences of varying degrees of atrial or ventricular overload that may be common to a number of defects. The basic patterns associated with congenital abnormalities in the adult are similar to those found in childhood, although in the adult they may be modified or obscured by conduction disturbances, arrhythmias, or other changes resulting from the wear and tear of chronic hemodynamic overload. These patterns can also be altered by the added effects of acquired heart disease.

Detailed descriptions of the specific electrocardiographic findings associated with each defect are presented in the chapters on the individual cardiac lesions. This chapter is organized around the electrocardiogram itself, attempting to point out its utility as a means of suspecting and diagnosing congenital heart disease in the adult.

Associations between common electrocardiographic features and a number of congenital heart defects are depicted in Table 1. The cardiac lesions are listed in their approximate order of prevalence among young to middle-aged adults who present to internists and cardiologists for evaluation.

RHYTHM AND CONDUCTION ABNORMALITIES

Atrial Fibrillation and Flutter

These two arrhythmias are characteristically seen in conditions in which the atria are enlarged or under stress, and are most commonly a result of volume overload or increased filling pressures secondary to ventricular abnormalities. Even with severe lesions resulting in marked atrial enlargement or hypertrophy, children seldom exhibit atrial fibrillation or flutter, unless they are under the added stress of surgery, and then only occasionally. In adults, however, these arrhythmias become more frequent with advancing age as ventricular decompensation increases and pressure overload is added to chronic dilatation of the atria.[1] Thus, all lesions which produce hemodynamically significant left-to-right shunting predispose to atrial arrhythmias, particularly when ventricular decompensation supervenes.

Atrial fibrillation is a common presenting arrhythmia in middle-aged adults with atrial

Table 1. Electrocardiographic patterns associated with congenital heart defects

Cardiac Defect	Abnormal Q Waves or Myocardial Infarction Pattern	Bi-ventricular Overload	Left Ventricular Pressure Overload	Left Ventricular Volume Overload	Right Ventricular Pressure Overload	Right Ventricular Volume Overload	Right Bundle Branch Block	Left Bundle Branch Block	Left Axis Deviation	Left Atrial Overload	Right Atrial Overload	Abnormal P Orientation	Pre-excitation Syndrome	Atrioventricular Block	Ventricular Arrhythmia	Supraventricular Tachycardia	Atrial Flutter/Fibrillation
Atrial Septal Defect (secundum)	0	0	0	0	+	+	+	0	0	+	+	+	0	+	0	+	++
Prolapsed Mitral Valve Syndrome	0	0	+	0	0	0	0	0	+	+	0	0	+	0	+	+	+
Aortic Stenosis	0	++	0	0	0	0	+	+	+	0	0	0	0	0	0	0	0
IHSS	++	++	0	0	0	0	+	+	0	+	+	0	0	0	+	0	+
Pulmonary Stenosis	0	0	0	0	+	0	0	0	+	0	+	0	0	0	0	+	0
Ventricular Septal Defect	0	+	0	++	0	+	0	+	0	0	0	0	0	0	0	0	0
Patent Ductus Arteriosus	0	0	+	++	0	0	+	+	+	+	0	0	0	0	0	0	0
Tetralogy of Fallot	0	0	0	0	+	0	+	0	0	0	+	0	0	0	+	0	0
Coarctation of Aorta	0	0	+	0	0	0	0	0	+	0	0	0	0	0	0	+	+
Eisenmenger's Syndrome	0	+	0	0	+	0	0	0	0	+	0	0	0	0	0	+	+
Atrial Septal Defect (primum)	0	+	0	+	0	+	+	+	++	+	+	0	0	0	0	++	++
Corrected Transposition*	+++	+	0	0	0	++	0	++	++	+	++	0	+	++	0	+	+
Ebstein's Anomaly	0	0	0	0	0	++	+	++	0	++	+	0	++	++	+	++	++
Tricuspid Atresia	+	0	+	0	+	0	+	++	++	+	0	0	0	0	+	+	+
Congenital Anomalies of Coronary Arteries	+++	0	0	0	0	0	+	+	++	0	0	0	0	0	0	0	0
Transposition of Great Arteries	0	0	+	0	+	0	0	0	0	0	0	0	0	0	0	++	0
Transposition of Great Arteries (postop)	0	0	0	+++	0	0	0	0	0	+	0	0	+	+	0	0	0

+ + + = Almost always seen (characteristic of defect)
+ + = Commonly seen with defect
+ = Sometimes seen with defect (especially with associated defects or advancing age)
0 = Rarely seen with defect

* The precordial QRS progression in corrected transposition may mimic left ventricular hypertrophy, usually with S-T abnormalities. True hypertrophy of the left-sided ventricle can occur in corrected transposition from associated left atrioventricular valvular insufficiency, ventricular septal defect, etc.

septal defect and is occasionally seen along with ventricular defect or patent ductus arteriosus accompanied by a large left-to-right shunt. Atrial flutter is less common than atrial fibrillation and may occur more frequently in lesions producing predominant enlargement of the right atrium such as atrial septal defect or Ebstein's anomaly of the tricuspid valve.[2-4] Atrial fibrillation also occurs in these lesions but appears to be more typical of shunts which enlarge the left atrium, e.g., ventricular septal defect and patent ductus arteriosus. As in the case of acquired mitral valve disease, congenital insufficiency of the left atrioventricular valve (which occurs in association with ostium primum atrial septal defect, corrected transposition of the great arteries, and prolapse of the mitral valve) may result in left atrial enlargement and atrial fibrillation. Atrial fibrillation is also common in idiopathic hypertrophic subaortic stenosis (IHSS), where its development will often dramatically increase symptoms. Atrial fibrillation and other atrial arrhythmias are not uncommon as an early or late postoperative complication following repair of congenital heart disease, particularly when the sinoatrial node and/or its blood supply are injured during cannulation or atriotomy. Arrhythmias resulting from such damage have been relatively frequent sequelae of Mustard's operation for transposition of the great arteries.[5]

Paroxysmal Supraventricular Tachycardia

Ebstein's anomaly, both in children and adults, commonly leads to supraventricular tachycardias.[4] Other lesions that may be associated with such arrhythmias include atrial septal defect, floppy mitral valve syndrome, corrected transposition of the great arteries, and tricuspid atresia. Especially in younger people, however, such arrhythmias are usually not associated with underlying structural heart disease, although they may result from bypass tracts leading to accelerated atrioventricular conduction, as in the Wolff-Parkinson-White syndrome.

Ventricular Arrhythmias

Ventricular arrhythmias in congenital heart disease are, for the most part, a nonspecific manifestation of marked ventricular enlargement and/or dysfunction. As such, they tend to occur in longstanding volume overload, decompensated semilunar valve stenosis, aortic regurgitation or atrioventricular valvular incompetence, as well as in IHSS. In our experience, ventricular arrhythmias have been particularly troublesome in postoperative patients where there has been extensive surgery on the ventricles, as with tetralogy of Fallot, and in conditions where there has been chronic combined volume and pressure overload of the left ventricle (as in aortic valve disease, patent ductus arteriosus, and palliative systemic–pulmonary arterial shunts). Arrhythmias may consist of only isolated ventricular extrasystoles, but more malignant forms of ventricular arrhythmia, including ventricular tachycardia and fatal ventricular fibrillation, may be a major problem, particularly when associated with severe left ventricular dysfunction.

Severe ventricular arrhythmias and sudden death may also occur in conditions without ventricular disease; this has been noted in several syndromes characterized by a long Q-T interval.[6] The combination of congenital deafness, prolonged Q-T interval, and repeated syncopal episodes which may lead to sudden death is known as the Jervell and Lange-Nielsen syndrome;[7] the Romano-Ward syndrome[8,9] presents a similar clinical picture except for the absence of deafness. Ventricular arrhythmias and sudden death are known to be associated with the mitral valve prolapse syndrome and recently a young man with the Jervell and Lange-Nielsen syndrome was found to have a floppy mitral valve.[10] It may well be that serious ventricular arrhythmias and sudden death in patients with only the mitral valve prolapse syndrome are similarly related to repolarization abnormalities.[11]

Atrioventricular Conduction Abnormalities

Congenital abnormalities of atrioventricular conduction are not rare in association with congenital heart defects or as isolated abnormalities. They tend not to be symptomatic in childhood but may be clinically significant in adult life. The most striking example of these abnormalities is congenital complete heart block. Usually appearing as an isolated abnormality, congenital complete heart block or high-grade second-degree atrioventricular block may be an important clue to corrected transposition of the great arteries (Fig. 1). The block in these patients presumably relates to the abnormal course of the His bundle secondary to atrioventricular discordance. First-degree heart block may occur in any congenital cardiac anomaly, but is most characteristically associated with endocardial cushion defects, and is less characteristically linked with other atrial defects and large ventricular defects.

Whether complete or partial, congenital atrioventricular block is caused by abnormal development of the atrioventricular node and/or its connections with the bundle of His.[12] The sequence of ventricular depolarization is therefore normal and the QRS will reflect the presence or absence of associated cardiac structural abnormalities in the same fashion as a normally conducted beat would reflect them.

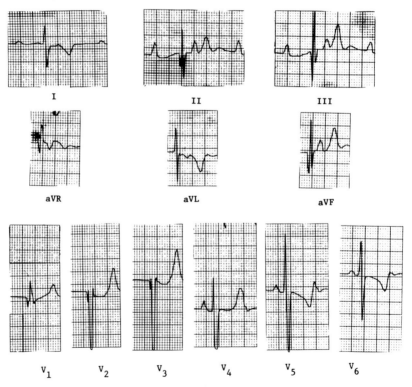

Figure 1. The electrocardiogram of a 19-year-old man with corrected transposition of the great arteries, ventricular septal defect, and severe pulmonary vascular disease. Complete heart block is present. The P wave is normally directed, indicating situs solitus of the atria; there is biatrial overload. Septal Q waves are seen in the right precordial leads, indicating ventricular inversion; the T wave progression is similarly inverted. There is evidence of biventricular hypertrophy.

Atrioventricular block has been a major problem following repair of congenital heart disease and will be discussed in this respect subsequently. Although the overall frequency of this complication has decreased markedly in recent years, it has been noted particularly following surgery for tetralogy of Fallot or other lesions with ventricular septal defect in the subaortic position, complex forms of endocardial cushion defect, corrected transposition, and complete transposition of the great arteries.[13-15] At particular risk for the late development of complete heart block (which has been noted to develop as late as 14 years following surgery[16]) are those individuals in whom there was evidence of bifascicular block postoperatively, and of this group, those individuals in whom there was a transient postoperative period of complete heart block are especially susceptible.[16-18]

Pre-excitation Syndrome

Although pre-excitation syndrome (Wolff-Parkinson-White or Lown-Ganong-Levine pattern) is usually found in the absence of associated cardiac structural abnormality, the syndrome may be an indication of congenital heart disease or an important associated manifestation. Wolff-Parkinson-White syndrome is most characteristically associated with Ebstein's anomaly of the tricuspid valve, and is thus possibly related to the persistence of muscular bridges between the atrium and ventricle that result from maldevelopment of the tricuspid annulus. With right ventricular pre-excitation, the syndrome is usually of the type B variety, with the delta wave directed posteriorly[19] (Fig. 2). Less commonly, Wolff-Parkinson-White syndrome occurs with other forms of congenital heart disease, including corrected transposition, atrial septal defect, certain cardiomyopathies, and, probably, mitral valve prolapse as well. The paroxysmal tachycardias due to Wolff-Parkinson-White syndrome may cause significant hemodynamic embarrassment, particularly in individuals with associated major congenital cardiac anomalies.

ABNORMALITIES OF THE P WAVE

Abnormal Site of Origin

An abnormally directed P wave may be an important clue to congenital abnormalities of the atrial situs, sinus node development, or atrial morphology. Marked right axis deviation of the P wave (negative P wave in lead I) is typical of atrial situs inversus. Coronary sinus rhythm (superior P wave vector) is not rare in normals, but when it is persistent (particularly at more rapid rates) should raise the suspicion of absence or malformation of the sinoatrial node, a defect seen most commonly in sinus venosus atrial septal defect and common atrium[20,21] (Fig. 3).

Evidence of Atrial Overload

Evidence of right, left, or combined atrial overload is common in hemodynamically significant congenital heart disease. Enlargement of either atrium may result from large shunt flow, atrioventricular valve disease, or abnormal ventricular compliance. *Right atrial enlargement* is common in atrial septal defect, where it is usually electrocardiographically mild; it is nearly always present when the right ventricle is functioning at systemic pressure, as in tetralogy of Fallot, pulmonary hypertension, and moderately severe pulmonary stenosis. It may be striking in severe pulmonary stenosis, Ebstein's anomaly, and tricuspid atresia. In adults, the differential diagnosis of right atrial enlargement includes chronic pulmonary disease, primary or secondary pulmonary hypertension, and acquired valvular heart disease.

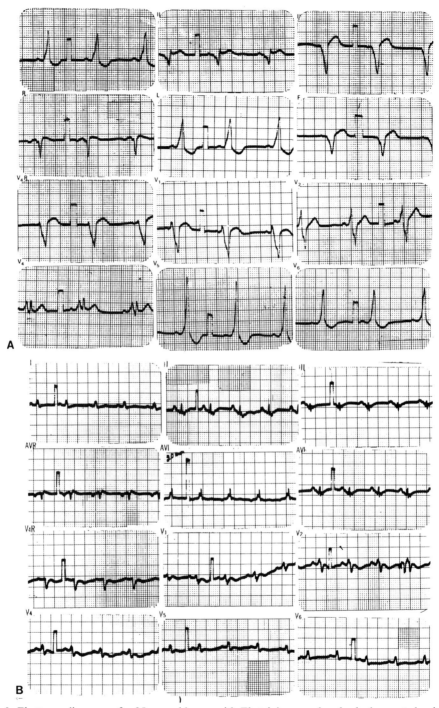

Figure 2. Electrocardiograms of a 25-year-old man with Ebstein's anomaly who had repeated episodes of supraventricular tachyarrhythmia. A, The electrocardiogram shows Wolff-Parkinson-White syndrome, type B: a short P-R interval, slurring of the initial inscription of the QRS producing a delta wave which is directed superiorly, posteriorly, and to the left. B, The electrocardiogram now shows typical findings of Ebstein's anomaly: peaked P waves indicating right atrial overload, low voltage "splintered" QRS complexes with right ventricular conduction delay.

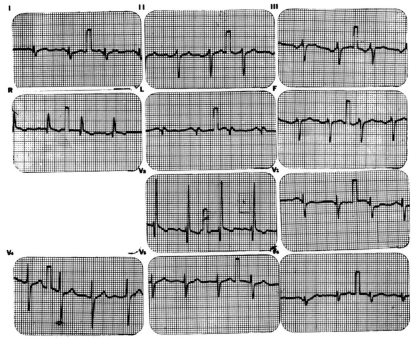

Figure 3. The electrocardiogram of an 18-year-old woman with common atrium associated with polysplenia syndrome. The P wave is directed superiorly, indicating an ectopic origin low in the atrium. The QRS forces are directed superiorly in the frontal plane, with the pattern of left anterior fascicular block. Combined right ventricular volume and pressure overload are best appreciated in lead V_2.

Left atrial enlargement is common in many forms of acquired heart disease in the adult, and is most typically and strikingly found with rheumatic mitral valve disease. Left atrial enlargement due to congenital heart disease is typically present where there is large left-to-right shunting because of patent ductus arteriosus or, less commonly, ventricular septal defect; it is also seen with the severe left ventricular pressure overload which accompanies congenital aortic stenosis and coarctation of the aorta, particularly when there is associated left ventricular dysfunction (Fig. 4). Other causes of left atrial enlargement include idiopathic hypertrophic subaortic stenosis, left atrioventricular valve dysfunction in corrected transposition or endocardial cushion defects, and left ventricular disease secondary to congenital abnormalities of the coronary arteries (the most common of these abnormalities being anomalous origin of the left coronary artery from the pulmonary artery).

ABNORMALITIES OF THE QRS COMPLEX

Abnormal Patterns of Depolarization

Abnormal patterns of ventricular depolarization are common in congenital heart disease and may be of considerable help in distinguishing one form from another. Corrected transposition may be diagnosed from the pattern of ventricular depolarization, since inversion of the ventricles results in right-to-left depolarization of the septum (septal Q waves over the right rather than the left precordium) and abnormal QRS progression in the precordial leads[22] (Fig. 1). *Superior deviation of the terminal QRS forces*, resulting from or mimicking left anterior fascicular block, is a char\arcteristic electrocardiographic finding in all forms of endocardial cushion defect[23] (Figs. 3 and 5).

125

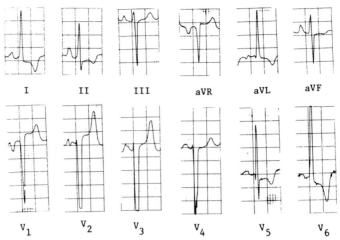

Figure 4. The electrocardiogram of a 24-year-old female college student with severe membranous subvalvar aortic stenosis (with a peak left ventricular systolic pressure of 270 mm. Hg). The electrocardiogram shows left atrial overload, with prominent terminal P wave negativity in V_1. There is minor left ventricular conduction delay and striking pressure overload left ventricular hypertrophy and strain.

It is occasionally seen as a "congenital" finding in almost every type of congenital heart disease, including ASD secundum,[24] isolated ventricular septal defect,[25] corrected transposition,[26] double outlet right ventricle,[27] and even valvar pulmonary stenosis.[28] It is common in conditions where the right ventricle is hypoplastic, such as single (left) ventricle and tricuspid atresia. In children, a superior axis (pathologic left axis deviation) is not a feature of left ventricular hypertrophy, even in extreme cases; however, it frequently occurs secondary to congenital aortic stenosis or coarctation of the aorta in adults, probably as a result of left anterior hemiblock.

Incomplete and complete left bundle branch block are nonspecific manifestations of left ventricular disease and are most commonly associated with severe decompensated aortic valve disease. The electrocardiogram in uncomplicated corrected transposition may resemble incomplete left bundle branch block because both septal and systemic ventricular free wall forces are directed to the left. Left bundle branch block is some-

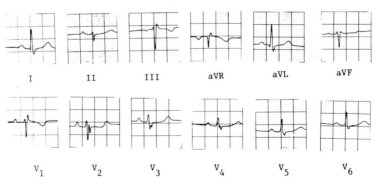

Figure 5. The electrocardiogram of a 36-year-old woman with ostium primum atrial septal defect, a large atrial left-to-right shunt with normal pulmonary pressures, and trivial mitral valve dysfunction. The electrocardiogram shows an upper-normal P-R interval. The P waves in the precordial leads show evidence of mild right atrial overload. There is a superior QRS axis and rather subtle evidence of volume overload right ventricular hypertrophy ("incomplete right bundle branch block" pattern).

times seen in IHSS (common postoperatively) and occasionally found in tricuspid atresia. Congenital coronary abnormalities can also exhibit this pattern.

Right ventricular conduction delay is a common manifestation of congenital heart disease in adults; the pattern of *incomplete right bundle branch block* is the characteristic electrocardiographic pattern in atrial septal defect (Figs. 5 and 6). A similar pattern may also be caused by right ventricular hypertrophy of any other cause, including mild pulmonary stenosis, ventricular septal defect with a moderate shunt, mild forms of pulmonary hypertension, etc. *Complete right bundle branch block* in adults may be a manifestation of right ventricular overload of any type. It is almost characteristic in atrial septal defect primum, but it is also quite common in the secundum type of defect. Right bundle branch block is less characteristic of lesions where there is right ventricular pressure overload and it is frequent in postoperative patients. It is most universally present following right ventriculotomy,[17] and may even occur after transatrial closure of a ventricular septal defect.[29]

Evidence of Ventricular Hypertrophy

Ventricular hypertrophy is the characteristic manifestation of volume or pressure overload of either ventricle and thus often serves as an accurate guide to differential diagnosis. As noted, *volume overload of the right ventricle* manifests itself most characteristically as the electrocardiographic pattern of "incomplete right bundle branch block," and usually produces moderate degrees of right axis deviation with an RSR′ in the right precordial leads (Figs. 5 and 6). Increases in right ventricular overload produce progressive increases in the terminal right ventricular forces which generate the R′ (Fig. 3). *Pressure overload of the right ventricle* is usually manifested by overt right ventricular hypertrophy: rightward and anterior displacement of the QRS forces without prolongation of ventricular depolarization results in right axis deviation with tall right precordial R waves, and deep S waves in the lateral leads. In an adult, an R/S ratio greater than 1 in lead V_1 is strongly suggestive of pressure overload of the right ventricle. A pure R wave in V_1 usually indicates that right ventricular systolic pressure is approaching that of the systemic circulation; this is a typical finding in severe pulmonary vascular obstructive disease (Eisenmenger's syndrome), tetralogy of Fallot, and severe pulmonary stenosis (Fig. 7). More severe degrees of right ventricular hypertrophy, with tall R waves in the right precordial leads preceded by Q waves and followed by deeply inverted T waves (right ventricular "strain"), is seen in pulmonary stenosis with suprasystemic right ventricular pressure (Fig. 8). We have also noted such

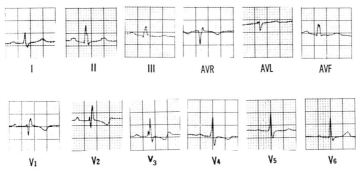

Figure 6. The electrocardiogram of a 52-year-old woman with a large left-to-right shunt via an ostium secundum atrial septal defect; pulmonary pressures are normal. The electrocardiogram shows borderline first-degree atrioventricular block; the P wave shows slight evidence of right atrial overload in the precordial leads. The QRS axis is normal; there are typical findings of volume overload right ventricular hypertrophy.

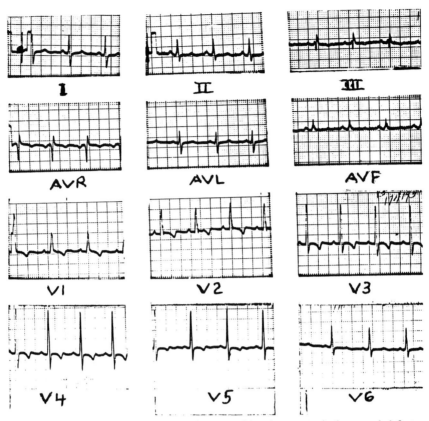

Figure 7. The electrocardiogram of a 33-year-old man with a large ventricular septal defect, pulmonary hypertension at systemic levels, and bidirectional shunting. There is mild right atrial overload seen in the precordial leads. The QRS pattern is that of marked right ventricular hypertrophy with concomitant T wave abnormalities; normal left ventricular forces are present.

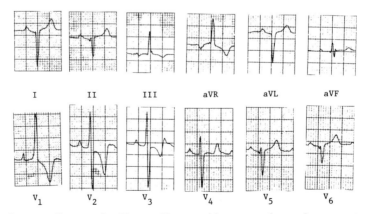

Figure 8. The electrocardiogram of a 21-year-old man with severe valvar pulmonary stenosis. The right ventricular peak systolic pressure is considerably in excess of systemic levels. The P wave reflects right atrial overload; the P-R interval is at the upper limit of normal. There is marked right axis deviation and right ventricular hypertrophy with "strain." Left ventricular forces are inapparent.

128

a pattern in association with marked right atrial enlargement, myocardial repolarization abnormality due to ventricular dysfunction, or severe hypoxemia. The more severe cases of right ventricular hypertrophy, regardless of etiology, are usually associated with evidence of right atrial overload because of diminished right ventricular compliance.

Differentiation between volume overload and pressure overload in right ventricular hypertrophy may be difficult when the patterns are mild; this situation is not uncommon in mild pulmonary stenosis and in small atrial shunts. In adults, it is important to differentiate anterior deviation of the initial QRS forces due to right ventricular hypertrophy from the similar pattern produced by posterior wall myocardial infarction. Posterior infarction is generally associated with inferior or lateral wall infarction and concomitant primary T wave abnormalities. When there is doubt, vectorcardiography may be helpful.

As with right ventricular hypertrophy, left ventricular overloads of volume or pressure tend to be associated with typical electrocardiographic manifestations, at least in uncomplicated cases. *Volume overload of the left ventricle* is usually manifested by increase in left ventricular potentials, large "septal" Q waves, and normal repolarization, often with large, normally inscribed T waves (Fig. 9). Mild forms of volume

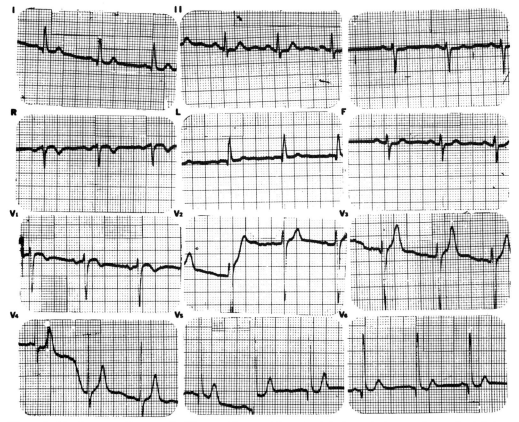

Figure 9. The electrocardiogram of a 57-year-old man with a patent ductus arteriosus and a moderately large left-to-right shunt who presented with mild congestive heart failure. There is left atrial enlargement with terminal P wave negativity in lead V_1. There are typical findings of volume overload left ventricular hypertrophy with a somewhat leftward QRS axis, large left ventricular potentials in the precordial leads with prominent septal Q waves, and normally directed T waves.

overload left ventricular hypertrophy are the rule in ventricular septal defect and in congenital (as well as acquired) mitral regurgitation. More marked degrees of left ventricular hypertrophy are unusual in these lesions, where the physiology includes a low impedance outlet for the left ventricle. Marked degrees of left ventricular diastolic overload pattern—often accompanied by left axis deviation and increase in the QRS duration—point to lesions where the overload is pumped out the aorta, an occurrence characteristic of large patent ductus arteriosus and other arteriovenous fistulae. A similar pattern can be produced by aortic regurgitation, whether congenital or acquired. With advancing age and the onset of ventricular disease, ST segment and T wave changes which are compatible with strain may appear; the QRS complex usually does not change until ventricular decompensation is well established. Varying degrees of left bundle branch block may be present.

The electrocardiographic pattern in tricuspid atresia is often similar to the previously cited patterns (Fig. 10). Septal forces may be increased or decreased, and a strain pattern is frequent, especially in older patients.[30]

Pressure overload of the left ventricle is manifested by a pattern of left ventricular hypertrophy in which initial anterior forces are reduced and septal forces become inconspicuous, with the predominant QRS forces being directed toward the free wall of the left ventricle, i.e., posteriorly and leftward (Fig. 4). In adults, pressure overload is typically accompanied by abnormalities of repolarization: anterior and rightward shift of the major T wave forces produce a discrepancy between the QRS and T axes. Pressure overload left ventricular hypertrophy is a characteristic electrocardiographic manifestation of left ventricular outflow tract obstruction, whether at valvar, supravalvar, or subvalvar level. The pattern is almost always present in adults with hemodynamically severe aortic stenosis, although there are rare exceptions and the pattern may be subtle in some individuals. Changes in the electrocardiographic pattern, particularly the development of T wave abnormalities, may provide a means of gauging changes in hemodynamics in aortic stenosis. Even in children and young people, congenital valvar aortic stenosis tends to be a progressive disease; calcification and other degenerative

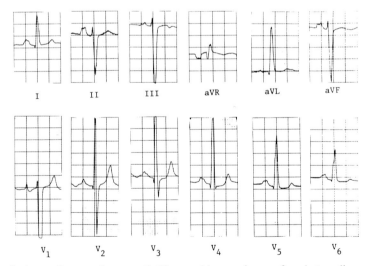

Figure 10. The electrocardiogram of a cyanotic 22-year-old man who was found at cardiac catheterization to have tricuspid atresia. There is biatrial overload. The QRS axis is deviated superiorly with a pattern identical to that of left anterior fascicular block; there is moderate prolongation of the QRS with left ventricular hypertrophy and diminished or absent right ventricular forces. The rightward displacement of the interventricular septum is reflected in the precordial QRS progression.

changes in the aortic valve make progression the rule in adult life. Development or worsening of a strain pattern may also reflect left ventricular disease of other causes, such as coronary artery disease. Coarctation of the aorta and, occasionally, left-to-right shunts (especially patent ductus arteriosus) may also produce a similar pattern.

Combined or biventricular hypertrophy is a relatively unusual manifestation of congenital heart disease in adults, and in adults most frequently results from rheumatic valvular heart disease. When due to congenital heart disease, biventricular hypertrophy most commonly indicates a left-to-right shunt with pulmonary hypertension (Fig. 11) or, less commonly, mild pulmonary stenosis. A fairly common syndrome of childhood, large ventricular septal defect with large shunt and pulmonary hypertension seldom persists as such into adult life; most patients develop progressive pulmonary vascular obstructive disease and the electrocardiographic pattern of pure or predominant right ventricular hypertrophy.

Patterns Suggesting Myocardial Infarction

Myocardial infarction, a common clinical and electrocardiographic syndrome in adults, may occasionally be mimicked, or even produced by congenital heart disease. Bizarre and large septal Q waves may be seen with hypertrophic cardiomyopathy, which is often congenital or familial, and, as mentioned previously, unusual Q waves are seen in corrected transposition. A typical pattern of infarction can also be seen in tricuspid atresia.[30] Congenital anomalies of the coronary arterial circulation, particularly anomalous origin of the left coronary artery from the pulmonary artery, may lead to actual infarction and present electrocardiographically as extensive anterior myocardial infarction. These anomalies may also present more subtly as left ventricular hypertrophy and/or ST segment and T wave abnormalities.[31,32]

ELECTROCARDIOGRAPHIC PATTERNS ASSOCIATED WITH SPECIFIC LESIONS

While most electrocardiographic abnormalities reflect a hemodynamic state which can be attributed to any of a number of possible etiologies, there are certain lesions which are accompanied by typical electrocardiographic manifestations.

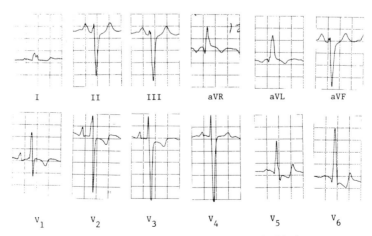

Figure 11. The electrocardiogram of a 45-year-old man who presented with the recent onset of cyanosis and congestive heart failure; catheterization revealed a large patent ductus arteriosus, pulmonary hypertension, and a bidirectional shunt. The tracing shows predominant right atrial and lesser left atrial overload. There is prolongation of the QRS complex with left anterior fascicular block and biventricular hypertrophy.

131

Ebstein's Anomaly

The typical electrocardiogram of Ebstein's anomaly consists of right atrial enlargement, often marked, and either a bizarre right ventricular conduction defect with a broad "splintered" right bundle branch block-like QRS complex, or Wolff-Parkinson-White syndrome, type B[33] (Fig. 2). This electrocardiogram is often diagnostic, particularly in an adult presenting with a large heart, cyanosis, and multiple heart sounds.

Endocardial Cushion Defect

The typical electrocardiogram in an endocardial cushion defect consists of a combination of (1) atrioventricular conduction abnormality (usually first degree atrioventricular block); (2) right ventricular conduction defect with or without right ventricular hypertrophy; (3) superior axis deviation simulating left anterior fascicular block; and (4) where there is a significant ventricular shunt or left atrioventricular valve incompetence, some degree of left ventricular hypertrophy.[23] These findings combined with a chest film showing a large heart and pulmonary plethora make the diagnosis of endocardial cushion defect highly probable (Figs. 3 and 5).

Corrected Transposition

The characteristic electrocardiogram of corrected transposition contains (1) abnormal atrioventricular conduction, often with high grade atrioventricular block (e.g., second-degree block or complete block); (2) abnormal QRS forces with evidence of right-to-left septal depolarization (initial forces directed toward the left); and, less often, (3) a QRS complex of left ventricular morphology over the right precordium and right ventricular complexes (e.g., RSR') in the left precordial leads[22,34] (Fig. 1).

Tricuspid Atresia

Tricuspid atresia produces right (and sometimes left) atrial enlargement associated with marked left ventricular hypertrophy, often with strain. There is a superior frontal axis, probably related to an abnormal course of the proximal portion of the left bundle branch[35] (Fig. 10).

ELECTROCARDIOGRAPHIC FEATURES OF THE POSTOPERATIVE PATIENT WITH CONGENITAL HEART DISEASE

Open heart surgery has drastically changed the course of the patient born with congenital heart disease. Palliative or, in most cases, corrective procedures are now available for most lesions, and operative mortality has dropped to low levels. As a consequence, increasing numbers of these patients are surviving into adult life.

The postoperative electrocardiogram departs from the preoperative tracing of a particular lesion in ways which reflect relief or alteration of hemodynamic overloads, injury to or interruption of impulse formation and conducting tissue, and alterations in the geometry of the heart, pericardium, and chest. Correlations between electrocardiographic features and hemodynamics are, in general, much poorer in the postoperative patient than in the patient who has not undergone surgery. While "improvement" in the electrocardiographic picture usually indicates a good surgical result, the failure of the electrocardiogram to approach normal does not necessarily indicate that surgery has been unsuccessful. Residual electrocardiographic abnormalities following adequate relief of the hemodynamic abnormality appear to be more prevalent among patients operated on at an older age, and presumably reflect irreversible myocardial changes (hypertrophy and fibrosis).[36]

Congenital Valvar Aortic Stenosis

The common operation for congenital valvar aortic stenosis in children is valvotomy, which, in general, should be considered as a palliative rather than a curative procedure. Some degree of residual stenosis is common, and restenosis frequently occurs post-operatively.[37] Consequently, significant residual or recurrent left ventricular outflow obstruction must always be considered in an adult patient with this defect, even if "successful" surgery had been performed previously.

Unfortunately, the electrocardiogram is not nearly so reliable in assessing severity in the postoperative patient as it is in assessing the preoperative patient.[28,38] Thus, while the return of the electrocardiogram to normal almost always indicates successful relief of the stenosis through surgery, persistence of some degree of left ventricular hypertrophy, or even a left ventricular strain pattern, does not necessarily indicate unsuccessful hemodynamic relief (Fig. 12).

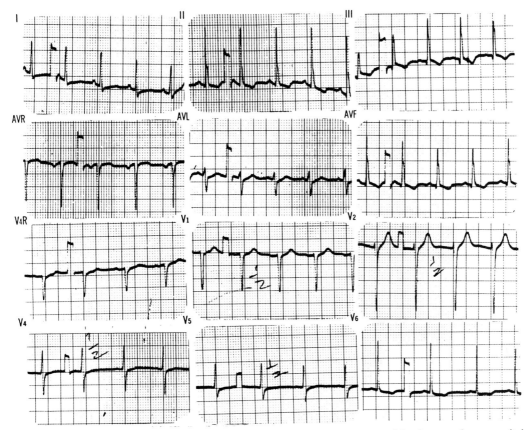

Figure 12. The electrocardiogram of a 24-year-old man who underwent successful valvotomy for congenital valvar aortic stenosis at 17 years of age. Preoperatively the aortic pressure gradient was 80 mm. Hg; at postoperative catherization four years later, the gradient had been reduced to 10 mm. Hg and very mild aortic regurgitation was noted. The electrocardiogram continues to show left ventricular hypertrophy and strain, with little change from the preoperative tracing.

Pulmonary Stenosis

Unlike the situation in aortic stenosis, pulmonary valvotomy performed during childhood is practically always a curative operation, insofar as relief of the right ventricular outflow obstruction is concerned.[39] Evidence of right ventricular hypertrophy decreases rapidly in the postoperative period,[40] although maximal regression of hypertrophy on the electrocardiogram may continue for up to three years postoperatively.[41] A pattern of mild right ventricular hypertrophy may persist indefinitely despite almost complete relief of stenosis.

Coarctation of the Aorta

The electrocardiogram becomes normal following resection of coarctation of the aorta in two thirds of patients who undergo surgery during childhood or early adult life; about one quarter of these patients continue to show left ventricular hypertrophy (with or without strain) which occasionally even progresses following adequate surgery.[42] Postoperative patients with a persistently abnormal electrocardiogram should be evaluated for residual or recurrent coarctation (especially if the original surgery was performed when the patient was young) as well as for associated aortic valve disease or systemic hypertension.

Atrial Septal Defect Secundum

Following corrective surgery for this lesion about 85% of patients have a decrease in the R' wave over the right precordium and a decrease in the S wave over the left precordium, evidence of regression of the right ventricular hypertrophy.[43] Failure to effect a significant decrease in right ventricular forces may indicate either persistence of the defect or the presence of pulmonary hypertension.[44] Atrial arrhythmias or conduction abnormalities are not uncommon in the adult patient who has undergone repair of an atrial defect.[45] These abnormalities reflect the extensive incision and manipulation of the atria and the sinoatrial node and its arterial supply, the latter being particularly a problem in patients with the sinus venosus type of atrial defect. The most common arrhythmias are atrial fibrillation and variants of the sick sinus syndrome: sinus exit block or bradycardia with ectopic atrial rhythm, with or without a variety of supraventricular tachyarrhythmias. Atrioventricular junctional rhythms are not uncommon, especially during the early postoperative period, and complete right bundle branch block may appear for the first time following surgery. Less often, disturbances of atrioventricular conduction may develop postoperatively.[43]

Atrial Septal Defect Primum

Left axis deviation persists after repair of a primum type of atrial septal defect, and left ventricular hypertrophy may be more prominent as right ventricular hypertrophy becomes less evident. The development of arrhythmias postoperatively parallels their development in secundum defects, except for an increased incidence of atrioventricular conduction disturbances. Complete heart block has been observed as late as ten years following surgery.[46]

Patent Ductus Arteriosus

When patent ductus arteriosus is divided surgically during early childhood, the electrocardiogram usually returns to normal.[47] For the rare adult patient who has a persisting patent ductus arteriosus, residual left ventricular hypertrophy, with or without strain, may be encountered.

Ventricular Septal Defect

The usual finding following transventricular surgical repair of ventricular septal defect is right bundle branch block. It occurs in most patients when the right ventriculotomy incision disrupts terminal branches of the right bundle.[48] This pattern is less common in the case of transatrial closure; when complete right bundle branch block occurs in these patients it probably reflects proximal damage to the right bundle at the site of the ventricular defect.[29] Until recently, between 5 and 15 percent of patients also showed the postoperative development of left axis deviation.[17,49] When this pattern represents bifascicular block from damage to the proximal His-Purkinje system, complete heart block may develop, although sometimes not for many years following surgery.[17,50]

Tetralogy of Fallot

Patients with tetralogy of Fallot undergo right ventriculotomy and extensive infundibular resection; the postoperative electrocardiogram shows right bundle branch block from disruption of distal branches of the right bundle.[51] Closure of the large ventricular defect may cause proximal interruption of the right bundle and the left anterior fascicle, resulting in the additional presence of left axis deviation and the possibility of future heart block.[16,18,52,53] Ventricular tachyarrhythmias are not uncommon,[18] and appear to be more frequent in patients with severe right or left ventricular dysfunction and enlargement from extensive ventriculotomy, previous large shunts for palliation, or incomplete repair (Fig. 13).

Transposition of the Great Arteries

With the advent of new surgical procedures, particularly the Mustard operation, many children with transposition of the great arteries should now survive into adult life.

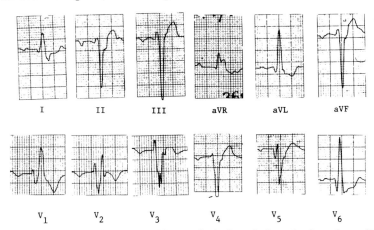

Figure 13. The electrocardiogram of a 30-year-old man who had surgical repair of tetralogy of Fallot in his late teens. A previous systemic-pulmonary shunt (Potts) had been performed in early childhood. He now has progressive heart failure; recent catheterization demonstrated severe biventricular dysfunction. The tracing shows atrial flutter with 3:1 atrioventricular block. There is marked intraventricular conduction delay with right bundle branch block and left anterior fascicular block.

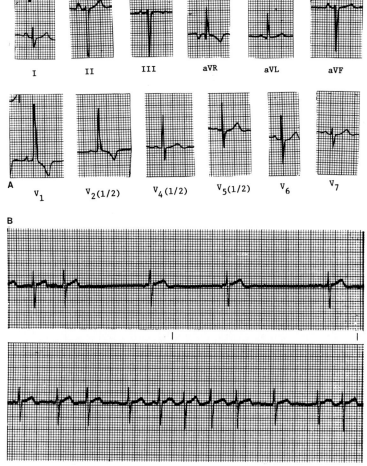

Figure 14. Electrocardiograms of a nine-year-old girl who has undergone Mustard's operation for transposition of the great arteries. A, The standard electrocardiogram discloses right atrial overload; there is superior deviation of the QRS axis in the frontal plane. The precordial leads disclose marked right ventricular hypertrophy; well-preserved left ventricular forces reflect a moderately increased left ventricular pressure secondary to residual pulmonary stenosis. B, Strips from a 24-hour Holter monitor disclose irregular supraventricular tachycardia interspersed with periods of marked sinus bradycardia, typical of the sick sinus syndrome.

Since the right ventricle continues to be the systemic ventricle following this procedure, these patients all have very marked right ventricular hypertrophy on the electrocardiogram. Unless there is pulmonary artery hypertension, the left ventricular influence should be small. Arrhythmias have been, and to some extent continue to be, the foremost problem of the postoperative patient.[5,15,54,55] Most appear to be related to sinus node dysfunction, giving the sick sinus syndrome with sinus arrest, sinus block, wandering atrial pacemaker, junctional rhythm, and a variety of supraventricular tachyarrhythmias (Fig. 14); complete heart block may also occur.[56]

REFERENCES

1. TIKOFF, G., SCHMIDT, A. M., AND HECHT, H. H.: *Atrial fibrillation in atrial septal defect.* Arch. Intern. Med. 121:402, 1968.

2. STERN, S., AND BORMAN, J. B.: *Atrial flutter associated with isolated pulmonic stenosis.* Circulation 36:313, 1967.

3. JOHNSON, J. C., FLOWERS, N. C., AND HORAN, L. G.: *Unexplained atrial flutter: A frequent herald of pulmonary embolism.* Am. J. Cardiol. 25:105, 1970.

4. KUMAR, A. E., FYLER, D. C., MIETTINEN, O. S., ET AL.: *Ebstein's anomaly: clinical profile and natural history.* Am. J. Cardiol. 28:84, 1971.

5. EL-SAID, G., ROSENBERG, H. S., MULLINS, C. E., ET AL.: *Dysrhythmias after Mustard's operation for transposition of the great arteries.* Am. J. Cardiol. 30:526, 1972.

6. SCHWARTZ, P. J., PERITI, M., AND MALLIANI, A.: *The long Q-T syndrome.* Am. Heart. J. 89:378, 1975.

7. JERVELL, A., AND LANGE-NIELSEN, F.: *Congenital deaf-mutism, functional heart disease with prolongation of the Q-T interval, and sudden death.* Am. Heart J. 54:59, 1957.

8. ROMANO, C., GEMME, G., AND PONGIGLIONE, R.: *Aritmie cardiache rare dell'età pediatrica.* Clin. Pediatr. 45:656, 1963.

9. WARD, O. C.: *New familial cardiac syndrome in children.* J. Ir. Med. Assoc. 54:103, 1964.

10. KALBIAN, V. V., PERLMAN, A., AND CHAR, F.: *The Jervell and Lange-Nielsen syndrome.* Birth Defects 8 (5):134, 1972.

11. MILLS, P., ROSE, J., HOLLINGSWORTH, J., ET AL.: *Long-term prognosis of mitral valve prolapse.* N. Engl. J. Med. 297:13, 1977.

12. LEV, M., BENJAMIN, J., AND WHITE, P.: *A histiopathic study of the conduction system in a case of complete heart block of 42 years' duration.* Am. Heart J. 55:198, 1958.

13. MCGOON, D. C., ONGLEY, P. A., DUSHANE, J. W., ET AL.: *Surgical induced heart block.* Ann. N.Y. Acad. Sci. 3:830, 1964.

14. MCGOON, D. C., AND RASTELLI, G. C.: *Operation for persistent atrioventricular canal.* In Feldt, R. H. (ed.): *Atrioventricular Canal Defects.* W. B. Saunders, Philadelphia, 1976, p. 119.

15. GILLETTE, P. G., EL-SAID, G. M., SIVARAJAN, N., ET AL.: *Electrophysiological abnormalities after Mustard's operation for transposition of the great arteries.* Br. Heart J. 36:186, 1974.

16. MOSS, A. J., KLYMAN, G., AND EMMANOUILIDES, G. C.: *Late onset complete heart block: newly recognized sequela of cardiac surgery.* Am. J. Cardiol. 30:884, 1972.

17. KULBERTUS, H. E., COYNE, J. J., AND HALLIDIE-SMITH, K. A.: *Conduction disturbances before and after surgical closure of ventricular septal defect.* Am. Heart J. 77:123, 1969.

18. WOLFF, G. S., ROWLAND, T. W., AND ELLISON, R. C.: *Surgically induced right bundle branch block with left anterior hemiblock: An ominous sign in postoperative tetralogy of Fallot.* Circulation 46:587, 1972.

19. ROBERTSON, P. G. C., EMSLIE-SMITH, D., LOWE, K. G., ET AL.: *The association of type B ventricular pre-excitation and right bundle-branch block.* Br. Heart J. 25:755, 1963.

20. HANCOCK, E. W.: *Coronary sinus rhythm in sinus venosus defect and persistent left superior vena cava.* Am. J. Cardiol. 14:608, 1964.

21. MUNOZ-ARMAS, S., GORRIN, J. R. D., ANSELMI, G., ET AL.: *Single atrium: embryologic, anatomic, electrocardiographic and other diagnostic features.* Am. J. Cardiol. 21:639, 1968.

22. ANDERSON, R. C., LILLEHEI, C. W., AND LESTER, R. G.: *Corrected transposition of the great vessels of the heart: a review of 17 cases.* Pediatrics 20:626, 1957.

23. ONGLEY, P. A., PONGPANICH, B., SPANGLER, J. G., ET AL.: *The electrocardiogram in atrioventricular canal.* In Feldt, R. H. (ed.): *Atrioventricular Canal Defects.* W. B. Saunders, Philadelphia, 1976, p. 51.

24. DUSHANE, J. W., WEIDMAN, W. H., BRANDENBURG, R. O., ET AL.: *Differentiation of interatrial communications by clinical methods. Ostium secundum, ostium primum, common atrium, and total anomalous pulmonary venous connection.* Circulation 21:363, 1960.

25. PRYOR, R., WOODWARD, G. M., AND BLOUNT, S. G., JR.: *The clinical significance of true left axis deviation. Left intraventricular blocks.* Am. Heart J. 72:391, 1966.

26. ROTEM, C. E., AND HULTGREN, H. N.: *Corrected transposition of the great vessels without associated defects.* Am. Heart J. 70:305, 1965.

27. NEUFELD, H. N., DUSHANE, J. W., WOOD, E. H., ET AL.: *Origin of both vessels from the right ventricle. I. Without pulmonary stenosis.* Circulation 23:399, 1961.

28. ELLISON, R. C., AND RESTIEAUX, N. J.: *Vectorcardiography in Congenital Heart Disease.* W. B. Saunders, Philadelphia, 1972.

29. OKOROMA, E. O., GULLER, B., MALONEY, J. D., ET AL.: *Etiology of right bundle branch block (RBBB) following closure of ventricular septal defect (VSD).* Pediatr. Res. 8:353/79, 1974 (abstract).

30. GAMBOA, R., GERSONY, W. M., AND NADAS, A. S.: *The electrocardiogram in tricuspid atresia and pulmonary atresia with intact ventricular septum.* Circulation 34:24, 1966.

137

31. BURCH, G. E., AND DePASQUALE, N.: *The anomalous left coronary artery. An experiment of nature.* Am. J. Med. 37:159, 1964.

32. NADAS, A. S., GAMBOA, R., AND HUGENHOLTZ, P. G.: *Anomalous left coronary artery originating from the pulmonary artery. Report of two surgically treated cases with a proposal of hemodynamic and therapeutic classification.* Circulation 29:167, 1964.

33. VAN LINGEN, B., AND BAUERSFELD, S. R.: *The electrocardiogram in Ebstein's anomaly of the tricuspid valve.* Am. Heart J. 50:13, 1955.

34. FRIEDBERG, D. Z., AND NADAS, A. S.: *A clinical profile of patients with congenital corrected transposition of the great arteries. A study of 60 cases.* N. Engl. J. Med. 282:1053, 1970.

35. GULLER, G., DuSHANE, J. W., AND TITUS, J. L.: *The atrioventricular conduction system in two cases of tricuspid atresia.* Circulation 40:217, 1969.

36. CUTILLETTA, A. F., RUDNIK, M., DOWELL, R. T., ET AL.: *Regression of myocardial hypertrophy.* Pediatr. Res. 8:348/74, 1974 (abstract).

37. WAGNER, H. R., ELLISON, R. C., KEANE, J. F., ET AL.: *Clinical course in aortic stenosis.* Circulation 56:I-47, 1977.

38. MORROW, A. G., GOLDBLATT, A., AND BRAUNWALD, E.: *Congenital aortic stenosis: II. Surgical treatment and the results of operation.* Circulation 27:450, 1963.

39. NUGENT, E. W., FREEDOM, R. M., NORA, J. J., ET AL.: *Clinical course in pulmonary stenosis.* Circulation 56:I-38, 1977.

40. SHAMS, A., KEITH, J. D., EDIBAM, B., ET AL.: *The rate of regression of ventricular hypertrophy in vectorcardiogram and electrocardiogram after surgery on congenital heart disease.* J. Electrocardiol. 6:243, 1973.

41. CAMPBELL, M., AND BROCK, R.: *The results of valvotomy for simple pulmonary stenosis.* Br. Heart J. 17:229, 1955.

42. SCHUSTER, S. R., AND GROSS, R. E.: *Surgery for coarctation of the aorta: A review of 500 cases.* J. Thorac. Cardiovasc. Surg. 43:54, 1962.

43. CLARK, D. S., HIRSCH, H. D., TAMER, D. M., ET AL.: *Electrocardiographic changes following surgical treatment of congenital cardiac malformations.* In Rosenthal, A., Sonnenblick, E. H., and Lesch, M. (eds.): *Postoperative Congenital Heart Disease.* Grune and Stratton, New York, 1975, p. 65.

44. SWAN, H., KORTZ, A. B., DAVIES, D. H., ET AL.: *Atrial septal defect, secundum.* J. Thorac. Cardiovasc. Surg. 37:52, 1959.

45. REID, J. M., AND STEVENSON, J. C.: *Cardiac arrhythmias following successful surgical closure of atrial septal defect.* Br. Heart J. 29:742, 1960.

46. McMULLAN, M. H., McGOON, D. C., WALLACE, R. B., ET AL.: *Surgical treatment of partial atrioventricular canal.* Arch. Surg. 107:705, 1973.

47. LANDTMAN, B.: *Postoperative changes in the electrocardiogram in congenital heart disease: II. Coarctation of the aorta and patent ductus arteriosus.* Circulation 10:871, 1954.

48. BRISTOW, J. D., KASSEBAUM, D. G., STARR, A., ET AL.: *Observations on the occurrence of right bundle-branch block following open repair of ventricular septal defects.* Circulation 22:896, 1960.

49. DOWNING, J. W., JR., KAPLAN, S., AND BOVE, K. E.: *Postsurgical left anterior hemiblock and right bundle-branch block.* Br. Heart J. 34:263, 1972.

50. SAYED, H. M.: *Complete heart block following open heart surgery.* J. Cardiovasc. Surg. 6:426, 1965.

51. GELBAND, H., WALDO, A. L., KAISER, G. A., ET AL.: *Etiology of right bundle-branch block in patients undergoing total correction of tetralogy of Fallot.* Circulation 44:1022, 1971.

52. POTTER, R. T., LIU, L., AND MAYNARD, E. P., JR.: *Post-surgical heart block: Report of a case with bilateral bundle-branch block and changing rhythms.* Br. Heart J. 33:412, 1971.

53. CHESLER, E., BECK, W., AND SCHRIRE, V.: *Left anterior hemiblock and right bundle branch block before and after surgical repair of tetralogy of Fallot.* Am. Heart J. 84:45, 1972.

54. KHOURY, G. H., SHAHER, R. M., FOWLER, R. S., ET AL.: *Preoperative and postoperative electrocardiogram in complete transposition of the great vessels.* Am. Heart J. 72:199, 1966.

55. ZUBERBUHLER, J. R., AND BAUERSFELD, S. R.: *Unusual arrhythmias after corrected surgery for transposition of the great vessels.* Am. Heart J. 73:752, 1967.

56. HALLER, J. A., CRISLER, C., BRAWLEY, R., ET AL.: *Operative correction and postoperative management of transposition of the great vessels in nine children.* Ann. Thorac. Surg. 7:212, 1969.

Evaluation of Older Children and Adults with Congenital Heart Disease by M-Mode and Cross-Sectional Echocardiography

Walter L. Henry, M.D.

There is a lower incidence of congenital malformations of the heart in older children and adults[1-5] than in infants and young children.[5-9] Although transposition of the great arteries, persistent truncus arteriosus, and tricuspid atresia account for approximately 12 percent of all congenital lesions of the heart in live newborns, these lesions account for only 3 percent of all congenital cardiac malformations in older children and adults. Campbell has summarized the work of several investigators[5] and noted that the percentage distribution of various malformations in children and adults are as follows: atrial septal defect—17.5 percent, ventricular septal defect—17 percent, patent ductus arteriosus—14.5 percent, tetralogy of Fallot—14.5 percent, pulmonic stenosis—13 percent, coarctation of the aorta—7 percent, aortic stenosis—5 percent, and all other defects—11.5 percent. When subdivided into cyanotic and acyanotic cases,[5] the overwhelming number of acyanotic malformations were either shunts (atrial septal defect, ventricular septal defect, patent ductus arteriosus) or obstruction to right or left ventricular ejection (pulmonic stenosis, aortic stenosis, coarctation of the aorta). Although these same lesions were found also in cyanotic patients, most (65 percent) had more complicated malformations (tetralogy of Fallot, transportation of the great arteries, tricuspid atresia, etc.).

These data are pertinent to echocardiography. For example, M-mode echocardiography provides important diagnostic information in many acyanotic patients.[10-13] While M-mode studies may be useful in patients with cyanosis, the techniques and diagnostic observations often are difficult to apply and can be used only by clinicians with considerable experience in M-mode echocardiography. Use of the newer cross-sectional echocardiographic systems[14-17] has simplified the diagnosis of cyanotic congenital heart disease. This chapter discusses the reasons underlying this simplification and the specific echocardiographic findings in various congenital malformations of the heart.

ACYANOTIC CONGENITAL HEART DISEASE

As already indicated, most children and adults with acyanotic congenital malformations of the heart have either shunts or obstruction to ventricular outflow. In all but a small percentage of cases, the overall morphology of the heart is normal. That is, there are two atria in the correct left-right orientation and each empties into the appropriate ventricle (right atrium into right ventricle and left atrium into left ventricle). Each ventricle then empties into the proper great artery and each great artery supplies the appropriate part of the body (pulmonary artery to lungs and aorta to the rest of the body). As a result, the problem in diagnosis of the acyanotic patient is not to elucidate overall morphology of the heart but rather to identify the improper cardiac and vascular communications or the abnormally narrowed valves, outflow areas, or great arteries.

M-mode echocardiography has not been very useful in directly visualizing intracardiac or extracardiac communications. Nor has it been possible in many cases to use M-mode echocardiography to directly visualize valvular stenosis. However, the effect of these lesions on cardiac chamber internal dimensions and wall thicknesses, and on the motion pattern of various cardiac structures, can be assessed by M-mode echocardiography. This information, although often indirect, has proven to be useful diagnostically.

An analysis of abnormal structure motion is largely qualitative. Although it is necessary to understand the motion patterns of all the cardiac structures, a complete familiarity with pulmonic valve motion is essential because of its importance in the diagnosis of congenital malformations.[18–20] In addition, this is the most recent valve to be studied by ultrasound and hence least likely to be understood. The key to understanding pulmonic valve motion is the hemodynamic fact that periodically the right atrial pressure exceeds the pulmonary artery end-diastolic pressure in normal subjects. Since the tricuspid valve is open when right atrial pressure exceeds pulmonary artery end-diastolic pressure, the pulmonic valve will open as blood flows in response to the pressure differential between right atrium and pulmonary artery. This particular condition exists in normal subjects when atrial systole occurs during inspiration. Thus, the combination of increased venous return and decreased pulmonary artery pressure during inspiration coupled with an increase in right atrial pressure due to right atrial contraction can produce a pressure that is sufficient to open the pulmonic valve in late diastole. This premature opening is seen on the pulmonic valve echocardiogram as a downward deflection that occurs before the QRS complex and hence before the downward opening of the valve during ventricular systole. This downward deflection before the QRS complex is known as the "a" kick and is produced by right atrial systole (Fig. 1).

Not only is it important to recognize that an "a" kick is present, it is also important to measure the magnitude of its downward motion. In normal subjects, the downward deflection of the "a" kick during inspiration is between 2 and 4 mm. Both the absence of "a" kick in a patient in sinus rhythm and the occurrence of "a" kick exceeding 5 mm. are important diagnostic aids. For example, if pulmonary hypertension is present, right atrial contraction can no longer produce a pressure sufficient to exceed pulmo-

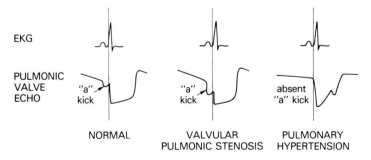

Figure 1. Diagrammatic sketch of the M-mode echocardiographic patterns of pulmonic valve motion in normal subjects (left panel), patients with valvular pulmonic stenosis (middle panel), and patients with pulmonary artery hypertension (right panel).

nary artery end-diastolic pressure, and the "a" kick will not be seen on the pulmonic echogram (Fig. 1). Experience indicates that the "a" kick is lost when pulmonary artery systolic pressure exceeds 35 to 40 mm. Hg. On the other hand, if pulmonary artery pressure is low but right ventricular and right atrial pressures are increased, right atrial pressure will exceed pulmonary artery pressure by a larger-than-normal amount and the magnitude of the "a" kick will be increased. This situation occurs in patients with valvular pulmonic stenosis, whose "a" kick typically exceeds 5 mm. (Fig. 1).

To determine whether a specific cardiac chamber or great artery is enlarged or thickened it is necessary to compare the echocardiographic measurement in a quantitative manner with those obtained in normal subjects. This comparison is complicated in infants and children because heart size increases considerably during normal growth and development. To account for this growth, echocardiographic measurements obtained from normal subjects are expressed as a function of either body weight or body surface area.[21-24]

Even though the body surface areas encountered in older children and adults fall within a fairly narrow range, body surface area (or weight) must be taken into account if the individual being studied is either small or large. An additional complicating factor in older adults is the effect of age on cardiac dimensions. Several studies, performed both at necropsy and with echocardiography, have demonstrated that the aorta and left atrium enlarge with age while the thickness of the left ventricular wall increases.[25-27] Hence, it is also necessary to include age in the consideration of echocardiographic measurements, particularly if the subject is over 40 years old.

To be applicable to a high percentage of adults and older children, normal echocardiographic data should take into account both body surface area and age. Such data

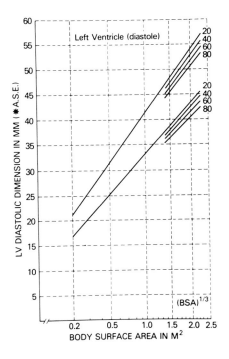

Figure 2. Plot of left ventricular dimension at end diastole in millimeters (vertical axis) versus body surface area in square meters (horizontal axis) for normal subjects from one month to 96 years of age. The two solid lines drawn from a body surface area of 0.2 to 2.2 square meters represent 95 percent prediction intervals for subjects from one month to 20 years of age. The sets of parallel lines shown between a body surface area of 1.4 and 2.2 square meters represent 95 percent prediction intervals for older normal subjects. These sets of lines are shown and labeled for individuals 40, 60, and 80 years of age. The data shown in this figure and in Figures 3 through 8 were derived using the measurement standards recommended by the American Society of Echocardiography.

141

have been compiled in our laboratory[24,27] (Figs. 2–9). In a study of younger normal subjects from birth to 23 years of age we noted that various echocardiographic parameters varied in a linear manner with certain root functions of the body surface area.[24] As a result, these figures are constructed using the root function that produced a linear regression with the specific echocardiographic parameter. Thus, left ventricular dimensions at end-diastole and end-systole, aortic root and left atrial dimensions, and mitral valve E-F slope are plotted versus the cube root of body surface area. Ventricular septal and left ventricular free wall thickness are plotted against the square root of body surface area while estimated left ventricular mass is plotted against the direct measurement of body surface area. Data from older normal subjects (collected by Jules Garden who was working in our laboratory) have been combined with the younger normal data and have been used to account for the effect of age.[27] In combining these two sets of data, the 95 percent prediction intervals were calculated using a percentage assumption. In the study of younger normal subjects the prediction intervals were best modeled using the assumption that data scatter varied as a percentage of the mean value. The older normal data were reanalyzed using this assumption. Since the percentage variability of the older and younger normal data were nearly identical for most parameters, the average of the two percentage variabilities was used. Therefore, in Figures 2 through 9, one pair of parallel lines is shown over the body surface area range from 0.2 to 2.2 meters squared. These represent the data for normals from birth to 20 years of age. Several pairs of lines are plotted for the range of body surface area from 1.4 to 2.2 meters squared. These pairs of parallel lines are labeled from 40 to 80 and correspond to the age decades. By knowing the age and body surface area of the subject

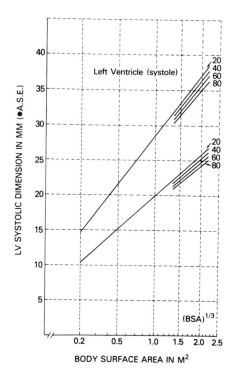

Figure 3. Plot of left ventricular dimension at end systole in millimeters (vertical axis) versus body surface area in square meters (horizontal axis) for normal subjects from one month to 96 years of age. See legend to Figure 2 for additional details.

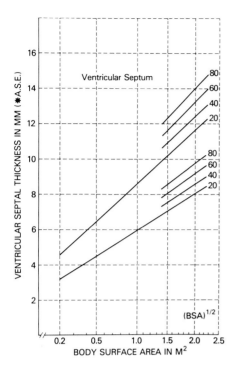

Figure 4. Diastolic ventricular septal thickness in millimeters is plotted on the vertical axis versus body surface area in square meters (horizontal axis) for normal subjects from one month to 96 years of age. See legend to Figure 2 for additional details.

being studied, it is possible to use these graphs to determine whether a given echocardiographic measurement falls within the normal range.

Various parameters of left ventricular systolic function were found to be independent of both body size and age. Thus, in normal subjects left ventricular ejection fraction varies between 65 and 85 percent (mean, 75), while fractional shortening of the left ventricle varied between 28 and 46 percent (mean, 37).[24,27] The percentage of systolic thickening of the ventricular septum varied from 14 to 48 (mean, 31), while that of the left ventricular free wall varied from 29 to 69 (mean, 49).

Right ventricular and right atrial dimensions have not been included in these figures. It has been our experience that right ventricular dimension is difficult to quantitate in normal subjects because of several factors: it is influenced by respiration which we do not routinely take into account, and it is altered by the position of the subject. For example, right ventricular dimension will be less when the subject is supine than when he or she is rolled onto the left side. Unless these factors are taken into account measurements will vary considerably. One useful rule of thumb is that the right ventricle is almost certainly dilated when its internal dimension exceeds that of the left ventricle. Also, other published normal data may be used.[10,21] Although right atrial size cannot be measured at present, the use of cross-sectional imaging may eventually provide a method for quantitation.[28]

With this knowledge of normal cardiac dimensions, it is possible to evaluate a number of congenital malformations with M-mode echocardiography by considering the effect these various lesions produce on cardiac dimensions and motion. Although this consideration of acyanotic lesions will center around M-mode echocardiographic findings, the use of cross-sectional echocardiography also will be discussed.

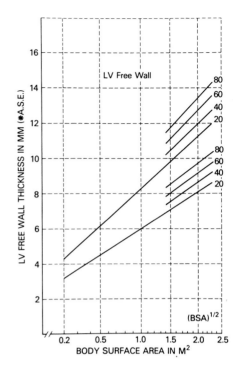

Figure 5. Plot of diastolic left ventricular free wall thickness in millimeters (vertical axis) versus body surface area in square meters (horizontal axis) for normal subjects. See legend to Figure 2 for additional details.

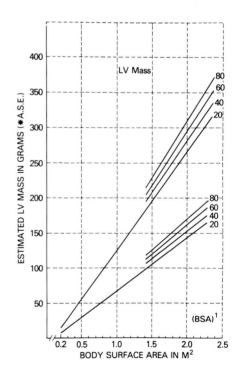

Figure 6. Plot of estimated left ventricular mass in grams (vertical axis) versus body surface area in square meters (horizontal axis) for normal subjects. See legend to Figure 2 for additional details.

144

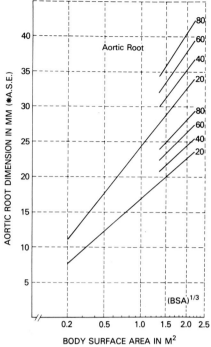

Figure 7. Diastolic aortic root dimension in millimeters is plotted on the vertical axis versus body surface area in square meters (horizontal axis) for normal subjects. See legend to Figure 2 for additional details.

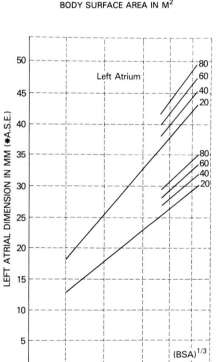

Figure 8. Plot of left atrial dimension at end systole (or onset of diastole) in millimeters (vertical axis) versus body surface area in square meters (horizontal axis) for normal subjects. See legend to Figure 2 for additional details.

145

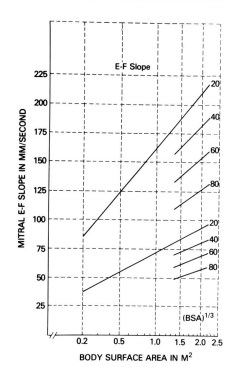

Figure 9. Velocity of closure of the anterior leaflet of the mitral valve in early diastole (E-F slope) (vertical axis) versus body surface area in square meters (horizontal axis) for normal subjects. See legend to Figure 2 for additional details.

Shunt Lesions

In acyanotic individuals an abnormal communication between the right and left sides of the heart allows blood to flow from the left side of the heart (where the pressures normally are higher) to the right side of the heart (where pressures usually are lower). As a result, more blood passes through some of the cardiac chambers and great arteries, which dilate to compensate for the additional volume of blood flow. This compensatory dilatation can be detected by echocardiography and used to deduce the site of the shunt.

Atrial Septal Defect

When the abnormal communication is through the atrial septum, the right atrium, body and outflow tract of the right ventricle, pulmonary artery, pulmonary veins, and part of the left atrium conduct the increased volume of blood flow. As a result, the right-sided chambers and pulmonary arteries and veins dilate (Fig. 10). The left atrium, however, is rarely dilated, presumably because the increased volume of blood flowing into the left atrium immediately moves either through the mitral valve into the left ventricle or through the defect into the right atrium. The left ventricle and aorta are not involved with the shunt; therefore, all left-sided structures usually are normal in size. Thus, the findings of a dilated right ventricle with normal left atrial and aortic root dimensions should lead one to consider the diagnosis of atrial septal defect (Table 1).

Several practical and clinical problems arise with this approach. One major problem is that lesions other than atrial septal defect can produce isolated right ventricular dilatation; these include tricuspid regurgitation, pulmonic valve regurgitation, and anamolous pulmonary venous drainage.[10,11,13] From a statistical point of view these other

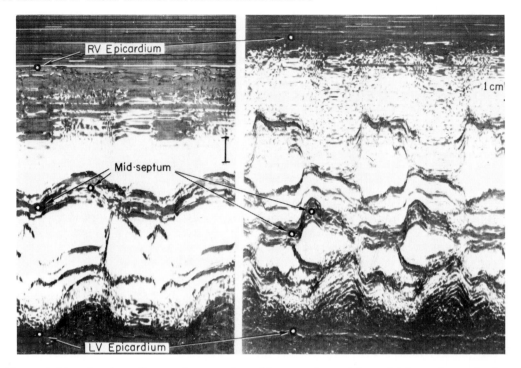

Figure 10. M-mode echocardiograms from a patient with a secundum atrial septal defect and normal pulmonary artery pressure (left panel) and a patient with idiopathic pulmonary hypertension (right panel). Note the abrupt anterior motion of the ventricular septum in early systole in the patient with elevated pulmonary artery pressure.

malformations are uncommon. However, definitive diagnosis cannot be made at present with M-mode echocardiography.

Another condition that can produce isolated right heart dilatation is pulmonary hypertension. M-mode echocardiography provides information that allows a reasonably accurate distinction between right ventricular dilatation due to either a volume load or to an elevation of pulmonary arterial pressure. This distinction is based on an evaluation of the motion of the base of the ventricular septum during systole. In the normal subject the internal dimension of the left ventricle is larger than that of the right ventricle. When the heart contracts, the ventricular septum moves toward the center of the left ventricle and hence *away from* the anterior chest wall.[10–13] In patients with right ventricular dilatation, however, the right ventricular internal dimension approaches and

Table 1. Typical echocardiographic findings

Defect	Right Ventricle Body	Left Atrium	Left Ventricle	Aortic Root	Septal Motion
Atrial septal defect	↑	normal	normal	normal	Paradoxic (continuous anterior motion throughout systole)
Ventricular septal defect	normal	↑	↑	normal	normal
Patent ductus arteriosus	normal	↑	↑	↑	normal
Pulmonary hypertension	↑	normal	normal	normal	Paradoxic (marked anterior motion in early systole)

may exceed that of the left ventricle. In this circumstance the ventricular septum moves toward the center of the right ventricular cavity and hence *toward* the anterior chest wall.[10-13] This abnormal motion toward the anterior chest wall has been referred to as "paradoxical septal motion." The association between paradoxical septal motion and right ventricular dilatation has been commented upon by several groups of investigators.[29-31] In addition, Pearlman has noted that although paradoxical septal motion occurs in right ventricular dilatation due to either an elevated pulmonary arterial pressure or volume overload, these two conditions produce different *patterns* of motion[30] (Fig. 10). Thus, in patients with volume overload the septum moves from beginning to end of systole in a gradual and continuous motion toward the anterior chest wall. In patients with an elevated pulmonary arterial pressure, however, the septum moves anteriorly very rapidly at the onset of systole and then moves either parallel to or away from the anterior chest wall during the remainder of systole. Experience in our laboratory has continued to confirm the usefulness of this observation: we have noted that the motion pattern seen in patients with an elevated pulmonary arterial pressure is best detected when the ultrasound beam is directed through the left ventricle at the tips of the mitral leaflets. Our preliminary Doppler blood flow studies suggest that the marked early systolic anterior motion of the ventricular septum seen in patients with pulmonary arterial hypertension results from rapid initial ejection of blood from the dilated right ventricle into the dilated pulmonary trunk.

In summary, the diagnostic features of an atrial septal defect are isolated right ventricular dilatation in association with the gradual and continuous anterior movement pattern of paradoxical septal motion. Although one cannot definitively diagnose an atrial septal defect from these criteria, the diagnosis is highly likely, particularly if a fixed split-second heart sound is heard on physical examination and the physical signs of tricuspid or pulmonic valve regurgitation are absent. In addition, if an atrial septal defect was previously documented or suspected clinically, the presence in early systole of a sudden anterior movement of the ventricular septum toward the anterior chest wall with subsequent motion away from the chest wall during systole suggests that pulmonary arterial hypertension has developed.

An early report suggested that the defect in the atrial septum could be directly visualized by cross-sectional echocardiography.[32] Subsequent experience has shown that numerous false positive diagnoses occur because the pattern described as diagnostic of atrial septal defect is seen in many normal subjects. A recent abstract has described the use of the echo-contrast technique in atrial septal defect and indicates that these false positives can be eliminated.[33] If this report is confirmed by additional data, it may well be possible to visualize the defects directly with cross-sectional echocardiography.

Ventricular Septal Defect

The most common site of an isolated ventricular septal defect is the region of the membranous septum. In this situation blood passes from the left ventricle into the right ventricular outflow tract. As a result, the pulmonary trunk and veins, the left atrium, and the left ventricle dilate in response to the increased volume of blood. The shunt flow does not involve the body of the right ventricle or the aorta which remain normal in size. Since it is difficult to measure the size of the pulmonary trunk by echocardiography, the major findings in patients with a ventricular septal defect are left ventricular and left atrial dilatation (Table 1). But these findings are not specific since they can be produced by other lesions including mitral regurgitation, aortic regurgitation, and patent ductus arteriosus.[10,11,13] However, one would expect to find high frequency fluttering of the mitral leaflets during diastole if aortic regurgitation was the primary lesion. Also, in aortic regurgitation and patent ductus arteriosus, the aorta conducts an increased volume of blood flow and, therefore, usually is enlarged. The finding of a normal aortic root dimension in association with left ventricular and left atrial dilatation would argue for either a ventricular septal defect or mitral regurgitation. Unfortunately, these clues are only useful in a statistical sense and are not definitive. However, physical examination is useful and can usually assist in distinguishing between these various diagnostic possibilities.

If it has been determined that a ventricular septal defect is present, echocardiographic measurements are useful in that they give an indication of the hemodynamic significance of the defect. For example, a large left ventricle and left atrium in association with a normal "a" kick on the pulmonic valve echogram would indicate that the left-to-right shunt is large and that pulmonary arterial pressures are relatively normal. Conversely, normal left ventricular and left atrial dimensions and normal pulmonic valve motion would indicate that the shunt is small. Finally, normal left ventricular and left atrial dimensions in association with an enlarged right ventricle and no "a" kick on the pulmonic valve echogram should suggest that pulmonary hypertension may have developed. These differential points have proved helpful and allowed echocardiography to be useful in determining whether and when operative intervention is indicated in infants and young children.[11] However, the technique is not useful as a method for following adults because spontaneous closure of the defect is unlikely and the finding of a large shunt indicates the need for operative repair. Hence, there has been little opportunity for careful serial evaluation of adults with isolated ventricular septal defect.

In a small percentage of patients with ventricular septal defect, prolapse of the aortic valve cusps occurs and results in varying degrees of aortic regurgitation. The prolapse of the aortic cusps can be directly visualized in some patients (Fig. 11). Normally, the

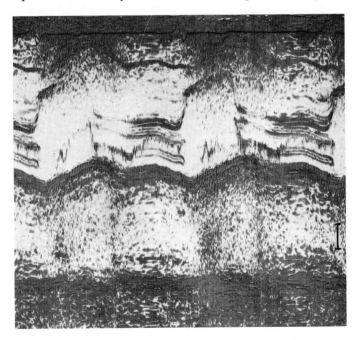

Figure 11. M-mode echocardiogram of the aortic valve obtained from a subject with a supracristal ventricular septal defect and aortic valve prolapse. Note the nonparallel motion and high-frequency fluttering of the aortic valve cusps in diastole.

aortic valve cusps coapt midway between the anterior and posterior wall of the aorta. As a result, the aortic valve echogram appears as a single line that parallels the motion of the aortic walls throughout diastole. In aortic valve cuspal prolapse, the prolapsed cusp may be seen to flutter and move in diastole in a nonparallel fashion relative to the aortic walls. Also, part of the cusp may be seen to move into the upper portion of the left ventricular outflow tract during diastole. Although not seen in all cases of aortic valve cuspal prolapse associated with ventricular septal defect, the echocardiographic findings, when present, are reasonably specific and should be searched for when the diagnosis is suspected.

An early report suggested that ventricular septal defect could be visualized directly by cross-sectional echocardiography.[34] Subsequent experience has indicated that membranous septal defects cannot be visualized reliably. However, defects involving a lack of continuity between the aorta and ventricular septum, such as tetralogy of Fallot and double outlet right ventricle, can be identified in many patients.[35]

Patent Ductus Arteriosus

If the ductus arteriosus fails to close shortly after birth, an abnormal communication exists between the aorta and left main pulmonary artery. As a result, an increased volume of blood flow must be conducted by the right and left pulmonary arteries, pulmonary veins, left atrium, left ventricle, and ascending aorta. Thus, the echocardiographic findings in this condition are dilatation of the left atrium, left ventricle, and aorta[11] (Table 1). This latter finding, aortic root dilatation, could provide a useful differentiating point, although studies have not been performed in adults to substantiate this observation. As in patients with a ventricular septal defect, echocardiography is useful in determining the hemodynamic significance of the defect. By assessing the amount of dilatation of the left-sided cardiac chambers and recording the pulmonic valve motion, it is often possible to determine whether the shunt is large or small and whether pulmonary hypertension has developed.

Recently, Sahn and coworkers reported that it is possible to visualize patent ductus arteriosus by contrast cross-sectional echocardiography.[36] As seen in Figure 12, the

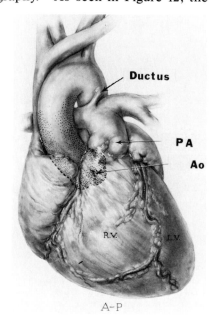

Ductus

PA

Ao

R.V.   L.V.

A-P

Figure 12. Drawing of the heart and great arteries of a normal subject. The remnant of the ductus arteriosus is seen as a fibrous structure extending from the bifurcation of the pulmonary trunk to the aorta.

ductus arteriosus can be thought of as a rudimentary continuation of the pulmonary trunk beyond the branch point of the right and left pulmonary arteries. Thus, by visualizing the bifurcation of the pulmonary trunk, one can locate the region where the origin of the ductus arteriosus would be seen. In infants this visualization was accomplished by injecting saline through an indwelling umbilical catheter into the aortic arch; this results in the appearance of microbubbles in the distal pulmonary artery. This approach is only practical in infants who have indwelling catheters in place. Whether a patent ductus arteriosus can be visualized in older children and adults without the injection of microbubbles remains to be determined.

Obstruction to Ventricular Outflow

Obstruction to ventricular outflow may occur at any of several locations between the body of the ventricle and the periphery of the great artery. In many cases the specific site of obstruction can be determined with M-mode echocardiography.[10] Each lesion, regardless of location, produces the same thickening effect on the ventricular wall and this effect can be measured with echocardiography. We will discuss the most common lesions, beginning with those that occur on the left side of the heart.

Obstruction at the Mitral Valve (IHSS or Obstructive ASH)

This lesion has been discussed in another chapter. However, it is worth re-emphasizing that this diagnosis can be made accurately by echocardiography. The characteristic features are asymmetric septal hypertrophy[37-39] (diagnosed when the ratio of ventricular septal thickness divided by left ventricular free wall thickness is greater than or equal to 1.3) and marked anterior motion of the anterior leaflet of the mitral valve during systole[40-42] (Figs. 13 and 14). The abnormal systolic motion of the mitral valve is probably a result of Venturi phenomenon[43-44] and results in apposition of the anterior mitral leaflet and ventricular septum. This apposition produces a pressure gradient between the body of the left ventricle and the left ventricular outflow tract which leads to secondary thickening of the left ventricular free wall.[45] The left ventricular transverse dimension is almost always normal or reduced, but the left atrium usually is enlarged. Cross-sectional echocardiography has been useful in elucidating the mechanism of obstruction in this disease[44] (Fig. 15). In most patients, however, it does not provide new diagnostic information beyond that available from M-mode echocardiography. Of note, recent reports from Japan suggest it might be useful in detecting unusual thickening of the apex and lateral walls of the left ventricle.

Obstruction in Left Ventricular Outflow Tract

Narrowing of the left ventricular outflow tract (i.e., the region between the basal attachment of anterior mitral leaflet and aortic valve) may be caused by a discrete fibrous membrane or diffuse tunnel-like narrowing, or a combination of both. When the narrowing is diffuse, it can be detected by slowly scanning the ultrasound beam from the tip of the anterior mitral leaflet to the aortic valve. Measurements of the outflow tract dimension in this condition are approximately one third of normal size. In patients with left ventricular outflow obstruction due to a discrete membrane it is difficult to visualize the membrane itself and impossible to evaluate the degree of narrowing. However, it has been our experience that the outflow tract on either side of the fibrous membrane is nearly always reduced. This reduction can be detected by M-mode echocardiography (Fig. 16). In most instances, the outflow tract dimension is decreased

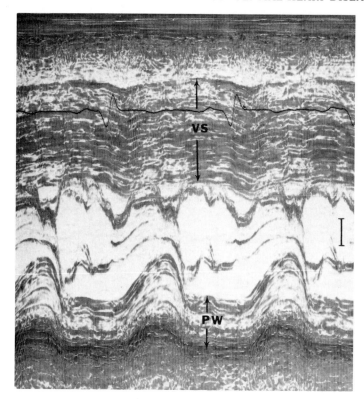

Figure 13. M-mode echocardiogram from a patient with asymmetric septal hypertrophy and left ventricular outflow obstruction (IHSS). This image was obtained with the ultrasound beam slightly below the tip of the mitral valve.

to approximately one-half of the normal dimension. The finding of a narrow outflow tract in both the diffuse and discrete type of obstruction suggests that these two apparently different entities may be part of the same disease spectrum. The finding of patients with abnormalities between these two extremes supports this concept. Differential diagnosis is facilitated by the use of cross-sectional echocardiography, with which the diffuse, tunnel-like narrowing can easily be seen and even the discrete membranes are usually visualized. Distinction between these two general types of outflow narrowing is important because the tunnel-like narrowing frequently is not successfully treated by operation[46] while the discrete membrane usually can be removed with good hemodynamic benefit.

In both types of outflow obstruction aortic valve motion may be abnormal; in some, only high frequency fluttering may be seen during systole, while in others the valve may open wide at onset of systole and then move quickly to a partially open position (Fig. 17). This early systolic spike on the aortic valve echogram is a useful clue that subaortic stenosis may be present.[47] Another useful finding is that the ventricular septum and left ventricular free wall are often increased in thickness.[11] Thickening suggests that the obstruction is hemodynamically significant. Echocardiography is also useful in evaluating the internal dimensions of the aorta and left ventricle as well as the opening distance between anterior and posterior mitral leaflets. This assessment is particularly important in patients with the tunnel-like narrowing since these structures may occasionally be hypoplastic.[46]

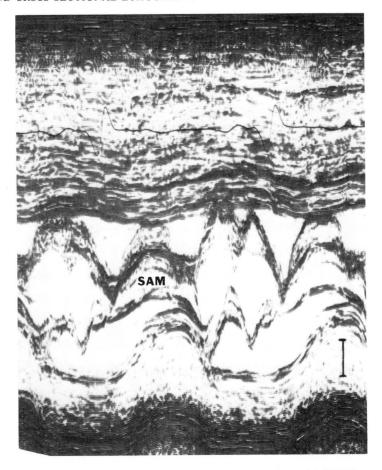

Figure 14. M-mode echocardiograms from a patient with IHSS. The patient with IHSS has marked anterior motion of the anterior mitral leaflet in mid-systole (SAM).

Obstruction at the Aortic Valve

Congenital malformations of the aortic valve may result in a valve with only one or two cusps instead of a normal tricuspid valve. When the valve is unicuspid, obstruction may be present from an early age and diagnosis is usually made well before adolescence. Whatever the ages, the echocardiographic picture in congenital aortic stenosis may be confusing.[10-13] The aortic valve on echogram often appears to open widely, and valvular stenosis is then thought unlikely. The reason for this confusion is that the malformed valve in many patients forms a dome during systole. If the ultrasound beam traverses the base of the dome the valve appears to open widely. Unfortunately, the apex of the dome (where the narrowed opening occurs) may be parallel to the ultrasound beam and not well seen. Use of the newer cross-sectional imaging devices frequently allows this dome-shaped appearance to be visualized and often provides an estimate of the severity of narrowing (Fig. 18). These valves have an abnormal appearance in diastole[48] (Fig. 19). When visualized by cross-sectional echocardiography, the normal aortic valve leaflets coapt in diastole and appear as a thin line parallel to and midway between the two walls of the aorta. In congenital aortic stenosis this parallel line is not seen; instead, the valve in diastole usually appears as a thick line perpendicu-

153

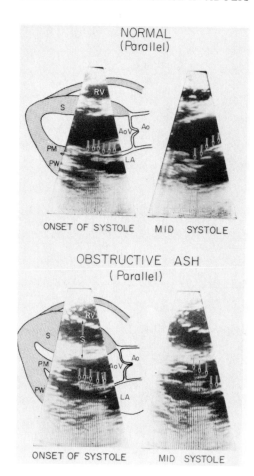

Figure 15. Cross-sectional echocardiograms of a normal subject and a patient with IHSS. In mid-systole the anterior mitral leaflet is seen to move toward the ventricular septum by bending at a right angle to both proximal portion of the anterior mitral leaflet and the papillary muscles.

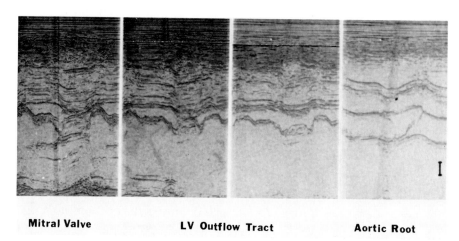

Figure 16. M-mode echocardiograms from a patient with tunnel subaortic stenosis obtained at the tip of the mitral valve (left panel), from the left ventricular outflow tract (center panels), and at the aortic valve (right panel). Note the narrowed outflow tract of the left ventricle at the onset of systole as well as the additional narrowing during systole due to systolic anterior motion (SAM) of the mitral valve (center panels).

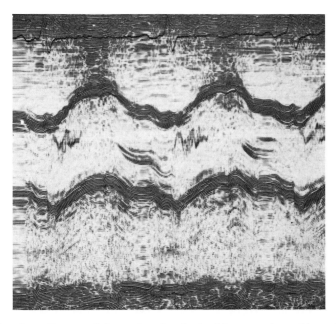

Figure 17. M-mode echocardiogram of the aortic valve obtained from a patient with a subaortic membrane. Note that the rapid initial opening of the aortic valve at the onset of systole is followed quickly by partial closure. This partial closure occurs much earlier than that seen in IHSS.

lar to and connecting the two walls of the aorta. This unusual coaptation visualized on cross-sectional echocardiography appears on M-mode echocardiography as multiple lines between the two walls of the aorta and is believed by many to be a useful diagnostic sign of congenital aortic stenosis.

As with the other forms of obstruction to left ventricular outflow, the thickness of the ventricular septum and left ventricular free wall are usually increased when the

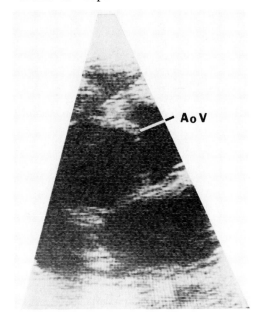

Figure 18. Cross-sectional echocardiogram of the aortic valve of a patient with congenital aortic valve stenosis. This stop-frame image was obtained in systole and demonstrates the dome-shaped appearance of the aortic valve seen in many patients with this congenital abnormality.

155

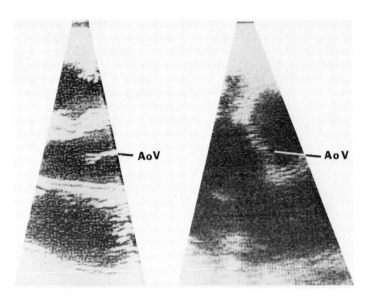

Figure 19. Cross-sectional echocardiograms of the aortic valve of a normal subject (left panel) and a patient with congenital aortic valve stenosis (right panel). During diastole in the normal subject the coapted aortic valve appears as a thin line *parallel* to the aortic walls; in the patient with congenital aortic valve stenosis the coapted aortic leaflets appear as a line *perpendicular* to the aortic walls during diastole.

obstruction is severe. Although post-stenotic dilatation of the aorta is common in patients with congenital aortic stenosis, the dilatation occurs above the level of the aortic cusps. Since the echocardiographic measurement of aortic root dimension is made with the ultrasound beam traversing the aorta at the level of the aortic valve, the aortic root dimension is normal in the great majority of patients with congenital aortic stenosis.

Obstruction Above the Aortic Valve

Obstruction to left ventricular outflow may occur either immediately above the aortic valve (supravalvular aortic stenosis) or at the aortic isthmus (coarctation of the aorta). The former is an uncommon congenital malformation and, when present, usually is recognized in childhood by the precordial murmur and elf-like facial appearance characteristic of this disease. Coarctation of the aorta is much more common and may be first detected in older children and adults. M-mode echocardiography is only useful in this disease as a tool for determining whether the left ventricular walls have thickened. When wall thickening is detected by echocardiography in a patient in whom the diagnosis of coarctation already has been made, the obstruction is very likely to be moderate or severe.

A recent report by Sahn and coworkers indicates that cross-sectional echocardiography may be useful in diagnosing patients with coarctation of the aorta.[49] These investigators used a mechanical sector-scanner placed in the suprasternal notch to directly visualize the arch of the aorta. With this approach, they were able to image the narrowing of the aorta in patients with coarctation. If confirmed by others this may prove an exciting noninvasive method for directly visualizing coarctation of the aorta and perhaps for determining the type and severity of narrowing.

Obstruction to Right Ventricular Outflow

In the acyanotic patient congenital obstruction to right ventricular outflow usually is caused by pulmonic valve stenosis. The recent eludication of pulmonic valve motion in normal subjects and in patients with heart disease allows pulmonic valve stenosis to be diagnosed by echocardiography[18-20] (Fig. 20). As indicated earlier the pulmonic valve in normal subjects moves away from the chest wall in late diastole before ventricular contraction. This "a" kick is synchronous with atrial systole and in normal subjects the maximum downward motion rarely exceeds 4 mm. In patients with valvular pulmonic stenosis the right ventricular and right atrial diastolic pressures are elevated and the pulmonary arterial pressure is low. As a result, right atrial contraction produces a pressure that exceeds pulmonary arterial end-diastolic pressure by a larger than normal amount; this creates a larger "a" kick on the pulmonic valve echogram. The magnitude of the "a" kick usually exceeds 5 mm. in patients with valvular pulmonic stenosis.[18-20]

Although the internal dimension of the right ventricle usually is normal, the right ventricular free wall thickness often is increased. Because of difficulty in measuring right ventricular free wall thickness this finding has not been carefully evaluated. Recent improvements in ultrasound receivers are allowing wall thickness measurements to be made more reliably and right ventricular wall thickening may soon become a useful echocardiographic marker of elevated right ventricular systolic pressure. Since the ventricular septum is also exposed to the increased right ventricular pressure, it too may thicken. In some patients this septal thickening may be marked. However, the left ventricular free wall does not thicken and the ventricular septal-left ventricular free wall thickness ratio may thus exceed 1.3.[50] Nonetheless, the ratio exceeds 1.3 in less than one half of patients with severe right ventricular hypertension.[51] Also, the absolute magnitude of ventricular septal thickness rarely exceeds 20 mm. in adults.

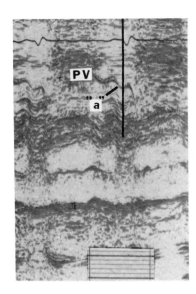
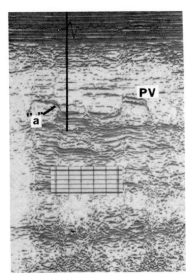

NORMAL   PULMONIC STENOSIS

Figure 20. M-mode echocardiograms of the pulmonic valve obtained from a normal subject (left panel) and a patient with severe valvular pulmonary stenosis (right panel). Note that in contrast to the normal subject, the pulmonic valve in the patient with pulmonic stenosis is completely opened by atrial systole and does not partially close before ventricular systole.

157

Cross-sectional echocardiography has recently been used in identifying patients with valvular pulmonic stenosis. A preliminary report suggests that the dome-shaped appearance of the pulmonic valve can be visualized with cross-sectional echocardiography and appears similar in configuration to the dome-shaped appearance of the congenitally stenotic aortic valve.[52] Until this report is confirmed by others, M-mode echocardiography remains the preferred method for identifying patients with valvular pulmonic stenosis.

CYANOTIC CONGENITAL HEART DISEASE

Most patients with cyanotic congenital heart disease have complex malformations of the heart. In these patients no assumptions can be made about the number or spatial position of the atria, ventricles, and great arteries. Several diagnostic techniques, including physical examination, electrocardiography, x-ray examination, and cardiac catheterization, are currently used to determine the underlying cardiac anatomy in patients with cyanosis. Echocardiography also has proved useful as a technique for obtaining this information. The first attempts to determine complex congenital malformations were made by investigators who used M-mode echocardiography. These studies required considerable expertise but often elucidated complex lesions.[53-57] However, the method had significant limitations for most clinicians. The introduction of cross-sectional imaging provided a technique that allowed marked improvement in visualization of the spatial relations of the chambers of the heart and simplified the evaluation of congenital malformations.[35,58-62]

One of the unique features of cross-sectional imaging is its ability to provide slices or cross-sectional views of the heart in almost any plane.[61] This capability permits the diagnosis of congenital heart disease to be made in a manner similar to that employed by pathologists at necropsy. Van Praagh has emphasized the advantages of a segmental approach to diagnosis.[63] In this approach the position, number, and orientation of the atria, ventricles, and great arteries are determined, as are their interrelations. A major advantage of this method is that complex lesions can be described in a straightforward manner. Cross-sectional echocardiography allows this same segmental approach to be applied clinically to the diagnosis of congenital heart disease. The remainder of this chapter is devoted to this topic.

Information about segmental anatomy can be obtained from several locations on the chest and with the imaging plane oriented in several directions. Either a linear-array imaging system[14] or a sector-scanner ultrasound system[15-17] can be used. In older children and adults, the sector-scanning approach has numerous advantages. Probably its major advantage is that it functions from a small spot on the chest wall and thereby avoids losing the signal through absorption and reflection by the sternum, ribs, and lungs.

The method that we have found most useful is to place the scanner in the third or fourth intercostal space near the left sternal border with the image plane oriented perpendicular to the long axis of the heart (Fig. 21). The images shown in this chapter were obtained in this way using a mechanical sector-scanner. It should be emphasized that experience with the application of this method is still relatively limited so that not every congenital malformation will be discussed. It does appear, however, that this approach can elucidate most, if not all, complex malformations of the heart.

Atrial Situs

Echocardiography has not been useful in distinguishing the right from the left atrium. There are, theoretically, differences that might allow this distinction to be made (i.e.,

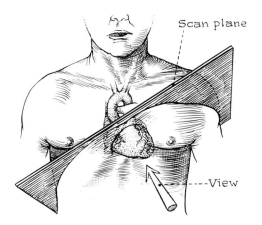

Scan plane

----View

Figure 21. Drawing of a supine subject showing the relation of the ultrasound scan plane to external landmarks of the body.

presence of pulmonary veins) but echocardiographic studies attempting to identify characteristic morphologic features of the atria have not yet been performed. Fortunately, the routine chest x-ray provides information about atrial situs that is correct with rare exception. This information is based on the anatomic observations that the right atrium is almost always on the same side as the liver and the left atrium on the same side as the spleen. The major exception to this rule that atrial situs is determined by visceral situs occurs in patients with asplenia, polysplenia, or midline livers. With these recognizable exceptions atrial situs can be deduced by determining visceral situs from a plain film of the chest.

Ventricular Situs

Cross-sectional echocardiography is useful in determining ventricular situs.[64] The approach is based on the anatomic observation that the mitral valve occurs in the morphologic left ventricle and the tricuspid valve in the morphologic right ventricle. Thus, if it can be determined that a ventricle contains a mitral valve, it can be identified as morphologic left ventricle. Likewise, the right ventricle can be identified if it can be determined that it contains a tricuspid valve. The mitral and the tricuspid valves can be identified by cross-sectional echocardiography by adjusting the position of the scanner to cross-section the heart at its base (Fig. 22). Identification is based on the fact that the mitral valve contains two leaflets and appears as an elliptically shaped structure in mid-diastole. The tricuspid valve never assumes this shape in mid-diastole. Thus, by visualizing the atrioventricular valve to the left of the ventricular septum and determining whether the valve has an elliptical shape in mid-diastole, it can be determined if the left-sided ventricle is a morphologic right or left ventricle.

This approach cannot be used in every malformation. For example, the shape of the mitral valve in mid-diastole is considerably distorted in patients with an ostium primum endocardial cushion defect because of the cleft in the mitral valve. Also, patients with complete endocardial cushion defects will have marked distortion of valve shape. The atrioventricular valves in these defects, however, have relatively characteristic shapes which allow them to be identified and a correct diagnosis established. It remains to be determined whether similar distinctions can be made in patients with single ventricles or double inlet ventricles.

Great Artery Relations

The number and spatial relations of the great arteries also can be identified with cross-sectional echocardiography.[61] Identification is accomplished by cross-sectioning

159

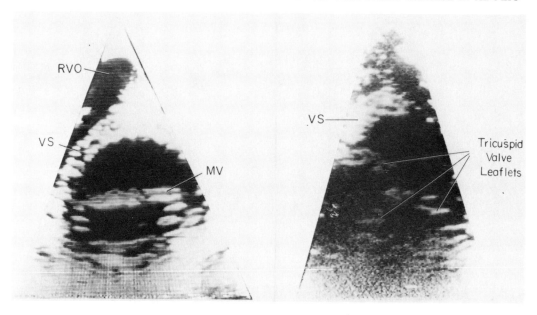

Figure 22. Cross-sectional echocardiograms of the atrioventricular valve to the left of the ventricular septum in a subject with normal ventricular situs (left panel) and a patient with ventricular inversion (right panel). In the subject with normal ventricular situs the mitral valve is to the left of the ventricular septum and appears as an elliptically shaped structure in mid-diastole. In the patient with ventricular inversion the tricuspid valve is to the left of the septum and never assumes an elliptical shape in mid-diastole.

the great arteries at their origin, i.e., where they exit from the heart (Fig. 23). When visualized in this manner, the great arteries can be grouped into three basic patterns: (a) two great arteries whose outflow tracts cross perpendicular to each other at their origin; (b) two great arteries that are parallel to each other at their origin; (c) one single great artery. These three patterns will be considered individually (Fig. 24).

Two Crossing Great Arteries. In this situation the right ventricular outflow tract crosses from right to left, anterior to the origin of the aorta, before connecting with the pulmonary trunk. If the great arteries are cross sectioned perpendicular to the aorta, the aorta will appear as a circle and the right ventricular outflow tract will appear as a sausage-shaped structure curving anterior and lateral to the aorta[61] (Fig. 24). This is the great artery relation found in normal subjects. This circle-sausage pattern also is seen in cyanotic patients with abnormal intracardiac communications (VSD, ASD) who have infundibular or valvular pulmonic stenosis or who have developed pulmonary hypertension and hence right-to-left shunting. It is also seen in patients with tetralogy of Fallot.

Two Parallel Great Arteries. In this situation two great arteries leave the heart parallel to each other and appear in cross-sectional images as two adjacent circles.[58,61] This situation of parallel great arteries is seen in the various types of transposition of the great arteries. In the most common type of transposition (complete or *d*-transposition) the two great arteries are in an anterior-posterior relation to each other with the aorta anterior and the pulmonary trunk posterior. Thus, the cross-sectional image in *d*-transposition of the great arteries is two adjacent circles with one anterior and usually slightly to the right of the other (Figs. 24 and 25). In corrected or *l*-transposition the two circles are nearly side by side with the aorta lateral and usually slightly anterior to the pulmonary trunk. A similar pattern of two side-by-side circles is also seen in patients with double outlet right ventricle[35] (Fig. 26). These two similar patterns can be distinguished from each other by identifying whether the medial great

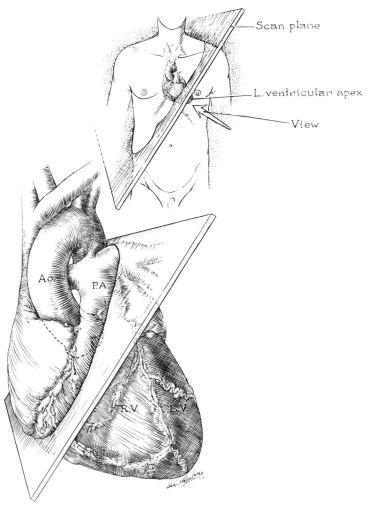

Figure 23. Drawing of a normal heart showing the ultrasound scan plane intersecting the heart perpendicular to the long axis of the aorta at the origin of the great arteries. Ao = aorta; PA = pulmonary artery; RV = right ventricle; LV = left ventricle.

artery is an aorta or pulmonary artery. If the medial great artery is a pulmonary artery, then the patient has corrected or *l*-transposition; if it is an aorta, then the patient has double outlet right ventricle. This identification is possible with cross-sectional echocardiography by angling the scanner in a superior direction (Fig. 26). During this angulation the pulmonary trunk usually can be seen to course in a posterior direction and then bifurcate into the right and left main pulmonary arteries.[35] Thus, in patients with double outlet right ventricle, the lateral great artery is seen to course in a posterior direction and bifurcate, whereas in patients with corrected or *l*-transposition of the great arteries the medial vessel follows this pattern.

SINGLE GREAT ARTERY. In this situation only one great artery leaves the heart. Therefore, only one circle will be visualized when the heart is imaged in cross section at the origin of the great arteries (Fig. 24). This single circle image is seen in either truncus arteriosus or pulmonic atresia.[61] In the latter condition a right ventricular

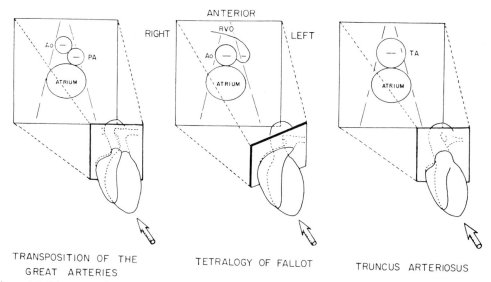

Figure 24. Diagrammatic summary of the three different patterns seen when cross-sectional echocardiograms are obtained at the origin of the great arteries in patients with congenital heart disease. These patterns indicate that (a) two great arteries leave the heart and cross perpendicular to each other (left panel); (b) two great arteries leave the heart and are parallel to each other (center panel); and (c) only one great artery leaves the heart (right panel).

outflow tract of varying size may be seen. Thus far, studies have not been performed to determine whether pulmonic atresia can be easily distinguished from truncus arteriosus or whether the various types of truncus arteriosus can be identified.

Experience in visualizing the great arteries in this fashion indicates that specific diagnoses often can be made from the great artery images alone. However, when other

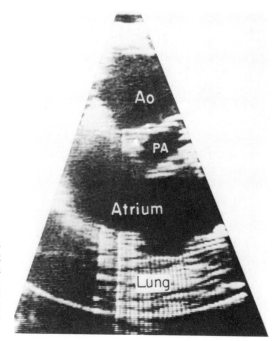

Figure 25. Cross-sectional echocardiogram obtained perpendicular to the long axis of the aorta at the origin of the great arteries in a patient with complete or *d*-transposition of the great arteries. The two circular images of the great arteries are nearly anterior-posterior to each other with the aorta anterior and slightly to the right of the pulmonary artery.

162

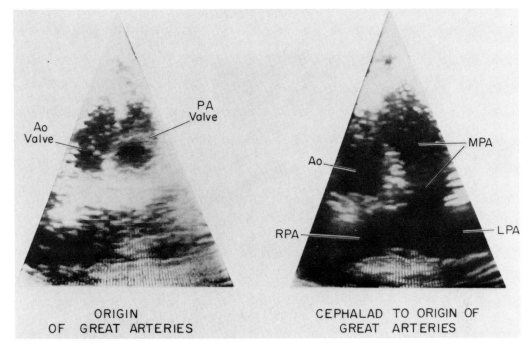

ORIGIN
OF GREAT ARTERIES

CEPHALAD TO ORIGIN OF
GREAT ARTERIES

Figure 26. Cross-sectional echocardiograms obtained from a patient with double outlet right ventricle. The left panel was obtained at the origin of the great arteries and demonstrates two side-by-side circles. The lateral great artery is identified as the pulmonary artery by its characteristic shape (right panel). The image shown in the right panel was obtained by angling the scan plane in a cephalad direction from the origin of the great arteries.

information from cross-sectional echocardiography is correlated with great artery patterns, diagnostic accuracy is improved considerably.

Septal–Great Artery Positions

In addition to identifying atrial situs, ventricular situs, and great artery relations, it is important to determine the connections between the great arteries and the ventricles.[35] This is accomplished by first cross sectioning the heart at the base of the left-sided ventricle, i.e., at the tip of the leaflets of the left-sided atrioventricular valve. At this level the scanner is angled either medially or laterally until the ventricular septum is visualized. The scanner is then angled in a cephalad direction until the origins of the great arteries are seen. These images are recorded on video tape and replayed for analysis. With the image of the ventricular septum on the video screen, the tape recorder is moved frame by frame until a late-diastolic frame is obtained. A transparent plastic sheet is taped in place over the video screen and the right and left surfaces of the ventricular septum are traced (Fig. 27). The tape recorder is then advanced until a late-diastolic image of the origins of the great arteries is seen. The outline of the ventricular septum on the plastic sheet is then compared to the image of the great arteries, thus allowing the spatial relationship between the great arteries and ventricles to be determined.[35]

In normal subjects the aorta originates posterior and to the left of the ventricular septum (Fig. 27). In tetralogy of Fallot the aorta is displaced anteriorly and to the right so that it overrides the ventricular septum, i.e., the anterior wall of aorta originates anterior to the right septal surface and the posterior wall of aorta originates posterior

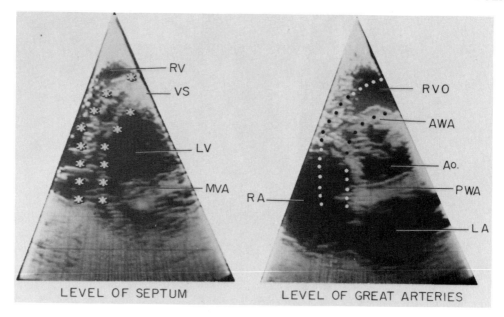

Figure 27. Cross-sectional echocardiograms of a normal subject obtained in late diastole. The ultrasound scan plane intersected the heart at the base of the ventricular septum (left panel) and at the origins of the great arteries (right panel). The right and left surfaces of the ventricular septum are outlined by asterisks in the left panel and superimposed on the image of the origin of the great arteries (right panel). In normal subjects the aorta originates posterior and to the left of the ventricular septum.

to the left septal surface (Fig. 28). In double outlet right ventricle both great arteries originate anterior and to the right of the ventricular septum, whereas in complete or *d*-transposition of the great arteries the aorta is located anterior and the pulmonary artery is visualized posterior to the ventricular septum. These orientations are summarized graphically in Figure 29 and related to the amount of twisting (or spiraling) of the great arteries and their outflow tracts.[35]

As with any method, certain pitfalls must be recognized and avoided.[35] For example, it is important to compare the position of the great arteries and the ventricular septum during late diastole. The aorta usually moves anteriorly during systole while the ventricular system moves in a posterior direction, so that a comparison of great artery–septal position during systole may produce false information about the degree of aortic overriding. In addition, it is important to place the scanner in the intercostal space that allows the tip of the left-sided atrioventricular valve to be imaged with the scanner perpendicular to the chest wall. If a higher or lower intercostal space is used, it is possible that scanner angulation may produce inaccurate information about the degree of aortic overriding. Even if these techniques are followed, patients with an aneurysmally dilated aortic root may be confusing. In this condition the aorta often dilates in an anterior and medial direction, and the walls of the aorta may then appear to override the ventricular septum. However, when these patients are imaged at or just slightly caudad to the aortic leaflets, it is obvious that the origin of the aorta does not override the ventricular septum.

Differential Diagnosis

Once atrial situs, ventricular situs, great artery relations, and septal–great artery positions have been identified, it is then possible to deduce the underlying cardiac

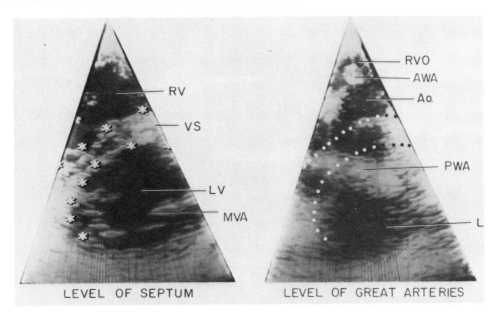

LEVEL OF SEPTUM   LEVEL OF GREAT ARTERIES

Figure 28. Cross-sectional echocardiograms of a patient with tetralogy of Fallot obtained in late diastole at the base of the ventricular septum (left panel) and the origins of the great arteries (right panel). In this condition the aorta is displaced anteriorly and to the right so that it overrides the outlined surfaces of the ventricular septum.

anatomy in most patients with cyanotic congenital heart disease. This information is summarized in Figure 30 and outlined briefly here.

INTRACARDIAC COMMUNICATIONS COEXISTING WITH PULMONIC STENOSIS OR PULMONARY HYPERTENSION. In these situations the basic anatomy of the heart is normal. Ventricular situs is normal so that an elliptically shaped atrioventricular valve is seen to the left of the ventricular septum. Two great arteries leave the heart and their outflow tracts cross so that the cross-sectional image of the great arteries is a circle and sausage. In addition, the circular aorta originates posterior and to the left of the ventricular septum. Common clinical examples of this situation include atrial or ventricular septal defect with secondary pulmonary arterial hypertension and membranous ventricular septal defect with coexistent valvular pulmonic stenosis.

TETRALOGY OF FALLOT. Ventricular situs is normal in this condition. Two great arteries leave the heart and their outflow tracts partially cross so that a circle and sausage pattern is seen. However, the circular aorta is dilated and displaced so that the origin of the aorta is seen to override the ventricular septum and narrow the right ventricular outflow tract.

DOUBLE OUTLET RIGHT VENTRICLE. In this situation ventricular situs is normal and two great arteries leave the heart. However, their outflow tracts do not cross and the two great arteries are parallel to each other at their origin. As a result, the great arteries appear in cross section as two side-by-side circles. Also, both great arteries originate from the right ventricle so that both circles appear to originate anterior and to the right of the ventricular septum. When scanning in a cephalad direction from the origin of the great arteries, the lateral great artery is seen to be the pulmonary trunk.

COMPLETE OR *D*-TRANSPOSITION OF THE GREAT ARTERIES. Ventricular situs is normal in this situation and two great arteries leave the heart. The outflow tracts do not cross and the great arteries are parallel. The great arteries appear in cross section as two circles located in an anterior-posterior relation to each other. The anterior circle is

165

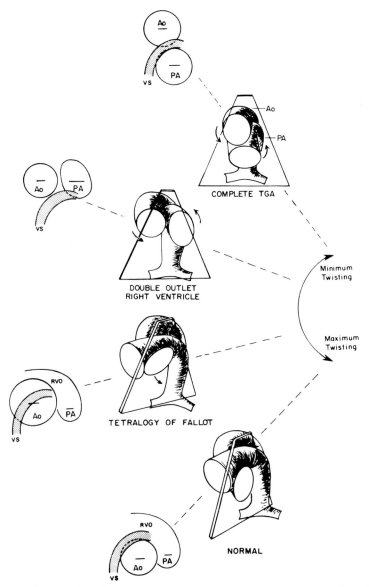

Figure 29. Diagram of the relationship between the ventricular septum and great arteries. The right side of the diagram illustrates the degree of twisting (or spiraling) of the great arteries and their outflow tracts relative to each other. The left side of the diagram contains sketches of the corresponding cross-sectional echocardiograms.

the aorta and is usually located slightly to the right of the posterior circle. As a result, the term dextro- or *d*-transposition of the great arteries is used. Since the aorta originates from the right ventricle, the anterior circle is located anterior to the ventricular septum. The pulmonary trunk originates from the left ventricle; therefore, the posterior circle is posterior to the ventricular septum and is seen to become a pulmonary trunk when the scanner is angled in a cephalad direction.

CORRECTED OR *L*-TRANSPOSITION OF THE GREAT ARTERIES. In this situation the ventricles are inverted so that the tricuspid valve is to the left of the septum. When the

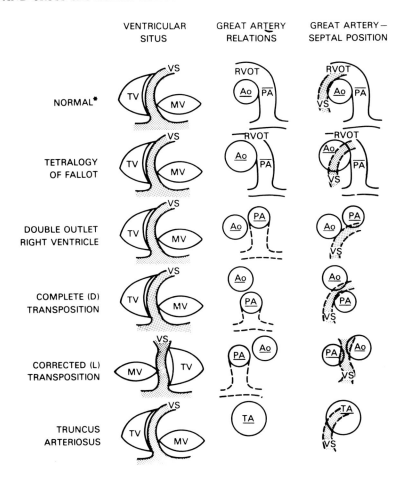

*ALSO SEEN IN CYANOTIC PATIENTS WITH INTRACARDIAC COMMUNICATIONS COEXISTING WITH EITHER PULMONIC STENOSIS OR PULMONARY ARTERY HYPERTENSION

Figure 30. Diagrammatic summary of the segmental approach to the diagnoses of congenital heart disease using cross-sectional echocardiography. The abnormalities summarized in this drawing are shown for the condition of normal visceral (and hence atrial) situs. TV = tricuspid valve; MV = mitral valve; VS = ventricular septum; RVOT = right ventricular outflow tract; Ao = aorta; PA = pulmonary artery; TA = truncus arteriosus.

heart is cross sectioned at the base, therefore, the atrioventricular valve to the left of the septum will not appear to be elliptically shaped in mid-diastole but will be seen to consist of three leaflets. Two great arteries leave the heart and their outflow tracts do not cross. As a consequence, the two great arteries appear in cross section as two side-by-side circles. The medial circle (pulmonary trunk) originates from the right ventricle and, hence, is anterior and to the right of the ventricular septum while the lateral circle (aorta) originates posterior and to the left of the septum, i.e., from the left ventricle. When scanning in a cephalad direction, the medial circle is seen to be the pulmonary trunk.

TRUNCUS ARTERIOSUS. Ventricular situs usually is normal in this situation. Only one great artery originates from the heart so that only a large single circle is seen in cross-sectional images. This single circle often overrides the ventricular septum. As discussed earlier, these patients may be confused with patients who have pulmonic atresia.

Other Views

This chapter has emphasized a segmental approach to the diagnosis of cyanotic congenital heart disease that relies on cross-sectional echocardiographic images obtained with the scanner oriented perpendicular to the long axis of the heart. Other views also provide important information and hence are useful diagnostically. For example, if the scanner is oriented parallel to the long axis of the heart, it is possible to detect discontinuity between the ventricular septum and the anterior wall of the aorta (overriding) in patients with either tetralogy of Fallot or double outlet right ventricle.[60] Also, the long axis view allows visualization of the course of the aorta and thus facilitates identification of the great arteries.[60] In our experience, however, it is occasionally difficult to distinguish patients with double outlet right ventricle from those with tetralogy of Fallot using only the parallel view of the heart at the base of the ventricular septum.

Another view that is proving useful in imaging congenital malformations of the heart is obtained with the scanner placed over the apical impulse. This view, known as the "hemiaxial" or "four-chamber" view, has been studied extensively by Schiller and Silverman[65] who have identified a number of congenital malformations. This view undoubtedly will be used widely in the diagnosis of congenital heart disease; at present, the images seen in Ebstein's malformation of the tricuspid valve are perhaps the most striking and diagnostically useful.

As previously indicated, a sector-scanner placed in the suprasternal notch also provides useful diagnostic information. Applications include visualization of coarctation of the aorta and of patent ductus arteriosus.[36,49] In addition to these views, other transducer locations, including the subxiphoid approach, are presently being explored.

SUMMARY

Echocardiography is proving to be an extremely valuable technique for diagnosing patients with congenital heart disease. Because the underlying anatomy is normal in all but a few acyanotic patients, M-mode echocardiography can be used and provides valuable information about cardiac chamber size and function. Cross-sectional echocardiography also provides additional and useful information in many acyanotic patients. However, its greatest use is in patients with cyanosis. In these individuals the underlying anatomy of the heart often is markedly abnormal. By providing information about the spatial orientations of cardiac structures, cross-sectional echocardiography allows complicated malformations to be elucidated in a manner superior to that of any other noninvasive technique, including M-mode echocardiography. In some patients it is possible to achieve an accurate and complete diagnosis with echocardiography alone. In other patients echocardiography provides information that allows invasive studies to be performed more expeditiously and hence with greater safety. In regard to future developments, the combination of a Doppler blood flowmeter with a cross-sectional imaging system[66] promises further diagnostic flexibility and accuracy.

REFERENCES

1. CAMPBELL, M.: *The frequency of different types of congenital heart disease.* Br. Heart J. 15:462,1953.
2. BLUMENTHAL, S.: *The incidence of congenital cardiac malformations.* Trans. Am.Coll.Cardiol. 3:209,1953.
3. WOOD, P.: *Diseases of the Heart and Circulation,* ed. 2. Eyre and Spottiswoode, London, 1956.

4. SCHRIRE, V.: *Experience with congenital heart disease at Groote Shuur Hospital, Cape Town*. S. Afr. Med. J. 37:1175,1963.

5. CAMPBELL, M.: *The incidence and later distribution of malformations of the heart*. In Watson, H. (ed.): *Paediatric Cardiology*. C. V. Mosby Co., St. Louis, 1968, pp. 71–83.

6. MACMAHON, B., MCKEOWN, T., AND RECORD, R. G.: *The incidence and life expectation of children with congenital heart disease*. Br. Heart J. 15:121,1953.

7. HARRIS, L. E., AND STEINBERG, A. G.: *Abnormalities observed during the first six days of life in 8716 live-born infants*. Pediatrics 14:314,1954.

8. CARLGREN, L. E.: *The incidence of congenital heart disease in children born in Gothenberg, 1941–1950*. Br. Heart J. 21:40, 1959.

9. MCINTOSH, R., MERRIT, K. K., RICHARDS, M. R., ET AL.: *The incidence of congenital malformations: a study of 5964 pregnancies*. Pediatrics 14:505,1954.

10. FEIGENBAUM, H.: *Echocardiography*, ed. 2. Philadelphia, Lea and Febiger, 1976.

11. GOLDBERG, S. J., ALLEN, H. D., AND SAHN, D. J.: *Pediatric and Adolescent Echocardiography: A Handbook*. Year Book Medical Publishers, Chicago, 1975.

12. GRAMIAK, R., AND WAAG, R.: *Cardiac Ultrasound*. C. V. Mosby Co., St. Louis, 1975.

13. WILLIAMS, R. G., AND TUCKER, C. R.: *Echocardiographic Diagnosis of Congenital Heart Disease*. Little, Brown and Co., Inc., Boston, 1977.

14. BOM, N., LANCEE, C. T., ZWIETEN, G., ET AL.: *Multiscan echocardiography. 1. Technical description*. Circulation 48:1066,1973.

15. GRIFFITH, J. M., AND HENRY, W. L.: *A sector scanner for real-time two-dimensional echocardiography*. Circulation 49:1147,1974.

16. HENRY, W. L., AND GRIFFITH, J. M.: *Sector-scanning echocardiography*. In Harrison, D. C., Sandler, H., and Miller, H. A. (eds.): *Cardiovascular Imaging and Image Processing—Theory and Practice 1975*. The Society of Photo-optical Instrumentation Engineers, Palos-Verdes Estates, Calif., 1975.

17. VON RAMM, D. T., AND THURSTONE, F. L.: *Cardiac imaging using a phased array ultrasound system*. Circulation 53:258,1976.

18. GRAMIAK, R., NANDA, N. C., AND SHAH, P. M.: *Echocardiographic detection of the pulmonary valve*. Radiology 102:153,1972.

19. WEYMAN, A. E., DILLON, J. C., FEIGENBAUM, H., ET AL.: *Echocardiographic patterns of pulmonic valve motion in pulmonic stenosis*. Am. J. Cardiol. 33:178,1974.

20. WEYMAN, A. E.: *Pulmonary valve echo motion in clinical practice*. Am. J. Med. 62:843,1977.

21. EPSTEIN, M. L., GOLDBERG, S. J., ALLEN, H. D., ET AL.: *Great vessel, cardiac chamber, and wall growth patterns in normal children*. Circulation 51:1124,1975.

22. ALLEN, H. D., GOLDBERG, S. J., SAHN, D. J., ET AL.: *A quantitative echocardiographic study of champion childhood swimmers*. Circulation 55:142,1977.

23. LUNDSTROM, N.: *Clinical applications of echocardiography in infants and children without heart disease*. Acta Paediatr. Scand. 63:23,1974.

24. HENRY, W. L., WARE, J. GARDIN, J. M., ET AL.: *Echocardiographic measurements in normal subjects: growth-related changes that occur between infancy and early adulthood*. Circulation 57(2):278,1978.

25. ROBERTS, W. C., AND PERLOFF, J. K.: *Mitral valve disease. A clinicopathologic survey of the conditions causing the mitral valve to function abnormally*. Ann. Intern. Med. 77:939,1972.

26. GERSTENBLITH, G., FREDERICKSEN, J., YIN, F. C. P., ET AL.: *Echocardiographic assessment of a normal adult aging population*. Circulation 56:273,1977.

27. GARDIN, J. M., HENRY, W. L., SAVAGE, D. D., ET AL.: *Echocardiographic measurements in normal subjects: evaluation of an adult population without clinically apparent heart disease*. J. Clin. Ultrasound (in press).

28. KUSHNER, F. G., LAM, W., KLUNDER, P., ET AL.: *The assessment of the right atrium using apex-sector echocardiography*. Am. J. Cardiol. 41:392,1978.

29. LAURENCEAU, J. L., AND DUMESNIL, J. G.: *Right and left ventricular dimensions as determinants of ventricular septal motion*. Chest 69:388,1976.

30. PEARLMAN, A. S., CLARK, C. E., HENRY, W. L., ET AL.: *Determinants of ventricular septal motion: influence of relative right and left ventricular size*. Circulation 54:83,1976.

31. WEYMAN, A. E., WANN, S., FEIGENBAUM, H., ET AL.: *Mechanism of abnormal septal motion in patients with right ventricular volume overload: a cross-sectional echocardiographic study*. Circulation 54:179,1976.

32. TANAKA, M., NEYAZAKI, T., KOSAKA, S., ET AL.: *Ultrasonic evaluation of anatomical abnormalities of heart in congenital and acquired heart diseases*. Br. Heart J. 33:686,1971.

169

33. WEYMAN, A. E., WANN, L. S., HURWITZ, R. A., ET AL.: *Negative contrast echocardiography: A new technique for detecting left-to-right shunts.* Circulation 56(Suppl. III):26,1977.

34. KING, D. L., STEEG, C., AND ELLIS, K.: *Visualization of ventricular septal defects by cardiac ultrasonography.* Circulation 48:1215,1973.

35. HENRY, W. L., MARON, B. J., AND GRIFFITH, J. M.: *Cross-sectional echocardiography in the diagnosis of congenital heart disease: Identification of the relation of the ventricles and great arteries.* Circulation 56:267,1977.

36. SAHN, D. J., SOBOL, R. G., AND ALLEN, H. D.: *Non-invasive direct imaging and measurement of the patent ductus arteriosus (PDA) using real-time cross-sectional echocardiography.* Circulation 56(Suppl. III):191,1977.

37. ABBASSI, A., MACALPIN, R. N., EBER, L. M., ET AL.: *Echocardiographic diagnosis of idiopathic hypertrophic cardiomyopathy without outflow obstruction.* Circulation 46:897,1972.

38. HENRY, W. L., CLARK, C. E., AND EPSTEIN, S. E.: *Asymmetric septal hypertrophy (ASH): echocardiographic identification of the pathognomonic anatomic abnormality of IHSS.* Circulation 47:225,1973.

39. HENRY, W. L., CLARK, C. E., AND EPSTEIN, S. E.: *Asymmetric septal hypertrophy (ASH): the unifying link in the IHSS disease spectrum: observations regarding its pathogenesis, pathophysiology, and course.* Circulation 47:827,1973.

40. SHAH, P. M., GRAMIAK, R., AND KRAMER, D. H.: *Ultrasound localization of left ventricular outflow obstruction in hypertrophic obstructive cardiomyopathy.* Circulation 40:3,1969.

41. POPP, R. L., AND HARRISON, D. C.: *Ultrasound in the diagnosis and evaluation of therapy of idiopathic hypertrophic subaortic stenosis.* Circulation 40:905,1969.

42. HENRY, W. L., CLARK, C. E., GLANCY, D. L., ET AL.: *Echocardiographic measurement of the left ventricular outflow gradient in idiopathic hypertrophic subaortic stenosis.* N. Engl. J. Med. 288:989,1973.

43. WIGLE, E. D., ADELMAN, A. G., AND SILVER, M. D.: *Pathophysiological considerations in muscular subaortic stenosis.* In Wolstenholme, G. E. W., and O'Connor, M. (eds.): *Hypertrophic Obstructive Cardiomyopathy.* J. & A. Churchill, London, 1971, pp. 63–76.

44. HENRY, W. L., CLARK, C. E., GRIFFITH, J. M., ET AL.: *Mechanism of left ventricular outflow obstruction in patients with obstructive asymmetric septal hypertrophy (idiopathic hypertrophic subaortic stenosis).* Am. J. Cardiol. 35:337,1975.

45. HENRY, W. L., CLARK, C. E., ROBERTS, W. C., ET AL.: *Differences in distribution of myocardial abnormalities in patients with obstructive and nonobstructive asymmetric septal hypertrophy (ASH): echocardiographic and gross anatomic findings.* Circulation 50:447,1974.

46. MARON, B. J., REDWOOD, D. R., ROBERTS, W. C., ET AL.: *Tunnel subaortic stenosis: left ventricular outflow tract obstruction produced by fibromuscular tubular narrowing.* Circulation 54:404,1976.

47. DAVIS, R. H., FEIGENBAUM, H., CHANG, S., ET AL.: *Echocardiographic manifestations of discrete subaortic stenosis.* Am. J. Cardiol. 33:277,1974.

48. WEYMAN, A. E., FEIGENBAUM, H., DILLON, J. C., ET AL.: *Cross-sectional echocardiography in assessing the severity of valvular aortic stenosis.* Circulation 52:828,1975.

49. SAHN, D. J., ALLEN, H. D., McDONALD, G., ET AL.: *Real-time cross-sectional echocardiographic diagnosis of coarctation of the aorta: a prospective study of echocardiographic-angiographic correlations.* Circulation 56:762,1977.

50. GOODMAN, D. J., HARRISON, D. C., AND POPP, R. L.: *Echocardiographic features of primary pulmonary hypertension.* Am. J. Cardiol. 33:438,1974.

51. MARON, B. J., CLARK, C. E., HENRY, W. L., ET AL.: *Prevalence and characteristics of disproportionate ventricular septal thickening in patients with acquired or congenital heart diseases: echocardiographic and morphologic findings.* Circulation 55:489,1977.

52. WEYMAN, A. E., HURWITZ, R. A., GIROD, D. A., ET AL.: *Cross-sectional echocardiographic visualization of the stenotic pulmonary valve.* Circulation 56:769,1977.

53. TAJIK, A. J., GAU, G. T., RITTER, D. G., ET AL.: *Illustrative echocardiogram. Echocardiogram in tetralogy of Fallot.* Chest 64:107,1973.

54. CHUNG, K. J., NANDA, N. C., MANNING, J. A., ET AL.: *Echocardiographic findings in tetralogy of Fallot.* Am. J. Cardiol. 31:126,1973.

55. MEYER, R. A., AND KAPLAN, S.: *Noninvasive techniques in pediatric cardiovascular disease.* Prog. Cardiovasc. Dis. 15:341,1973.

56. SOLINGER, R., ELBL, F., AND MINHAS, K.: *Deductive echocardiographic analysis in infants with congenital heart disease.* Circulation 50:1072,1974.

57. SOLINGER, R. E.: *Ultrasound in congenital heart disease.* In Gramiak, R., and Waag, R. (eds.): *Cardiac Ultrasound.* C. V. Mosby Co., St. Louis, 1975, p. 185.

58. KING, D. L., STEEG, C. N., AND ELLIS, K.: *Demonstration of transposition of the great arteries by cardiac ultrasonography.* Radiology 107:181,1973.

59. SAHN, D. J., TERRY, R., O'ROURKE, R., ET AL.: *Multiple crystal echocardiographic evaluation of endocardial cushion defect.* Circulation 50:25,1974.

60. SAHN, D. J., TERRY, R., O'ROURKE, R., ET AL.: *Multiple crystal cross-sectional echocardiography in the diagnosis of cyanotic congenital heart disease.* Circulation 50:230,1974.

61. HENRY, W. L., MARON, B. J., GRIFFITH, J. M., ET AL.: *Differential diagnosis of anomalies of the great arteries by real-time two-dimensional echocardiography.* Circulation 51:283,1975.

62. HENRY, W. L., SAHN, D. J., GRIFFITH, J. M., ET AL.: *Evaluation of atrioventricular valve morphology in congenital heart disease by real-time cross-sectional echocardiography.* Circulation 52(Suppl. II):120,1975.

63. VAN PRAAGH, R.: *The segmental approach to diagnosis in congenital heart disease.* In Bergsma, D. (ed.): *Fourth Conference on the Clinical Delineation of Birth Defects. Birth Defects: Original Article Series.* Williams and Wilkins, Baltimore, 1972.

64. HENRY, W. L., SAHN, D. J., GRIFFITH, J. M., ET AL.: *Cross-sectional echocardiography in the diagnoses of congenital heart disease: Determination of ventricular situs,* submitted for publication.

65. SCHILLER, N. B., AND SILVERMAN, N. H.: *Apex echocardiography: a two-dimensional technique for evaluating congenital heart disease.* Circulation 57:503,1978.

66. GRIFFITH, J. M., AND HENRY, W. L.: *An ultrasound system for combined cardiac imaging and Doppler blood flow measurement in man.* Circulation 57:925,1978.

Cardiac Catheterization in Adults
with Congenital Heart Disease*

J. Michael Criley, M.D., and William J. French, M.D.

Over the past decade there has been an increasing emphasis on the study of patients with ischemic heart disease in many cardiovascular laboratories. A large part of this attention is the result of the current enthusiasm for coronary bypass operations. Because of this emphasis catheterization procedures have become streamlined and somewhat steretoyped, focusing on visualization of the coronary anatomy and evaluation of left ventricular wall motion. This specialization on a single disease entity puts the laboratory and the investigator at a disadvantage when the patient under investigation has congenital heart disease (CHD).

The approach to the patient with suspected CHD requires considerable planning and familiarity with a wide range of laboratory techniques and, most importantly, individualization. Each patient poses a unique challenge, and the investigator has an obligation to achieve a definitive diagnosis at minimal risk to the patient. Not all catheterization laboratory investigators possess the training and experience, nor are all laboratories properly equipped to provide an optimal diagnostic study in these potentially complex and technically challenging patients.

The adult with CHD has survived because the lesions involved may be mild or surgically palliated, or because unique adaptive or compensatory mechanisms have taken place. At the same time, adverse complications also may have occurred which confuse the picture further. Thus, the adult may present a clinical and laboratory picture quite different from the infant or child with CHD.

The laboratory investigator must therefore define the anatomical and hemodynamic alterations caused by the inborn abnormalities as well as the modifications imposed by adaptive mechanisms and complications in the long-term survivor. Advances in surgical procedures are rendering more and more patients with CHD operable but require increased precision in diagnosis. It is a serious disservice to the patient to perform a study which fails to accurately define the anatomical and hemodynamic abnormalities, particularly if the patient is cyanotic and has a potentially correctable malformation. According to Mary Allen Engle, "physical disability and premature death are the lot of the cyanotic person, unless his condition can be relieved by surgery and complications prevented or ameliorated by medical measures. . . . Only a few anomalies are still beyond (surgical) help."

It is estimated that 0.07 to 0.16 percent of all adults have some form of CHD. The cardiologist may be confronted by a patient with a previously unsuspected or undiag-

*Supported in part by N.I.H. grant HL 14717 and by an Investigative Group Support Award from the American Heart Association, Greater Los Angeles Affiliate.

nosed heart condition, or by a patient with a previously studied or surgically modified malformation. In our experience the diagnosis carried by previously studied patients is frequently incomplete or incorrect, and management has been less than optimal as a result.

The purpose of this chapter is to outline a rational approach to the investigative study of adults with CHD which emphasizes individualization through a thorough pre-catheterization assessment. Because of space limitations it is not possible to cover the full range of congenital malformations, but commonly encountered problems will be dealt with in sufficient detail to permit a basis for the study of most defects.

CLINICAL APPROACH TO THE PATIENT SUSPECTED OF HAVING CONGENITAL HEART DISEASE

It is not always obvious that a patient has CHD since the presentation can simulate acquired heart disease or pulmonary disorders, or may present as a neurological, hematological, or orthopedic problem. The clinician can correctly identify most patients with rheumatic heart disease by the history and the predominance of mitral valve involvement; and cardiomyopathies are identified by the four-chamber enlargement, gallop rhythm, and lack of significant murmurs. Echocardiography has further enhanced our ability to identify these forms of acquired disease and can sometimes disclose congenital lesions. CHD should be suspected, therefore, whenever the patient's findings cannot be readily explained by an acquired disease.

A significant congenital defect will present two or more of the following findings: (1) precordial murmur, (2) chamber enlargement or hypertrophy, (3) abnormal pulmonary vascular pattern, (4) abnormal cardiac silhouette, and (5) cyanosis. The presence of congenital noncardiac lesions or a family history of CHD can further enhance the suspicion that a cardiac disorder is congenital. It is our philosophy that a patient suspected of CHD on the basis of 2 or more of the aforementioned findings is in a low risk/high benefit category when being considered for cardiac catheterization—regardless of his disability—provided that the study is performed by an experienced team. The presence of a continuous murmur without any other findings also qualifies a patient to be considered for cardiac catheterization, provided that this auscultatory finding is not caused by a venous hum or mammary souffle.

Planning the Catheterization Study

A thorough clinical evaluation of the patient with suspected CHD usually will yield a specific diagnosis or a narrow range of diagnostic possibilities. The experienced investigator will plan the catheterization procedure to focus on the suspected entity, to establish or eliminate commonly associated defects or complications, and will, at the same time, be vigilant of the possibility that the clinical impression was in error. The goals of a cardiac catheterization study for suspected CHD are as follows:

1. Establish the anatomical diagnosis
2. Quantitate lesions and their (a) severity of obstruction, (b) pulmonary vascular resistance, and (c) magnitude of shunts involved
3. Perform serial studies to follow course of disease, i.e., natural history and post-surgical intervention

The first two categories are self-explanatory, but the third category may require elucidation. CHD is often a dynamic and evolving process since it may be affected by a number of factors. These include:

1. Growth of the patient
2. Changing pulmonary and systemic vascular resistances
3. Progressive chamber hypertrophy
4. Increasing hematocrit (increased viscosity)
5. Arrhythmias
6. Progressive ventricular outflow tract obstruction
7. Progressive valvular incompetence
8. Complications such as thromboembolism, infective endocarditis, intercurrent rheumatic fever, arrhythmias, and surgical alterations or misadventures

Thus, in selected patients serial studies permit the cardiologist to make better decisions regarding the need for or timing of surgery, and also whether surgery should be a single or multistage undertaking.

Cardiac Catheterization Procedure

There are two phases of the catheterization study, the hemodynamic phase (pressure, flow, shunt detection, resistance, etc.) and the angiographic phase. We believe that a thorough hemodynamic study should precede the angiographic injections, because the results often will influence the selection of injection sites. Moreover, the injection of contrast substance affects virtually all of the hemodynamic parameters.

Table 1 summarizes our investigative hemodynamic approach to the acyanotic patient with suspected CHD. Since virtually all patients with acyanotic CHD have a left-to-right shunt and/or a ventricular outflow tract obstruction, the hemodynamic investigation should be designed to locate and quantitate these lesions.

Table 2 summarizes our investigative approach to the patient with cyanotic CHD. Since cyanosis is a result of right-to-left shunting, the site of the shunt and why it is

Table 1. Hemodynamic studies in acyanotic congenital heart disease

Problem	*Diagnostic Technique*
1. Is there a left-to-right shunt?	
a. Locate recipient site	Serial H_2 curves
	Serial oximetry
b. Locate site of origin	Selective left heart or pulmonary venous injections of indicator with sampling in recipient site or peripheral artery may be necessary in some cases
c. Quantification	Determine ratio of pulmonary to systemic blood flow and magnitude of left-to-right shunt by Fick principle (Table 4)
2. What is the status of the pulmonary vasculature?	
a. Pressure/flow relationship	Determine pulmonary vascular resistance (PVR) (Table 4)
b. Reactivity of pulmonary vascular bed	Repeat PVR determination after 100% O_2 inhalation, drugs (isoproterenol, tolazoline, aminophylline, etc.)
3. What is the status of the outflow tract?	Measure pressure gradient and localize site of obstruction by catheter withdrawal; estimate outflow orifice area by Gorlin formula (Table 4)

175

Table 2. Hemodynamic studies in cyanotic congenital heart disease

Problem	Diagnostic Technique
1. Is there a right-to-left shunt?	
a. Site of communication	Serial right heart indicator dilution curves
b. Quantification	Determine ratio of pulmonary to systemic blood flow and magnitude of shunt by Fick principle (Table 4)
2. What is location of resistance downstream from communication?	
a. Pulmonary hypertension	Determine pulmonary vascular resistance (PVR) (Table 4)
b. Right ventricular outflow obstruction	Measure pressure gradient and localize
or	obstruction by catheter withdrawal
c. Right ventricular inflow obstruction	
3. Is there obligatory venous admixture?	
a. Transposition of great vessels	Lateral x-ray of catheters positioned in aorta and pulmonary artery
b. Systemic venous drainage into left atrium	Selective venous indicator dilution curves
c. Pulmonary A–V fistula	Selective pulmonary arterial indicator dilution curves and pulmonary angiography

present must be defined. The usual explanation for reversed shunting is a combination of a communication (e.g., septal defect) and a *downstream* obstruction or resistance, although in some patients the venous admixture is *obligatory* because of abnormal anatomical continuity (e.g., transposition of the great vessels).

Catheterization Site and Technique

In our laboratory we generally perform the catheterization procedure by the percutaneous transfemoral approach. The advantages to this approach in right heart catheterization are: (1) there is a greater likelihood of traversing the atrial septum via an atrial septal defect or patent foramen ovale: (2) transseptal technique can be used if the left ventricle must be entered; (3) the vein is not sacrificed, and (4) large bore catheters can be used without inducing spasm. The disadvantages to this approach are a potentially greater likelihood of thromboembolism and the occasional absence of the inferior vena cava which requires catheterization via the arm. To minimize the potential for thromboembolic complications after a long procedure, we administer low-dose heparin for 48 to 72 hours.

Platinum electrode catheters with one or more electrodes are introduced through a sheath for initial screening of left-to-right shunts; these can be replaced later by appropriate catheters for optimal pressure recording and angiography. To enter the pulmonary trunk through a stenotic or tortuous outflow tract, a positive torque control catheter or balloon-tipped flotation catheter often is utilized. It is possible to introduce small (4 French) platinum electrodes or micromanometers through end-hole catheters, and we have also adapted an endomyocardial biopsy technique to the percutaneous transfemoral approach.

Pressure Recording

Fluid-filled catheter-transducer systems are used by most laboratories to monitor pressure. When used properly such systems can be relied upon to provide accurate recordings of the magnitude and contour of cardiac pressures. However, the investigator must be aware of potential artifacts which may cause faulty and misleading data.

Optimal pressure recordings provide quantitation of the magnitude of pressures, gradients, localization of stenotic areas, and diagnostic contours of the pressure waves. Catheter withdrawal recordings from end-hole or bird's-eye (pair of side holes near the end-hole) catheters can indicate valvular, supravalvular, or subvalvular location of an obstruction (Fig. 1). The slow rising contour of the low pressure region confirms the pressure of an anatomical (discrete) proximal stenosis.

We prefer to record simultaneous pressures above and below stenotic areas whenever possible, so that the effects of interventions (e.g., exercise, pharmacologic agents) can be accurately followed. It is essential to measure cardiac output in conjunction with pressure data in order to determine the pulmonary vascular resistance and/or estimate the magnitude of outflow tract obstruction, particularly if interventions are employed which alter pressure and flow.

Some laboratories employ micromanometer catheters which permit high-fidelity recording of pressure events. We do not routinely employ these, however, as they are quite expensive, relatively inflexible, fragile, and prone to undergo shifts in baseline and/or calibration.

High-frequency differentiation of the electrical signal from micromanometers or external pressure transducers can be used to record murmurs. Although the frequency response of fluid-filled catheters limits the fidelity of these intracardiac phonocardiograms, they can be useful in localizing the site of origin of murmurs or sounds (Fig. 2).

Flow Studies

Flow is measured in the cardiovascular system by indicator dilution technique (indocyanine green dye or cold saline) or direct Fick determination (Tables 3 and 4). Quantitative indicator dilution determinations by the Stewart–Hamilton method require that the calibrated injectate be homogeneously mixed in the flowing blood before distribution through divergent pathways (e.g. shunts) and that the initial downslope of the primary circulation curve be plotted. For these reasons the direct Fick technique is usually preferable in the presence of large shunts. However, in the presence of extremely large shunts, the Fick principle is prone to inaccuracy because of the small pulmonary arteriovenous difference. Thus, calculations of flow based on dye curves are often more useful.

This chapter concerns only those techniques used in our laboratory to determine pulmonary and systemic flows. Direct Fick measurement of pulmonary blood flow is made by simultaneous determination of oxygen consumption and the pulmonary arteriovenous oxygen content difference (Table 4 and Fig. 3). Oxygen consumption is measured over a 3-minute period; it utilizes a collection bag attached to a mouthpiece and valve apparatus that allows the patient to inhale room air and exhale only into the bag. The difference in oxygen content between room air and exhaled air is also measured. During the second minute of exhaled air collection, heparinized blood samples are withdrawn from a mixed venous site (usually the pulmonary artery) and a peripheral artery, unless a pulmonary vein can be catheterized directly. The two blood samples plus another aliquot of blood equilibrated with atmospheric air are subjected to Van Slyke analysis of oxygen content. If a left-to-right shunt is present, an additional venous sample is taken upstream from the shunt and analyzed for oxygen content. The Fick formula utilizes oxygen consumption in the numerator and arteriovenous oxygen difference in the denominator.

Direct Fick cardiac output determinations are most accurate in low or normal flow states; in the presence of high flow states minor measurement errors of the small A-V

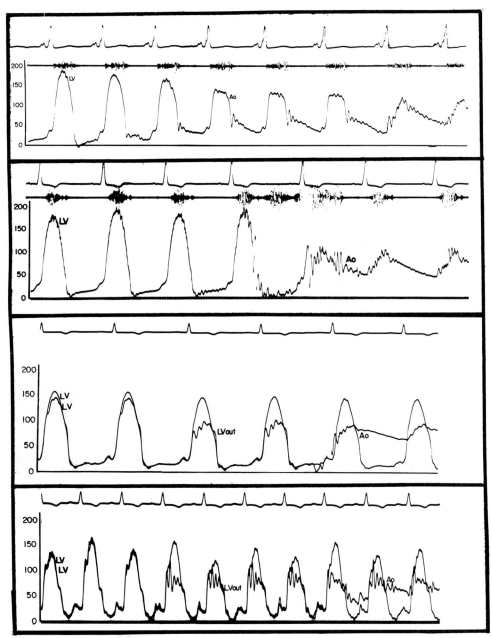

Figure 1. Catheter withdrawals in left ventricular outflow obstruction. Each panel represents a pressure withdrawal tracing from a retrograde catheter pulled slowly through the outflow tract of the left ventricle. The top panel represents *supravalvular aortic stenosis* and demonstrates a systolic pressure of 180 mm. Hg in the left ventricle and 110 mm. Hg in the ascending aorta (far right). Although there is a pressure drop as the catheter enters the aorta, the first three aortic pulses demonstrate a rapid upstroke, while the last two demonstrate a slow upstroke. The second panel from the top demonstrates *valvular aortic stenosis* in which there is an abrupt systolic pressure change from 180 mm. Hg in the left ventricle to 100 mm. Hg in the aorta; the aortic pressure pulse demonstrates a slow upstroke. The third panel from the top represents *discrete subvalvular aortic stenosis*. Two catheters are in the body of the left ventricle, and one is slowly withdrawn through the outflow tract and demonstrates a pressure transition within the left ventricle. A pressure pulse distal to the discrete obstruction demonstrates a slow upstroke. The bottom panel represents *hypertrophic cardiomyopathy*. Two catheters have been placed in the body of the left ventricle, and one is slowly withdrawn through the outflow tract. There is a pressure transition in the left ventricular outflow tract, but the pulse pressure in the outflow tract and aorta retains a rapid upstroke in contrast to the pulse contour of the other three withdrawal tracings.

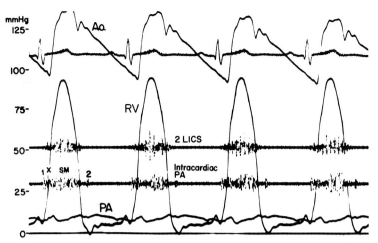

Figure 2. "Intracardiac phonocardiography" in pulmonic stenosis. Pulmonary arterial (PA), right ventricular (RV), and aortic (Ao) pressures are displayed along with an external phonocardiogram from the second left intercostal space (2 LICS) and an intracardiac sound recording from the pulmonary artery. This was generated by high frequency differentiation of the signal from the external transducer recording pulmonary artery pressure. The systolic murmur (SM), ejection sound (X), and pulmonic closure sound (2) are recorded from the intracardiac sound tracing. The right ventricular pressure exhibits a peaked appearance and the pulmonary artery tracing has an early imperceptible upstroke followed by a mid-systolic dip, probably representing a Venturi phenomenon.

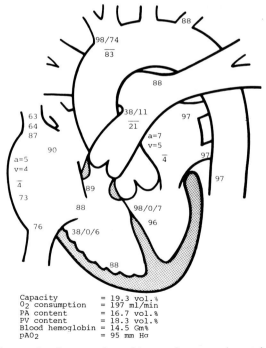

```
Capacity          = 19.3 vol.%
O2 consumption    = 197 ml/min
PA content        = 16.7 vol.%
PV content        = 18.3 vol.%
Blood hemoglobin  = 14.5 Gm%
pAO2              = 95 mm Hg
```

Figure 3. Pressure and oximetry data from a patient with an ostium secundum atrial septal defect. These data form the basis for the calculations in Tables 3 and 4. The two-digit numbers in the cardiac diagram represent oximetry readings in percent saturation, and the other numbers represent phasic and mean pressures in the various chambers (body surface area = 1.6 M²).

179

Table 3. Oxygen determinations in cardiac catheterization

Term	Definition	Technique for Determination	Sample (from Fig. 3)
O_2 Capacity	Quantity of O_2 (ml) contained in 100 ml (vol %) sample of blood equilibrated with room air a. Measured directly or b. Estimated: $1.34 \times$ blood Hb concentration	Van Slyke apparatus or Lex-O-Con*	Measured capacity = 19.3 vol. % or estimated capacity 1.34×14.5 ({Hb}) = 19.4 vol. %
O_2 Content	Quantity of O_2 (vol %) in a sample of blood a. Measured directly or b. Estimated: % saturation $\times$ capacity	Van Slyke apparatus or Lex-O-Con and/or oximeter	Measured P.A. content = 16.7 vol. % Estimated P.A. content: 88% (P.A. saturation) $\times$ 19.3 (capacity) = 16.98 vol. %
O_2 Saturation (%)	Percentage of O_2 capacity in a sample of blood a. Measured directly: O_2 content/O_2 capacity or b. Determined by reflectance or c. Estimated from pO_2 and oxyhemoglobin dissociation curve at appropriate pH	Van Slyke apparatus or Lex-O-Con (2 samples) Oximeter Oxygen Electrode, pH electrode, and nomogram	Measured P.A. saturation: $\dfrac{16.7 \text{ (P.A. content)}}{19.3 \text{ (capacity)}}$ = 87% 88%
O_2 Consumption (VO_2)	Amount of O^2 (ml.) extracted from inspired air in a minute a. Measured directly or b. Estimated: 130 ml./min./M^2	Collection bag, spirometer, oxygen analyzer (Scholander)	Measured O_2 consumption = 197 ml./min. Estimated O_2 consumption 130×1.6 (BSA) = 208 ml./min.

Measurement	Method	Description	Calculation
Oxygen partial pressure (pO_2)	Oxygen electrode	Pressure (mm. Hg) exerted by oxygen in a sample of blood or inspired air, measured directly	Systemic arterial pO_2 $pAO_2 = 95$ mm. Hg
Pulmonary arteriovenous O_2 difference (pulmonary A–V O_2)	Van Slyke apparatus or Lex-O-Con (2 samples)	Increase in O_2 content across pulmonary vascular bed; difference between pulmonary venous and pulmonary artery O^2 content in vol. % a. Measured directly or b. Pulmonary venous O_2 content ($P.V.O_2$) may be estimated as: 1. $P.V.O_2$ = systemic arterial O_2 (if no R-L shunt) 2. $P.V.O_2 = 95\%$ × capacity	Measured pulmonary A–V O_2 $= P.V.O_2 - P.A.O_2$ $= 18.3 - 16.7 = 1.6$ vol. % Estimated pulmonary A–V O_2 = (est. P.V. sat. – P.A. sat) × capacity $= (95\% - 88\%) \times 19.3$ $= 1.4$ vol. %
Systemic arteriovenous O_2 difference (systemic A–V O_2)	Van Slyke apparatus or Lex-O-Con Oximeter	Decrease in O_2 content across systemic vascular bed; difference between systemic arterial and mixed venous O_2 content in vol. % a. Measured directly mixed venous $O_2 = P.A.O_2$ (if no L-R shunt) or b. Mixed venous ($M.V.O_2$) may be estimated: $$M.V.\ sat. = \frac{2\,IVC + SVC}{3}$$ $M.V.\ O_2 = M.V.\ sat.$ × capacity	Measured systemic A–V O_2 $= Ao - MVO_2$ contents $= 18.3 - 13.9 = 4.4$ vol. % $$M.V.\ sat. = \frac{2 \times 76\% + 63\%}{3} = 71.7\%$$ $M.V.O_2 = 71.7\% \times 19.3 = 13.8$ vol. % Estimated systemic A–V O_2 = (Ao – MV) × capacity $= (97 - 71.7) \times 19.3 = 4.9$ vol. %

*Lexington Instruments Corp., 241 Crescent St., Waltham, Mass.

Table 4. Cardiac catheterization measurements—examples based on data in Figs. 3 and 9

1. Flow

    A. Pulmonary blood flow (PBF, Qp)

        Formula:
        (direct
        Fick)

$$PBF = \frac{O_2 \text{ consumption}}{\text{pulmonary A} - \text{V O}_2} = \frac{O_2 \text{ consumption}}{\text{P.V.} - \text{P.A. content}}$$

        Example:
        (Fig. 3)

$$PBF = \frac{197 \text{ ml./min.}}{18.3 - 16.7 \text{ vol.\%} \times 10^*} = 12.3 \text{ L/min.}$$

    B. Pulmonary/systemic flow ratio (PBF/SBF, Qp/Qs)

        Formula:

$$\frac{PBF}{SBF} = \frac{\dfrac{O_2 \text{ consumption}}{\text{pulmonary A} - \text{V O}_2}}{\dfrac{O_2 \text{ consumption}}{\text{systemic A} - \text{V O}_2}} = \frac{\text{systemic A} - \text{V O}_2}{\text{pulmonary A} - \text{V O}_2} = \frac{\text{Ao} - \text{M.V. sat.}}{\text{PV} - \text{P.A. sat.}}$$

        Example:
        (Fig. 3)

$$\frac{PBF}{SBF} = \frac{97 - 71.7}{97 - 88} = \frac{2.8}{1}$$

    C. Systemic blood flow (SBF, Qs)**
        alternate method based on known PBF and PBF/SBF ratio

        Formula:

$$SBF = \frac{1}{PBF/SBF} \times PBF \text{ (direct Fick)}$$

        Example:

$$SBF = \frac{1}{2.8/1} \times 12.3 = 4.4 \text{ L/min.}$$

    D. Systemic blood flow (SBF, Qs)

        Formula:
        (indirect
        Fick)

$$SBF = \frac{O_2 \text{ consumption}}{\text{systemic A} - \text{V O}_2} = \frac{O_2 \text{ consumption}}{\text{Ao} - \text{M.V. content}}$$

$$\text{M.V. content} = \frac{2 \times IVC + SVC}{3} \times \text{ capacity}$$

        Example:
        (Fig. 3)

$$\text{Ao content} = 97\% \times 19.3 = 18.7 \text{ vol.\%}$$

$$\text{M.V. content} = \frac{2 \times 76\% + 63\%}{3} \times 19.3 = 71.7\% \times 19.3 = 13.8 \text{ vol.\%}$$

$$SBF = \frac{197 \text{ ml./min.}}{18.7 - 13.8 \text{ vol.\%} \times 10^*} = 4.02 \text{ L/min.}$$

2. Shunts

    A. L−R = PBF − SBF
        Example: L−R = 12.3 − 4.4 = 7.9 L/min.
        (from 1 A & C)

    B. Percent L−R = $\dfrac{\text{L−R}}{PBF}$

        Example: % L−R = $\dfrac{7.9}{12.3}$ = 64%
        (From 1A and 2A)

Table 4. *Continued*

C. R−L = SBF − PBF

      Example:
      (Fig. 9)

$$SBF = \frac{220 \text{ ml./min}}{(27.8 - 25.6 \text{ vol.}\%) \times 10} = 10 \text{ L/min.}$$

$$\frac{PBF}{SBF} = \frac{Ao - M.V. \text{ sat.}}{P.V. - P.A. \text{ sat.}} = \frac{82 - 76}{97 - 76} = \frac{1}{3.5}$$

$$PBF = PBF/SBF \quad \times \quad SBF = \frac{1}{3.5} \times 10$$

$$= 2.9 \text{ L/min.}$$

$$R-L = SBF - PBF = 10 - 2.9 = 7.1 \text{ L/min.}$$

D. Percent R−L shunt $= \dfrac{R-L}{SBF}$

      Example:
      (from 2A)
$$\%R-L = \frac{7.1}{10} = 71\%$$

3. Resistance

A. Systemic vascular resistance (SVR) $= \dfrac{\text{Mean Ao pressure} - \text{mean RA pressure}}{\text{SBF (L/min.)}}$

      Example:
      (Fig. 3)
$$SVR = \frac{83 - 4}{4.4\dagger} = 18.0 \text{ units}$$

B. Pulmonary vascular resistance (PVR) $= \dfrac{\text{mean PA pressure} - \text{mean LA pressure}}{\text{PBF (L/min.)}}$

      Example:
      (Fig. 3)
$$PVR = \frac{21 - 4}{12.3} = 1.4 \text{ units}$$

C. Total pulmonary resistance (TPR) $= \dfrac{\text{mean PA pressure}}{\text{PBF (L/min.)}}$

      Example:
      (Fig. 3)
$$TPR = \frac{21}{12.3} = 1.7 \text{ units}$$

D. Resistance (units) $\times$ 80 = resistance (dynes sec. cm.$^{-5}$)

      Example: SVR = 18 units $\times$ 80 = 1440 dynes sec. cm.$^{-5}$

4. Valve area (Gorlin)

A. Aortic or pulmonic

    Valve flow (VF) $= \dfrac{\text{C.O. (ml./min.)}}{\text{systolic ejection period (SEP)}}$

    SEP (sec./min.) = systolic time $\dfrac{\text{sec.}}{\text{beat}} \times$ hr. $\left(\dfrac{\text{beat}}{\text{min.}}\right)$

    Valve area (VA) $= \dfrac{\text{VF (ml./sec.)}}{44.5 \sqrt{\text{mean valvular gradient}}}$

Table 4. *Continued*

Example: aortic stenosis (Fig. 4)
Left ventricular pressure (4a)
SEP   = 0.27 sec. × 100 beats/min.

= 27 sec./min.

$$AVF = \frac{5500 \text{ ml./min.}}{27 \text{ sec./min.}}$$

= 204 ml./sec.

$$AVA = \frac{204}{44.5 \sqrt{114}}$$

= 0.43 cm.^{2}

Aortic pressure (Fig. 4b)
SEP   = 0.27 sec. × 100 beats/min.

= 27 sec./min.

$$AVF = \frac{5500 \text{ ml./min.}}{27 \text{ sec./min.}}$$

= 203 ml./sec.

$$AVA = \frac{203}{44.5 \sqrt{75}}$$

= 0.53 cm.^{2}
Average AVA = 0.48 cm.^{2}

B. Mitral

$$\text{Mitral valve flow (MVF)} = \frac{\text{C.O. (ml./min.)}}{\text{diastolic filling period (DFP)}}$$

$$\text{DFP (sec./min.)} = \text{diastolic time } \frac{\text{sec.}}{\text{beat}} \times \text{hr. } \left(\frac{\text{beat}}{\text{min.}}\right)$$

$$\text{Mitral valve area (MVA)} = \frac{\text{MVF (ml./sec.)}}{37.9 \sqrt{\text{mean MV gradient}}}$$

---

*vol.% × 10 = ml./L, permits calculation of flow in L/min.

**We utilize this method to calculate SBF in the presence of a L−R shunt, since the PBF is accurately measured by direct Fick method, and the PBF/SBF ratio is based on a single technique (oximetry). It is therefore preferable to converting % saturation to O_2 content for calculation of SBF (indirect Fick, see part 1D of this table.

†See part 1C of this table.

oxygen difference can lead to large errors in flow calculations. Another disadvantage of the Fick method is that steady-state conditions are necessary for the 3-minute measurement period.

Indicator dilution curves require the rapid injection of a known quantity of indicator into the central circulation. Dilution is then measured from the time-concentration curve at a site downstream with one or more intervening "mixing chambers" (ventricles) interposed. Thermodilution curves are not distorted by recirculation, and are therefore ideal for rapid calculation by dedicated minicomputers interfaced with the measuring thermistor. Indocyanine green dye recirculates and thus distorts the downslope of the time density curve recorded from the densitometer. Since flow calculations require the measurement of dilution in a single passage through the circulation, a semilogarithmic replotting of the nonexponential terminal portion of the downslope is required for calculation. Although dedicated minicomputers can perform this task with reasonable accuracy, manual processing requires only a few minutes. The inscription of indicator dilution curves requires less than 30 seconds of steady-state conditions, and as a result, dye curves are more readily used in the measurement of responses to interventions (e.g., exercise) than the Fick method. In low flow states or in large volume hearts (e.g., incompetent valves), the long, low dye curves may lead to significant error in calculation of cardiac output.

Pressure-Flow Relationships

Simultaneous measurement of pressure and flow permits calculation of *resistance* across a vascular bed or estimation of *valve area* in a stenotic valve, both of which may be of prime importance in evaluation of a patient with CHD.

Resistance is the pressure drop across a vascular bed divided by the flow (Table 4) and is a crucial determinant of operative risk. The "reactivity" or ability to decrease the elevated pulmonary vascular resistance in response to pulmonary vasodilators (oxygen, tolazoline, isoproterenol, etc.) is an essential measurement if operation is contemplated in a patient with pulmonary hypertension.

In our experience a pulmonary vascular resistance that cannot be lowered to less than 5 units (400 dyne sec. cm.$^{-5}$) precludes a successful operation for closure of a shunt in an adult, since significant pulmonary hypertension usually persists. It should be mentioned that patients with "fixed" elevated pulmonary vascular resistance cannot tolerate profound decreases in systemic pressure or venous return in response to potent vasodilators; so extreme caution and systemic arterial pressure monitoring should be employed when studying patients with pulmonary hypertension.

We report resistance in Woods units (*m*), expressed in mm. Hg/L./min. Wood units carry the same information content as the more formal dyne sec. cm.$^{-5}$ units, which are derived merely by multiplying Wood units by 80 (Table 4).

Valve area calculations using the Gorlin formula (Table 4) require simultaneous or closely sequential measurement of transvalvular gradients and flow (Fig. 4). It should be noted that the transvalvular gradient increases as the square of a flow increase, so that doubling the flow can increase a gradient fourfold. Because pressure gradients are extremely dependent on flow, a patient with pulmonic or aortic stenosis should be evaluated under normal conditions as well as during exercise. A heavily sedated patient may generate a seemingly insignificant gradient if the cardiac output is depressed.

Occasionally, a patient with aortic stenosis will have significant systemic hypertension (e.g. aortic systolic pressure > 150 mm. Hg), and this apparent increase in systemic vascular resistance may modify the magnitude of the transvalvular gradient. We prefer to repeat gradient and flow measurements after decreasing systemic resistance with a vasodilator (e.g., sodium nitroprusside) in hypertensive patients with aortic stenosis.

Detection, Localization and Quantification of Shunts

Shunts may be detected by several methods and the investigator should be familiar with the usefulness and limitations of each. Since it is imperative to define both the recipient site and the site of origin, it may be necessary to employ more than one method of shunt detection.

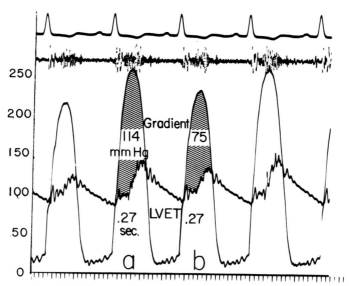

Figure 4. Left ventricular and aortic pressure in a patient with severe valvular aortic stenosis. These pressure data form the basis for the calculations of valve area in Table 4. Pulsus alternans is exhibited, so that the pressure gradient is 114 and 75 mm. Hg on the large and small beats, respectively. The left ventricular ejection time is 0.27 second (time lines = 0.04 second).

LEFT-TO-RIGHT (L-R) SHUNTS

Hydrogen Curves. Hydrogen gas (H_2) inhalation is the most sensitive way of detecting a L-R shunt. This indicator substance is injected into the pulmonary veins by inhalation and the appearance time is detected by a platinum-tipped electrode placed in the bloodstream. In practice, an electrode catheter is passed to the pulmonary artery to determine if a shunt is present at any proximal site. In our laboratory, saline saturated with hydrogen gas is initially injected through the electrode catheter to test its ability to detect hydrogen. If the electrode is responsive, the patient may then inhale a single breath of H_2 through a bag mask. If there is a L-R shunt, an electrode downstream from the recipient site will detect a change in potential in less than 5 seconds. The resulting deflection resembles a qualitative indicator dilution curve (Fig. 5).

If no L-R shunt is present, the indicator passes through the left side of the heart and systemic circulation before returning to the right side of the heart, and a low amplitude deflection is recorded from the electrode after 5 to 15 seconds (Fig. 6, R.A.).

If hydrogen is detected in less than 5 seconds following delivery of H_2 (the onset can be marked manually or detected by a moistened platinum electrode placed in a nostril), serial H_2 curves are recorded as the electrode is withdrawn to more proximal chambers in the right heart. The site immediately proximal to the recipient site of the shunt is indicated by a delayed appearance time. Triple electrode catheters are available* which permit simultaneous recording of the appearance time in three chambers (e.g., PA, RV, and RA) (Fig. 6).

There are potential hazards in using the hydrogen technique. Hydrogen is explosive if ignited, particularly when mixed with oxygen. Small quantities in a suitably ventilated room with well-grounded electrical equipment are therefore advisable. We prefer to use a lecture bottle or small tank as a reservoir, transferring only a small quantity to the bag mask immediately before use. In addition, intra-cardiac electrodes, if improperly

---

*Levy Triple Electrode Catheter manufactured by U.S.C.I., a division of C.R. Bard, Inc., Billerica, Mass.

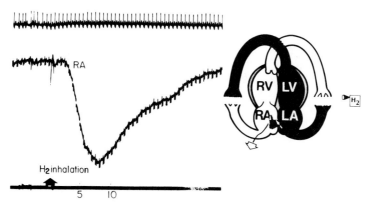

Figure 5. Hydrogen inhalation study in a patient with atrial septal defect. A platinum electrode in the right atrium records the appearance of hydrogen (downward deflection) three seconds after inhalation. The resulting curve resembles an inverted indicator dilution curve. An electrocardiographic signal can be seen superimposed on the tracing from the hydrogen electrode.

grounded, can permit current leakage from the recorder to the patient. In the senior author's 18 years of personal experience with the technique, no mishaps have occurred. Dickerson has established the relative safety of hydrogen as compared with other flammable gases in medical use.

Oximetry. The serial determination of oxygen saturation, content, or partial pressure

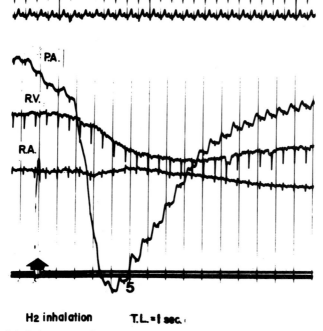

Figure 6. Hydrogen inhalation curves from a tripolar catheter in a patient with patent ductus arteriosus and pulmonic valve regurgitation. Simultaneous recordings from the pulmonary artery, right ventricle, and right atrium reveal an abrupt downward deflection in the pulmonary artery two seconds after inhalation (arrow at bottom left) followed by a more gradual decline in the right ventricular curve. A slow decline of the right atrial curve begins nine seconds after inhalation and represents detection of recirculating hydrogen. The hemodynamic and angiographic studies in this patient revealed a large left-to-right shunt through a patent ductus, mild pulmonary hypertension, and pulmonic valve regurgitation.

187

in the cardiac chambers and great vessels permits detection, localization, and quantitation of shunts. Saturation and content can be readily interconverted (Table 3). The partial pressure (Po_2) can be converted to saturation by use of nomograms based on oxyhemoglobin dissociation curves at the appropriate blood pH.

The recipient site of a shunt is defined as the most proximal chamber in which a significant increase (or step-up) in blood oxygen is detected. Because of the heterogeneity of oxygen content in the unmixed blood entering the right atrium from the venae cavae and coronary sinus, a larger step-up is needed to reliably detect a shunt at atrial level than is needed to detect shunts at downstream sites, where there is better mixing of venous blood. In our laboratory the following thresholds for shunt detection are used:

Presumed Recipient Site of L–R Shunt	Oxygen Step-up Required to Detect Shunt Reliably (content/saturation)
right atrium	1.5 vol.%/7.5%
right ventricle	1.0 vol.%/5%
pulmonary artery	0.5 vol.%/3%

In practice, the significance of small or equivocal step-ups in oxygen content is best confirmed by other methods of shunt detection (hydrogen inhalation, angiography, or selective dye curves).

Quantitation of left-to-right shunts is estimated from oximetry data. The Fick principle is used to measure the pulmonary blood flow directly, and the systemic blood flow and shunt flows are derived from oximetry as shown in Table 4.

Since the Fick principle is based on steady state conditions and representative sampling from known locations, sequential samples for shunt determination should be taken by strict protocol rather than by random acquisition in order to minimize errors. In our laboratory, oximetry blood samples are obtained immediately after collection of data for direct Fick determination of pulmonary blood flow. Samples are taken in rapid sequence under steady-state conditions. To minimize time delays and effects of arrhythmias induced by catheter manipulation, samples are taken in the pulmonary artery and right ventricle on *withdrawal*. Samples from venae cavae and right atrium are taken on *withdrawal* from the superior cava (if catheterized from below) or inferior cava (if catheterized from above). The location of each sampling site is documented by fluoroscopy and pressure monitoring, and sampling from transitional or questionable sites is avoided. For example, between right atrial samples the catheter should be withdrawn along the lateral atrial wall but not advanced; this avoids inadvertently entering an atrial septal defect, pulmonary vein, or coronary sinus ostium. Inferior vena caval samples should not be taken from hepatic veins.

If the patient's status changes during sequential sampling (i.e., tachycardia, anxiety, O_2 administration), the entire oximetry sequence is repeated as soon as steady-state conditions are achieved.

Indocyanine Green Dye Dilution Technique. Indocyanine green dye can be used both to detect and to localize shunts. Quantitation of shunt size from dye curves has been attempted by various investigators, but unless rigorous criteria are met (i.e., thorough mixing of the indicator before its passage through a shunt) the calculations are, at best, only rough estimates. Oximetry is more reliable for quantification, indicator dilution curves for detecting and localizing shunts.

Downstream arterial sampling during injection of dye demonstrates a left-to-right shunt by an interruption of the exponential downslope of the primary curve which is caused by early recirculation through the shunt. If the dye injection is made in the right side of the heart, a shunt of 25 percent or more of the pulmonary blood flow will cause a distinct break in the downslope. However, these injections will not demonstrate the site of shunting. Localization of the shunt can be achieved by selectively injecting the left side of the heart. In the case of anomalous pulmonary venous connection, selective pulmonary arterial or pulmonary venous injections are made with downstream sampling. If the injection is made distal to the origin of the shunt, the curve will be monophasic and have a normal downslope. An intracardiac shunt can then be localized as coming from the most distal chamber from which an early recirculation break occurs (Fig. 7).

There are, however, several potential pitfalls with the downstream sampling method. If there is valvular incompetence involving the chamber containing the shunt (e.g., mitral regurgitation and atrial septal defect), an injection in the downstream chamber (the left ventricle) will reflux dye into the left atrium. The resulting dye curve will simulate that of a ventricular septal defect. Similarly, a left ventricular dye curve from a left ventricular to right atrial shunt will be indistinguishable from that of a ventricular septal defect (Fig. 8).

Upstream sampling from a right-sided cardiac chamber, with injection in the left side of the heart, permits the most precise localization of left-to-right shunts with dye curves. This technique is particularly useful in localizing shunts from the systemic circulation into the right-sided cardiac chambers, or documenting left ventricular to right atrial shunts (Fig. 8).

Angiography. Although high quality angiocardiography or cineangiocardiography will permit precise anatomical shunt localization and an estimate of shunt size, we precede contrast medium injections with at least one other form of shunt detection to help select angiographic injection sites and obviate unnecessary injections.

RIGHT-TO-LEFT (R–L) SHUNTS

Oximetry. The presence of significant desaturation of systemic arterial blood (≥ 94

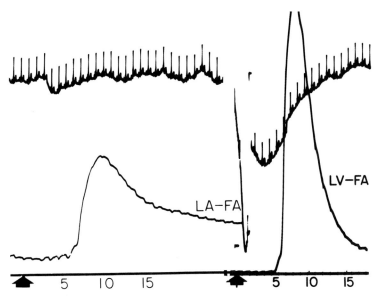

Figure 7. Indicator dilution curves in atrial septal defect (Case 1). Indocyanine green dye has been injected into the left atrium (LA) and left ventricle (LV) while the density of the blood withdrawn from the femoral artery (FA) is continuously recorded. A left atrial curve displays a break in the exponential downslope which is not seen on the left ventricular curve; thus, a left-to-right shunt is demonstrated at atrial level which is not present at ventricular level and the presence of an atrial septal defect is confirmed.

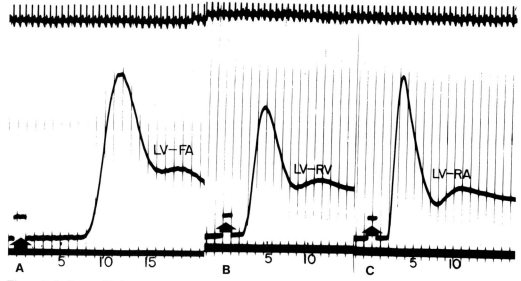

Figure 8. Indicator dilution curves in left ventricular to right atrial shunt. A, The curve recorded from a left ventricular (LV) injection reveals a break on the downslope indicating a left-to-right shunt at or beyond the left ventricle, compatible with a ventricular septal defect, left ventricular to right atrial shunt, patent ductus, etc. Repeat injections with sampling from the right side of the heart define the origin and recipient sites of the shunt. FA = femoral artery. B, Left ventricular injection with right ventricular (RV) sampling through a densitometer demonstrates a break on the downslope, compatible with a shunt at or proximal to the right ventricle. C, A repeat injection in the left ventricle, with right atrial (RA) sampling indicates a shunt at or proximal to the right atrium. Cineangiographic studies demonstrated a left ventricular right atrial shunt (Fig. 13C).

percent saturation) suggests the presence of a right-to-left shunt, and if serial samples can be obtained from the pulmonary veins, left atrium, left ventricle, and aorta, the site of "step-down" will localize the site of shunt. The method of quantitation of right-to-left shunts is demonstrated in Table 4 and Figure 9. Since oximetry is relatively insensitive to small shunts, and because access to these left-sided cardiac structures is not always possible or justifiable in a given patient, dye dilution curves are more widely utilized for confirmation and localization of R–L shunts.

Indocyanine Green Dye Dilution Technique. Selective injections into the right side of the heart with downstream sampling in a peripheral artery confirms the presence of very small shunts and permits their precise localization (Fig. 10). Injection into a right-sided cardiac chamber proximal to a shunt will cause earlier appearance of indicator at the sampling site than an injection downstream from the shunt site. In our laboratory an inferior caval injection is chosen as the first "screening" dye curve when a R–L shunt is suspected, since it is upstream to any potential right-sided cardiac shunting site and it is more likely to traverse an atrial septal defect or patent foramen ovale than a superior caval injection. Occasionally, an injection after the patient releases a sustained Valsalva maneuver will permit detection of a potential interatrial communication as systemic venous return momentarily exceeds pulmonary return.

Angiographic Technique. Although angiography may permit direct visualization of a right-to-left shunt, cumulatively deleterious doses of contrast medium are not justified for the purpose of ruling in or out the presence of a shunt. Furthermore, rapid injections of large volumes of contrast medium may cause spurious shunting. Therefore, angiography is not employed as a primary method of shunt detection in our laboratory.

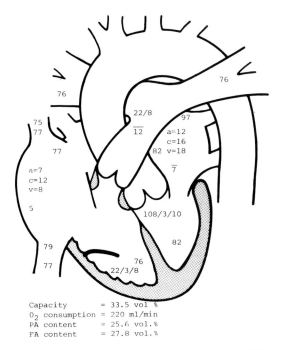

```
Capacity        = 33.5 vol %
O₂ consumption  = 220 ml/min
PA content      = 25.6 vol.%
FA content      = 27.8 vol.%
```

Figure 9. Pressure and oximetry data in a patient with Ebstein's anomaly of the tricuspid valve. These data provide the basis for the calculations in Table 4 (body surface area = 1.63 M²).

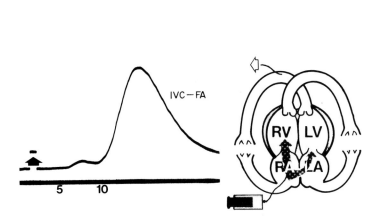

Figure 10. Indicator dilution curve in right-to-left shunt. Indocyanine green dye is injected into the inferior vena cava (IVC) in a patient with valvular pulmonic stenosis and a patent foramen ovale. An early appearance of dye, 6 seconds after injection, confirms the presence of a right-to-left shunt. A curve from the left atrium (not shown) revealed no break in the downslope, indicating only a right-to-left shunt at atrial level. FA = femoral artery.

191

Electrophysiologic Recording

Recording of electrical signals from intracardiac sites can be performed relatively rapidly, and can enhance the diagnostic potential of cardiac catheterization. We have obtained intracardiac electrocardiograms using a catheter electrode as an exploring lead (V lead) in conjunction with blood samples and pressure recordings from "unknown" ventricular sites in patients with complex forms of congenital heart disease. For example, in catheterizing a cyanotic patient who might have transposition complexes, common ventricle, or double outlet right ventricle, the pressure is the same at all ventricular sites and it may not be clear from which ventricle the oximetry samples and pressure recordings have been obtained. In such cases we record an intracardiac electrocardiogram and pressure recording immediately before each oximetric sample so that the ventricle can be more accurately characterized.

If normal conduction is present, the initial septal depolarization is toward the right ventricle: an "rS" complex is recorded in the right ventricle and a "qS" in the left. Although these conduction patterns may be altered somewhat unpredictably in transposition and common ventricle complexes, the morphology of the intracardiac electrocardiogram serves as a "signature" for a specific site and permits correct grouping of samples (Fig. 11).

In a complex cyanotic condition it is not unusual to enter a region with ventricular pressure antegrade through one or both atrioventricular valves and retrograde from the aortic valve, and the portal of entry does not necessarily establish the identity of the chamber entered. For example, a catheter passed retrograde through the aortic valve may enter either ventricle in tetralogy of Fallot and Eisenmenger's complex, and catheters may move freely among all 4 chambers in patients with A-V cushion defects.

His Bundle Electrogram. Conduction abnormalities and rhythm disturbances can be further evaluated by study of the specialized cardiac conduction system. His bundle recordings use a bipolar or tripolar pacing catheter passed percutaneously through the right femoral vein and advanced across the tricuspid valve, so that the tip lies in the right ventricle (Fig. 12). The normal values are summarized in Table 5.

Angiography–Cineangiography

Contrast angiography can establish a definitive anatomical diagnosis if performed expertly. The selection of optimal injection sites and radiographic projections usually requires a thorough knowledge of the clinical and hemodynamic findings, so we defer angiographic injections until all pressures, flows, and shunt determinations have been made.

Biplane angiographic equipment records more information per injection of contrast medium than single plane apparatus, a feature that is particularly important in complex forms of CHD. However, many laboratories do not have biplane equipment and therefore require considerable planning to record from each injection the maximum amount of information.

In most laboratories cineangiography has supplanted serial film angiography because of its convenience and greater potential for recording moving structures. However, the reduced image-intensifier-field size (maximum 9- to 10-in. diameter) limits diagnostic accuracy in some instances. We employ serial film angiograms when the entire pulmonary arterial tree or major systemic-pulmonary vascular channels must be demonstrated for operative repair (as in suspected truncus).

Choice of Injection Site. Contrast medium is injected into the chamber which will best demonstrate a particular lesion (Tables 6 and 7). It is important to be cognizant of

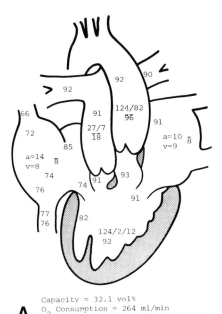

Capacity = 32.1 vol%
O_2 Consumption = 264 ml/min

A

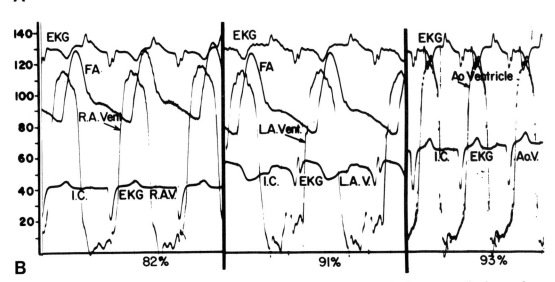

B

Figure 11. The use of intracardiac electrocardiography in localizing the site of oximetry sampling in complex congenital heart disease. A, Data from a patient with common ventricle, transposition of the great vessels, and pulmonic stenosis underwent cardiac catheterization; B, The intracardiac electrocardiogram (I.C. EKG) from three areas in the ventricle, all of which had nearly identical pressures but different oxygen saturations and different intracardiac electrocardiographic complexes. The ventricle entered via the right atrium (R.A.V.) demonstrates a QS intracardiac electrocardiogram, and the sample from that area had an 82 percent saturation. The ventricle entered from the left atrium (L.A.V.) demonstrates a QRS intracardiac electrocar-diogram, and the blood had a saturation of 91 percent. A retrograde catheter passed into the ventricle (Ao.V.) demonstrated a QS intracardiac electrocardiogram and a 93 percent oximetry saturation. These electrocar-diograms aided in characterizing these zones in the ventricle from which samples were taken, since the pressures were identical in all three areas.

193

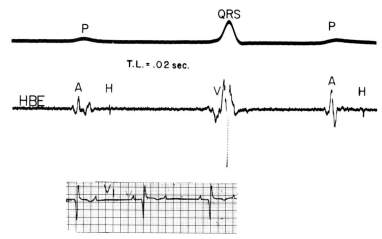

Figure 12. A His bundle electrogram (HBE) in a patient who acquired complete heart block 16 years after closure of a ventricular septal defect demonstrates a conduction time of 130 msec. between the atrium (A) and His spike (H). There was no relationship between the His spike and the ventricular complex (V). The origin of the ventricular rhythm is, therefore, in the ventricle or bundle branch. Inset at bottom shows a lead V₁ electrocardiogram.

frequently associated lesions so that complete anatomical information is provided and a secondary site can be chosen if necessary.

Primary Lesion	Frequently Associated Lesion	Secondary Injection Site
ASD, secundum type	mitral valve prolapse	left ventricle
ASD, primum type	mitral valve deformity with cleft and regurgitation; ventricular septal defect	left ventricle
coarctation of aorta	bicuspid aortic valve	aortic root

The primary lesion is often well characterized by the catheterization study. For example, in studying a patient with atrial septal defect the site and magnitude of shunt are established. Therefore, we frequently perform our first angiographic injection in the *left ventricle* to visualize the mitral valve and rule out a possible left ventricular to right atrial communication or unsuspected partial cushion defect (Fig. 13).

CHOICE OF PROJECTION. Tables 6 and 7 summarize injection sites and projections used in our laboratory to demonstrate congenital cardiac lesions, and Figure 14 diagrammatically depicts the cardiac chambers in the standard projections.

With rare exceptions, we favor the *oblique* projections over the frontal and lateral views. The heart is obliquely oriented in the thorax and optimal display of anatomical features is obtained when projections are selected which effect separation of overlapping structures. The frontal and lateral projections overlap the various chambers; in addition, the frontal projection superimposes the spine on the central axis of the heart. This obscures key features and adds undesirable radiographic problems, such as scatter, and prevents optimal radiographic conditions for angiography.

Several forms of CHD present unusual anatomical planes of chamber separation which are *not* well defined in the oblique projections. When we encounter or suspect such a case, we *do* employ the frontal and lateral projections because of the reproducibility of these standard projections. Included in this category are *l*-transposition complexes such as corrected transposition of the great vessels and complex dextrocar-

Table 5. Normal values and pressures

Normal values	
O_2 consumption (VO_2)	$110 - 150$/ml./min./ M^2
Pulmonary A–V O_2 difference	$3.5 - 4.7$ vol. %
Systemic A–V O_2 difference	$3.5 - 4.7$ vol. %
Systemic O_2 saturation	$\geqslant 94\%$
Cardiac index (C.I.)	$2.5 - 4.0$ L/min./ M^2
Systemic vascular resistance (SVR)	$8.0 - 15.0$ units
Pulmonary vascular resistance (PVR)	$0.2 - 1.2$ units
Total pulmonary resistance (TPR)	$1.0 - 3.0$ units
Aortic valve area (AVA)	$2.6 - 3.5$ cm.^{2}
Mitral valve area (MVA)	$4.0 - 6.0$ cm.^{2}
LV end-diastolic volume	< 90 ml./ M^2
Ejection fraction	$55 - 70\%$
His bundle electrogram	
A–H interval	$60 - 115$ msec.
H–V interval	$35 - 55$ msec.
Normal pressures (mm. Hg)	
Right atrium (RA), mean	$1 - 8$
Right ventricle (RV) systolic	$15 - 28$
End-diastolic (RVEDP)	$0 - 8$
Pulmonary artery (PA)	
Systolic	$15 - 28$
Diastolic	$5 - 16$
Mean	$10 - 22$
Pulmonary artery wedge (PAW)	
Mean	$4 - 12$
Left atrium (LA)	
Mean	$4 - 12$
Left ventricle (LV)	
Systolic	$85 - 150$
End-diastolic (LVEDP)	$4 - 12$
Aortic (AO)	
Systolic	$85 - 150$
Diastolic	$60 - 90$
Mean	$70 - 105$

dias. We also employ the frontal projection to define discrete subvalvular aortic stenosis because the septal plane in the region of the lesion is less foreshortened; an axial tilt left anterior oblique (LAO) projection, when possible, also defines the lesion well (Fig. 14).

The amount of contrast medium injected should provide adequate opacification for diagnostic purposes, but a total dose should not exceed 2.5 to 3.0 ml./kg. during the catheterization study. If an injection is made into a normal-sized chamber with neither valvular regurgitation or shunt, an injection of 0.5 to 0.8 ml./kg. in 2 to 3 seconds will usually provide adequate opacification. If an atrial septal defect is present, we inject 0.5 ml./kg. into the left ventricle. On the other hand, a left atrial injection in a patient with atrial septal defect will opacify all 4 chambers within 1 to 2 cardiac cycles, and an injection of 1 to 1.5 ml./kg. is required to produce films of diagnostic quality. A suspected ventricular septal defect with aortic regurgitation also requires a large aortic injection (1 to 1.5 ml./kg.) for adequate visualization. To opacify an anomalously draining pulmonary or systemic vein, we prefer automatic (power) injections of 10 to 15 ml. in 1 to 2 seconds because the rate of blood flow will dilute the opacity of a slower manual

Table 6. Cineangiography in acyanotic congenital heart disease

Type	Injection Site	Projection
1. Aortic stenosis		
Supravalvular	Left ventricle	RAO
	Aortic root	LAO
Valvular	Left ventricle	RAO
	Aortic root	LAO
Subvalvular	Left ventricle	Frontal or LAO—axial tilt
	Aortic root	LAO
2. Hypertrophic cardiomyopathy (IHSS)	Left ventricle	RAO
		LAO—axial tilt
3. Coarctation of aorta	Aortic root or arch	LAO
4. Pulmonic stenosis		
Supravalvular	Pulmonary artery	Frontal—axial tilt
Valvular	Right ventricle	RAO, LAO
Subvalvular	Right ventricle	RAO, LAO
5. Ventricular septal defect		
Supracristal	Left ventricle	Frontal or RAO
Others	Left ventricle	LAO
6. Atrial septal defect		
Ostium Primum	Left ventricle	RAO, LAO
Secundum	Left atrium	30-degree LAO
	Left ventricle	LAO or RAO
7. Patent ductus arteriosus	Aortic arch	LAO

RAO = right anterior oblique; LAO = left anterior oblique and is equivalent to 45 to 60 degrees unless otherwise indicated; axial tilt = (angle view) elevation of head 30 degrees.

Table 7. Cineangiography in cyanotic congenital heart disease

Type	Injection Site	Projection
1. Tetralogy of Fallot	Right ventricle	15-degree RAO
		LAO
2. Ebstein's anomaly	Right ventricle	RAO
	Right atrium	RAO
3. Transposition of great vessels	Venous and arterial ventricles	LAO
4. Truncus arteriosus	Aortic root	Frontal (cut films)
		Left lateral (cut films)
	Selective PA	
5. Double outlet		
Right ventricle	Right ventricle	RAO, LAO
	Left ventricle	Left lateral
6. Anomalous pulmonary venous connection	Right and left pulmonary arteries	Frontal
	Selective pulmonary view	Frontal
7. Tricuspid atresia	Left ventricle	LAO
	Right atrium	Frontal
8. Common atrium	Atrium	
9. Common ventricle	Ventricle	RAO, LAO
10. Eisenmeger's syndrome	Angiography entails high risk to patient; diagnosis and site of shunt best detected by other methods	
11. Dextrocardia	Systemic and pulmonary ventricles, pulmonary artery	Frontal, lateral
12. Other complex congenital defects	Must individualize each case	

RAO = right anterior oblique; LAO = left anterior oblique and is equivalent to 45 to 60 degrees unless otherwise indicated.

196

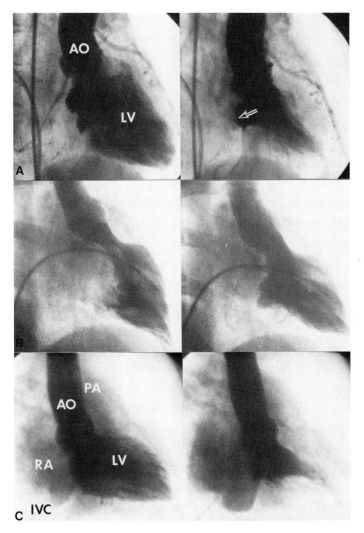

Figure 13. Left ventriculography in three patients with left-to-right shunts at atrial level. A, Ostium secundum atrial septal defect with mitral leaflet prolapse. A right anterior oblique left ventriculogram in early systole (left) and late systole (right) in patient SS (Case #1) demonstrates prolapse of the inferior scallop of the posterior leaflet with trivial mitral regurgitation. B, Right anterior oblique (RAO) left ventriculogram in ostium primum atrial septal defect. Mid-diastolic (left) and mid-systolic (right) frames demonstrate a "gooseneck deformity" of the subaortic region of the left ventricle caused by abnormal placement of the anterior mitral leaflet. Significant mitral regurgitation is seen. C, RAO left ventriculograms in left ventricular to right atrial shunt. Early (left) and late (right) systolic frames in a patient demonstrating reflux into an atrial chamber considerably inferior to the expected location of the left atrium (Fig. 15). A catheter in the inferior vena cava (lower left) can be seen to enter this chamber, which proved to be the right atrium. The dye curves from this patient demonstrated a left ventricular to right atrial communication (Fig. 8).

injection of the same quantity of contrast. Injections into small, low-flow pulmonary vascular beds (e.g., tetralogy of Fallot) require only 10 to 20 ml. in 2 seconds.

The use of angled or axial tilt views for angiography provides better separation or definition of some structures than conventional views. Since many laboratories do not have the necessary angiographic apparatus to achieve all of the "compound" projections (cranial or caudal tilt combined with oblique rotation), some flexibility of

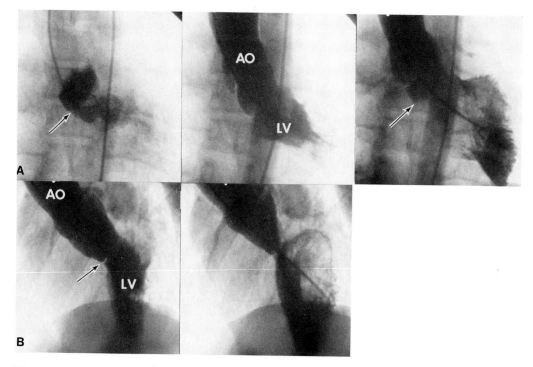

Figure 14. Discrete subvalvular aortic stenosis. A, Frontal left ventriculograms demonstrate a discrete membrane (arrow) best seen at the beginning of the injection (left). B, Axial tilt left anterior oblique angiograms demonstrate the discrete membrane below the aortic valve. The conical narrowing shown in diastole (right) is caused by the forward excursion of the anterior mitral leaflet.

angulation can be achieved by placing a wedge pillow* under the patient. A wedge pillow permits cephalad angulation of the angiographic axis which can be combined with a frontal projection to decrease foreshortening of the pulmonary trunk and its branches; with LAO projections the wedge provides better definition of the ventricular septum (Fig. 15). The disadvantage of angled or axial tilt projections is the superimposition of the diaphragm (and underlying liver) upon cardiac structures; this superimposition tends to increase radiographic scatter and decrease resolution. Therefore, we prefer conventional views and only employ the compound views when a critical anatomical feature is not adequately defined in the conventional view.

The two case summaries which follow illustrate the importance of thorough preparation for the catheterization and highlight pitfalls which may occur if the catheterization procedure is entered into without optimal preparation and experience on the part of the catheterization team.

Case 1

S.S., a 63-year-old woman, claimed that childhood pneumonia caused her to have a deformed heart, but was not told of a heart murmur. During adulthood she had recurrent episodes of pneumonia and bronchitis associated with pleural effusions and intermittent systemic hypertension for 20 years. In 1963 she underwent cardiac catheterization at another hospital because of nonexertional chest pain; the study revealed mild

---

*Grollman Wedge for Arteriography, Stanco Medical, Inc., Goleta, Calif.

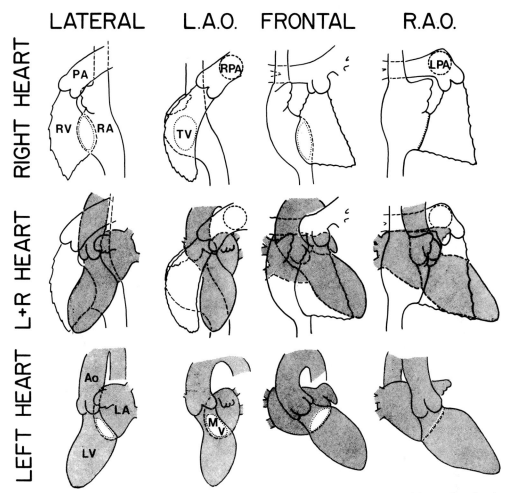

LATERAL   L.A.O.   FRONTAL   R.A.O.

RIGHT HEART

L+R HEART

LEFT HEART

Figure 15. Angiographic projections of the right and left sides of the heart. Diagrams of the cardiac chambers in the right side of the heart (top row) and left side of the heart (bottom row) are shown in lateral, LAO, frontal, and RAO projections. The right- and left-sided cardiac silhouettes are combined in the middle row, and demonstrate the plane of the lower ventricular septum in the LAO projection and the separation of the great vessels in the frontal and RAO projections. The position of the atrioventricular valves are shown by dotted lines. The RAO projection displays the atrioventricular valves on edge, while the LAO projection displays the orifice of the atrioventricular valves.

mitral regurgitation, an unexplained oxygen step-up at the right ventricular level (71 to 82 percent), no mitral gradient, and normal coronary arteries. During the past 2 years she had noted easy fatigability, dyspnea on walking 2 flights of stairs, paroxysmal nocturnal dyspnea, ankle swelling, and orthopnea. She was started on digoxin and diuretics. Six months later she had another episode of "bronchitis." A chest x-ray showed cardiomegaly and pulmonary edema and she was begun on procainamide for an atrial arrhythmia.

On physical examination, blood pressure was 130/90, pulse 96 and regular, and respirations 18 per minute. Fundi showed mild hypertensive changes. The carotids were brisk and the jugular veins were normal. Pectus excavatum was present and there were scattered rales in her lungs. The point of maximal impulse was within the midclavicular line with an apical systolic thrill. S_1 was normal and S_2 was widely and fixedly split. A

199

systolic ejection click and an S $_4$ were present at the left sternal border. A grade 3/6 ejection murmur was heard in the second left intercostal space, and a grade 4/6 harsh, holosystolic murmur was audible at the apex. There was no clubbing, cyanosis or edema. Peripheral pulses were normal.

The electrocardiogram showed sinus rhythm, an axis of 100 degrees, an rSR' V_1 with a duration of 0.11 second, and an RV_6 of 2.5 mv. suggesting left ventricular hypertrophy (Fig. 16). The chest x-ray demonstrated right atrial and ventricular enlargement, dilated pulmonary arteries with increased vascularity, and left pleural scarring. An echocardiogram demonstrated right ventricular enlargement, reduced septal motion, some thickening of the mitral leaflets, and holosystolic, posterior "hammocking" of the mitral leaflets.

This history of recurrent pulmonary infections and increased vascularity on x-ray indicated a probable left-to-right shunt which in association with a murmur of mitral regurgitation, suggested an ostium secundum atrial septal defect with mitral valve prolapse. The approach was to locate and quantitate the shunt, determine pulmonary vascular resistance, and assess the mitral lesion by angiography. The right axis deviation mitigated against an ostium primum defect.

A percutaneous transfemoral venous catheter entered a right superior pulmonary vein (RSPV) on initial entry into the right side of the heart. The oxygen saturation was 92 percent.

PROBLEM #1. Is the catheter in an anomalous pulmonary vein?

Approach. Perform dye curves from the vein and compare with dye appearance time from injection into the right side of the heart (Fig. 17).

Results. Dye appearance times at the femoral artery for the right superior pulmonary vein, inferior vena cava, and right pulmonary artery were 5.0, 7.0, and 6.0 seconds, respectively.

Conclusion. Dye appeared from the right superior pulmonary vein 2 seconds earlier

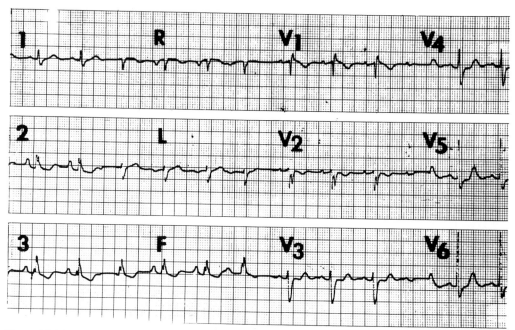

Figure 16. Electrocardiogram from Case #1. A 12-lead electrocardiogram demonstrates right axis deviation, right atrial enlargement, an rSR' in V_1, and voltages in V_6 suggestive of left ventricular hypertrophy.

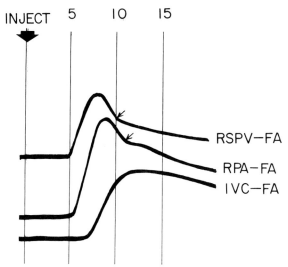

Figure 17. Indicator dilution curves from Case #1. Superimposed dye curves from injections in the right superior pulmonary vein (RSPV), right pulmonary artery (RPA) and inferior vena cava (IVC) with sampling through a densitometer from the femoral artery (FA). The earliest appearance time (5.0 sec.) occurs in the RSPV, followed by the RPA and IVC at 6 and 7 sec. respectively. The arrows indicate the break on the exponential downslope denoting early recirculation. These curves confirm normal drainage from the RSPV into the left atrium, and a left-to-right shunt at or beyond atrial level.

than it did from the inferior vena cava, confirming drainage into the *left* atrium. "Early recirculation" break on downslope confirmed a left-to-right shunt, and later appearance from the inferior vena cava ruled out a right-to-left shunt. The desaturation of the pulmonary venous sample was thought to be the result of torrential pulmonary blood flow.

From its position in the right superior pulmonary vein, the catheter was twisted counterclockwise and then advanced into the left atrium and ventricle, where pressures were recorded and blood samples for oximetry were obtained (Fig. 18 and Table 8). Injections of indocyanine green dye at the left atrium appeared at the femoral artery in 6.0 seconds; dye injected at the left ventricle appeared in 5.0 seconds. There was an earlier break in the downslope of the left atrial curve than the left ventricular curve.

PROBLEM #2. Where is the site of left-to-right shunting?

Approach. Analysis of the dye curves (Figs. 17 and 7).

Conclusion. The normal downslope of the left ventricular curve ruled out a shunt at ventricular level as well as massive mitral regurgitation into the left atrium with atrial shunting. The break on the atrial curve downslope confirmed the atrial origin of the shunt.

The systolic pressures in the left ventricle and aorta (Fig. 19) were mildly elevated, and there were no significant gradients across either the mitral or aortic valve. Withdrawal of the catheter from the left atrium to right atrium revealed distinctly different pressure magnitude and contours (Fig. 20), with a prominent "a" wave and higher mean pressure in the left atrium reflecting the higher end-diastolic pressure in the left ventricle. The different pressures in the atria suggested a "restrictive" atrial septal defect.

Right ventricular and pulmonary arterial systolic pressures were mildly elevated (32 mm. Hg). Oximetry revealed a step-up from 70 percent (mixed vena caval O_2) to between 75 and 77 percent at atrial level; at ventricular lever this increased to between 86 and 87 percent.

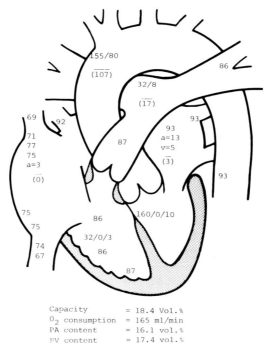

Capacity = 18.4 Vol.%
O$_2$ consumption = 165 ml/min
PA content = 16.1 vol.%
PV content = 17.4 vol.%

Figure 18. Cardiac catheterization data from Case #1. Oximetry valves are denoted by double digit numbers and demonstrate an increase in oxygen saturation at atrial level, with a larger increment at ventricular level. The decreased systemic arterial saturation (93 percent) is apparently caused by low saturation in the pulmonary vein and not by right-to-left shunting. A significant right-to-left shunt was ruled out by indicator dilution curves (Fig. 17A). These data provide the basis for the calculations shown in Table 8 (body surface area = 1.37 M²).

Table 8. Cardiac catheterization data, Case 1 (see Fig. 18)

A. Flow and shunt studies (see Table 4 for formulae)

$$\text{PBF} = \frac{165 \text{ ml./min.}}{(17.4 - 16.1 \text{ vol.\%})10} = 12.7 \text{ L/min.}$$

$$\frac{\text{PBF}}{\text{SBF}} = \frac{93 - 70}{93 - 87} = \frac{3.8}{1}$$

$$\text{SBF} = \frac{1}{3.8/1} \times 12.7 \text{ L/min.} = 3.3 \text{ L/min.}$$

$$\text{L-R} = 12.7 - 3.3 \text{ L/min.} = 9.4 \text{ L/min.}$$

$$\%\text{L-R} = \frac{9.4 \text{ L/min.}}{12.7 \text{ L/min.}} = 74\%$$

B. Resistance

$$\text{SVR} = \frac{107 - 0 \text{ mm. Hg.}}{3.3 \text{ L/min.}} = 32 \text{ units}$$

$$\text{PVR} = \frac{17 - 3 \text{ mm. Hg}}{12.7 \text{ L/min.}} = 1.1 \text{ units}$$

C. LV ejection fraction = 75%

202

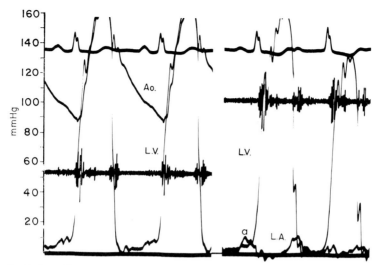

Figure 19. Left-sided cardiac pressures and phonocardiogram (2 LICS) from Case #1. Left ventricular, aortic, and left atrial pressures demonstrate elevated systemic systolic pressure and a prominent "a" wave in the left ventricle. The second complex in the right panel demonstrates a premature atrial contraction, with the "a" wave occurring before mitral valve opening.

PROBLEM #3. Oximetry reveals the major step-up to be at the ventricular level. Is there a ventricular shunt as well?

Approach. Examine dye curves (see Problem #2 of this case).

Conclusion. The possibility of a ventricular septal defect is excluded by the normal downslope of the left ventricular dye curve. "Streaming" of oxygen-rich shunted blood from an atrial defect through the tricuspid valve simulates a "ventricular" oxygen step-up.

Oxygen consumption was normal at rest, and a direct Fick measurement (Table 8) of

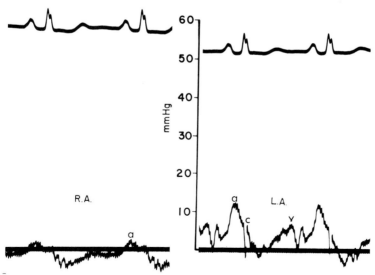

Figure 20. Right and left atrial pressures from Case #1. Pressures in the right and left atria are markedly dissimilar, with prominent "a" waves in the left atrium and a significantly higher pressure throughout the cardiac cycle. These pressures suggest a restrictive atrial septal defect.

203

pulmonary blood flow was 12.7 L/min. There was a 3.8/1 pulmonary/systemic flow ratio. The pulmonary vascular resistance was normal, but the systemic vascular resistance was quite high (32 units).

PROBLEM #4. There is a large (9.4 L/min.) left-to-right shunt despite the apparently restrictive atrial septal defect (suspected because of different atrial pressures). What might be responsible for the large magnitude?

Approach. The direction and magnitude of atrial shunting depends on the size of the atrial septal defect, the differences in compliance of the two ventricles, and any factor that tends to elevate one atrial pressure higher than the other (e.g., valvular stenosis or regurgitation).

Conclusion. Since the left ventricular dye curves had a normal downslope and the "v" waves were not elevated in the left atrium, significant mitral regurgitation is unlikely. Similarly, the lack of a left atrial to left ventricular pressure gradient rules out mitral stenosis. The markedly elevated systemic vascular resistance and the elevated left ventricular end-diastolic pressure (as reflected in the large atrial "a" waves) suggests that reduced left ventricular compliance due to hypertrophy or failure is primarily responsible for the large shunt.

PROBLEM #5. In planning the cineangiographic study, which chambers should be injected and in what order?

Approach. Since two abnormalities of left ventricular function (reduced compliance and failure) and a mitral valve abnormality (possible prolapse) are suspected, and since the presence of a restrictive atrial septal defect is well documented by other means, we studied the *left ventricle* first.

Conclusion. A right anterior oblique (RAO) left ventriculogram was chosen to provide an optimal determination of ejection fraction as well as delineation of the mitral valve.

The left ventricle was small (end-diastolic volume = 90 ml., or 67 ml./M ^{2}) and its ejection fraction was 75 percent. Moderate prolapse of the posterior leaflet was demonstrated, with minor mitral regurgitation into a small left atrium (Fig. 13A). A left atriogram in a 30-degree LAO projection demonstrated a small left atrium with jetting opacification through a 1.5-cm., mid-atrial septal defect (Fig. 21). Coronary arteriograms revealed patent but tortuous coronary arteries.

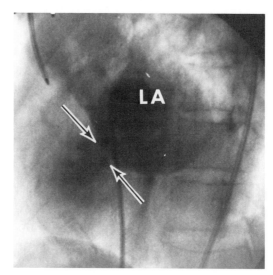

Figure 21. Left atriogram (30-degree LAO) from Case #1. A left atriogram demonstrates a small, rounded left atrium with jetting of contrast medium into the right side of the heart. See Figure 15 for orientation.

DISCUSSION. The catheterization demonstrated an unexpectedly large left-to-right shunt (74 percent) through a small (1.5-cm.) ostium secundum defect, thought to be a result of a hypertrophic, relatively noncompliant left ventricle. The small degree of mitral regurgitation did not appear to be a major contributory factor.

The patient was operated upon and found to have a fenestrated fossa ovalis defect which was closed by sutures. The left atrial pressure was 12 to 15 mm. Hg after closure, and minimal mitral regurgitation was palpated. Her recovery was slow but uneventful. She had a persistent apical systolic murmur but was well 2 years postoperatively. Her blood pressure has remained under good control with antihypertensive therapy.

Case 2

B.Y., a 27-year-old woman, had been followed in several hospitals for cyanotic CHD presumed to be tetralogy of Fallot. Two attempts to perform a Blalock-Taussig anastomosis were unsuccessful: in 1949 a left thoracotomy revealed a right-sided aortic arch and a moderate-size left pulmonary artery, and in 1951 a right thoracotomy demonstrated large bronchial collateral vessels and a small right pulmonary artery. A diagnosis of "pseudotruncus" (pulmonary atresia with ventricular septal defect) was made following cardiac catheterizations in 1959 and 1960. The pulmonary trunk was never entered. During the next 10 years, exertional dyspnea worsened progressively and she markedly restricted her activities. In the past six months she had several episodes of exercise-induced syncope and was considered to be in New York Heart Association Class IV.

She was intensely cyanotic and had severely clubbed fingers and toes. A prominent "a" wave was present in the neck. The lungs were clear. A prominent right ventricular lift was palpated. S $_2$ was single. A grade 3/6 continuous murmur, maximal over the right upper anterior chest wall, was heard over the entire precordium. A grade 3/6 systolic ejection murmur was audible at the second left intercostal space.

The electrocardiogram showed sinus rhythm, right axis deviation, and right ventricular hypertrophy. Chest x-ray revealed a 54 percent cardiothoracic ratio, a straight left cardiac border without a visible main pulmonary artery shadow, and an upwardly tipped cardiac apex. There was a right-sided aortic arch and a prominent right pulmonary artery. The pulmonary vascular markings were slightly increased on the right and slightly decreased on the left. The hematocrit was 60 percent.

She obviously had cyanotic congenital heart disease, probably pseudotruncus arteriosus or severe tetralogy of Fallot with bronchial collateral flow to the lungs. Because of progressive clinical deterioration a repeat study was deemed necessary to clarify the condition of her right ventricular outflow tract, the size of the pulmonary arteries, and the source of pulmonary blood flow.

A percutaneous transfemoral venous catheter easily traversed the atrial septum permitting pressure recording and oximetry sampling from the left sided cardiac chambers. The pressures in the right and left ventricle were identical. The left atrial pressure was 2 mm. Hg higher than right atrial pressure. The pulmonary trunk could not be entered by a conventional catheter, but it was entered with a positive torque control catheter.* The pressure in the pulmonary artery was normal (Fig. 22) but exhibited a slow pressure rise. Repeated, slow catheter withdrawals and insertions revealed an abrupt pressure transition occurring between pulmonary trunk and systemic ventricle; this suggested valvular stenosis with a pressure gradient of 103 mm. Hg.

PROBLEM #1. Do the systemic level of right ventricular pressure, the magnitude of

---

*Positrol, USCI, a division of C.R. Bard, Inc., Bilerica, Mass.

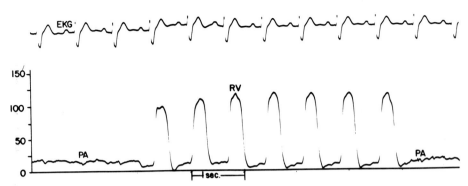

Figure 22. Pulmonary arterial and right ventricular pressures from Case #2 obtained on slow withdrawal and advance of the catheter. There is a pressure gradient of 100 mm. Hg between the right ventricle and pulmonary artery. On slow withdrawal tracings there was no apparent intermediate pressure zone denoting an infundibular chamber. Angiography demonstrated tight valvular pulmonic stenosis and significant infundibular narrowing. Note the "square-topped" pressure contour in the right ventricle as contrasted with the peaked pressures in Figure 2. This "isotonic" pressure configuration is characteristic of the right ventricle in the presence of a ventricular septal defect and pulmonic stenosis, and in contrast to the "isometric" appearance seen with pulmonic stenosis and intact ventricular septum (Fig. 2).

the pressure gradient, and the abrupt pressure transition permit assessment of the severity and anatomical site of outflow tract obstruction?

Approach. In tetralogy of Fallot (as well as pseudotruncus or ventricular septal defect with pulmonic atresia), the ventricular septal defect is sufficiently large to ensure equalization of left and right ventricular pressures; all patients with tetralogy will therefore have systemic pressure in the right ventricle. Similarly, the pulmonary arterial pressure level is usually low to normal (10 to 20 mm. Hg), so that there is very little difference in the magnitude of the outflow tract gradient regardless of the severity of obstruction.

Catheter withdrawals through the outflow tract may provide misleading information regarding the site of obstruction, since a critical valvular stenosis may mask the expected gradient across a proximal area of stenosis. Cardiac movement relative to the catheter tip and side-hole pressure sampling artifacts also can contribute to imprecision in localization and quantitation.

Conclusion. The systemic level of right ventricular pressure and gradient of 103 mm. Hg confirm the presence of significant stenosis, probably at the valvular level. The severity and localization of stenosis should be assessed by alternative methods (angiography and magnitude of right-to-left shunt).

Oximetry (Fig. 23) revealed heterogeneous samples in the right atrium (60 to 73 percent) and ventricle (65 to 70 percent), but no significant oxygen step-up until the pulmonary artery was reached; here a sharp rise to 81 to 84 percent oxygen saturation occurred. Retrograde percutaneous transfemoral arterial catheterization revealed a right aortic arch and a step-down in oxygen saturation in the left ventricle between the inflow portion (97 percent) and outflow tract (80.5 percent), confirming the presence of a right-to-left shunt at ventricular level. Aortic samples were 90 percent.

PROBLEM #2. What is the explanation for the pulmonary arterial oxygen step-up?

Approach. A higher oxygen saturation in the branches than in the proximal pulmonary artery tends to discount a left-to-right shunt at ventricular level.

Conclusion. The peripheral pulmonary arterial oxygen step-up and the continuous murmur suggest an aortic-to-pulmonary communication, either a patent ductus or bronchial arterial collateral circulation.

PROBLEM #3. What cineangiographic injections and projections should be employed to demonstrate the anatomical abnormalities?

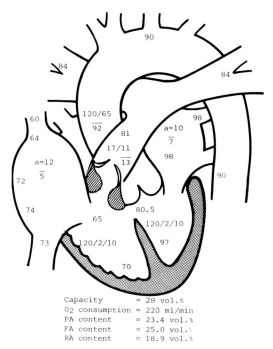

Capacity = 28 vol.%
O₂ consumption = 223 ml/min
PA content = 23.4 vol.%
FA content = 25.0 vol.%
RA content = 18.9 vol.%

Figure 23. Cardiac catheterization data from Case #2. Oximetry values are shown as double digit numbers, and the pressures are recorded in the appropriate chambers. These data provide the values for the calculations in Table 9. There is systemic right ventricular pressure, and a low pulmonary arterial pressure indicating pulmonic stenosis (Fig. 22). There is no apparent left-to-right shunt at atrial or ventricular level, but there is a pronounced step-up in oxygen saturation at the pulmonary arterial level. There is an oxygen step-down at left ventricular level, indicating a right-to-left shunt (body surface area = 1.57 M²).

Approach. The catheterization data suggest tetralogy of Fallot (systemic pressure in right ventricle, pulmonic stenosis, and right-to-left shunt at ventricular level) with an aortopulmonary communication causing a left-to-right shunt into the pulmonary artery. The outflow tract and pulmonary arteries should be visualized, therefore, to assess the prospects for reconstruction. The relative sizes of the two ventricles should be demonstrated and the septal defect visualized. Lastly, angiographic demonstration of systemic-pulmonary communication is important since operative correction would be hampered by persistent shunting while the heart was on bypass unless the shunt is located.

Conclusion. A pulmonary arteriogram (frontal, 21 ml. injection) was obtained before the catheter was withdrawn from the pulmonary trunk. A low dose (0.4 ml./kg.) was selected because of the anticipated low flow in the pulmonary artery and to conserve contrast medium for the upcoming right ventriculograms. Right ventricular injections of 50 ml. (1 ml./kg.) were performed in the right anterior oblique (to delineate the outflow tract) and in the left anterior oblique (to separate the ventricles). An aortic root injection was planned to visualize the site of aortopulmonary communication.

The pulmonary arteriogram demonstrated a small (1-cm. diameter) pulmonary trunk with a domed valve, as well as good opacification and slow washout of the main left pulmonary artery. There was no filling of the main right pulmonary artery.

PROBLEM #4. Why did the right pulmonary artery fail to opacify?

Approach. Unilateral absence of the pulmonary artery can occur in tetralogy of Fallot but it was possible to advance a catheter into the right pulmonary artery and obtain a

Table 9. Cardiac catheterization data, Case 2 (see Fig. 23)

1. Flow and shunt studies (see Tables 3 and 4 for formulae)

$$PBF = \frac{O_2 \text{ consumption}}{(PV - PA \ O_2 \text{ content})10} = \frac{228 \text{ ml./min.}}{(0.98 \times 28 - 0.84 \times 28)10} = 5.8 \text{ L/min.}$$

$$\text{Mixed venous } O_2 = \frac{2 IVC + SVC}{3} = \frac{2(73) + 60}{3} = 69\%$$

$$SBF = \frac{O_2 \text{ consumption}}{(Ao - M.V. \ O_2 \text{ content})10} = \frac{228 \text{ ml./min.}}{(0.90 \times 28 - 0.69 \times 28)10} = 3.9 \text{ L/min.}$$

$$\frac{PBF}{SBF} = \frac{5.8 \text{ L/min.}}{3.9 \text{ L/min.}} = \frac{1.5}{1}$$

$$R-L = PBF \times \frac{(PV - Ao \ O_2 \text{ content}) \ (PA - PV \ O_2 \text{ content})}{(Ao - M.V. \ O_2 \text{ content}) \ (M.V. - PV \ O_2 \text{ content})}$$

$$= 5.8 \times \frac{(0.98 \times 28 - 0.90 \times 28) \ (0.81 \times 28 - 0.98 \times 28)}{(0.90 \times 28 - 0.69 \times 28) \ (0.69 \times 28 - 0.98 \times 28)} = 1.3 \text{ L/min.}$$

$$\%R-L = \frac{R-L}{SBF} = \frac{1.3 \text{ L/min.}}{3.9 \text{ L/min.}} = 33\%$$

$$L-R = PBF \times \frac{M.V. - PA \ O_2 \text{ content}}{M.V. - PV \ O_2 \text{ content}}$$

$$= 5.8 \times \frac{(0.69 \times 28 - 0.81 \times 28)}{(0.69 \times 28 - 0.98 \times 28)} = 2.4 \text{ L/min.}$$

$$\%L-R = \frac{L-R}{PBF} = \frac{2.4 \text{ L/min.}}{5.8 \text{ L/min.}} = 41\%$$

2. Resistance

$$SVR = \frac{92 - 5 \text{ mm. Hg}}{3.9 \text{ L/min.}} = 22.3 \text{ units}$$

$$PVR = \frac{13 - 7 \text{ mm. Hg}}{5.8 \text{ L/min.}} = 1.0 \text{ unit}$$

3. Gradient

RV − PA (peak) = 103 mm. Hg

sample (84 percent) to rule out this possibility. The other possible explanation is competing flow from an aortopulmonary communication into the right lung.

The right ventriculograms demonstrated a domed pulmonic valve, a narrowed (< 1 cm.) infundibular area, and a large ventricular septal defect with an "overriding" and large (4.5-cm.) aorta.

The retrograde catheter was manipulated in the aortic arch in an attempt to enter a patent ductus or a bronchial collateral vessel. The catheter tip hung up in a recess on the right anterior aspect of the descending aorta, and manual injections of contrast medium washed out rapidly into the right pulmonary artery. A power injection (30 ml./2 sec.) faintly opacified a tortuous, dilated (8 to 10 mm.) vessel which coursed diagonally downward and rightward to anastomose with the right pulmonary artery and subsequently the pulmonary trunk and left pulmonary artery.

PROBLEM #5. What is the nature of the aortopulmonary communication?

Approach. The length, course, and tortuosity of the vessel suggested that it was not a patent ductus, but rather, an enlarged bronchial artery which expanded in response to the high flow into the low pressure pulmonary artery. Although the vessel was not well defined by cineangiography in only one plane, more than 3 ml./kg. of contrast medium had been used for angiography, so it was not advisable to perform additional injections.

Conclusion. It was decided to terminate the catheterization study but to do a separate aortic catheterization at another time which would employ large injections and serial film angiography to define the aortopulmonary communication.

Percutaneous transfemoral retrograde catheterization of the aorta was performed at a later date and the region of the aortic arch and proximal descending aorta was explored with a catheter. The previously engaged collateral vessel was the only one found. Injections (30 ml./sec.) were performed in this vessel in frontal (Fig. 24) and lateral projections which demonstrated rapid opacification and washout of a single convoluted bronchial collateral vessel. From this vessel, opacification proceeded first to the right lower lobe pulmonary artery and then to the upper lobe branch, pulmonary trunk, and left main pulmonary artery.

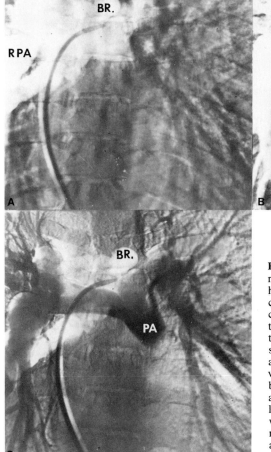

Figure 24. Subtraction films from a bronchial arterial injection (Case #2). A, A retrograde catheter has been placed in the ostium of an enlarged bronchial artery and an injection reveals rapid opacification of a tortuous bronchial collateral vessel and the right pulmonary artery (RPA). B, 1.5 sec. later, the enlarged right pulmonary artery and the smaller pulmonary trunk and left main pulmonary arteries are opacified from the bronchial collateral vessel. C, Superimposed subtraction views of the bronchial collateral vessel (BR) and the pulmonary artery (PA) demonstrate the enlarged bronchial collateral vessel coursing inferiorly and to the right with subsequent opacification of the entire pulmonary arterial tree. This bronchial collateral served as a "Blalock-Taussig" anastomosis for this patient with tight pulmonic stenosis.

209

DISCUSSION. The findings suggest severe tetralogy of Fallot with a large ventricular septal defect, severe pulmonic valvular and infundibular stenosis, and a right-sided aortic arch. The interatrial communication did not lead to a step-up at right atrial level or desaturation of left atrial blood, and therefore represented a patent foramen ovale.

The extracardiac systemic to pulmonary shunt was thought to represent an enlarged bronchial collateral vessel which provided pulmonary blood flow adequate for survival to adulthood, a mechanism analogous to the one effected by a Blalock-Taussig operation.

A repair of her defects was undertaken by utilizing a large bore suction catheter in the left atrium (to control the pulmonary venous return from the bronchial vessel during cardiopulmonary bypass) while the infundibular resection, valvotomy, and septal defect repair were performed. Next, a single large convoluted bronchial artery was ligated near its origin from the aorta.

The patient became acyanotic and has noted a significant improvement in exercise tolerance for over 7 years. Recently, she was catheterized again because of chronic fatigue and frequent respiratory infections, with the following findings:

	Pressure (mm. Hg)	Saturation (%)
Right atrium	a = 14 (mean 10)	72
Right ventricle	40/0/14	72
Pulmonary trunk	35/0/14	72
Right pulmonary artery	27/8 (mean 17)	72
Femoral artery	125/68 (mean 91)	97

Pulmonary vascular resistance was 1.8 units, oxygen consumption was 4.2 L/min., and stroke volume was 68 ml. Cineangiograms of the pulmonary artery and the right ventricle revealed the following: 2 + pulmonic regurgitation and branch stenosis at the origin of the right pulmonary artery; dilated, heavily trabeculated right ventricle with a wide outflow tract and a thickened pulmonic valve which moved poorly. There was 2 + tricuspid regurgitation into a dilated right atrium.

ACKNOWLEDGMENTS

The authors are indebted to Joy Morgridge, who typed the manuscript; Lambert Walker, Maggie Chacon, and Robert Knouse, who assisted with the technical aspects of the cardiac catheterization studies; Paul Cooper, who assisted in preparing the medical illustrations; and Steve Criley, who prepared the photographs.

BIBLIOGRAPHY

BETRIU, A., WIGLE, E. D., FELDENHOF, C. H., ET AL.: *Prolapse of the posterior leaflet of the mitral valve associated with secundum atrial septal defect.* Am. J. Cardiol. 35:363,1975.

BLOOMFIELD, D. A.: *Dye Curves.* University Park Press, Baltimore, 1974.

CASTAÑEDA, A. R., AND ROSENTHAL, A.: *Persistent abnormalities after repair of congenital heart defects.* Adv. Cardiol. 20:110,1977.

CARTER, S. A., BAJEC, D. F., YANNICELLI, E., ET AL.: *Estimation of left-to-right shunts from arterial dilution curves.* J. Lab. Clin. Med. 55:77,1960.

CLARK, L. C., JR., AND BARGERON, L. M., JR.: *Left-to-right shunt detection by an intravascular electrode with hydrogen as an indicator.* Science 130:709,1959.

COHEN, M. V., AND GORLIN, R.: *Modified orifice equation for mitral valve area.* Am. Heart J. 84:839,1972.

CRAIG, R. J., AND SELZER, A.: *Natural history and prognosis of atrial septal defect.* Circulation 37:805,1968.

CRILEY, J. M., AND ROSS, R. S.: *Cardiovascular Physiology.* Tampa Tracings, Oldsmar, Florida, 1971.

DICKERSON, R. B., JENSEN, W. L., JR., AND HOLLISON, R. V.: *The safety of hydrogen in shunt detection.* Circulation 31:705,1965.

ENGLE, M. A.: *Cyanotic congenital heart disease.* Am. J. Cardiol. 37:283,1976.

FELLOWS, K. E., KSAUR, J. F., AND FREED, M. D.: *Angled views in cineangiography of congenital heart disease.* Circulation 56:485,1977.

FRY, D. L.: *Physiologic recording by modern instruments with particular reference to pressure recording.* Physiol. Rev. 40:753,1960.

GENOVESE, B., RONAN, J. A., JR., APPLEFELD, M. D., ET AL.: *Effect of hypertension on the clinical assessment of severity in aortic stenosis.* Circulation 56(Suppl. III):69,1977.

GROSSMAN, W.: *Cardiac Catheterization and Angiography.* Lea and Febiger, Philadelphia, 1976.

GROVER, R. F., REEVES, J. T., AND BLOUNT, S. G., JR.: *Tolazoline hydrochloride (Priscoline): an effective pulmonary vasodilator.* Am. Heart J. 61:5,1961.

HELFANT, R. H., AND SCHERLAG, B. J.: *His Bundle Electrocardiography.* Medcom Press, New York, 1974.

HYMAN, A. L., HYMAN, E. S., QUINOZ, A. C., ET AL.: *Hydrogen platinum electrode system in detection of intravascular shunts.* Am. Heart J. 61:53,1961.

JARMAKANI, J. M.: *Cardiac catheterization.* In Moss, A. J., Adams, F. H., and Emmanouilides, G. C. (eds.): *Heart Disease in Infants, Children, and Adolescents.* Williams and Wilkins, Baltimore, 1977.

KAPLAN, S.: *Long-term results after surgical treatment of congenital heart disease.* Mod. Concepts Cardiovasc. Dis. 46:1,1977.

KROVETZ, L. J., AND GESSNER, I. H.: *A new method utilizing indicator dilution techniques for the estimation of left to right shunts in infants.* Circulation 32:772,1965.

LEACHMAN, R. D., COKKINOS, D. V., AND COOLEY, D. A.: *Association of ostium secundum atrial septal defects with mitral valve prolapse.* Am. J. Cardiol. 38:167,1976.

NADAS, A. S., ELLISON, R. C., AND WEIDMAN, W. H.: *Pulmonary stenosis, aortic stenosis, ventricular septal defect: clinical course and indirect assessment.* Circulation 56 (Suppl. I):1,1977.

NARULA, O. S.: *His Bundle Electrocardiography and Clinical Electrophysiology.* F. A. Davis, Philadelphia, 1975.

NEILL, C. A., AND HAROUTUNIAN, L. M.: *The adolescent and young adult with congenital heart disease.* In Moss, A. J., Adams, F. H., and Emmanouilides, G. (eds.): *Heart Disease in Infants, Children and Adolescents.* Williams and Wilkins, Baltimore, 1977.

PERLOFF, J. K.: *The changing population of congenital heart disease.* Trans. Assoc. Life Ins. Med. Dir. Am. 58:132,1975.

PERRY, L. W., HEMKOFF, L. M., AND FINDLAN, C.: *The prevalence of congenital heart disease in United States college freshmen, 1956–1965.* J. Pediatr. 75:876,1969.

ROWE, G. G., CASTILLO, C. A., MAXWELL, G. M., ET AL.: *Atrial septal defect and the mechanism of shunt.* Am. Heart J. 61:369,1961.

SHAPIRO, G. G., AND KROVETZ, L. J.: *Damped and undamped frequency responses of underdamped catheter manometer systems.* Am. Heart J. 80:226,1970.

SHETTIGAR, V. R., HULTGREN, H. N., SPECTER, M., ET AL.: *Primary pulmonary hypertension. Favorable effect of isoproterenol.* N. Engl. J. Med. 295:1414,1976.

SONNENBLICK, E. H., AND LESCH, M. (eds.): *Symposium: Postoperative congenital heart disease.* Prog. Cardiovasc. Dis. 17 and 18:401,1975.

SWAN, H. J. C., BURCHELL, H. B., AND WOOD, E. H.: *The presence of venoarterial shunts in patients with interatrial communications.* Circulation 10:705,1954.

TAKETA, R. M., SAHN, D. J., SIMON, A. L., ET AL.: *Catheter positions in congenital cardiac malformations.* Circulation 51:749,1975.

VEREL, D., GRAINGER, R. G., AND McMICHAEL, J.: *Clinical angiocardiographic investigations.* In *Cardiac Catheterization and Angiocardiography.* Williams and Wilkins, Baltimore, 1969.

WILSON, M. R., FONTANA, M. E., AND WOOLEY, C. F.: *Routine use of the hydrogen platinum electrode system in shunt detection.* Cathet. Cardiovasc. Diagn. 1:207,1975.

YANG, S. S., BENTIVOGLIO, L. G., MARANHÃO, V., ET AL.: *From Cardiac Catheterization Data to Hemodynamic Parameters.* F. A. Davis, Philadelphia, 1978.

Prolapsed Mitral Leaflet Syndrome*

J. Michael Criley, M.D., and Joel Heger, M.D.

The prolapsed mitral leaflet syndrome (PMLS) was first identified as a clinical pathologic entity in the mid 1960s[1,2] when the characteristic mid-systolic click and late systolic murmur were found to correlate with angiographic demonstrations of billowing of the mitral leaflets into the left atrium and late systolic regurgitation. The auscultatory findings had for over 50 years been ascribed to extracardiac causes,[3] and the symptoms often attributed to neuroses or neurocirculatory asthenia.[4]

Although it is not usually considered a form of congenital heart disease, PMLS has been documented as having familial occurrence[5-7] and is frequently associated with various forms of congenital heart disease (Table 1) as well as with connective tissue disorders.[8,9] PMLS has also been found in association with acquired cardiac disorders—principally rheumatic[5] and ischemic[10] heart disease—a relationship which may be the result of coincidence in some cases and cause-and-effect in others.

Although the condition was initially thought to be relatively rare and benign, the increased recognition of the disorder in seemingly healthy people[11,12] and the documentation of catastrophic complications such as life threatening arrhythmias,[13,14] progressive mitral regurgitation,[15,16] infective endocarditis,[17-19] embolic cerebral vascular accidents,[20] and sudden death,[10,21-25] have catapulted PMLS into the forefront of clinical cardiological interest.

Clinical or laboratory evidence of PMLS has been found in 6 to 20 percent of apparently normal females.[11,12] It has become a condition of considerable medical importance and economic impact, and despite intensive investigative work many questions have been raised about PMLS for which we have no satisfactory answers.

ETIOLOGY

Because PMLS has been linked to an autosomal dominant mode of inheritance in some kindreds,[6,7,18,23,24,26] is found in over one third of patients with ostium secundum atrial septal defects,[27] and has more recently been found in patients with hypertrophic cardiomyopathy[28,29] and Ebstein's anomaly of the tricuspid valve,[30,31] it is in some instances a form of congenital heart disease (Table 1). However, its association with ischemic and rheumatic heart disease (Table 2) and its discovery by left ventriculography in the course of diagnostic studies of patients with chest pain suggests that it can

*The clinical research support for the studies described in this manuscript was provided by the American Heart Association, Greater Los Angeles Affiliate, Investigative Group Support Award 427IG7.

Table 1. Congenital abnormalities
associated with mitral valve prolapse

Ostium secundum atrial septal defect[27]
Hypertrophic cardiomyopathy*[29]
Marfan's syndrome*[8]
Erdheim's medial necrosis*[41]
Ehlers-Danlos syndrome*[9]
Ebstein's anomaly of the tricuspid valve[30, 31]
Turner's syndrome[77]
Wolff-Parkinson-White syndrome*[62]
Corrected transposition of the great vessels[105]

*May also be familial

be acquired, or, alternatively, that chance association can occur between common types of heart disease.

Another confounding factor is the lack of a universally agreed upon standard for the diagnosis of PMLS, and the apparent lack of specificity of laboratory methods. Recent two-dimensional echocardiographic studies have suggested that false positive or "pseudoprolapse"[32] patterns can be recorded in conventional M mode (one dimension) echocardiograms, and a recent angiographic study of 336 consecutive patients—not selected for primary cardiac diagnosis[33]—revealed end-systolic posterior leaflet bulging in 43 percent; only a small percentage of these patients revealed diagnostic changes of PMLS when studied subsequently by echocardiography, but a small subgroup with prior diagnosis of click-murmur syndrome was found to have angiographic and echocardiographic evidence of prolapse. Thus, considerable confusion confronts the clinician who wishes to use objective methods to document the diagnosis of PMLS.

In an attempt to clarify some aspects of the confusion over PMLS, we have classified the disorder into *primary* and *secondary* forms.[34] The term primary is reserved for those patients with the click-murmur syndrome and mitral (and frequently tricuspid)[35-37] leaflet prolapse not associated with other forms of congenital heart disease or connective tissue entities, and preceding the onset of acquired heart disease. This classification is not without its deficiencies, since primary PMLS is frequently associated with abnormalities of the skeletal[26,38-40] and connective tissues,[8,9] and it is not always possible to distinguish causation from coincidence in a given case. However, we believe that the classification has some merit in that PMLS that accompanies the Marfan syndrome, ostium secundum atrial septal defects, or ischemic heart disease has significantly different implications than that occurring as an isolated entity.

In 1965, Read[41] described a symptomatic valvular myxomatous transformation ("the floppy valve syndrome") in nine patients; it involved the mitral valve alone in four, the

Table 2. Acquired conditions reported
to be associated with mitral valve prolapse

Ischemic heart disease[10]
Rheumatic heart disease[5]
  (also post-valvulotomy)
Relapsing polychondritis[106]
Periarteritis[34]
Trauma[2]

mitral and aortic valves in two, and the aortic valve in three. Erdheim's medial necrosis was found in three, and two had ruptured mitral chordae tendineae. The report suggested that these patients had a *forme fruste* of the Marfan syndrome, although none exhibited the characteristic abnormalities of body habitus. The valvular pathology and various musculoskeletal abnormalities in the patients and their close relatives were used as evidence for the *forme fruste* Marfan concept. It is difficult to explain Read's findings of aortic valve involvement in what has been assumed to be PMLS, when the large body of literature about the disease fails to mention aortic valve disease. The current authors believe that Read was indeed describing patients with *forme fruste* Marfan's, or Erdheim's medial necrosis, in the five with aortic valve involvement, while the four with isolated mitral valve disease probably had PMLS, which at the time of his report was not well described as a clinical pathologic entity.

Several clues to the embryological pathology of PMLS are furnished by its frequent association with tricuspid prolapse,[35-37] thoracic skeletal[26,38-40] and dermatoglyphic (fingerprint) abnormalities.[42] A more recent discovery is its association with Ebstein's anomaly of the tricuspid valve.[30,31] The differentiation of the atrioventricular valves, the chondrification and ossification of the vertebral column and thoracic cage, and the appearance of the primordia of the dermal ridges (the volar fetal pads) all occur in the fifth to sixth gestational week.[42] Ebstein's anomaly is thought by Van Mierop[43] to represent an abnormal diverticulation of the right ventricular wall with downward displacement of the tricuspid valve origin, and Swartz[42] has discussed the possibility that a related defect in A-V valve formation might explain the elongated chordae and redundant valve of mitral valve prolapse. Thus, the recent discovery of concurrence of Ebstein's anomaly and PMLS lends credence to Swartz' concept.

PATHOPHYSIOLOGY

Gross anatomical and histologic abnormalities have been found in the mitral and tricuspid valve in PMLS, the principal ones being redundancy ("hooding," "ballooning") and myxomatous degeneration of the involved leaflets,[44] dilatation of the mitral anulus,[45] and variable chordal pathology[10,17,24,45,46] (thin and elongated as well as thickened chordae have been described); but these findings are not specific for PMLS. The valvular pathology has been seen in accelerated "wear and tear" situations such as ruptured chordae and mitral regurgitation from a variety of causes, as well as from advanced age.[47] Anular dilatation has been described angiographically[48] and from postmortem examinations of patients with severe mitral regurgitation and "floppy valves" (presumably PMLS),[45] and it appears to be disproportionate to the ventricular dilatation; anular circumference is larger in PMLS than in any other form of mitral regurgitation, except the Marfan syndrome.

It appears to us that a mitral valve can maintain reasonable structural and functional integrity as long as the two leaflets have a broad zone of systolic apposition and can be maintained in an ideal subanular position within the ventricle during systole. The cause may be chordal or leaflet laxity, papillary muscle or left ventricular dysfunction, anular dilatation or calcification, hypercontractility of the ventricle, etc.; slippage of either leaflet exposes the leaflets and chordae to increasing stresses. This is the result of the La Place relationship between the intraventricular pressure and the expanding radius of curvature of the leaflet. The prolapsing leaflet behaves as an unfurled sail catching the "wind" of ventricular systole, and subjecting itself, its supporting chordae, papillary muscle, and the underlying ventricular wall to abnormal and destructive stress.[49-51] The mitral apparatus is subjected not only to "systolic stretch," but also to "diastolic dumping," as the blood-laden leaflet abruptly unloads itself and its contents into the relaxing ventricle.[52] The endothelial integrity of the leaflet may be disrupted by slipping and sliding against its opposing leaflet, by excessive expansion, or by the diastolic dumping phenomenon. The traumatized endothelium of the valve may provide a nidus for sterile vegetations[44] which could lead to embolization.[20] When infective endocarditis afflicts the PMLS, embolization is a frequent complication and is possibly the result of excessive rubbing together and violent excursions of the leaflets.

Although left ventricular dysfunction has been suggested by hemodynamic and angiographic studies as well as the propensity for arrhythmias, there has been a paucity of satisfactory anatomical histologic findings[53] to substantiate a myopathic process. Similarly, no consistent pathologic abnormalities have been found to explain the chest pain syndromes—often suggesting ischemia—which have been noted frequently in PMLS. It is not known whether the anular dilatation found in severe mitral regurgitation associated with PMLS is a cause or a result of the leaflet prolapse.

Subendocardial injury patterns (ST segment depression) have been provoked by exercise or amyl nitrite inhalation;[22] chest pain, ECG changes, and myocardial lactate production have been induced in various combinations by investigators using phenylephrine[54] and atrial pacing.[55,56] However, the vast majority of patients with clinically recognized PMLS who undergo coronary arteriographic studies for chest pain syndromes have widely patent major coronary vessels[22] and endomyocardial biopsies have not revealed disease of the small vessels.[53] It has been suggested that Prinzmetal's angina, or major coronary artery spasm, might be responsible for myocardial infarctions in patients with PMLS;[57] one case report has demonstrated the coexistence of PMLS and angiographically demonstrated segmental spasm of the right coronary artery.[58] Unfortunately, considerable confusion has resulted from reporting angiographic evidence of mitral prolapse in patients with obstructive coronary arterial disease, since it seems to be well established that mitral leaflet prolapse can result from ischemic heart disease,[59-61] and, conversely, that bypass surgery can reverse mitral prolapse when it is on an apparently ischemic basis.[60]

Cobbs has championed the possibility that papillary muscle ischemia could result from the powerful pull exerted by a prolapsing leaflet;[49-51] he also suggests that the angiographic contraction abnormalities and certain arrhythmias might also be caused by this pull. Other investigators have found evidence of pre-excitation (WPW) bypass tracts in patients with PMLS,[62] but this association does not satisfactorily explain the vast majority of arrhythmias encountered in PMLS. Several published and unpublished observations note that replacement or repair of the mitral valve has ameliorated arrhythmias.[51,63,64] There are three functional/anatomical bases for the valvulogenic origin of the arrhythmias: (1) The mitral leaflets contain myocardium which, under conditions of stretch or catecholamine excess, are capable of spontaneous phase 4 depolarization (pacemaker activity).[65] (2) The pull exerted on the papillary muscles and underlying muscle may render them ischemic and "irritable."[49-51] (3) The diastolic dumping action of the blood-laden leaflets may act as a tactile stimulus to the impact regions in the left ventricle.[52]

FUNCTIONAL ANATOMY

Although PMLS has been associated with a number of disease entities, the common denominator which best explains the abnormality is a *valvuloventricular disproportion* in which the valve is "too big" for the ventricle, or the ventricle is "too small" for the valve.[34] This concept is, admittedly, an oversimplification, but it serves to explain the response to the various postural and pharmacological interventions which have profound effects on the clinical manifestations of PMLS (Fig. 1).

Angiocardiographic and echocardiographic studies have documented a close correlation between ventricular size and the timing of valve prolapse,[66-69] so that in a given

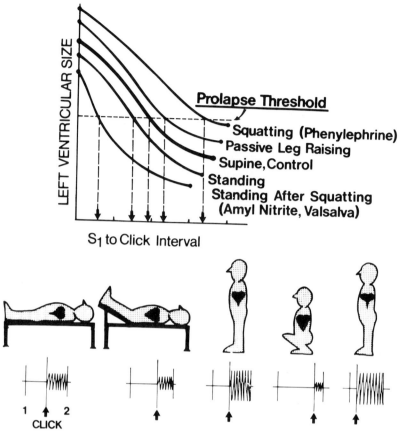

Figure 1. Diagram of the effects of postural changes on ventricular size and the timing of the click and murmur of PMLS. Postural (and pharmacologic) changes affect the filling volume (preload) and resistance to ejection (afterload) resulting in changes in ventricular geometry which affect the timing and extent of mitral leaflet prolapse. The graph depicts an arbitrary "prolapse threshold" at which the valvuloventricular disproportion leads to prolapse. Left ventricular size, on the vertical axis, is plotted against the interval between the first sound and click on the horizontal axis. When the ejecting ventricle reaches the prolapse threshold, the valve prolapses, leading to inscription of the click and late systolic murmur. If the prolapse threshold is crossed early in systole as a result of decreased preload and/or afterload—as occurs in the standing position—the click occurs closer to S_1 and the murmur is longer and louder. An increase in preload and afterload results from squatting, the prolapse threshold is crossed later, and the click and murmur are moved to the right. Standing up after squatting causes an abrupt and profound decrease in preload and afterload, which leads to an earlier click and loud murmur.

individual interventions which decrease end-diastolic ventricular dimensions lead to prolapse earlier in systole. The dimension at which prolapse occurs might be termed the "prolapse threshold." When that threshold is crossed during systole, a leaflet is no longer able to maintain a subanular position within the ventricle; it inflates excessively and prolapses toward the atrium. If sufficient slippage occurs the valve becomes incompetent in mid or late systole (Fig. 1).

The disproportion in PMLS results in seemingly paradoxical responses to intervention as compared to those of conventional (e.g., rheumatic) mitral regurgitation. The latter syndrome may be ameliorated by decreasing the preload or afterload so that the murmur becomes softer after the Valsalva maneuver and louder with handgrip.

CLINICAL FEATURES

Patients with PMLS are often referred for cardiac examination because an unusual murmur was detected on a routine physical examination, or because of presenting symptoms such as palpitations, chest pain, syncope, fatigue, or apparently neurotic symptoms (Table 3). Occasionally, the detection of an arrhythmia by the patient or referring generalist may initiate a cardiac consultation. Although PMLS occurs in both sexes, there appears to be a nearly 2:1 predominance in females[10] possibly because the smaller ventricle in females is more likely to make the condition manifest.[70] Although PMLS is found in patients of every body habitus, the "typical" patient has a thin, gracile habitus, often exhibiting subtle or overt thoracic cage deformities (pectus excavatum, loss of normal kyphosis, scoliosis, etc.), a high-arched palate, and increased dorsal mobility of the fingers.[71]

The pulse is often normal at rest and accelerates excessively on standing; it may also exhibit marked sinus arrhythmia or more striking arrhythmias. The carotid pulse may be hyperactive and the jugular pulse is usually unremarkable. The precordial examination usually reveals a heart of normal size, and careful palpation may bring out a

Table 3. Clinical features suggestive or diagnostic of PMLS

___

History

Palpitations, syncope, fatigue, or chest pain, typically in a young, thin female. May be thought to have "anxiety neurosis."

Physical Examination
   Skeletal (may have some of the following features):
      High-arched palate
      Chest wall deformity (pectus excavatum, straight back, scoliosis)
      Hyperextensible index fingers
      "Double-jointed"
   Precordium:
      Mid-systolic cardiac apical retraction
      Mobile mid-systolic click at left sternal edge
      Variable mid or late systolic apical murmur, may transmit to aortic area
      Occasionally widely split S-2 or "opening snap"

Noninvasive Laboratory
   a. ECG: prolonged Q-T, inferior-lateral T wave changes, atrial and
      ventricular arrhythmias, pre-excitation (rare), occasional "positive" treadmill
   b. Phonocardiogram: nonejection click and late systolic murmur
      which vary with postural and pharmacological interventions
      (Figs. 1 and 2); midsystolic retraction of apexcardiogram
   c. Echocardiography: M mode late systolic dorsal dipping (Fig. 3);
      more specific than "holosystolic hammocking"; high opening
      excursion of anterior leaflet which may impinge on septum
   d. Two-dimensional echocardiography
      (1) Posterior displaced coaptation of the leaflets
      (2) Systolic superior movement of one or both leaflets

Cardiac Catheterization

Rarely required for diagnosis. May be indicated in patients with chest pain or severe mitral regurgitation. Billowing of scallops of posterior leaflet causing variable sagging of anterior mitral leaflet (Fig. 6). Often associated with LV contraction abnormalities and variable mitral regurgitation.

Coronary arteries usually normal, but may exhibit concurrent atherosclerosis. Prinzmetal's angina with coronary artery spasm has been reported.

___

mid-systolic retraction of the apex beat.[72-74] Auscultation may reveal the classic diagnostic features of PMLS discussed later in this chapter, but often the findings are subtle and require a certain amount of "tuning up." The clinician who is alerted to the possibility of PMLS may be able to bring out diagnostic features which could otherwise be missed, even on careful examination.

The *click* of PMLS is usually described as mid-systolic, or "nonejection" in timing, but it may be early in systole and even fuse with the first sound, or it may occur sufficiently late to simulate a split second heart sound. The key to proper identification is the predictable *mobility* of the click (Figs. 1 and 2). Postural or pharmacological interventions can decrease the ventricular dimensions and move the click toward the first sound, and conversely toward the second sound when ventricular dimensions are increased. There may be multiple clicks, occurring in staccato fashion; we consider these to be as diagnostic of PMLS as a single mobile click. Occasionally the click may be absent or buried in a holosystolic murmur. The click is often heard best along the left sternal border, where the murmur may be more subdued.

The *murmur* of PMLS may be variably present and require manipulations to bring it out. Classically, it is late systolic in timing and initiated by the click, though it may be holosystolic. As with the click, the response to postural and pharmacologic perturbations can provide diagnostic information. The intensity of the murmur varies: on occasion it is sufficiently loud to be detected by others at a considerable distance. We examined a patient on several occasions who had no murmur at rest, nor was it provocable with any postural maneuver. But after exercising on the treadmill for several minutes he developed a murmur loud enough to be heard without a stethoscope. When he stopped exercising, the loud whooping murmur disappeared in a few seconds.

The character of the murmur is quite variable, even when an individual is examined serially. It is often more harsh or musical than conventional mitral regurgitation, although it can be blowing in character. The murmur may be best heard at the apex or left midprecordium, and its transmission to other areas varies. Occasionally the murmur is well heard at the base and into the neck, possibly a reflection of the superior direction of the intense regurgitant jet. As already noted, the murmur may be "whooping" or "honking" in character.[75,76] The second sound may be widely split; this has been attributed to early aortic closure[51] (Fig. 3).

We believe that PMLS cannot be ruled out on clinical examination without putting the patient through the appropriate postural maneuvers diagrammed in Figure 1. If there is no click or murmur at rest, the best "tuneup" can be achieved by repeated squatting and standing. Squatting causes a large increase in left ventricular volume; standing causes a profound decrease and, often, tachycardia. Occasionally, mild to moderate exercise or a pharmacological challenge (e.g., amyl nitrite inhalation) is needed to produce a murmur. If a murmur is present, passive leg-raising or squatting may alter its time of onset or intensity (Fig. 1). It should be mentioned that the various maneuvers may not always yield the expected result, in part explainable by variations in performance of the maneuvers by the patient. For example, if leg-raising is not completely passive and the patient attempts to assist the physician, a Valsalva maneuver or tachycardia can be effected, and thus negate the volume-loading effects of the leg-raising. Response to sustained isometric handgrip varies with the degree of tachycardia counteracting the pressor effect of the maneuver, and with the patient's tendency to perform an involuntary Valsalva maneuver while gripping (Fig. 2).

LABORATORY STUDIES

The *chest roentgenogram* in PMLS is of little diagnostic value, except to confirm the thoracic skeletal abnormalities. Also, depending on the degree of mitral regurgitation,

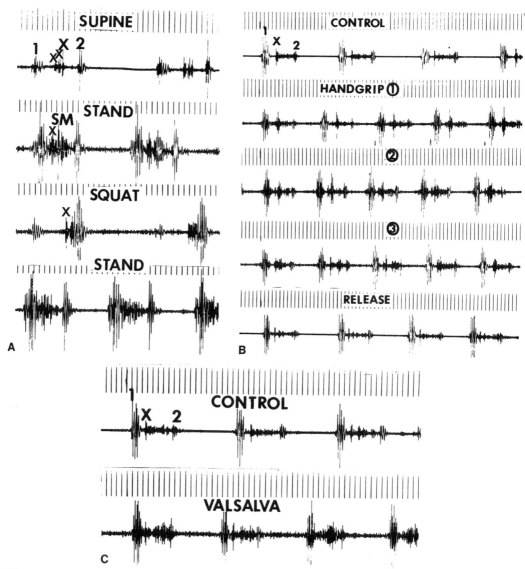

Figure 2. Phonocardiogram of PMLS. The effects of postural and physiologic interventions on the apical phonocardiogram are demonstrated in a 27-year-old male (A) and a 30-year-old female (B and C) with typical PMLS confirmed by echocardiography. Each panel was excerpted from a continuous phonocardiogram recorded at constant amplification with time lines at 0.04 sec. (40 msec.). A, Postural maneuvers. A cluster of staccato clicks (X) is seen beginning 180 msec. after the first sound (1), but there is no murmur when the patient is *supine. Standing* causes clicks to occur earlier, and induces a crescendo-decrescendo systolic murmur (SM). *Squatting* causes the click and murmur to occur later. *Standing up after squatting* produces a nearly holosystolic murmur, and clicks are not consistently seen, presumably because they are incorporated into S_1 or the early part of the murmur. B, The effect of handgrip (isometric exercise). At rest there is an early systolic click followed by a soft mid to late systolic murmur. With initiation of *handgrip,* ①, the click is louder and later in systole, but with sustained handgrip, ② and ③, the heart rate increased and the click occurs earlier, while the murmur increases in intensity. After *release* the initial click occurs closer to the first sound. These variable changes with handgrip are thought to result from a combination of early increased afterload, ①, followed by later involuntary Valsalva, ② and ③, as the handgrip is sustained. Upon release the abupt decrease in afterload causes the click to occur earlier. C, The Valsalva maneuver. During the strain phase the click occurs earlier and the murmur is augmented.

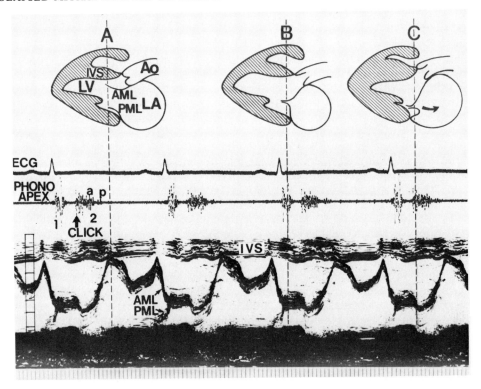

Figure 3. An M mode echocardiogram and apical medium frequency phonocardiogram of PMLS are displayed with diagrammatic depictions of the left heart for anatomical reference. A, High-opening excursion of the anterior mitral leaflet (AML) is seen in early diastole with apparent impingement on the interventricular septum (IVS). B, In early systole the anterior (AML) and posterior (PML) mitral leaflets coapt as the anterior leaflet swings dorsally to meet the posterior leaflet, which arches upward to form a shelf (Fig. 5) against which the anterior leaflet abuts. C, In midsystole an abrupt dorsal excursion of the mitral leaflets occurs, and a concomitant midsystolic click (X) and late systolic murmur (SM) are recorded. Although the anterior mitral leaflet echo is seen continuously during the cardiac cycle, the posterior leaflet echo "drops out" because of several factors: it is shorter in length, its systolic position is largely parallel with the echo beam, and the heart is moving caudally and ventrally during systole so that the fixed echo beam traverses the heart progressively more cephalad during systolic ejection. The longer anterior leaflet remains nearly perpendicular to the echo beam through all phases of the cardiac cycle, and although the echo beam "climbs" up the leaflet during systole, an ideal reflecting surface is maintained. In three dimensions, the anterior leaflet changes from diastolic convexity (Fig. 4) to systolic concavity (Fig. 5) relative to the left ventricular outflow tract, so that during systole it forms the posterolateral boundary of the nearly columnar outflow tract (Fig. 5C). Time lines = 0.04 sec.

it may indicate enlargement of the left atrium and ventricle. Typically, the heart is not enlarged and the only abnormal contour is a slight straightening of the left atrial border contour.

The *electrocardiogram* may be normal, but often reveals ST segment or T wave abnormalities and a variety of arrhythmias. The most common repolarization abnormalities are prolongation of the QT interval[77] and T wave inversion in the inferolateral leads (II, III, aVF, and V_{4-6}).[5,76,77] If these changes are not apparent on a resting ECG, they may emerge with exercise, amyl nitrite inhalation, or ambulatory (Holter) monitoring which may also bring out subendocardial injury current patterns.[22]

Cardiac rhythm disturbances are common, particularly with exercise or following exertion, and consist of: marked sinus arrhythmia (often suggesting sinoatrial Wenckebach), frequent premature atrial contractions (PACs), atrial tachycardias, and premature ventricular contractions (PVCs) which may be multifocal or paired, or occur in salvoes.[34,78,79] In older patients, we have noted recurrent atrial fibrillation and varying degrees of heart block.

Various bradyarrhythmias are associated with PMLS, though not as commonly as the tachyarrhythmias. We observed a 69-year-old man with confirmed PMLS and a bradycardia-tachycardia syndrome consisting of alternating sinus bradycardia (40 to 52 beats per minute) and atrial flutter with 2:1 to 8:1 ventricular response. Liechtman[7] studied eleven members of a family with a high incidence of mitral valve prolapse; three of the seven with bradycardia had PMLS, while two others with PMLS did not have bradycardia. Electrophysiologic studies suggested that the bradycardia and observed atrioventricular block with atrial pacing resulted from increased vagal tone, and two of the patients with syncope responded favorably to permanent transvenous pacing.

Phonocardiography can be helpful in documenting the characteristic mobility of the nonejection click and variation of the murmur with postural or pharmacological interventions. The characteristic murmur usually begins with the click, and extends up to or through the aortic closure sound[51] (Fig. 2). The intensity (amplitude) may be uniform or crescendo-decrescendo; on occasion it may gradually increase to a peak in late systole. The murmur may be difficult to differentiate from the murmur of hypertrophic cardiomyopathy (HCM), since these murmurs may have the same timing, exhibit the same responses to alterations in preload and afterload, and produce nonejection clicks. The apexcardiogram may reveal a mid-systolic retraction, synchronous with the click, which is thought to be caused by the sudden tension release of valve prolapse.[72–74] This dip is not always present; when it is it may simulate or be simulated by the systolic notch seen in left atrial myxoma. The carotid pulse tracing often reveals a brisk upstroke, but there are no diagnostic features.

Echocardiography in PMLS[80–84] often reveals a characteristic systolic dorsal movement of the posterior and/or the anterior leaflets of the mitral valve (Fig. 3) and the tricuspid valve,[37] although the potential for false positive and false negative results from this technique should be appreciated.[6,32,84]

The conventional echocardiogram presents information in only one spatial dimension, while the mitral valve is a three-dimensional structure which undergoes intricate contortions in the act of normal closure. In order for the mitral valve to reflect the ultrasound beam and register an echocardiographic image it must approximate a right angle relationship to the oncoming ultrasound beam. Rather than representing an "icepick" of ultrasound, the beam actually diverges into a cone as it penetrates the cardiac structures, and thus impacts upon and reflects waves from structures which are not truly on the central axis. To compound the confusion, there are great variations in patterns of "normal" mitral closure among individuals as well as at different times in the same individual and in different parts of the same mitral valve. Two-dimensional echocardiography is now possible with multibeam mechanical sector scanning and phased-array electronic sector scanning instruments, but even these devices share many of the previously noted limitations of the conventional echocardiographs. Experience with these new devices is still needed to establish how they differentiate cases of PMLS from normal mitral closure in various instances.[32,85]

The two leaflets of the mitral valve are quite different in structure and function (Figs. 4 and 5), and in their ability to reflect ultrasound.[86–90] The anterior leaflet is an ideal echocardiographic target, since its large curtain-like structure performs relatively simple motions—more-or-less toward and away from the chest wall—and almost always presents a broad right-angle interface to ultrasound waves. Although the anterior mitral leaflet changes from a diastolic convexity to a systolic concavity (relative to the left ventricle) as it swings across the left ventricular outflow tract, its movements are relatively simple and ideally suited to ultrasound reflection. The posterior leaflet is more complex. It surrounds nearly two thirds of the mitral circumference and consists of

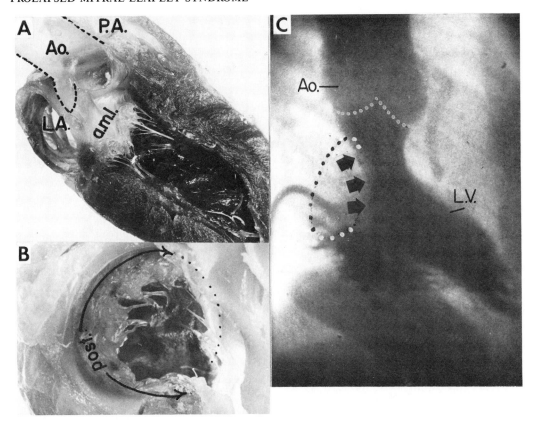

Figure 4. Anatomic and angiographic demonstrations of the normal mitral valve in diastole. A, A right anterior oblique view, equivalent to 45 degrees, of the left heart in diastole demonstrates the broad reflecting surface of the convexly bowed anterior mitral leaflet (a.m.l.) and its continuity with the left coronary and noncoronary (cut) leaflets of the aortic valve. B, A right posterior oblique view from the left atrial aspect demonstrates the long circumferential anular attachment of the posterior leaflet (solid line), and the lack of an anular structure corresponding to the anterior leaflet (dotted line). C, A 75-degree RAO transseptal left ventriculogram of a normal heart demonstrating the opened anterior leaflet (three arrows) and the position of posterior anulus (dotted C-shaped structure) which forms the basal attachment of the posterior leaflet. The closed aortic valve (Ao) is indicated by white dots.

three separate functional units (cusps or scallops and their chordae) which, during systole, engulf the anterior leaflet and form a C-shaped gasket against which the convex curtain-like leaflet abuts (Fig. 5B). Instead of swinging like a curtain during diastole, the posterior scallops hang down into the ventricle like a basketball net from the atrioventricular anulus (Fig. 4B); during systole they arch upward as they "inflate" to form the C-shaped gasket. The distance from basal to chordal attachment is considerably shorter for the posterior scallops than for the anterior leaflet; the former are thus less capable of reflecting ultrasound. This is particularly evident during systole, when inflation places a major portion of their surface in a shelf parallel to the echocardiographic beam (Fig. 3). To compound the difficulty, the mitral anulus contracts[91] to decrease the mitral circumference, causing the lobular structure of the posterior leaflet to "wrinkle" even more (Fig. 5B). The systolic descent of the base causes the mitral valve to move apically and ventrally in a twisting motion during systolic ejection. Space limitations prevent a more accurate and detailed account of the convoluted movements of the mitral leaflets during systole, but it should be clear from this brief account that

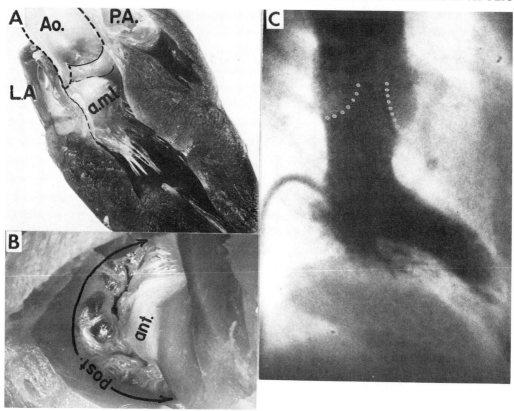

Figure 5. Anatomic and angiographic demonstrations of the normal mitral valve in systole. A, A 45-degree RAO view of the left heart in systole reveals the broad reflecting surface of the concavely bowed anterior mitral leaflet. B, A right posterior oblique view from the atrial aspect reveals the inflated and quilted C-shaped gasket formed by the posterior leaflet which engulfs the hemicylindrical anterior leaflet. Even though the anterior "curtain" remains nearly parallel to the major axis of the outflow tract, the posterior leaflet has less echo-reflecting potential because of its shorter length and inflated systolic position. C, A 75-degree RAO transseptal left ventriculogram during systole demonstrates the columnar outflow tract leading to the open aortic leaflets (white dots); the posterior aspect is formed by the concavely bowed anterior mitral leaflet. The posterior leaflet is nearly obscured in this view, except for the inflated posteromedial commissural scallop visible below the transseptal catheter.

trying to differentiate normal closure from PMLS with a one-dimensional, narrowly collimated beam through a moving target is difficult under the best of circumstances.

It is our feeling that the late systolic dorsal dipping pattern ("question mark on its side") of either leaflet (Fig. 3) is a more reliable sign of PMLS than "holosystolic hammocking,"[84] which may merely represent increasing concavity of the anterior mitral leaflet as it is engulfed by the C-shaped posterior leaflet and constricting anulus (Fig. 5B).

Cardiac catheterization and angiocardiography are rarely necessary to confirm the diagnosis in a "typical" patient with PMLS, since the clinical findings are clear-cut and noninvasive studies can provide adequate confirmation. The hemodynamic values obtained at catheterization are normal unless the degree of mitral regurgitation is significant. Although a number of investigators suspect that PMLS represents a disorder of the myocardium as well as the valve,[13,35,92–94] there is no consistent and agreed upon category of hemodynamic abnormality.

Contrast ventriculography in a typical case of PMLS demonstrates a protrusion of the mitral apparatus across the plane of the atrioventricular anulus. This protrusion may persist through all phases of the cardiac cycle, but more commonly develops during systole (Fig. 6). When the protrusion progresses to the point that apposition between adjacent leaflets is no longer adequate, varying degrees of mitral regurgitation may be demonstrated. Often the regurgitant jet can be seen to impact on the inferior or dorsal wall of the atrium; it may also move in a clockwise direction (in the RAO projection) along the inferior and dorsal atrial wall, apparently impacting on the atrial-aortic surface.

Tricuspid valve prolapse has been seen in approximately 40 percent of patients with PMLS.[35]

Various "contraction abnormalities" of the left ventricle have been described in patients with PMLS and some of these may seem contradictory. For example, some investigators have reported *hyper*contractility of the basal part of the left ventricle,[92,95] while others have reported *hypo*contractility of this region.[48,96] The "ballerina foot"[35] deformity caused by inferior indentation is a frequent finding; it has been thought by some to represent the cause of prolapse, by others as the result of tugging on the papillary muscle by the prolapsing leaflet. Cobbs has demonstrated absence of the inferior indentation following mitral valve replacement.[51]

Opinions differ considerably as to what constitutes PMLS and what is "normal" inflation of the posterior leaflet scallops. Much of the confusion centers around the correct identification of the anterior commissural scallop (frequently and erroneously called the anterior leaflet)[22,28,97] as it forms a "hump" anterior to and beneath the aortic valve on RAO ventriculograms (Fig. 6).[98] Investigators should cautiously avoid overinterpretation of left ventriculograms—particularly if mitral valve prolapse is seen only with ectopic beats during contrast injections—and primary and secondary forms of PMLS should be as clearly differentiated as possible. For example, if PMLS is seen in a patient with advanced coronary arterial obstructive disease, the mitral valve abnormality could be secondary to the ventricular damage and contraction abnormalities could be the result of the other disease process. In differentiating mitral valve prolapse from exaggerated inflation of the posterior leaflet, therefore, the investigator would be wise to err toward conservatism when interpreting a left ventriculogram which demonstrates

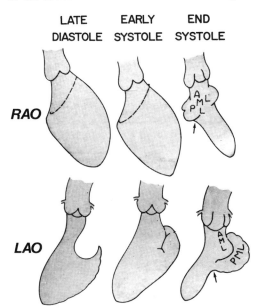

LATE EARLY END
DIASTOLE SYSTOLE SYSTOLE

RAO

LAO

Figure 6. Angiographic silhouettes of PMLS. Diastolic, early systolic, and late systolic silhouettes of left ventriculograms in 45-degree RAO and 60-degree projections. In the LAO projection the position of the open leaflets can be seen in diastole, and the nearly normal systolic position of the hemicylindrical anterior leaflet and the encircling scallops of posterior leaflet can be seen in early systole. In late systole the overinflated and prolapsing posterior leaflet can be seen in both projections. The "anterior hump" seen in the right upper figure represents the anterior commissural scallop of the posterior leaflet. The inferior indentation in the region of the posteromedial papillary muscle is indicated by arrows.

225

equivocal mitral prolapse in a patient who does not exhibit the expected clinical or echocardiographic findings.

NATURAL HISTORY

The available data on long-term prognosis in PMLS are sketchy and beclouded by biased methods of case selection. A study done in an arrhythmia or stroke clinic population will obviously have a higher long-term morbidity and mortality than a followup study of patients found to have PMLS on routine examination for school, military service, or insurance purposes.

A British study[99] excluded patients with any preceding complications except ventricular ectopic beats; of 62 patients followed for between 9 and 22 years 5 developed infective endocarditis, 1 patient developed chordal rupture, and 1 died at age 75 of severe mitral regurgitation. A more recent American study[100] was based on 53 patients, followed for 10 to 22 years. All patients had phonocardiographic evidence of click and/or murmur; of the 3 with infective endocarditis 1 died; of 5 who developed significant mitral regurgitation, 1 died suddenly (48 hours after starting quinidine), and 1 patient was resuscitated after spontaneous ventricular fibrillation. Thus, a total of 15 percent developed significant complications in a mean followup period of 14 years.

Although there are no clear-cut predictive features for significant complications, morbidity seems to be more common in females, familial cases, and patients with mental instability.[101]

Cardiac catheterization and angiography are often indicated if the degree of mitral regurgitation is thought severe enough to consider mitral valve replacement, or if disabling chest pain is present. In the young patient with PMLS the coronary arteries are usually angiographically normal, while in the older patient coronary obstructive disease may be present and it may be difficult to differentiate coexistence from causation. As previously noted, several documented myocardial infarctions have occurred in patients with PMLS and normal coronary arteriograms,[57] and the suggestion that coronary artery spasm might be responsible has received confirmation in at least one reported instance.[58]

THERAPY

Since relatively few patients with PMLS develop significant mitral regurgitation warranting valve replacement, therapy is primarily medical in the majority of cases of PMLS (Table 4).

The *asymptomatic patient* who is discovered to have PMLS on the basis of a routine examination or evaluation of an unrelated problem poses some difficult dilemmas for the physician. Should he inform the patient of a condition that leads to sudden death in an unknown percentage of patients? Should he prescribe antibiotic prophylaxis for dental procedures or potentially contaminated surgical procedures or childbirth? Should he treat prophylactically with propranolol in the hope of preventing progressive wear and tear of the mitral apparatus?

Our philosophy is to not inform the patient of sudden death potential, and to downplay it on the basis of its rarity when a previously informed patient inquires. Anxiety over an apparently uncommon complication which—if it does occur—is a painless and peaceful demise can do nothing but increase its likelihood. We had one patient with PMLS who had an episode of ventricular fibrillation from which he was successfully resuscitated; he reported that he felt that he had "just dozed off." There is evidence which suggests that the anxious or psychiatrically unstable patient is a more likely candidate for life-threatening arrhythmias.[101]

Table 4. Suggested approach to management of patients with PMLS

Clinical Setting	*Authors' Suggestions*
All patients with confirmed PMLS, with or without mitral regurgitation, with or without symptoms	1. Counseling as to nature of mitral valve abnormality, possibility of arrhythmias and syncope 2. Antibiotic prophylaxis (A.H.A. recommendation, Schedule A)* 3. Consider prohibiting commercial piloting
Symptomatic patients A. Fatigue, dyspnea, chest pain	1. Reassurance; monitored, progressive, mild exercise 2. Treat arrhythmias if present 3. Consider propranolol, 40 to 160 mg. per day
B. Arrhythmias Infrequent PVCs	1. Reassurance 2. Serial ambulatory ECGs at yearly intervals or if symptoms increase
Frequent (> 300/hr.) or multifocal PVCs	1. Propranolol, 80 to 400 mg. per day (occasionally 400 to 1000 mg. when needed for control) 2. Dilantin, 300 to 400 mg. per day 3. Other antiarrhythmic agents if drugs listed above prove ineffective (disopyramide, quinidine, etc.)
Documented ventricular tachycardia or fibrillation	1. Antiarrhythmic drugs (listed above) 2. If drugs are ineffective, consider adding atrial overdrive pacing or valve replacement
Paroxysmal atrial tachyarrhythmias	1. Propranolol, 40 to 400 mg. per day
Symptomatic bradycardia or bradycardia-tachycardia syndromes	1. Consider transvenous atrial, ventricular or sequential pacing
C. Congestive failure	1. Digitalis glycosides 2. Valve replacement for severe mitral regurgitation
D. Cerebral vascular accidents	1. Consider coumadin anticoagulation (life-long therapy) 2. Consider aspirin and dipyridamole

*Circulation 56:139A, 1977.

We do believe that the potential for infective endocarditis warrants the use of antibiotic prophylaxis for dental procedures in all patients with PMLS, whether or not a murmur is present. The "stress" of sitting in a dental chair, combined with the legs-down posture, tendency to isometric handgrip exercise, etc., is likely to convert a click-only patient into a click-murmur patient during the period of iatrogenic bacteremia. But we do not feel that our knowledge of the long-term effects of propranolol or our lack of information about its possible role in preventing progressive PMLS justifies the use of the drug in an asymptomatic patient.

The *symptomatic patient* with PMLS also poses a challenge to the physician. The most common symptoms are palpitations, syncope, chest pain, and undue fatigue. The palpitations and syncope are usually caused by arrhythmias, and it behooves the physician to document this by ambulatory ECG monitoring or to try to uncover other arrhythmic episodes and assess their potential for morbidity. We believe that symptomatic arrhythmias should be treated, as should potentially life-threatening arrhythmias, even when they are "silent," and proposed treatment regimens are given in Table 4. The chest pain, which is not typically anginal in nature, may respond to propranolol, but the medication should be supplemented by reassurance that the pain is (usually) of no physiological significance. Typical anginal pains should be investigated by exercise ECG and by coronary arteriography if they are debilitating or unresponsive to medications. The possibility that Prinzmetal's angina, or major coronary artery spasm, may be operative in patients with PMLS should be investigated further before any pronouncements can be made about management of this condition with agents such as alpha adrenergic receptor blocking drugs or nifedipine which have shown considerable promise in the management of Prinzmetal's angina.[102] Fatigue, often referred to as "the blahs" by patients with PMLS, is common, but the mechanism creating it is poorly understood. Propranolol (40 to 160 mg./day) and considerable reassurance may be beneficial. "Mood elevators," particularly those with sympathomimetic mechanisms of action, should be avoided.

Embolic cerebral vascular accidents have recently been described in 12 relatively young patients found to have PMLS,[20] but the overall incidence of this complication is unknown. Either coumadin-type anticoagulation or platelet aggregation inhibitor therapy (aspirin, dipyridamole) would seem to be indicated in those cases of cerebral emboli in which bacterial endocarditis is ruled out by appropriate procedures.

Mitral valve replacement for life-threatening arrhythmias refractory to medical management has been suggested based on the belief that the mitral valve is responsible for the arrhythmias (see Pathophysiology). There have been some encouraging results,[51,63,64] but we know of two patients with PMLS, one with Marfan's syndrome and the other with a repaired ostium secundum atrial septal defect (and therefore "secondary" PMLS), who died suddenly in the late postoperative period despite technically satisfactory valve replacement in both instances; there was attempted overdrive coronary sinus pacing[103] in the patient with Marfan's syndrome.

UNANSWERED QUESTIONS

This treatise emphasizes the ubiquity of PMLS, the potential for both under- and over-diagnosis, and some of the dilemmas facing the physician caring for patients with PMLS. Perhaps the greatest dilemma is posed by the apparently asymptomatic individual who is found to have PMLS in the course of a routine examination for insurance, employment, etc.

Should he or she be fully informed about the potentially morbid complications of PMLS? Should the patient be told to avoid strenuous exertion? Should he be prohibited from flying commercial aircraft? Should he be forced to pay prohibitively high insurance premiums for health insurance? What is the likelihood of developing a significant complication that will affect productivity or lifespan? Since there may be dominant inheritance of PMLS, should genetic counseling be given?

These questions cannot be answered despite the recent profusion of scientific communications regarding PMLS. Our current responses to these questions are only partially supported by objective data. In discussing the significance of PMLS with a patient or family it is important to be candid and informative, but not alarming. We do believe that the patient should be told of the deformity, and that with appropriate followup care (including antibiotic prophylaxis for dental procedures, etc.), significant complications can usually be avoided. Unless asked specifically about the more morbid complications, we do not believe that the physician should outline them to the asymptomatic patient, but we do mention the remote possibility of syncope or symptomatic arrhythmias, and stress the importance of reporting them to the physician. We would recommend that a patient with well established PMLS (e.g., click, murmur, and echocardiographic confirmation) not perform exhaustive or highly competitive physical exercise, since arrhythmias are likely to be provoked under these circumstances and it could be speculated that the likelihood of syncope or sudden death might be enhanced. We do not believe that insurance companies have the necessary supporting data to consider an asymptomatic patient with PMLS a "high risk case," and are therefore not justified in charging significantly higher premiums. On the other hand, since there is a remote possibility of enhanced incidence of a disabling arrhythmia occurring in a stressful profession upon which many other lives are dependent, we believe that individuals with *confirmed* PMLS should not be commercial pilots. We do not recommend genetic counseling, if for no other reason based on the knowledge that many leaders of the scientific and medical community have established PMLS.

The socioeconomic impact of these important questions and our tenuously supported answers is considerable, so it is of great importance that large scale, multicenter prospective studies be undertaken. We recommend that a national registry be established in which asymptomatic and symptomatic patients with PMLS could be followed. The incidence of significant complications could then be determined from a more appropriate sampling of data than is currently available.

ACKNOWLEDGMENT

The authors thank Joy Morgridge, who typed the manuscript, and Paul Cooper, who assisted in preparing the illustrations.

REFERENCES

1. BARLOW, J. B., AND BOSMAN, C. K.: *Aneurysmal protrusion of the posterior leaflet of the mitral valve: An auscultatory–electrocardiographic syndrome.* Am. Heart J. 71:166,1965.
2. CRILEY, J. M., LEWIS, K. B., HUMPHRIES, J. O., ET AL.: *Prolapse of the mitral valve: Clinical and cineangiographic findings.* Br. Heart J. 28:488,1966.
3. GALLAVARDIN, L.: *Pseudo-dedoublement du deuxieme bruit du coeur, etc.* Lyon Med. 121:409,1913.
4. WOOLEY, C. F.: *Where are the diseases of yesterday? DaCosta's syndrome, soldiers heart, the effort syndrome, neurocirculatory asthenia and the mitral valve prolapse syndrome.* Circulation 53:749,1976.
5. BARLOW, J. B.: *The significance of late systolic murmurs and non ejection clicks.* J. Chronic Dis. 18:665,1965.
6. WEISS, A. N., MIMBS, J. W., LUDBROOK, P. A., ET AL.: *Echocardiographic detection of mitral valve prolapse. Exclusion of false positive diagnosis and determination of inheritance.* Circulation 52:1091,1975.
7. LEICHTMAN, D., NELSON, R., GOBEL, F. L., ET AL.: *Bradycardia with mitral valve prolapse (A potential mechanism of sudden death).* Ann. Intern. Med. 85:453,1976.
8. SEGAL, B. L., AND LIKOFF, W.: *Late systolic murmur of mitral regurgitation.* Am. Heart J. 66:443,1964.
9. McKUSICK, V. A.: *Heritable Disorders of Connective Tissue,* ed. 4. C.V. Mosby, St. Louis, 1972.
10. BARLOW, J. B., BOSMAN, C. K., POCOCK, W. A., ET AL.: *Late systolic murmurs and nonejection ("mid late") systolic clicks: An analysis of 90 patients.* Br. Heart J. 30:203,1968.
11. MARKIEWICZ, W., STONER, J., LONDON, E., ET AL.: *Mitral valve prolapse in one hundred presumably healthy young females.* Circulation 53:464,1976.
12. PROCACCI, P. M., SAVRAN, S. V., SCHREITER, S. L., ET AL.: *Prevalence of clinical mitral-valve prolapse in 1169 young women.* N. Engl. J. Med. 294:1086,1976.
13. GOOCH, A. S., VICENCIO, F., MARANHO, V., ET AL.: *Arrhythmias and left ventricular asynergy in prolapsing mitral leaflet syndrome.* Am. J. Cardiol. 29:611,1972.
14. WINKLE, R. A., LOPES, M. G., AND FITZGERALD, J. W.: *Arrhythmias in patients with mitral valve prolapse.* Circulation 52:73,1975.
15. GOODMAN, D., KIMBIRIS, D., AND LINHART, J. W.: *Chordae tendinae rupture complicating the systolic click-late systolic murmur syndrome.* Am. J. Cardiol. 33:681,1974.
16. HILL, D. G., DAVIES, M. J., AND BRAINBRIDGE, M. V.: *The natural history and surgical management of the redundant cusp syndrome (floppy mitral valve).* J. Thorac. Cardiovasc. Surg. 67:519,1974.

17. McKay, R., and Yacoub, M. H.: *Clinical and pathologic findings in patients with "floppy" valves treated surgically.* Circulation 48(Suppl. III):63,1973.

18. Barlow, J. B., and Pocock, W. A.: *The problem of non-ejection systolic clicks and associated mitral systolic murmurs: Emphasis on the billowing mitral leaflet syndrome.* Am. Heart J. 90:636,1975.

19. Lachman, A. S., Bramwell-Jones, D. M., Lakier, J. B., et al.: *Infective endocarditis in the billowing mitral leaflet syndrome.* Br. Heart J. 37:326,1975.

20. Barnett, H. J., Jones, M. W., Boughner, D. R., et al.: *Cerebral ischemic events associated with prolapsing mitral valve.* Arch. Neurol. 33:777,1976.

21. Marchand, P.: *Late systolic murmurs and non-ejection ("mid-late") systolic clicks: An analysis of 90 patients.* Br. Heart J. 30:203,1968.

22. Jeresaty, R. M.: *Mitral valve prolapse–click syndrome.* Prog. Cardiovasc. Dis. 25:623,1973.

23. Shappell, S. D., Marshall, C. E., Brown, R. E., et al.: *Sudden death and the familial occurrence of mid-systolic click, late systolic murmur syndrome.* Circulation 48:1128,1973.

24. Marshall, C. E., and Shappell, S. D.: *Sudden death and the ballooning posterior leaflet syndrome.* Arch. Pathol. 98:134,1974.

25. Jeresaty, R. M.: *Sudden death in the mitral valve prolapse–click syndrome.* Am. J. Cardiol. 37:317,1976.

26. Fontana, M. E., Pence, H. L., Leighton, R. F., et al.: *The varying clinical spectrum of the systolic click—late systolic murmur syndrome.* Circulation 41:807,1970.

27. Betriu, A., Wigle, E. D., Felderhof, C. H., et al.: *Prolapse of the posterior leaflet of the mitral valve associated with secundum atrial septal defect.* Am. J. Cardiol. 35:363,1975.

28. Jeresaty, R. M.: *The syndrome associated with midsystolic click and/or late systolic murmur.* Chest 59:643,1971.

29. Chandraratna, P. A. N., Tolentino, A. O., Mutucumarana, W., et al.: *Echocardiographic observations on the association between mitral valve prolapse and asymmetric septal hypertrophy.* Circulation 55:622,1977.

30. Baba, K., Yoshikawa, J., Owaki, T., et al.: *Tricuspid and mitral echocardiogram of Ebstein's anomaly with complication of mitral valve prolapse syndrome.* J. Cardiography 6:87,1976.

31. Roberts, W. C., Glancy, D. L., Seningen, R. P., et al.: *Prolapse of the mitral valve (floppy valve) associated with Ebstein's anomaly of the tricuspid valve.* Am. J. Cardiol. 38:377,1976.

32. Sahn, D. J., Wood, J., Allen, H. D., et al.: *Echocardiographic spectrum of mitral valve motion in children with and without mitral valve prolapse: the nature of false positive diagnosis.* Am. J. Cardiol. 39:422,1977.

33. Smith, E. R., Fraser, D. B., Purdy, J. W., et al.: *Angiographic diagnosis of mitral valve prolapse: correlation with echocardiography.* Am. J. Cardiol. 40:165,1977.

34. Criley, J. M., and Kissel, G. L.: *Prolapse of the mitral valve—the click and late systolic murmur syndrome.* Prog. Cardiol. 4:23,1975.

35. Scampardonis, G., Yang, S. S., Maranhao, V., et al.: *Left ventricular abnormalities in prolapsed mitral leaflet syndrome.* Circulation 48:287,1973.

36. Chandraratna, P. A. N., Lopez, J. M., Fernandez, J. J., et al.: *Echocardiographic detection of tricuspid valve prolapse.* Circulation 51:823,1975.

37. Werner, J. A., Schiller, N. B., and Prasquier, R.: *Occurrence and significance of echocardiographically demonstrated tricuspid valve prolapse.* Circulation 54:913,1976.

38. DeLeon, A. C., and Ronan, J. A.: *Thoracic bony abnormalities with the click and late systolic murmur syndrome.* Circulation 43(Suppl. II):157,1971.

39. Bon Tempo, C. P., Ronan, J. A., Jr., De Leon, A. C., et al.: *Radiographic appearance of the thorax in systolic click-late systolic murmur syndrome.* Am. J. Cardiol. 36:27,1975.

40. Salomon, J., Shah, P. M., and Heinle, R. A.: *Thoracic skeletal abnormalities in idiopathic mitral valve prolapse.* Am. J. Cardiol. 36:32,1975.

41. Read, R. C., Thal, A. P., and Vernon, E. W.: *Symptomatic valvular myxomatous transformation (the floppy valve syndrome); a possible forme fruste of the Marfan syndrome.* Circulation 32:897,1965.

42. Swartz, M. H., Herman, M. V., and Teicholz, L. E.: *Dermatoglyphic patterns in patients with mitral valve prolapse: A clue in pathogenesis.* Am. J. Cardiol. 38:588,1976.

43. Van Mierop, L. H. S.: *Embryology.* In Netter, F. H. (ed.): *CIBA Collection of Medical Illustrations,* Vol. 5, *Heart.* New York, CIBA Pharmaceutical, 1969, pp. 143–144.

44. Pomerance, A.: *Ballooning deformity (mucoid degeneration) of atrioventricular valves.* Br. Heart J. 31:343,1969.

45. Bulkley, B. H., and Roberts, W. C.: *Dilatation of the mitral anulus. A cause of mitral regurgitation?* Ann. Intern. Med. 59:457,1975.

46. SHERMAN, E. B., CHAR, F, DUNGAN, W. T., ET AL.: *Myxomatous transformation of the mitral valve producing mitral insufficiency.* Am. J. Dis. Child. 119:191,1970.

47. POMERANCE, A.: *Aging changes in human heart valves.* Br. Heart J. 29:222,1967.

48. LEACHMAN, R. D., DEFRANCHESCHI, A., AND ZAMALLOS, O.: *Late systolic murmurs and clicks associated with abnormal mitral valve ring.* Am. J. Cardiol. 23:679,1969.

49. COBBS, B. W.: *Clinical recognition and medical management of rheumatic heart disease and other acquired valvular disease.* In Hurst, J. W., and Logue, R. B. (eds.): *The Heart,* ed. 2. McGraw-Hill, New York, 1970.

50. COBBS, B. W.: *Rheumatic heart disease and other acquired valvular disease.* In Hurst, J. W. (ed.): *The Heart,* ed. 3. McGraw-Hill, New York, 1974.

51. COBBS, B. W., AND KING, S. B.: *Ventricular buckling: A factor in the abnormal ventriculogram and peculiar hemodynamics associated with mitral valve prolapse.* Am. Heart J. 93:741,1977.

52. CRILEY, J. M., ZEILENGA, D. W., AND MORGAN, M. T.: *Mitral dysfunction. A possible cause of arrhythmias in prolapsed mitral leaflet syndrome.* Trans. Am. Clin. Climatol. Assoc. 85:44,1973.

53. KOCH, F. H., BILLINGHAM, M. E., MASON, J. W., ET AL.: *Pathogenesis of the click-murmur-prolapse syndrome: Biopsy evidence supporting an underlying cardiomyopathic process.* Am. J. Cardiol. 39:272,1977.

54. LEWINTER, M. M., HOFFMAN, J. R., SHELL, W. E., ET AL.: *Phenylephrine-induced atypical chest pain in patients with prolapsing mitral leaflets.* Am. J. Cardiol. 34:12,1974.

55. KHULLAR, S. C., AND LEIGHTON, R. F.: *Mitral valve prolapse syndrome (MVPS): Left ventricular function and myocardial metabolism.* Am. J. Cardiol. 35:149,1975.

56. NATARAJAN, G., NAKHJAVAN, F. K., KAHN, D., ET AL.: *Myocardial metabolic studies in prolapsing mitral leaflet syndrome.* Circulation 52:1105,1975.

57. CHESLER, E., MATISONN, R. E., LAKIER, J. B., ET AL.: *Acute myocardial infarction with normal coronary arteries: a possible manifestation of the billowing mitral leaflet syndrome.* Circulation 54:203,1976.

58. AWDEH, M., AND GHOLSTON, D. E.: *Mitral valve prolapse and coronary artery spasm.* Circulation 56:329,1977.

59. CHENG, T. O.: *Late systolic murmur in coronary artery disease.* Chest 61:346,1972.

60. ARANDA, J. M., BEFELER, B., LAZZARA, R., ET AL.: *Mitral valve prolapse and coronary artery disease.* Circulation 52:245,1975.

61. CRAWFORD, M. H.: *Mitral valve prolapse due to coronary artery disease.* Am. J. Med. 62:447,1977.

62. GALLAGHER, J. J., GILBERT, M., SVENSON, R. H., ET AL.: *Wolff-Parkinson-White syndrome.* Circulation 51:767,1975.

63. ROSS, A. M., DEWEESE, J. A., AND YU, P. N.: *Mitral valve prolapse. Personal communication.*

64. KAY, J. H.: *Personal communication.*

65. WIT, A. L., FENOGLIO, J. J., WAGNER, B. M., ET AL.: *Electrophysiological properties of cardiac muscle in the anterior mitral valve leaflet and the adjacent atrium in the dog. Possible implications for the genesis of atrial dysrhythmias.* Circ. Res. 32:731,1973.

66. FONTANA, M. E., WOOLEY, C. F., LEIGHTON, R. F., ET AL.: *Postural changes in left ventricle and mitral valve dynamics in the systolic click-late systolic murmur syndrome.* Circulation 51:165,1975.

67. FONTANA, M. E., KISSEL, G. L., AND CRILEY, J. M.: *Functional anatomy of mitral valve prolapse.* Am. Heart Assoc. Monograph: *Physiologic Principles of Heart Sounds and Murmurs,* p. 126,1975.

68. WINKLE, R. A., GOODMAN, D. J., AND POPP, R. L.: *Simultaneous echocardiographic–phonocardiographic recordings at rest and during amyl nitrite administration in patients with mitral valve prolapse.* Circulation 51:522,1975.

69. MATHEY, D. G., DECODT, P. R., ALLEN, H. N., ET AL.: *The determinants of mitral valve prolapse in the systolic click late systolic murmur syndrome.* Circulation 51, 52(Suppl. II):77,1975.

70. DEVEREUX, R. B., PERLOFF, J. K., REICHEK, N., ET AL.: *Mitral valve prolapse.* Circulation 54:3,1976.

71. EVANS, P., HUGES, D., SMITH, S., ET AL.: *Joint laxity associated with the mitral valve prolapse syndrome.* Circulation 53, 54(Suppl. II):104,1976.

72. SPENCER, W. H., BEHAR, V. S., AND ORGAIN, E. S.: *The apexcardiogram in patients with prolapsing mitral valves.* Circulation 43, 44(Suppl. II):106,1971.

73. EPSTEIN, E. J., AND COULSHED, N.: *Phonocardiogram and apexcardiogram in systolic click–late systolic murmur syndrome.* Br. Heart J. 35:260,1973.

74. TOWNE, W. D., RAHIMTOOLA, S. H., ROSEN, K.M., ET AL.: *The apexcardiogram in patients with systolic prolapse of the mitral valve.* Chest 63:569,1973.

75. LEON, D. F., LEONARD, J. J., KROETZ, F. A., ET AL.: *Late systolic murmurs, clicks and whoops arising from the mitral valve.* Am. Heart J. 72:325,1966.

76. POCOCK, W. A., AND BARLOW, J. B.: *Etiology and electrocardiographic features of the billowing posterior leaflet syndrome; analysis of a further 130 patients with a late systolic murmur or nonejection click.* Am. J. Med. 51:731,1971.

77. HANCOCK, W. E., AND COHN, K.: *The syndrome associated with midsystolic click and late systolic murmur.* Am. J. Med. 41:183,1966.

78. SLOMAN, G., WONG, M., AND WALKER, J.: *Arrhythmias on exercise in patients with abnormalities of the posterior leaflet of the mitral valve.* Am. Heart J. 83:312,1972.

79. DEMARIA, A. N., AMSTERDAM, E. A., VISMARA, L. A., ET AL.: *Arrhythmias in the mitral valve prolapse syndrome; prevalence, nature, and frequency.* Ann. Intern. Med. 84:656,1976.

80. SHAH, P. M., AND GRAMIAK, R.: *Echocardiographic recognition of mitral valve prolapse.* Circulation 42(Suppl. III):45,1970.

81. DILLON, J. C., HAINE, C. L., CHANG, S., ET AL.: *Use of echocardiography in patients with prolapsed mitral valve.* Circulation 43:503,1971.

82. KERBER, R. E., ISAEFF, D. M., AND HANCOCK, E. W.: *Echocardiographic patterns in patients with the syndrome of systolic click and late systolic murmur.* N. Engl. J. Med. 284:691,1971.

83. POPP, R. L., BROWN, O. R., SILVERMAN, J. F., ET AL.: *Echocardiographic abnormalities in the mitral valve prolapse syndrome.* Circulation 49:428,1974.

84. DEMARIA, A. N., KING, J. F., BOGREN, H. G., ET AL.: *The variable spectrum of echocardiographic manifestations of the mitral valve prolapse syndrome.* Circulation 50:33,1974.

85. GILBERT, D. W., SCHATZ, R. A., VON RAMM, O. T., ET AL.: *Mitral valve prolapse—two-dimensional echocardiographic and angiographic correlation.* Circulation 54:716,1970.

86. DUPLESSIS, L. A., AND MARCHAND, P.: *The anatomy of the mitral valve and its associated structures.* Thorax 19:221,1964.

87. WALMSLEY, R., AND WATSON, H.: *The outflow tract of the left ventricle.* Br. Heart J. 28:435,1966.

88. SILVERMAN, M. E., AND HURST, J. W.: *The mitral complex.* Am. Heart J. 76:399,1968.

89. LAM, J. H. C., RANGANATHAN, N., WIGLE, E. D., ET AL.: *Morphology of the human mitral valve: I. Chordae tendinae: A new classification.* Circulation 41:449,1970.

90. RANGANATHAN, N., LAM, J. H. C., WIGLE, E. D., ET AL.: *Morphology of the human mitral valve: II. The valve leaflets.* Circulation 41:459,1970.

91. TSAKIRIS, A. G., VON BERNUTH, G., RASTELLI, G. C., ET AL.: *Size and motion of the mitral valve annulus in anesthetized intact dogs.* J. Appl. Physiol. 30:611,1971.

92. EHLERS, K. H., ENGLE, M. A., LEVIN, A. R., ET AL.: *Left ventricular abnormality with late mitral insufficiency and abnormal electrocardiogram.* Am. J. Cardiol. 26:333,1970.

93. GULOTTA, S. J., GULCO, L., PADMANABAN, V., ET AL.: *The syndrome of systolic click, murmur, and mitral valve prolapse—a cardiomyopathy?* Circulation 49:717,1974.

94. JERESATY, R. M.: *Etiology of the mitral valve prolapse–click syndrome.* Am. J. Cardiol. 36:110,1974.

95. GROSSMAN, H., FLEMING, R. J., ENGLE, M. A., ET AL.: *Angiocardiography in the apical systolic click syndrome. Left ventricular abnormality, mitral insufficiency, late systolic murmur and inversion of T waves.* Radiology 91:898,1968.

96. LIEDTKE, A. J., GAULT, J. H., LEAMAN, D. M., ET AL.: *Geometry of left ventricular contraction in the systolic click syndrome. Characterization of a segmental myocardial abnormality.* Circulation 47:27,1973.

97. JERESATY, R. M.: *Ballooning of the mitral valve leaflets.* Radiology 100:45,1971.

98. RANGANATHAN, N., SILVER, M. D., ROBINSON, T. I., ET AL.: *Idiopathic prolapsed mitral leaflet syndrome.* Circulation 54:707,1976.

99. ALLEN, H., HARRIS, A., AND LEATHAM, A.: *Significance and prognosis of an isolated late systolic murmur: A 9 to 22 year follow-up.* Br. Heart J. 36:525,1974.

100. ROSE, J. D., MILLS, P., HOLLINGSWORTH, B. A., ET AL.: *Long term prognosis of mitral valve prolapse— 53 patients followed for 10–22 years (mean 14 years).* Am. J. Cardiol. 39:272,1977.

101. SHAPPELL, S. D., ORR, W., AND GUNN, C. G.: *The ballooning posterior leaflet syndrome: Minnesota multiphasic personality inventory profiles in symptomatic and asymptomatic groups.* Chest 66:690,1974.

102. ENDO, M., KANDA, I., HOSODA, S., ET AL.: *Prinzmetal's variant form of angina pectoris.* Circulation 52:33,1975.

103. RITCHIE, J. L., HAMMERMEISTER, K. E., AND KENNEDY, J. W.: *Refractory ventricular tachycardia and fibrillation in a patient with the prolapsing mitral leaflet syndrome: Successful control with overdrive pacing.* Am. J. Cardiol. 37:314,1976.

104. LEACHMAN, R. D., COKKINOS, D. V., AND COOLEY, D. A.: *Association of ostium secundum atrial septal defects with mitral valve prolapse.* Am. J. Cardiol. 38:167,1976.

105. COWLEY, M. J., COGHLAN, H. C., MANTLE, J. A., ET AL.: *Chest pain and bilateral atrioventricular valve prolapse with normal coronary arteries in isolated corrected transposition of the great vessels*. Am. J. Cardiol. 40:458,1977.

106. HEMRY, D. A., MOSS, A. J., AND JACOX, R. F.: *Relapsing polychondritis, a "floppy" mitral valve, and migratory polytendinitis*. Ann. Intern. Med. 77:576,1972.

Congenital Aortic Stenosis in Adults*

*William F. Friedman, M.D., Valerie Novak, and
Allen D. Johnson, M. D.*

The bicuspid aortic valve is the most frequent congenital malformation of the heart, with a prevalence estimated at between 0.7 and 2 percent of the United States population.[1] Its occasional association with other cardiovascular anomalies, such as coarctation of the aorta, patent ductus arteriosus, ventricular septal defect and isolated pulmonic stenosis, is well established.[2-5] Additionally, a recently described association of bicuspid aortic valve, short left main coronary artery, and left coronary artery dominance, [6,7] suggests that the bicuspid aortic valve may be one component of an abnormal developmental complex yet to be elucidated. Nora and Nora[8] have reported a 3.9 percent incidence of congenital bicuspid aortic valve in children who have one parent with this malformation.

The bicuspid aortic valve may be discovered at any age; it may even be an incidental finding in the elderly at autopsy. This discussion will be limited to the problems and presentation of isolated valvar aortic stenosis in the adolescent and adult to the exclusion of other discrete forms of left ventricular outflow tract obstruction, such as subvalvar and supravalvar aortic stenosis. In considering congenital aortic stenosis in these two age groups we will focus on the available information in three major areas: (1) the natural history of the bicuspid aortic valve that is either stenotic or nonstenotic at birth, (2) myocardial adaptation to significant aortic stenosis, and (3) the "unnatural" history of the patient with congenital aortic stenosis following valvotomy or valve replacement.

ANATOMICAL HISTORY OF THE CONGENITALLY ABNORMAL AORTIC VALVE

Fenoglio and coworkers [9] have suggested that about one third of patients beyond age 20 born with nonstenotic bicuspid aortic valves will go on to develop aortic stenosis; one third will develop aortic insufficiency; and the remainer will be free of any hemodynamically significant problem. The incidence of stenosis appears to increase with age. By age 60, 53 percent of bicuspid aortic valves have become stenotic; by age 70 this figure has risen to 73 percent. Roberts'[10] autopsy series in patients from ages 15 to 88 revealed that 72 percent of the patients with isolated aortic stenosis and 26 percent of those with aortic regurgitation had congenitally malformed valves. Why significant

*Supported by U. S. Public Health Service Grants HL 12373, HL 05846, and HL 17334.

stenosis develops in some bicuspid aortic valves and not others remains poorly understood.

The valve that is stenotic from birth is most often bicuspid, with a single fused commissure and an eccentric orifice. False commissures may be located on one of the cusps. In rare instances the valve is unicuspid and dome-shaped with no lateral attachments to the aorta. Subtle inequalities among individual cusps of a tricuspid aortic valve may exist and are presumably part of this congenital spectrum. Edwards[11] has conjectured that only the unicuspid valve is stenotic intrinsically; stenosis in other anatomic situations progresses with time. Thickening and increased rigidity of valve tissue with varying degrees of commissural fusion comprise the basic malformation of aortic stenosis in childhood and adolescence; secondary calcification of the valve is rare in this age group. The minimum age at which calcification occurs is not clear, although it has been reported occasionally in teenagers.[12,13] In adults, however, commissural fusion is rare; the stenotic valve is uniformly calcified, and the frequency with which calcification occurs increases with age.[9] To encounter stenosis without some degree of calcification after age 40 is uncommon; conversely, heavy deposits of calcium are minimal or absent in purely incompetent or normally functioning bicuspid valves.[1,9]

The mechanism responsible for progressive calcification leading to stenosis is unclear. The "wear and tear" theory describes a gradual progression from focal to diffuse fibrous thickening and, ultimately, to calcification as a result of improper contact between the two unequal valve leaflets of a malformed bicuspid valve.[14] Tricuspid aortic valves with minimally unequal but misaligned cusps are candidates for the same process.[10] Other investigators believe that calcification occurs in the region of turbulent blood flow as blood elements interact with the valve surface.[15] The cascade of events which ensues involves hemolysis, ADP release, platelet aggregation and microthrombi that ultimately organize and calcify. Calcific deposits appear to be nodular and lie above the surface of the valve cusps, a pattern consistent with an inflammatory process.[9] Once initial thickening and calcification are present, a vicious cycle exists whereby the restriction in valve mobility results in further calcification and obstruction to left ventricular outflow.

MYOCARDIAL ADAPTATION TO SIGNIFICANT AORTIC STENOSIS

The usual response of the left ventricle to a chronic pressure overload is concentric hypertrophy with an increase in both left ventricular mass and wall thickness. Light and electron microscopic studies of left ventricular myocardium in patients with aortic stenosis disclose hypertrophied muscle cells surrounded by small amounts of fibrous tissue.[16] Experimental left ventricular outflow tract obstruction in animals creates hypertrophy that is most prominent in the subendocardium.[17]

It has been suggested that hypertrophy is associated with an intrinsic impairment in myocardial contractility.[18,19] Recent papillary muscle studies of cats indicate that this depression in contractile state is reversible,[20,21] but it is difficult to extrapolate these data to human subjects with aortic stenosis in whom the pressure load is more chronic and uncontrolled. However, in a recent study of 15 patients with valvar aortic stenosis, ejection phase indices of left ventricular contractility showed that five patients had elevated values of mean wall stress and depressed contractility, whereas the remaining ten subjects maintained normal ventricular function and wall stress.[22] Both animal and human studies conclude tentatively that gradual concentric hypertrophy may be beneficial insofar as it serves to maintain wall stress and systolic myocardial performance within normal limits.

Concentric hypertrophy may also have deleterious effects upon cardiac function. Clinical symptoms of congestive heart failure, angina, syncope, and sudden death, and symptoms associated with high pulmonary venous pressures are observed in patients with aortic stenosis. Hypertrophy-induced increases in chamber "stiffness" and an increase in left atrial and ventricular end-diastolic pressures occurs despite normal heart size and normal left ventricular systolic function. It is more likely that the reduction in myocardial compliance is secondary to the increase in muscle mass rather than to a change in the intrinsic properties of the myocardial cell.[22]

The increase in left ventricular mass and wall tension in aortic stenosis requires an increase in myocardial oxygen supply. The increase in diastolic left ventricular intramural pressure and shortening of diastolic time oppose adequate delivery of oxygen to the myocardium. Consequently, coronary blood flow in diastole may fall conspicuously and result in subendocardial ischemia. Subendocardial ischemia may be estimated by relating the diastolic pressure time index (DPTI)—the area between the aortic and left ventricular pressures in diastole—to the systolic pressure time index (SPTI)—a measure of myocardial oxygen demands in patients with significant aortic stenosis. Inadequate subendocardial oxygen delivery is reflected by a ratio (DPTI $\times$ arterial O_2 content/SPTI) below 10.[23]

Thus, it is clear that the adaptation to aortic stenosis by concentric hypertrophy may, on the one hand, preserve left ventricular systolic function, and on the other hand, contribute to the development of myocardial ischemia. Subendocardial ischemia may also play a central role in syncope, ventricular arrhythmias, and sudden death in patients with aortic stenosis. Syncope and sudden death have also been attributed to a lack of reflex vasoconstriction in nonexercising muscles,[24] or to reflex peripheral vasodilatation secondary to activation of left ventricular baroreceptors.[25]

Significant myocardial disease with an overt decrease in myocardial performance and left ventricular dilatation develops in end-stage aortic valve disease; electron micrographs in this setting show muscle fiber degeneration rather than the findings of hypertrophy.

NATURAL HISTORY OF THE ADOLESCENT WITH AORTIC STENOSIS

The natural history of both the adolescent and adult with aortic stenosis is related to an understanding of the anatomic progression of the valvar lesion and to the process of adaptation to pressure overload discussed previously. In managing the adolescent with isolated aortic stenosis the major problem facing the clinician is to correctly identify the patient with severe aortic stenosis; the risk of sudden death in this age group is a major indication for hemodynamic study and surgical intervention.[26] In the child or adolescent severe or critical aortic stenosis is arbitrarily defined as a peak systolic pressure gradient from the left ventricle to the aorta greater than 75 mm. Hg in association with a normal cardiac output, or an effective aortic orifice area of less than 0.5 cm.²/M² body surface area.[27]

The reported incidence of sudden death, from aortic stenosis has varied from 1 to 19 percent, with an accepted average incidence of 7.5 percent.[2,28-34] More recent studies by Glew and coworkers[35] and Peckham and coworkers[36] reported an incidence of only 1 percent; but the risk of sudden demise is not accurately reflected here since observations were made over short time periods and patients with severe aortic stenosis were operated upon promptly. Aortic stenosis was the most common cause of sudden death in Lambert's international cooperative study of all forms of cardiovascular disease in children.[37] Overall, sudden death was most common less than one hour after the onset of acute signs and symptoms; warning syncope occurred in only 16 percent of patients and the majority of children were inactive at the time. However, half of the cases of sudden death which occurred shortly after engaging in strenuous athletics occurred in patients with severe aortic stenosis. Postmortem studies support the association of sudden death and anatomically severe stenosis;[34] the majority of patients who died suddenly had pre-existing symptoms of exertional dyspnea, syncope, chest pain, fatigue, and an electrocardiogram showing a left ventricular "strain" pattern. Nonetheless, sudden death may also occur in the asymptomatic patient or in the presence of a normal electrocardiogram.[38] Thus, the absence of symptoms or an abnormal electrocardiogram by no means excludes the possibility of severe obstruction or the threat of sudden death.

The adolescent with aortic stenosis also runs the risk of developing infective endocarditis. An incidence of 1.8 cases/1000 patient years has been reported,[39] and no correlation appears to exist between the severity of stenosis and the risk of endocarditis. Adequate antibiotic prophylaxis is necessary for oral and other indicated surgical procedures.

Clues have been sought to assess the severity of obstruction in the adolescent by the history and physical examination, chest x-ray, resting and exercise electrocardiogram, and single crystal and cross-sectional echocardiograms. The reliability of individual parameters varies. Careful attention must be directed to the patient's history, for although severe stenosis may be present without clinical symptoms, the presence of fatigability, exertional dyspnea, angina, or syncope strongly suggests that severe left ventricular outflow obstruction exists.[2]

On physical examination the presence of a fourth heart sound in the absence of P-R interval prolongation suggests the presence of severe aortic stenosis.[2] A left ventricular lift and systolic precordial thrill are associated with peak systolic gradients across the aortic valve of greater than 25 mm. Hg, but their presence does not necessarily indicate severe obstruction.[2] A systolic murmur peaking during the last 60 percent of ventricular systole suggests a gradient of at least 75 mm. Hg.[2,28,40,41] A short musical ejection murmur that peaks during the first third of systole usually suggests mild obstruction.

Typically, the radiologic examination of adolescents with congenital valvar aortic stenosis shows poststenotic dilatation of the ascending aorta and a normal or only minimally enlarged heart size. Concentric left ventricular hypertrophy is manifested by rounding of the cardiac apex in the frontal projection and posterior displacement in the lateral view. Left atrial enlargement suggests severe stenosis.

In severe stenosis, the resting electrocardiogram may reveal evidence of left ventricular hypertrophy and "strain," consisting of S-T segment depression and T wave inversion in the left precordial leads, although some patients with critical obstruction have a normal tracing.[2,27,34] The exercise electrocardiogram may be useful in unmasking ischemic S-T segment changes in patients with at least moderate obstruction,[42,43] although not all patients with severe aortic stenosis will be detected by stress testing, Hugenholtz[44] observed 21 such patients with a measured peak systolic gradient of greater than 40 mm. Hg, and 5 had a normal exercise tracing.

Single crystal echocardiographic findings include diminished systolic valve echo excursions toward the aortic wall, multiple diastolic echoes, eccentric diastolic closure lines, and an increased dimension of the aortic root.[45,46] The aortic eccentricity index—one-half the internal diameter of the aortic root divided by the shortest distance to the aortic wall in diastole—has been used to identify the presence of a bicuspid aortic valve[47,48] (Fig. 1). The index for normal values is usually 1.0 to 1.2; in bicuspid valves this value ranges from 1.5 to 4.5. A correlation has been shown by cross-sectional echo methods between the peak systolic pressure gradient and the rate of maximal aortic cusp separation/aortic root diameter, although refinements in measurement technique are required.[49] Also, the validity of cusp separation measurements remains in doubt.[50] An increase in the left ventricular wall thickness by echocardiography implies severe obstruction, and estimates of left ventricular pressure have been derived from measurements of posterior left ventricular wall thickness in end-systole

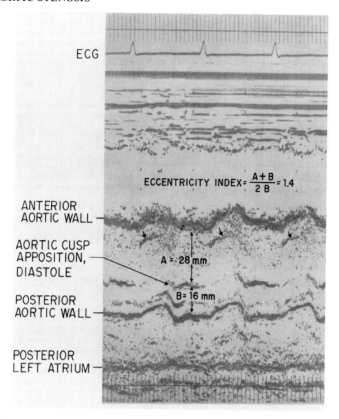

Figure 1. Echocardiogram of aortic cusps and aortic root in a patient with a bicuspid aortic valve. The eccentricity index is determined as shown in the illustration and explained in text. A = distance from anterior aortic wall to apposed aortic cusps in diastole. B = distance from posterior aortic wall to apposed aortic cusps in diastole. A + B = internal diameter of aortic root.

divided by end-systolic diameter × 225. The difference between the echo-derived left ventricular pressure and the cuff-measured arterial blood pressure provides an estimate of the transvalvar aortic gradient.[51]

Efforts to develop a noninvasive technique for estimating accurately the severity of left ventricular outflow obstruction continue. Recently, a collaborative study group compiled criteria to detect a small pressure gradient in order to avoid unnecessary cardiac catheterization in children and adolescents.[52] After multivariate analysis, an equation was derived to estimate the peak systolic pressure gradient based on the intensity of the systolic murmur on a scale of I to VI and the amplitude of the Q and R waves in lead V_6 of the electrocardiogram. Corrections were made for the presence or absence of the early diastolic murmur of aortic insufficiency. Murmur intensity is, of course, a less than perfect quantitative index and the overall correlation coefficient was only +0.50; of 147 patients with an estimated gradient less than 45 mm. Hg, 6 had a measured peak systolic gradient greater than 80 mm. Hg.

Cardiac catheterization is the definitive technique for assessing the severity of obstruction to left ventricular outflow. Right heart catheterization helps in detecting associated pulmonary hypertension or other cardiac malformations, while retrograde left heart catheterization allows withdrawal pressure recordings across the site of stenosis. Left ventricular angiography permits an evaluation of left ventricular function and mitral valve competency; it can also determine cavity size, wall thickness, and the diameter of the aortic root and ascending aorta, as well as the presence or absence of coexisting levels of outflow obstruction. Cardiac output, measured by indicator dilution or Fick techniques, should be related to the transvalvar gradient to calculate the orifice area of the aortic valve.[53]

We recommend that hemodynamic evaluation be performed every five to eight years in asymptomatic children with mild to moderate aortic stenosis because of the possibility of progression of the stenosis. As already mentioned, calcific deposits in the aortic valve are rarely encountered in patients under the age of 20. In most children and adolescents the valve has a relatively fixed effective orifice area which does not increase with growth; progression of the transvalvar gradient results from an increase in cardiac output associated with increased body growth.[54] Serial catheterization studies indicate that in some patients progression of stenosis with a decrease in valve area may occur early in life, even if the patient originally presented with mild stenosis.[54-61] In one of our prospective longitudinal studies an increase was noted in the average peak systolic pressure gradient across the aortic valve from 26 mm. Hg to 44 mm. Hg over an average four-year period in 12 of 15 initially asymptomatic children with isolated congenital aortic stenosis.[61] Figure 2 provides a composite of the serial hemodynamic data existing in the literature and illustrates the intensification of obstruction experienced by children and adolescents with aortic stenosis.

NATURAL HISTORY OF THE ADULT WITH AORTIC STENOSIS

The adult with a congenitally bicuspid aortic valve which has become stenotic usually presents to the cardiologist for evaluation of a murmur, or with symptoms that have developed insidiously over the course of several years. The cardinal symptoms include congestive heart failure, angina, and syncope or presyncope. All may be related to progression of stenosis and the myocardial adaptations discussed earlier. The risk of sudden death in the asymptomatic adult suspected of having severe aortic stenosis does not appear to be as high as it is for the adolescent.[62] The onset of symptoms in adults usually occurs in the fifth decade. Average life expectancy after the onset of symptoms is 4.8 years; it appears to be even less if congestive heart failure is the dominant symptom. The simultaneous presence of more than one symptom worsens the prognosist.[63] In a recent study of 15 adult patients with severe aortic stenosis who did not undergo valve replacement, the 5-year mortality rate was 52 percent; after 10 years it was 90 percent.[63]

In dealing with the adult patient the clinician faces four basic problems: (1) to establish that the uncomplaining patient with suspected severe aortic stenosis is truly asymptomatic; (2) to decide whether the symptoms of angina pectoris or exertional syncope arise from valvar aortic stenosis rather than from other cardiac or noncardiac causes; (3) to adequately evaluate the patient with congestive heart failure in the setting of aortic stenosis, as the low cardiac output state may make the assessment of clinical findings difficult; and (4) to outline management guidelines that take into consideration the patient's individual needs once severe aortic stenosis has been identified.

"Significant" aortic stenosis has been defined as a peak systolic pressure gradient greater than 50 mm. Hg and/or an aortic valve area index less than 0.7 cm.^{2}/M^2 body surface area.[62,63] However, in catheterized patients documented as having significant aortic stenosis by these criteria, measurements of peak systolic gradient, calculated valve orifice area, cardiac index, and left ventricular end-diastolic pressure did not distinguish the survivors from the nonsurvivors.[63] Careful attention should be directed to the interpretation of the peak systolic aortic valve gradient, as it will vary directly with the square of the systolic blood flow across the valve per unit of time; thus, a low

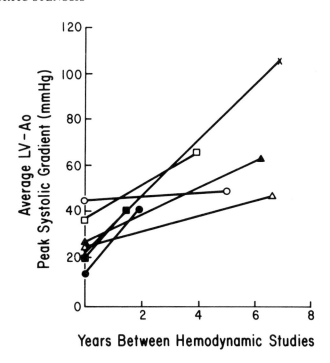

REFERENCE	NUMBER OF PATIENTS	AVERAGE AGE (yrs.)	
		1st CATH	2nd CATH
■ HOHN, et al.	4	6,10,10,45	N.A.
● BENTIVOGLIO, et. al.	1	27	29
□ EL-SAID, et. al.	18	7	11
○ HURWITZ	19	9	14
▲ FRIEDMAN, et. al.	9	6.8	13.1
△ COHEN, et. al.	15	8.5	15.1
X BANDY and VOGEL	1	5	12

Figure 2. Composite of serial hemodynamic studies in the literature showing the relationship between time and the left ventricular (LV)—aortic (Ao) pressure gradients in patients with congenital aortic stenosis.

cardiac output could be associated with a low gradient in the setting of a severely stenotic aortic valve.

The importance of a carefully taken history cannot be overemphasized when evaluating the adult patient with aortic stenosis; the history of the patient who claims to be asymptomatic is especially important. A subtle increase in fatigue and dyspnea or gradual curtailment of activities may suggest the presence of latent heart failure. A precipitating event such as thyrotoxicosis or anemia may impose an extra hemodynamic burden which narrows the margin of cardiac compensation.

The exercise electrocardiogram may be helpful in exposing symptoms associated with aortic stenosis. Patients with a history of exertional syncope have responded to supine leg exercise with an abnormal forearm vasodilator response and increased blood flow.[24] Thus, during treadmill testing, careful blood pressure monitoring which fails to show a rise in forearm blood pressure may provide a useful clue to severe obstruction. The presence of early-stage fatigue and dyspnea, and pulmonary rales is also signifi-

241

cant. Treadmill testing should not be conducted at a workload greater then the patient's maximum daily activity level.

If the patient is truly asymptomatic, close followup is indicated to detect any early signs and symptoms suggesting progression of obstruction. Although valve replacement in the asymptomatic patient has been recommended by some,[64] we do not currently believe valve replacement is indicated until the appearance of symptoms.

Aortic stenosis was once considered to have a protective effect on the development of coronary artery disease.[65,66] However, more recent studies conclude that aortic stenosis and coronary artery disease may, in fact, occur simultaneously. Paquay[67] reported a 39 percent prevalence of coronary artery disease in patients with aortic stenosis, and increasing prevalence with age. The reliability of angina as an indicator of coronary artery disease in the presence of aortic stenosis has been questioned. Some investigators believe that the absence of chest pain or ECG evidence of an infarct in the patient with aortic stenosis indicates small likelihood of associated coronary artery disease.[67,68] However, Hancock[69] found that in patients with aortic stenosis, 64 percent who had angina and 33 percent without angina had significant coronary artery disease. Thus, the absence of angina does not imply the absence of coronary artery disease and, conversely, the presence of angina does not necessarily indicate that coronary artery disease exists. Hence, in evaluating the adult patient who presents with angina and an outflow tract murmur, both hemodynamic and coronary angiographic studies are usually necessary to diagnose aortic stenosis and/or coronary artery disease, especially since the latter greatly influences long-term survival after aortic valve replacement.[70,71]

Syncope in adults with aortic stenosis is rare as an isolated symptom or at rest and is typically exertional or postexertional; thus, it may be exposed by exercise testing. Proposed mechanisms for syncopal episodes include ventricular arrhythmias secondary to subendocardial ischemia, inadequate reflex vasoconstriction of nonexercising muscles, and reflex activation of left ventricular baroreceptors resulting in peripheral vasodilation. Syncope may also be caused by dysrhythmias or intermittent heart block due to extension of calcification from the aortic valve to the region of the cardiac conduction system, in which case valve replacement may not be indicated.

Once symptoms of significant aortic stenosis are identified clearly, no role exists for medical management; the patient is a candidate for cardiac catheterization and aortic valve replacement.

Many parameters have been used to estimate the severity of aortic stenosis in the adult. The clinical history may reveal the presence of latent congestive heart failure, angina, or exertional syncope, as discussed previously. The chest wall configuration and underlying chronic lung disease of the elderly patient may disallow the identification of a palpable presystolic impulse and left ventricular lift. The presence of a fourth heart sound on auscultation is not as helpful in the adult as it is in the adolescent, where it suggests the presence of a severe gradient, since an S_4 is not uncommon in patients approaching age sixty. Furthermore, 15 percent of patients with critical obstruction have no audible S_4.[72,73] In significant aortic stenosis, the systolic ejection murmur persists through most of systole and peaks in the latter half of systole. Severe stenosis is often associated with a time interval greater than 0.19 sec. between the Q wave of the electrocardiogram and the peak of the systolic murmur.[74]

Hemodynamically significant aortic stenosis modifies the carotid pulse, a finding which can be appreciated at the bedside and by indirect recording techniques. The carotid pulse exhibits an anacrotic rise, interrupted by an anacrotic notch or shoulder and followed by a rounded or delayed peak, often with superimposed systolic vibrations and a delayed incisura. The ejection period (time interval on the carotid tracing from the onset of the anacrotic rise to the incisura) and the upstroke time (time interval from the onset of the anacrotic rise to the peak) are prolonged (Fig. 3). A maximum rate of

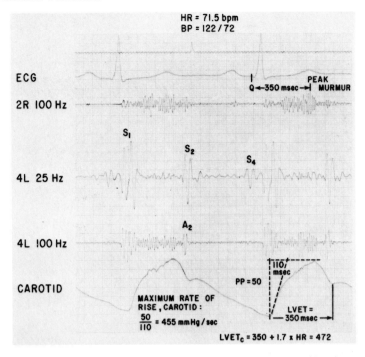

Figure 3. Simultaneous electrocardiogram (ECG), phonocardiogram, and carotid pulse tracing in an adult with congenital aortic stenosis. The carotid upstroke time is prolonged (horizontal line). The sex and heart rate corrected left ventricular ejection time (LVETc) is markedly prolonged, as is the peak of the systolic murmur recorded at the second right interspace (2R). PP = pulse pressure obtained with a sphygmomanometer in mm. Hg; A2 = aortic closure sound; S1 = 1st heart sound; S4 = atrial diastolic gallop; 4L = 4th left interspace; HR = heart rate; BP = blood pressure.

rise of the arterial pulse greater than 500 mm. Hg/second and a left ventricular ejection time greater than 420 msec. corrected for heart rate and sex, suggest a peak systolic gradient greater than 50 mm. Hg.[74] Unfortunately, recording indirect carotid pulse tracings may be technically difficult in the elderly patient. Moreover, because digitalis shortens the ejection time, its administration invalidates the use of this variable to assess the severity of stenosis.

Radiologic examination of the adult often shows no evidence of left ventricular enlargement although plain chest roentgenograms may show calcium in the region of the aortic valve (Fig. 4). Careful fluoroscopy is a reliable method of demonstrating valve calcification.

The resting electrocardiogram is a poor indicator of the severity of obstruction in the adult although the appearance on serial tracings of left ventricular hypertrophy and T wave changes may indicate progression to a high pressure gradient.[75] While the exercise electrocardiogram may expose symptoms associated with aortic stenosis, the possibility of pre-existing coronary artery disease makes the interpretation of ischemic S-T segment changes unreliable.

Thickened and calcified aortic valves often have a characteristic echocardiographic appearance (Fig. 5). Increased left ventricular wall thickness implies severe stenosis.

Cardiac catheterization remains the most definitive technique to assess the severity of aortic stenosis. Gradman and Hancock[76] described 12 patients, 22 to 71 years old—mean age 53 years—in whom the measured aortic valve gradient increased from 31 to 81 mm. Hg over an average of four years (range 2 to 10 years). Eleven of these patients developed severe aortic stenosis requiring valve replacement; in 8 of these 11, this

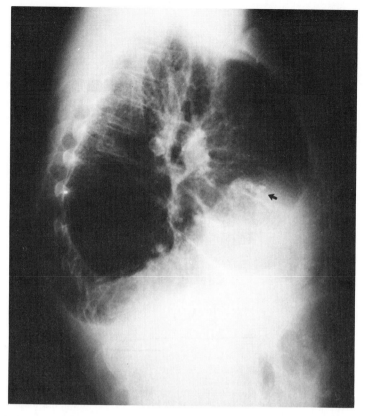

Figure 4. Lateral chest roentgenogram in an adult with valvar aortic stenosis and congestive failure (note bilateral pleural effusions). The arrow points to dense calcifications in the region of the aortic valve.

occurred in less than 5 years. Initial symptoms in 11 of the 12 were mild and usually atypical, and all but one developed more severe and typical symptoms with progressive aortic stenosis. Electrocardiographic signs of increased left ventricular hypertrophy and/or ischemia developed in 8 of the 10 patients in whom comparison was possible. In 11 patients aortic valve replacement was carried out; all had advanced calcific valvar disease, 7 had a congenital unicommisural or bicuspid valve and 3 had a tricuspid valve. In one case the underlying anatomy was not determined. Valvar calcification was initially present in at least 8, but its development was noted only once. The authors concluded that progressive calcific aortic stenosis in mildly symptomatic patients with small gradients occurs frequently and is associated with increasing symptoms and electrocardiographic changes. Some patients experience a rapidly progressive phase in the development of critical aortic outflow obstruction.

The serial cardiac catheterization studies by Cheitlin of 29 adults with calcific aortic stenosis followed over an average interval of 43.5 months indicate that the peak systolic pressure gradient may increase approximately 1.5 mm. Hg per month and, in some cases, the average monthly increment may be as high as 3 or 4 mm. Hg.[75] Progression, defined as a 50 percent increase in peak systolic pressure gradient between catheterizations, occurred in 16 of the 29 patients. The remaining patients had approximately the same low or high gradient at initial and followup study. Figure 6, supplied kindly by Cheitlin, illustrates the progressive intensification of obstruction in this group of adults.

In adults, as contrasted to adolescents, progression of the gradient is caused by

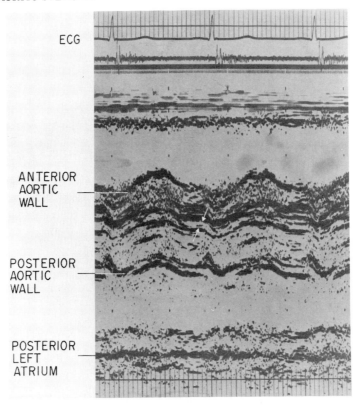

ECG

ANTERIOR
AORTIC
WALL

POSTERIOR
AORTIC
WALL

POSTERIOR
LEFT
ATRIUM

Figure 5. Aortic root echocardiogram from an adult with aortic stenosis. The arrows indicate dense echoes in the region of aortic leaflets, compatible with the presence of thickened aortic cusps.

increased valve calcification and decreased valve orifice area. The critical point in time at which the rapidly progressive stage of aortic stenosis is reached has yet to be defined.

"UNNATURAL" HISTORY OF AORTIC STENOSIS—ADOLESCENTS

In the adolescent the chief indication for valvotomy is the presence of severe left ventricular outflow obstruction, with or without associated symptoms.[2,26] Surgery is performed with peak systolic pressure gradients of 75 mm. Hg or a valve orifice area of less than 0.5 cm.^{2}/M^2. If there is evidence of left ventricular "strain" on the electrocardiogram, surgery is considered at a peak systolic pressure gradient of 40 to 50 mm. Hg or a valve orifice area in the range of 0.7 cm.^{2}/M^2 body surface area. Operation is carried out under direct vision after institution of cardiopulmonary bypass, and the fused valves are opened. The valve is not rendered anatomically normal by the procedure and the need for antibiotic prophylaxis continues after surgery.

Long-term studies on valvotomy have concluded that the procedure is both safe and effective, with an operative mortality of less than two percent. An increase in valve orifice area and a decrease in the peak systolic pressure gradient persists postoperatively.[77-80] Figure 7 illustrates the hemodynamic results of valvotomy in three longitudinal studies. Cardiac indices, normal before operation, remained unchanged. Most impressive is the relief of pre-existing symptoms by surgery.

Complications associated with aortic valvotomy include aortic regurgitation, residual stenosis, endocarditis, and the possibility of restenosis and calcification later in life. In

245

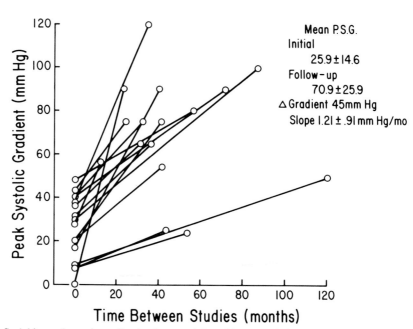

PEAK SYSTOLIC GRADIENT vs. TIME
Progression
n = 16

Mean P.S.G.
Initial
25.9 ± 14.6
Follow-up
70.9 ± 25.9
△ Gradient 45mm Hg
Slope 1.21 ± .91 mm Hg/mo

Figure 6. Serial hemodynamic studies in sixteen adults with congenital aortic stenosis. PSG = peak systolic gradient. The slope indicates the progression in severity of obstruction with time. (Courtesy of Dr. Melvin Cheitlin.)

42 patients studied by Jack and Kelly,[80] aortic regurgitation was present in 80 percent postoperatively, compared to 10 percent preoperatively. In 25 percent of all postoperative patients, aortic insufficiency was moderate or severe; one patient with severe regurgitation died suddenly; three required valve replacement, and in another three valve replacement was anticipated. Restenosis attributed to inadequate valvotomy was responsible for residual gradients greater than 60 mm. Hg in 6 of 15 patients who were catheterized serially. One 39-year-old patient developed calcification in his aortic valve 11½ years after valvotomy. The study did not answer the question of whether valvotomy hindered or led to the development of valve calcification.

"UNNATURAL" HISTORY OF AORTIC STENOSIS—ADULTS

Many investigators have attempted to identify preoperative predictors of successful aortic valve replacement in the adult. Preoperative functional class II patients (N.Y.H.A. criteria) have been shown to have a five-year postsurgical survival rate of 70 percent in contrast to 40 percent for patients in class III or IV.[81] A higher surgical mortality is associated with preoperative myocardial disease, coexisting angina, and coronary artery disease.[71] Patients with a dominant left coronary artery have a higher risk of myocardial infarction during valve replacement, especially in the presence of coronary arteriosclerosis.[7]

Postoperative complications appear to occur most often in patients in whom the cardiothoracic ratio does not decrease after surgery. However, Hirschfeld and cowork-

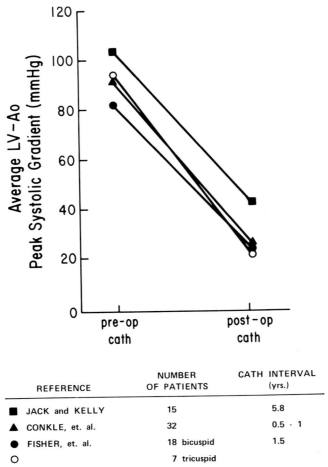

REFERENCE	NUMBER OF PATIENTS	CATH INTERVAL (yrs.)
■ JACK and KELLY	15	5.8
▲ CONKLE, et. al.	32	0.5 - 1
● FISHER, et. al.	18 bicuspid	1.5
○	7 tricuspid	

Figure 7. A composite of hemodynamic studies before and after aortic valvotomy in three clinical series.

ers[81] unexpectedly found that patients with normal-sized hearts before surgery (cardiothoracic ratio less than 0.45) were more likely candidates for sudden postoperative death than those with persistent cardiomegaly; perhaps an exceedingly thickened myocardium predisposed the former group to arrhythmias.

Aortic valve replacement carries an early operative mortality (up to 30 days) of 5 to 15 percent. Early deaths have been attributed to cardiac and noncardiac complications, including technical problems, hemorrhage, thromboembolism, arrhythmias and low cardiac output. Endocarditis occurs in 4 percent of patients after aortic valve replacement. The occurrence of endocarditis soon after operation is associated with a 79 percent mortality rate; after 60 days this drops to 35 percent.[82]

Postoperative mortality is highest in the first two years after surgery. The leading cause of late mortality is sudden death. A 27 percent, nine-year mortality in patients who underwent aortic valve replacement was reported by Barnhorst and coworkers,[83] versus a 78 percent mortality after nine years of medical treatment, reported by Rapaport.[64] Surgical survival also exceeds medical survival in those patients with severe myocardial fiber degeneration secondary to aortic stenosis. In addition to prolonged survival, surgery results in a significant improvement in functional class. Most of the 113 patients operated upon by Behrendt and Austen[84] were class III preoperatively; after operation 72 percent were class I and 28 percent were in class II.

Schuler and associates[85] have recently evaluated temporal changes in left ventricular function and hypertrophy after aortic valve replacement for pressure overload. Serial echocardiograms were obtained before and after aortic valve replacement on 22 subjects with no significant coronary atherosclerosis. Early followup was at 1 week, late followup between 2 and 6 months, and long-term followup at 7 to 20 months. Left ventricular muscle cross-sectional area was calculated from end-diastolic diameter and posterior wall thickness. Before surgery posterior wall thickness and cross-sectional area averaged 1.3 ± 0.09 cm. and 26.0 ± 2.1 cm.², respectively, and were not significantly different at early followup, while Δ D/end diastolic dimension (EDD) and ejection fraction fell insignificantly from 38 ± 4 percent and 66 ± 6 percent to 32 ± 4 percent and 59 ± 5 percent, respectively, and velocity of circumferential fiber shortening was unchanged at 1.2 circumferences per second. By late followup posterior wall thickness had fallen to 1.1 ± 0.06 cm. (p < 0.05), cross-sectional area to 20.8 ± 1.3 (p < 0.05), and Δ D/EDD, ejection fraction, and circumferential fiber shortening returned to preoperative levels. At the long-term followup posterior wall thickness and cross-sectional area had not changed significantly from late followup measurements, but Δ D/EDD (48.5 ± 4.2 percent), mean circumferential fiber shortening (1.5 ± 0.07 circumferences/second), and ejection fraction (75.6 ± 2.3 percent) had improved (p < 0.05) with respect to preoperative values.

The study concluded that significant regression of hypertrophy is confined to the first six months after aortic valve replacement, and although Δ D/EDD and ejection fraction tend to decline immediately postoperatively, by later long-term followup there is improvement in left ventricular function. Thus, intervention should be undertaken when myocardial performance is still normal and left ventricular hypertrophy is reversible. Further investigation in the area of myocardial adaptation is necessary and may help assure optimal surgical results following aortic valve replacement.

REFERENCES

1. ROBERTS, W C: *The congenitally bicuspid aortic valve—a study of 85 autopsy cases.* Am. J. Cardiol. 26:72,1970.

2. BRAUNWALD, E. GOLDBLATT, A. AYGEN, M. M., ET AL.: *Congenital aortic stenosis. I: Clinical and hemodynamic findings in 100 patients.* Circulation 27:426,1963.

3. LEES, M. H., HAUCH, A. J., STARKEY, G. B., ET AL.: *Congenital aortic stenosis. Operative indications and surgical results.* Br. Heart J. 24:31,1962.

4. NADAS, A. S., HAUWERT, L., VAN DER HAUGH, A. J., ET AL.: *Combined aortic and pulmonic stenosis.* Circulation 25:346,1962.

5. TAWES, R. L. JR., BERRY, C. L., AND ABERDEEN, E.: *Congenital bicuspid aortic valve associated with coarctation of the aorta in children.* Br. Heart J. 31:127,1969.

6. HIGGINS, E. B., AND WEXLER,, L.: *Reversal of dominance of the coronary arterial system in isolated ortic stenosis and bicuspid aortic valve.* Circulation 52:292,1975.

7. MURPHY, E. S., ROSCH, J., AND RAHIMTOOLA, S. H.: *Frequency and significance of coronary arterial dominance in isolated aortic stenosis.* Am. J. Cardiol. 39:505,1977.

8. NORA, J. J., AND NORA, A. H.: *Recurrence risks in children having one parent with a congenital heart disease.* Circulation 53:701,1976.

9. FENOGLIO, J. J., McALLISTER, H. A., JR., DeCASTRO, C. M., ET AL.: *Congenital bicuspid aortic valve after age 20.* Am. J. Cardiol 39:164,1977.

10. ROBERTS, W. C.: *Anatomically isolated aortic valvular disease—the case against its being of rheumatic etiology.* Am. J. Med. 49:151,1970.

11. EDWARDS, J. E.: *Calcific aortic stenosis: pathologic features.* Proc. Mayo Clin. 36:444,1961.

12. BERNHARD, W. F., KEANE, J. F., FELLOWS, K. E., ET AL.: *Progress and problems in the surgical management of congenital aortic stenosis.* J. Thorac. Cardiovasc. Surg. 66:404,1973.

13. CAMPBELL, M.: *The natural history of congenital aortic stenosis.* Br. Heart J. 30:514,1968.

14. EDWARDS, J. E.: *The congenital bicuspid aortic valve.* Circulation 23:485,1961.

15. STEIN, P. D., SABBAH, H. N., AND PITHA, J. V.: *Continuing disease process of calcific aortic stenosis—role of microthrombi and turbulent flow.* Am. J. Cardiol. 39:159,1977.

16. MARON, B. J., FERRANS, V. J., AND ROBERTS, W. C.: *Myocardial ultrastructure in patients with chronic aortic valve disease.* Am. J. Cardiol. 35:725,1975.

17. BISHOP, S., FRANKLIN, D., ROSS, J., FR., ET AL.: *Ultrastructural alterations of hypertrophied canine left ventricular subendocardium.* Circulation 50 (Suppl. III):13,1974.

18. SIMON, H., KRAYENBUEHL, H. P., RUTISHAUSER, W., ET AL.: *The contractile state of the hypertrophied left ventricular myocardium in aortic stenosis.* Am. Heart J. 79:587,1970.

19. SPANN, J. F., BUCCINO, R. A., SONNENBLICK, E. H., ET AL.: *Contractile state of cardiac muscle obtained from cats with experimentally produced ventricular hypertrophy and heart failure.* Circ. Res. 21:341,1967.

20. SASAYAMA, S., ROSS, J., JR., FRANKLIN, D., ET AL.: *Adaptations of the left ventricle to chronic pressure overload.* Circ. Res. 38:172,1976.

21. WILLIAMS, J. F., JR., AND POTTER, R. D.: *Normal contractile state of hypertrophied myocardium after pulmonary artery constriction in the cat.* J. Clin. Invest. 54:1266,1974.

22. JOHNSON, A. D., ENGLER, R. L., LeWINTER, M., ET AL.: *The medical and surgical management of patients with aortic valve disease—A symposium—University of California, San Diego, and San Diego Veteran's Administration Hospital (Specialty Conference).* West. J. Med. 126:460,1977.

23. LEWIS, A. L., HEYMANN, M. A., STANGER, P., ET AL.: *Evaluation of subendocardial ischemia in valvar aortic stenosis in children.* Circulation 49:978,1974.

24. MARK, A. L., KIOSCHOS, J. M., ABBOUD, F. M., ET AL.: *Abnormal vascular response to exercise in patients with aortic stenosis.* J. Clin. Invest. 52:1138,1973.

25. JOHNSON, A. M.: *Aortic stenosis, sudden death and left ventricular baroreceptors.* Br. Heart J. 33:1,1971.

26. FRIEDMAN, W. F., AND PAPPELBAUM, S. J.: *Indications for hemodynamic evaluation and surgery in congenital aortic stenosis.* Pediatr. Clin. North Amer. 18:1207,1971.

27. FRIEDMAN, W. F., AND KIRKPATRICK, S. E.: *Congenital aortic stenosis: valvular, discrete subvalvular, idiopathic hypertrophic subaortic, and supravalvular.* In Moss, A. J., AND ADAMS, F. H. (EDS.): *Heart Disease in Infants, Children, and Adolescents,* ed. 2. Williams & Wilkins, Baltimore, in press.

28. FRIEDMAN, W. F.: *Congenital aortic valve disease: natural history, indications and results of surgery,* In GOLDBERG, H., AND MORSE, D. (EDS.): *Important Topics in Congenital, Valvular, and Coronary Artery Disease.* Futura Publishing, Mt. Kisco, N. Y., 1975, p. 43.

29. BRAVERMAN, I. B., AND GIBSON, S.: *The outlook for children with congenital aortic stenosis.* Am. Heart J. 53:478,1957.

30. DOWNING, D. F.: *Congenital aortic stenosis: Clinical aspects and surgical treatment.* Circulation 14:188,1956.

31. MARQUIS, R. M., AND LOGAN, R.: *Congenital aortic stenosis and its surgical treatment.* Br. Heart J. 17:373,1955.

32. MORROW, A. G., GOLDBLATT, A., AND BRAUNWALD, E.: *Congenital aortic stenosis, II. Surgical treatment and the results of operation.* Circulation 27:426,1963.

33. ONGLEY, P. A., NADAS, A. S., PAUL, M. H., ET AL.: *Aortic stenosis in infants and children.* Pediatrics 21:207,1958.

34. REYNOLDS, J. L., NADAS, A. S., RULDOLPH, A. M., ET AL.: *Critical congenital aortic stenosis with minimal electrocardiographic changes.* N. Engl. J. Med. 262:276,1960.

35. GLEW, R. H., VARGHESE, P. J., KROVETZ, L. J., ET AL.: *Sudden death in congenital aortic stenosis.* Am. Heart J. 78:615,1969.

36. PECKHAM, G. B., KEITH, J. D., AND EVANS, J. R.: *Congenital aortic stenosis: Some observations on the natural history and clinical assessment.* Can. Med. Assoc. J. 91:639,1964.

37. LAMBERT, E. C., MENON, V. A., WAGNER, H. R., ET AL.: *Sudden unexpected death from cardiovascular disease in children. A cooperative international study.* Am. J. Cardiol. 34:89,1974.

38. DOYLE, E. F., ARUMUGHAM, P., LARA, E. ET AL.: *Sudden death in young patients with congenital aortic stenosis.* Pediatrics 53:481,1974.

39. GERSONY, W. M., AND HAYES, C. J.: *Bacterial endocarditis in patients with pulmonary stenosis, aortic stenosis, or ventricular septal defect.* Circulation 56 (Suppl. I):84,1977.

40. GAMBOA, R. HUGENHOLTZ, P. G., AND NADAS, A. S.: *Accuracy of the phonocardiogram in assessing severity of aortic and pulmonic stenosis.* Circulation 30:35,1964.

41. GLANCY, D. L., AND EPSTEIN, S. E.: *Differential diagnosis of type and severity of obstruction to left ventricular outflow.* Prog. Cardiovasc. Dis. 14:153,1971.

42. CHANDRAMOULI, B., EHMKE, D. A., AND LAUER, R. M.: *Exercise-induced electrocardiographic changes in children with congenital aortic stenosis.* J. Pediatr. 87:725,1975.

43. HALLORAN, K. H.: *A telemetered exercise electrocardiogram in congenital aortic stenosis.* Pediatrics 47:31,1971.

44. HUGENHOLTZ, P. G., LEES, M. M., AND NADAS, A. S.: *The scalar electrocardiogram, vectorcardiogram, and exercise electrocardiogram in the assessment of congenital aortic stenosis.* Circulation 26:79,1962.

45. NANDA, N. C., GRAMIAK, R., SHAH, P. M., ET AL.: *Echocardiography in the diagnosis of idiopathic hypertrophic subaortic stenosis coexisting with aortic valve disease.* Circulation 50:752,1974.

46. WILLIAMS, D. E., SAHN, D. J., AND FRIEDMAN, W. F.: *Cross-sectional echocardiographic localization of the sites of left ventricular outflow tract obstruction.* Am. J. Cardiol. 37:250,1976.

47. NANDA, N. C., GRAMIAK, R., MANNING, J., ET AL.: *Echocardiographic recognition of the congenital bicuspid aortic valve.* Circulation 49:870,1974.

48. RADFORD, D. J., BLOOM, K. R., IZUKAWA, T., ET AL.: *Echocardiographic assessment of bicuspid aortic valves: angiographic and pathological correlates.* Circulation 53:80,1976.

49. WEYMAN, A. E., FEIGENBAUM, H., HURWITZ, R. A., ET AL.: *Cross-sectional echocardiographic assessment of the severity of aortic stenosis in children.* Circulation 55:773,1977.

50. CHANG, S., CLEMENTS, S., AND CHANG, W.: *Aortic stenosis: echocardiographic cusp separation and surgical description of the aortic valve in 22 patients.* Am. J. Cardiol. 39:499,1977.

51. GLANZ, S., SELLENBRAND, W. E., BERMAN, M. A., ET AL.: *Echocardiographic assessment of the severity of aortic stenosis in children and adolescents.* Am. J. Cardiol. 38:620,1976.

52. ELLISON, R. C., WAGNER, H. R., WEIDMAN, W. H., ET AL.: *Congenital valvular aortic stenosis: Clinical detection of small pressure gradient.* Am. J. Cardiol. 37:757,1976.

53. GORLIN, R., AND GORLIN, S. G.: *Hydraulic formula for calculation of area of stenotic mitral valve, other cardiac valves, and central circulatory shunts.* Am. Heart J. 41:1,1951.

54. EL-SAID, G., GALIOTO, F. M., JR., MULLINS, C. E., ET AL.: *Natural hemodynamic history of congenital aortic stenosis in childhood.* Am. J. Cardiol. 30:6,1972.

55. BANDY, G. E., AND VOGEL, J. H. K.: *Progressive congenital valvular aortic stenosis.* Chest 60:189,1971.

56. BENTIVOGLIO, L. G., SAGARMINAGA, J., URICCHIO, J., ET AL.: *Congenital bicuspid aortic valve: A clinical and hemodynamic study.* Br. Heart J. 22:321,1960.

57. HOHN, A. R., VANPRAAGH, S., MOORE, A. A. D., ET AL.: *Aortic stenosis.* Circulation 31–32 (Suppl. III): 4,1965.

58. HURWITZ, R. A.: *Valvar aortic stenosis in childhood: Clinical and hemodynamic history.* J. Pediatr. 82:228,1973.

59. MODY, M. R., AND MODY, G. T.: *Serial hemodynamic observations in congenital valvular and subvalvular aortic stenosis.* Am. Heart J. 89:137,1975.

60. FRIEDMAN, W. F., MODLINGER, J., AND MORGAN, J.: *Serial hemodynamic observations in asymptomatic children with valvar aortic stenosis.* Circulation 43:91,1971.

61. COHEN, L. S., FRIEDMAN, W. F., AND BRAUNWALD, E.: *Natural history of mild congenital aortic stenosis elucidated by serial hemodynamic studies.* Am. J. Cardiol. 30:1,1972.

62. ROSS, J., FR., AND BRAUNWALD, E.: *Aortic stenosis.* Circulation 61 (Suppl. V): 37,1968.

63. FRANK, S., JOHNSON, A., AND ROSS, J., JR.: *Natural history of valvular aortic stenosis.* Br. Heart J. 35: 41,1973.

64. RAPAPORT, E.: *Natural history of aortic and mitral valve disease.* Am. J. Cardiol. 35: 221,1975.

65. ANDERSON, M. W., KELSEY, J. R., JR., AND EDWARDS, J. E.: *Clinical and pathological considerations in cases of calcific aortic stenosis.* JAMA 149:9,1952.

66. NAKIB, A., LILLEHEI, C. W., AND EDWARDS, J. E.: *The degree of coronary atherosclerosis in aortic valvular disease.* Arch. Pathol. 80:517,1965.

67. PAQUAY, P. A., ANDERSON, G., DIEFENTHAL, H., ET AL,: *Chest pain as a predictor of coronary artery disease in patients with obstructive aortic valve disease.* Am. J. Cardiol. 38:863,1976.

68. HARRIS, C. N., KAPLAN, M. A., PARKER, D. P., ET AL.: *Aortic stenosis, angina and coronary artery disease.* Br. Heart J. 37:656,1975.

69. HANCOCK, E. W.: *Clinical assessment of coronary artery disease in patients with aortic stenosis.* Am. J. Cardiol. 35:142,1975.

70. BERNDT, T. B., HANCOCK, E. W., SHUMWAY, N. E., ET AL.: *Aortic valve replacement with and without coronary artery bypass surgery.* Circulation 50:967,1974.

71. LINHART, J. W., DE LA TORRE, A., RAMSEY, H. W., ET AL.: *The significance of coronary artery disease in aortic valve replacement.* J. Thorac. Cardiovasc. Surg. 55:811,1968.

72. CAULFIED, W. H., DeLON, A. C., JR, PERLOFF, J. K., ET AL.: *The clinical significance of the fourth heart sound in aortic stenosis*. Am. J. Cardiol. 38:179,1971.

73. KAVALIER, M. A., STEWART, J., AND TAVEL, M. E.: *The apical A wave versus the fourth heart sound in assessing the severity of aortic stenosis*. Circulation 51: 324,1975.

74. BONNER, A. J., JR., SACKS, H. N., AND TAVEL, M. E.: *Assessing the severity of aortic stenosis by phonocardiography and external carotid pulse recordings*. Circulation 48:247,1973.

75. CHEITLIN, M., GERTZ, E., BRUNDAGE, B., ET AL.: *The rate of progression of aortic stenosis in the adult*. Personal Communication.

76. GRADMAN, A. H., AND HANCOCK, E. W.: *Progressive aortic stenosis*. Circulation 53–54 (Suppl. II):104,1976.

77. CONKLE, D. M., JONES, M., AND MORROW, A. G.: *Treatment of congenital aortic stenosis. An evaluation of the late results of aortic valvotomy*. Arch. Surg. 107: 649,1973.

78. FISHER, R. D., MASON, D. T., AND MORROW, A. G.: *Results of operative treatment in congenital aortic stenosis*. J. Thorac. Cardiovasc. Surg. 59:218,1970.

79. SHACKLETON, J. EDWARDS, F. R., BICKFORD, B. J. ET AL.: *Long-term followup of congenital aortic stenosis after surgery*. Br. Heart J. 34:47,1972.

80. JACK, W. D., AND KELLY, D. T.: *Long-term followup of valvulotomy for congenital aortic stenosis*. Am. J. Cardiol. 38:231,1976.

81. HIRSCHFELD, J. W., JR., EPSTEIN, S. E., ROBERTS, A. J., ET AL.: *Indices predicting long-term survival after valve replacement in patients with aortic regurgitation and patients with aortic stenosis*. Circulation 50:1190,1974.

82. KLOSTER, F. E.: *Diagnosis and management of complications of prosthetic heart valves*. Am. J. Cardiol. 35:872,1975.

83. BARNHORST, D. A., OXMAN, H. A., CONNELLY, D. C., ET AL.: *Isolated replacement of the aortic valve with the Starr-Edwards prosthesis*. J. Thorac. Cardiovasc. Surg. 70:113,1975.

84. BEHRENDT, D. M., AND AUSTEN, W. G.: *Current status of prosthetics for heart valve replacement*. Prog. Cardiovasc. Dis. 15:369,1973.

85. SCHULER, G., PETERSON, K., FRANCIS, G., ET AL.: *Temporal changes in left ventricular function and hypertrophy post-aortic valve replacement for pressure overload*. Am. J. Cardiol. 39:300,1977.

Clinical Course of Patients
with Hypertrophic Cardiomyopathy

Barry J. Maron, M.D., and Stephen E. Epstein, M.D.

Hypertrophic cardiomyopathy is a disease of cardiac muscle that is usually genetically transmitted as an autosomal-dominant trait[1] and characterized by disproportionate thickening of the ventricular septum with respect to the left ventricular free wall.[2-7] Several studies from institutions in the United States, Canada, and England have provided a vast amount of information regarding the clinical course and natural history of patients with this disease.[8-14] However, recent advances in diagnosis (particularly by echocardiography)[2-4,7] and in the medical[15-23] or operative treatment[24-27] of hypertrophic cardiomyopathy reveal that the "natural history" of this disease is more complex than previously thought. This chapter reviews the prognosis of hypertrophic cardiomyopathy and the more recent concepts of the clinical course of the disease in adults.

AVAILABLE DATA ON THE CLINICAL COURSE
OF PATIENTS WITH HYPERTROPHIC CARDIOMYOPATHY

It is worthwhile to emphasize at the onset a number of points concerning published data on the clinical course of hypertrophic cardiomyopathy. First, because of the introduction of β-adrenergic blocking agents (particularly propranolol) and septal myotomy-myectomy (or myotomy) in the treatment of hypertrophic cardiomyopathy we can no longer speak of the "natural history" of this disease, and can refer only to its *clinical course*. In addition, the widespread utilization of these modes of therapy since the mid-1960s has often made it difficult to separate the natural consequences of the disease from the effects of therapy. Indeed, the only available comprehensive study concerned primarily with the true natural history of hypertrophic cardiomyopathy is that of Frank and Braunwald[14] from the National Institutes of Health, which was assembled before the time of widespread use of propranolol in the treatment of this disease.

Second, the advent of echocardiography in the early 1970s as a routine diagnostic procedure provided an extremely powerful noninvasive method of identifying patients with hypertrophic cardiomyopathy.[2-4] Echocardiography has also alerted us to the fact that a comprehensive understanding of the clinical course of hypertrophic cardiomyopathy cannot be based solely on information derived from patients diagnosed in the 1960s. The reason for this is that echocardiography has made it possible to detect many patients within the disease spectrum of hypertrophic cardiomyopathy who otherwise would not have been recognized, i.e., primarily those patients without obstruction to left ventricular outflow and with minimal symptoms or no symptoms at all.[3] The clinical course of these patients will not be known for many years since they have been followed for a maximum of only five years. In this regard it is important to emphasize that the available studies on the clinical course of hypertrophic cardiomyopathy (which were all based on data derived before the advent of echocardiography) have either excluded patients without obstruction to left ventricular outflow by design[8,9,11] or include only a few such patients.[12,14] Hence, our current knowledge of the clinical course of hypertrophic cardiomyopathy pertains in large measure to those patients with marked obstruction to left ventricular outflow, i.e., typical idiopathic hypertrophic subaortic stenosis (IHSS).

Third, an attempt has been made in this review to amalgamate the data on the clinical course of patients with hypertrophic cardiomyopathy from several studies.[8-14] Such an analysis of a large number of patients has the theoretical advantage of enhancing the reliability of the observations made in each of the individual studies. However, this approach is limited by the fact that the clinical data has been drawn from six medical centers, each with inherently different patient referral patterns and different approaches to the medical and operative management of patients. For example, the five largest published studies on the clinical course of hypertrophic cardiomyopathy include one from the National Institutes of Health,[14] one from Toronto General Hospital,[11] two from Hammersmith Hospital (two years apart),[8,12] and one which is a collaborative study[9] including updated information from both Hammersmith and Toronto as well as from the University of Rochester and the University of Minnesota.

Finally, it should be pointed out that in none of these studies on the clinical course of hypertrophic cardiomyopathy did the average period of followup exceed five years. Hence, a relatively short period of observation forms our current concepts of the clinical course of this disease.

CLINICAL COURSE OF UNOPERATED PATIENTS WITH HYPERTROPHIC CARDIOMYOPATHY

Symptomatic Progression

As suggested earlier, assessment of the natural history of surviving patients with hypertrophic cardiomyopathy has become difficult because of the use of propranolol and operation in the treatment of these patients. Nevertheless, judging from available data, the true natural history of such patients is best described as *variable*. Although some patients progressively deteriorate or die, most remain essentially stable for many years; only rarely will a patient manifest spontaneous improvement.

The series reported by Frank and Braunwald[14] (assembled before the advent of propranolol) and that of Parker[13] both suggest that hypertrophic cardiomyopathy is a disease usually characterized by a relatively benign clinical course and slow progression. However, about 25 percent of the patients reported by Frank and Braunwald either deteriorated or died (Fig. 1). In contrast, Adelman and coworkers[11] considered hypertrophic cardiomyopathy to be more often a progressive disease; over 75 percent of their *untreated* patients either deteriorated or died and two thirds of the entire study group progressed to functional classes III or IV. These authors believed that left ventricular outflow obstruction and associated mitral regurgitation were the principal causes of symptoms early in the course of hypertrophic cardiomyopathy, but that the underlying myocardial disorder present in the disease was the major determinant of symptoms in the later stages. Goodwin[28-30] also showed that in a minority of patients, progression of disease may be associated with spontaneous loss of left ventricular outflow obstruction. Hence, it is evident that while hypertrophic cardiomyopathy is a

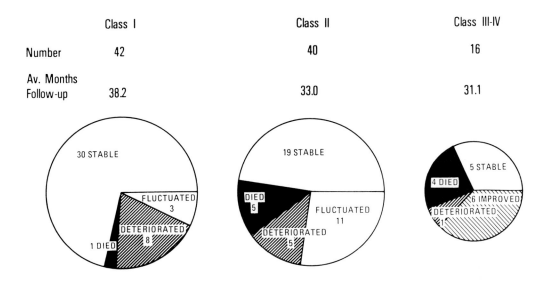

Figure 1. The clinical course of 98 patients with hypertrophic cardiomyopathy shown with regard to the functional classifications at the time of entry into the study. (From Frank and Braunwald,[14] by permission of the American Heart Association, Inc.)

disease which may result in symptomatic deterioration or sudden death, meaningful generalizations concerning the clinical course of such patients are, at this time, exceedingly difficult to make.

Although atrial fibrillation is a relatively uncommon complication in patients with hypertrophic cardiomyopathy, it is usually poorly tolerated and associated with clinical deterioration.[8,14,31,32] Whether such a rhythm disturbance reflects irreversible left ventricular dysfunction that ultimately causes death (i.e., progressive inflow resistance leading to left atrial enlargement which predisposes to atrial fibrillation), or is itself a primary cause of death, remains to be determined. However, regardless of which of these possibilities is most likely, atrial fibrillation appears to be an indicator of advanced disease in patients with hypertrophic cardiomyopathy.

Premature Death in Patients with Hypertrophic Cardiomyopathy

Premature cardiac death is not uncommon in patients with hypertrophic cardiomyopathy. Such deaths are usually sudden (87 percent of all cardiac deaths in one study[9]); however, death may also occur in the setting of chronic, progressive congestive heart failure.

The frequency of premature cardiac death in unoperated patients (diagnosed before the use of echocardiography) with hypertrophic cardiomyopathy has been reported by certain centers as about 3 percent per year[8,9] (Fig. 2). Our experience with 35 patients whose hypertrophic cardiomyopathy was first identified during childhood was similar.[10] Almost one third of these patients died suddenly after an average followup period of 7.4 years (annual mortality of about 4 percent per year); another 30 percent had deteriorated during this period (Fig. 3).

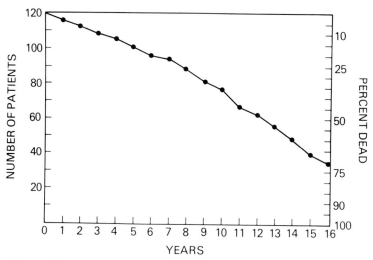

Figure 2. Mortality rate of 119 patients with hypertrophic cardiomyopathy plotted as a function of time in the study. (Adapted from Hardarson et al.[8])

Since sudden death is a relatively common sequela of hypertrophic cardiomyopathy, it is obviously important to identify those patients who are at risk for premature death. Unfortunately, no clinical parameter (i.e., age at onset of symptoms, sex, family history, symptomatic status, magnitude of left ventricular outflow gradient or left ventricular end-diastolic pressure, or electrocardiographic abnormalities) has proved consistently useful in this regard. Hardarson and coworkers[8] suggested that patients who were symptomatic at younger ages (<20 years) had higher mortality earlier in life than those patients who became symptomatic later in life, but this has not been confirmed by other investigators.[11,14] Swan and coworkers[12] suggested that elevated left ventricular end-diastolic pressure (LVEDP) was a poor prognostic sign in patients with hypertrophic cardiomyopathy, particularly in children without outflow obstruction. However, their data does not strongly support this conclusion since LVEDP was normal in one of the five patients in the study who died and was only mildly elevated in another. Also,

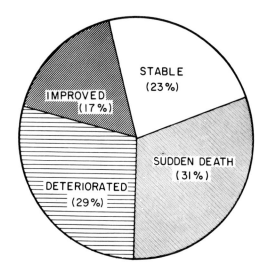

Figure 3. Clinical course of 35 patients with hypertrophic cardiomyopathy initially identified during childhood. (From Maron et al.[10] by permission of the American Heart Association, Inc.)

256

poor prognosis for patients with elevated LVEDP per se has not been confirmed by other studies.[10,33]

Recent studies have suggested that moderate to marked ventricular septal thickening measured by echocardiography or at necropsy, particularly when it is associated with a distinctly abnormal electrocardiogram, may identify patients at increased risk for sudden death whether or not they are symptomatic. We have evaluated 26 patients with hypertrophic cardiomyopathy in whom death was the first manifestation of cardiac disease.[33] Ages ranged from 8 to 49 years (mean 18 years) and 23 patients were under 25. All of the patients whose hearts could be examined had disproportionate thickening of the ventricular septum with respect to the left ventricular free wall; septal-free wall thickness ratios were markedly abnormal and ranged from 1.3 to 2.7 (median 1.9) (Fig. 4). Absolute ventricular septal thicknesses ranged from 17 to 55 mm. (median 25 mm.); in all but two patients septal thickness was ≥ 20 mm.—an 11-year-old (17 mm.) and a 12-year-old (18 mm.). Furthermore, the electrocardiogram was distinctly abnormal in each of the 19 patients studied before death and most commonly showed, alone or in combination, left ventricular hypertrophy, S-T segment and T wave abnormalities, and deep Q waves. Of the 26 patients, 13 had died during or immediately after moderate or severe physical exertion. No particular hemodynamic state was characteristic of the study group. In 6 of 12 patients studied hemodynamically, left ventricular outflow gradients of ≥ 50 mm. Hg were present under basal conditions (Fig. 5). In the remaining 6 patients, either no outflow gradient or a small gradient of ≤ 20 mm. Hg was present. Left ventricular end-diastolic pressure was elevated (> 12 mm. Hg) in 9 patients and normal in 3 others.

In another study we found that premature death occurred with particular frequency in certain families with hypertrophic cardiomyopathy,[34] suggesting that they have a

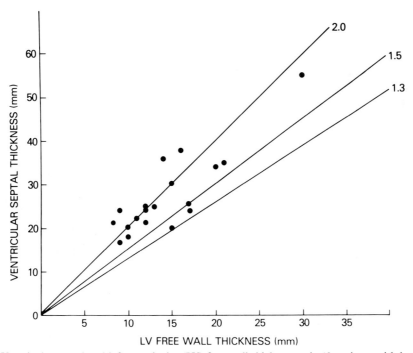

Figure 4. Ventricular septal and left ventricular (LV) free wall thicknesses in 19 patients with hypertrophic cardiomyopathy whose only manifestation of cardiac disease was death. Identity lines define septal–free wall ratios of 1.3, 1.5, and 2.0. (From Maron et al.[33] with permission of the American Journal of Cardiology.)

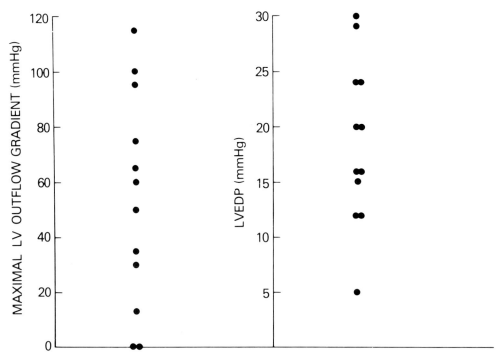

Figure 5. Left ventricular (LV) outflow gradients (maximal under basal conditions or with provocation) and left ventricular end-diastolic pressures (LVEDP) in patients with hypertrophic cardiomyopathy whose initial manifestation of cardiac disease was sudden death. (From Maron et al.[33] with permission of the American Journal of Cardiology.)

particularly virulent expression of the disease. To date, eight such families with "malignant" hypertrophic cardiomyopathy have been identified (Fig. 6). A total of 69 first-degree relatives in these families were studied; 41 relatives had evidence of hypertrophic cardiomyopathy and 31 (75 percent) of these subjects died from their heart disease (Fig. 7). Of these 31 patients 18 were under 25 years of age, and 23 experienced

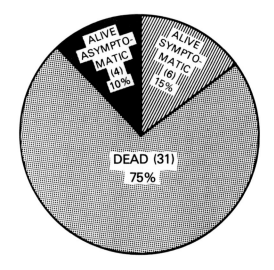

Figure 6. Diagram summarizing clinical outcome of 41 first-degree relatives in eight families with "malignant" hypertrophic cardiomyopathy. Number of patients in each subgroup are shown in parentheses. (From Maron et al.[34] with permission of the American Journal of Cardiology.)

258

FAMILY C.

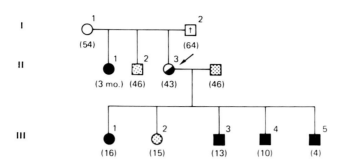

FAMILY Mo.

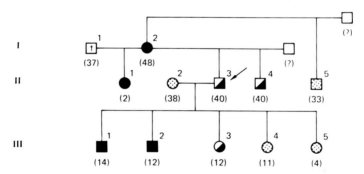

Figure 7. Pedigrees of two families with "malignant" hypertrophic cardiomyopathy (C. and Mo.). † = propositus; solid symbols = death probably or definitely due to hypertrophic cardiomyopathy; half-filled symbols = alive with an echocardiogram that was diagnostic of hypertrophic cardiomyopathy (i.e., showed asymmetric septal hypertrophy, ASH); clear symbols = echocardiogram was not obtained; † = death from noncardiac cause or cardiac disease other than hypertrophic cardiomyopathy; stippled symbols = alive, ASH not present on echocardiogram; round symbols = female; square symbols = male. Patient ages are shown in parentheses below symbols. (From Maron et al.[34] with permission of the American Journal of Cardiology.)

sudden death. The remaining eight patients died of chronic cardiac illnesses characterized by congestive heart failure, atrial fibrillation, or thromboembolic events. Of note: ventricular septal thickness in those family members who died was, on the average, significantly greater than in surviving family members: 26 ± 2 mm. versus 19 ± 1 mm.; $p < 0.02$ (Fig. 8). Furthermore, 11 of the 13 patients with ventricular septal thickness of ≥ 20 mm. died and the two surviving patients are symptomatic. Conversely, only 4 of 11 relatives with septal thickness of < 20 mm. died. Hence, *premature (particularly sudden) death may occur at almost any age, in either sex, and regardless of whether or not symptoms have been present.* Moderate to marked ventricular septal thickening may identify patients at increased risk for sudden death, particularly when associated with a distinctly abnormal electrocardiogram and a family history of multiple premature deaths.

259

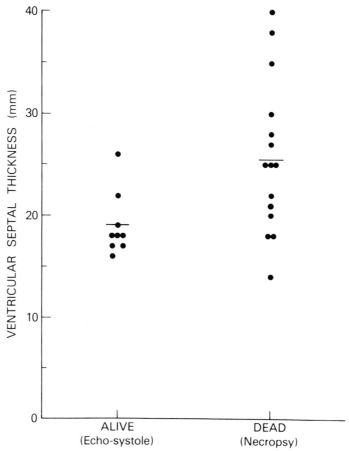

Figure 8. Ventricular septal thicknesses obtained in 9 surviving affected family members by echocardiography (echo) compared to those obtained at necropsy in 15 relatives who had died. Echocardiographic measurements shown were obtained in systole to permit comparison with necropsy measurements. Short horizontal lines indicate mean values for each group. (From Maron et al.[34] with permission of the American Journal of Cardiology.)

Role of Propranolol in the Treatment of Patients with Hypertrophic Cardiomyopathy

β-adrenergic blockers were introduced in the mid-1960s for the treatment of hypertrophic cardiomyopathy and have been used extensively in such patients over the past decade.[15-23] Administered acutely to patients with hypertrophic cardiomyopathy, β-adrenergic blocking agents such as propranolol reduce left ventricular outflow obstruction when sympathetic activity is high, i.e., during exercise or with the infusion of isoproterenol, but have little or no effect on left ventricular outflow tract obstruction at rest.[17,18,35,36] These differences are readily understood when it is recalled that under basal conditions sympathetic tone is absent or minimal[37] and therefore blocking sympathetic activity to the heart is without effect. On the other hand, an increase in sympathetic activity augments left ventricular outflow obstruction; hence, blocking sympathetic activity under these circumstances will reduce the outflow obstruction. Although propranolol does relieve symptoms in patients with hypertrophic cardiomyopathy [13,15-17,23] there are, unfortunately, no reliable studies regarding the efficacy of propranolol in altering the long-term symptomatic course of patients with hypertrophic cardiomyopathy. In addition, it is clear that β-adrenergic blockade does not *prevent* symptomatic deterioration; some patients who show an early impressive benefit from propranolol experience symptomatic deterioration months to years later.[21,22]

Nevertheless, while propranolol may not prevent disease progression in patients with hypertrophic cardiomyopathy, it is at this time the most effective agent available for symptomatic therapy. Thus, an adequate therapeutic trial of propranolol should be employed in any severely symptomatic patient with marked left ventricular outflow obstruction before surgery is recommended.

The utilization of propranolol prophylactically in the hope of preventing progression of the disease process or the occurrence of sudden death in asymptomatic or mildly symptomatic patients with hypertrophic cardiomyopathy has also been considered. Goodwin and Oakley[29] have recommended the use of β-adrenergic blockers for all patients with hypertrophic cardiomyopathy as soon as the diagnosis is made and regardless of the degree of symptomatic limitation or the presence or absence of outflow obstruction. It should be emphasized, however, that patients may die suddenly and unexpectedly while taking apparently adequate dosages of propranolol. Indeed, in one study[9] over 15 percent of patients reported to be taking propranolol died suddenly, although many of those patients (and others cited in the literature) received dosages that would now be considered inadequate.

The collaborative study by Shah and coworkers[9] showed no difference between the prevalence of sudden death in those patients treated with propranolol and those who were untreated. However, well controlled prospective studies have not, as yet, been performed to determine definitively how many patients at risk of sudden death do not die *because* they are taking propranolol. Therefore, the available data are inconclusive regarding the potential efficacy of propranolol in preventing or delaying disease progression in patients with hypertrophic cardiomyopathy. Hence, we prefer to limit our prophylactic use of propranolol to asymptomatic or mildly symptomatic patients who are members of families with "malignant" hypertrophic cardiomyopathy, and to patients who demonstrate marked ventricular septal thickening (by echocardiography) and a distinctly abnormal electrocardiogram.

CLINICAL COURSE OF OPERATED PATIENTS WITH HYPERTROPHIC CARDIOMYOPATHY

The role of operation in the management of severely symptomatic patients with obstructive hypertrophic cardiomyopathy is a controversial issue. The theoretical objections to operation in this disease have been proposed by Parker[13] and by Goodwin and Oakley:[29,38]

1. The primary cause of functional limitation is the cardiomyopathic component of the disease and operation will not alter the basic pathology or natural history of the condition.

2. Poor left ventricular compliance, as indicated by elevated left ventricular end-diastolic pressure, plays a major role in the patient's disability. Since operative procedures are designed primarily to relieve left ventricular outflow tract obstruction, the left ventricular end-diastolic pressure may not be altered or may actually increase.

3. Reduction of the left ventricular outflow obstruction through operation is really the result of further compromise of left ventricular function, a mechanism that has been noted in some patients during the natural progression of their disease.

4. Abolition of the left ventricular outflow gradient may result from damage inflicted on the left ventricle as a result of operation; hence, reduction of the gradient actually reflects reduced left ventricular contractile force and increased failure.

261

Despite these considerations a number of operative procedures have been proposed for patients with obstructive hypertrophic cardiomyopathy.[39-46] The most successful of these techniques has been ventricular septal myotomy-myectomy[25-27] or myotomy.[24] The published results from four medical centers[24,25,27,47] using septal myotomy-myectomy or myotomy over the past 15 years have been excellent, i.e., the vast majority of patients have shown distinct symptomatic and hemodynamic benefit following operation. Such experience demonstrates a useful role for operation in the management of patients with hypertrophic cardiomyopathy.

The group of patients assembled at the National Heart, Lung, and Blood Institute (NHLBI) is the largest available series and as such is probably the most useful from the standpoint of evaluating the effect of operation on the long-term clinical course of patients with hypertrophic cardiomyopathy. Recently, the long-term postoperative status of all 124 patients who were operated on at NHLBI between 1960 and 1975 was reviewed (average period of followup, 5.2 years).[48] The vast majority of these patients were operated on for severe symptoms refractory to medical therapy. Eight percent of the patients died of causes related to operation. Postoperatively, the majority of survivors (about 90 percent) reported distinct symptomatic improvement during the first years, and virtually all patients in the study group manifested a marked reduction in left ventricular outflow gradient under basal conditions. However, operation did not entirely prevent progression of symptoms or fatal events; 12 percent of the patients had persistent (6 percent) or recurrent (6 percent) severe functional limitation and 9 percent died between seven months and 13 years after operation of causes related to hypertrophic cardiomyopathy (Fig. 9). Of the 11 late postoperative deaths, 6 were sudden (presumably due to a ventricular arrhythmia) and 5 occurred after chronic illnesses characterized by congestive heart failure. Such observations indicate that the car-

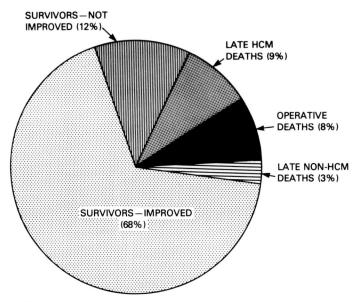

CLINICAL OUTCOME IN PATIENTS AFTER OPERATION FOR OBSTRUCTIVE HYPERTROPHIC CARDIOMYOPATHY

SURVIVORS—NOT IMPROVED (12%)

LATE HCM DEATHS (9%)

OPERATIVE DEATHS (8%)

LATE NON-HCM DEATHS (3%)

SURVIVORS—IMPROVED (68%)

Figure 9. Long-term clinical results in patients after operation for hypertrophic cardiomyopathy (HCM). (From Maron et al.[48] with permission of the American Heart Association, Inc.)

diomyopathic process inherent in all patients with hypertrophic cardiomyopathy can be one of the critical factors in determining ultimate prognosis. Hence, symptomatic deterioration, sudden death, and death from progressive congestive heart failure are not entirely eliminated by operative relief of the ventricular outflow tract obstruction, and may occur in a relatively small percentage of patients.

The overall annual mortality rate for the study group was 3.5 percent (including operative deaths and late postoperative deaths due to hypertrophic cardiomyopathy), but for late deaths alone it was only 1.8 percent. The latter statistic is lower than the average mortality rate (about 3 percent) reported for unoperated patients with obstructive hypertrophic cardiomyopathy.[8,9] Shah and coworkers[9] also noted a lower mortality rate in their patients who survived operation than in untreated patients and patients treated with propranolol. The conclusion implicit in these comparisons is that operation does not increase and may decrease long-term mortality. However, unoperated patients and operated patients can not be compared directly since those who undergo operation undoubtedly constitute a subgroup different from the unoperated patients. Hence, it is not possible at this time to determine definitively whether operation alters the longevity of patients with obstructive hypertrophic cardiomyopathy.

No preoperative or postoperative clinical, hemodynamic, or electrocardiographic parameter could identify those patients at risk for late postoperative death or poor long-term symptomatic result. However, virtually no severely symptomatic patients at the NHLBI with hypertrophic cardiomyopathy are excluded as operative candidates as long as obstruction to left ventricular outflow is present and the patient has not responded adequately to propranolol therapy. Therefore, some patients with important associated medical and cardiovascular problems are operated on. We have noted that those who died late postoperatively or were still severely symptomatic at long-term postoperative evaluation had significantly more of these associated medical or cardiovascular problems (e.g., chronic pulmonary disease, obesity, systemic hypertension, coronary heart disease, history of ventricular fibrillation, atrial fibrillation, habitual alcoholism, or severe congestive heart failure associated with pulmonary edema) than patients who survived and improved postoperatively. Hence, even better long-term postoperative results than those of our *total* population could be expected in symptomatic patients without any of the aforementioned preoperative complicating factors.

Further evidence that operation can objectively improve left ventricular function in patients with hypertrophic cardiomyopathy comes from two recent studies performed at our institution.[49,50] In an echocardiographic study of patients with obstructive hypertrophic cardiomyopathy before and after septal myotomy-myectomy, a significant decrease in left atrial size was noted in younger patients (under age 40).[49] In another study, enhanced cardiac performance during intense upright exercise—substantial increases in exercise capacity and peak oxygen consumption—was demonstrated in a majority of patients who had undergone septal myotomy-myectomy. These considerations strongly support our belief that operation is indicated for patients with obstructive hypertrophic cardiomyopathy who are severely symptomatic and whose symptoms do not respond satisfactorily to medical treatment with propranolol.

REFERENCES

1. CLARK, C. E., HENRY, W. L., AND EPSTEIN, S. E.: *Familial prevalence and genetic transmission of idiopathic hypertrophic subaortic stenosis.* N. Engl. J. Med. 289:709,1973.

2. HENRY, W. L., CLARK, C. E., AND EPSTEIN, S. E.: *Asymmetric septal hypertrophy (ASH): Echocardiographic identification of the pathognomonic anatomic abnormality of IHSS.* Circulation 47:225,1973.

3. EPSTEIN, S. E., HENRY, W. L., CLARK, C. E., ET AL.: *Asymmetric septal hypertrophy.* Ann. Intern. Med. 81:650,1974.

4. ABBASI, A. S., MACALPIN, R. N., EBER, L. M., ET AL.: *Left ventricular hypertrophy diagnosed by echocardiography.* N. Engl. J. Med. 289:118,1973.

5. MENGES, H., BRANDENBURG, R. O., AND BROWN, A. L.: *The clinical, hemodynamic and pathologic diagnosis of muscular subvalvular aortic stenosis.* Circulation 24:1126,1961.

6. ROBERTS, W. C.: *Valvular, subvalvular and supravalvular aortic stenosis: morphologic features.* Cardiovasc. Clin. 5(1):104,1973.

7. ABBASI, A. S., MACALPIN, R. N., EBER, L. M., ET AL.: *Echocardiographic diagnosis of idiopathic hypertrophic cardiomyopathy without outflow obstruction.* Circulation 46:897,1972.

8. HARDARSON, T., DE LA CALZADA, C. S., CURIEL, R., ET AL.: *Prognosis and mortality of hypertrophic obstructive cardiomyopathy.* Lancet 2:1462,1973.

9. SHAH, P. M., ADELMAN, A. G., WIGLE, E. D., ET AL.: *The natural (and unnatural) course of hypertrophic obstructive cardiomyopathy. A multicenter study.* Circ. Res. 34 and 35(Suppl. II):179,1973.

10. MARON, B. J., HENRY, W. L., CLARK, C. E., ET AL.: *Asymmetric septal hypertrophy in childhood.* Circulation 53:9,1976.

11. ADELMAN, A. G., WIGLE, E. D., RANGANATHAN, N., ET AL.: *The clinical course in muscular subaortic stenosis. A retrospective and prospective study of 60 hemodynamically proven cases.* Ann. Intern. Med. 77:515,1972.

12. SWAN, D. A., BELL, B., OAKLEY, C. M., ET AL.: *Analysis of the symptomatic course and prognosis and treatment of hypertrophic obstructive cardiomyopathy.* Br. Heart J. 33:671,1971.

13. PARKER, B. M.: *The course in idiopathic hypertrophic muscular subaortic stenosis.* Ann. Intern. Med. 70:903,1969.

14. FRANK, S., AND BRAUNWALD, E.: *Idiopathic hypertrophic subaortic stenosis. Clinical analysis of 126 patients with emphasis on the natural history.* Circulation 37:759,1968.

15. COHEN, L. S., AND BRAUNWALD, E.: *Amelioration of angina pectoris in idiopathic hypertrophic subaortic stenosis with β-adrenergic blockade.* Circulation 35:847,1967.

16. ROSENBLUM, R., FRIEDEN, J., DELMAN, A. J., ET AL.: *Long-term propranolol therapy in patients with idiopathic hypertrophic subaortic stenosis.* Circulation 36(Suppl. II):226,1967.

17. CHERIAN, G., BROCKINGTON, I. F., SHAH, P. M., ET AL.: *β-adrenergic blockade in hypertrophic obstructive cardiomyopathy.* Br. Med. J. 1:895,1966.

18. HARRISON, D. C., BRAUNWALD, E., GLICK, G., ET AL.: *Effects of β-adrenergic blockade on circulation with particular reference to observations in patients with hypertrophic subaortic stenosis.* Circulation 29:84,1964.

19. HUBNER, P. J. B., ZIADY, G. M., LANE, G. K., ET AL.: *Double-blind trial of propranolol and practolol in hypertrophic cardiomyopathy.* Br. Heart J. 35:1116,1973.

20. ADELMAN, A. G., SHAH, P. M., GRAMIAK, R., ET AL.: *Long-term propranolol therapy in muscular subaortic stenosis.* Br. Heart J. 32:804,1970.

21. SLOMAN, G.: *Propranolol in management of muscular subaortic stenosis.* Br. Heart J. 29:783,1967.

22. STENSON, R. E., FLAMM, M. D., HARRISON, D. C., ET AL.: *Hypertrophic subaortic stenosis. Clinical and hemodynamic effects of long-term propranolol therapy.* Am. J. Cardiol. 31:763,1973.

23. SCHEU, H., BOLLINGER, A., AND WIRZ, P.: *Medical treatment of idiopathic hypertrophic subaortic stenosis.* Cardiologia 49(Suppl. 2):43,1966.

24. BIGELOW, W. G., TRIMBLE, A. S., AUGER, P., ET AL.: *The ventriculomyotomy operation for muscular subaortic stenosis. A reappraisal.* J. Thorac. Cardiovasc. Surg. 52:514,1966.

25. MORROW, A. G., REITZ, B. A., EPSTEIN, S. E., ET AL.: *Operative treatment in hypertrophic subaortic stenosis: Techniques and the results of pre- and postoperative assessment in 83 patients.* Circulation 52:88,1975.

26. MORROW, A. G., FOGARTY, T. J., HANNAH, H., ET AL.: *Operative treatment in idiopathic hypertrophic subaortic stenosis. Techniques and the results of preoperative and postoperative clinical and hemodynamic assessments.* Circulation 37:589,1968.

27. AGNEW, T. M., BARRATT-BOYES, B. G., BRANDT, P. W. T., ET AL.: *Surgical resection in idiopathic hypertrophic subaortic stenosis with a combined approach through aorta and left ventricle.* J. Thorac. Cardiovasc. Surg. 74:307,1977.

28. GOODWIN, J. F.: *Prospects and predictions for the cardiomyopathies.* Circulation 50:210,1974.

29. GOODWIN, J. F., AND OAKLEY, C. M.: *The cardiomyopathies.* Br. Heart J. 34:545,1972.

30. GOODWIN, J. F.: *Clarification of the cardiomyopathies.* Mod. Concepts Cardiovasc. Dis. 41:41,1972.

31. GOODWIN, J. F.: *Congestive and hypertrophic cardiomyopathies: A decade of study.* Lancet 1:731,1970.

32. GLANCY, D. L., O'BRIEN, K. P., GOLD, H. K., ET AL.: *Atrial fibrillation in patients with idiopathic hypertrophic subaortic stenosis.* Br. Heart J. 32:652,1970.

33. MARON, B. J., ROBERTS, W. C., EDWARDS, J. E., ET AL.: *Sudden death in hypertrophic cardiomyopathy: Characterization of patients without previous functional limitation.* Am. J. Cardiol. 41:803,1978.

34. MARON, B. J., LIPSON, L. C., ROBERTS, W. C., ET AL.: *"Malignant" hypertrophic cardiomyopathy: Identification of a subgroup of families with unusually frequent premature deaths.* Am. J. Cardiol. 41:1133,1978.

35. GOODWIN, J. F., SHAH, P. M., OAKLEY, C. M., ET AL.: *The clinical pharmacology in hypertrophic obstructive cardiomyopathy.* In Wolstenholme, G. E. W., and O'Connor, M. (eds.): *CIBA Foundation Symposium: Cardiomyopathies,* Churchill, London, 1964, p. 189.

36. FLAMM, M. D., HARRISON, D. C., AND HANCOCK, E. W.: *Muscular subaortic stenosis. Prevention of outflow obstruction with propranolol.* Circulation 38:846,1968.

37. ROBINSON, B. F., EPSTEIN, S. E., BEISER, G. B., ET AL.: *Control of heart rate by the autonomic nervous system: Studies in man on the interrelation between baroreceptor mechanisms and exercise.* Circ. Res. 19:400,1966.

38. OAKLEY, C. M.: *Hypertrophic obstructive cardiomyopathy—patterns of progression.* In Wolstenholm, G. E. W., and O'Connor, M., (eds.): *CIBA Foundation Study Group No. 37: Hypertrophic Obstructive Cardiomyopathy,* Churchill, London, 1971, p. 9.

39. BENVENUTO, R., AND SERRATTO, M.: *Surgical aspects of idiopathic hypertrophic subaortic stenosis.* J. Cardiovasc. Surg. (Torino)7:389,1966.

40. JULIAN, O. G., DYE, W. S., JAVID, H., ET AL.: *Apical left ventriculotomy in subaortic stenosis due to a fibromuscular hypertrophy.* Circulation 31(Suppl. I):44,1965.

41. MEIJNE, N. G., AND LOSFKOOT, G.: *The surgical approach to the idiopathic hypertrophic subaortic stenosis via the left atrium.* J. Cardiovasc. Surg. (Torino) 8:284, 1967.

42 SHUMACKER, H.B., JR., AND KING, H.: *New operative approach in the management of hypertrophic subaortic stenosis.* J. Thorac. Cardiovasc. Surg. 49:497, 1965.

43. COOLEY, D. A., BLOODWELL, R. D., HALLMAN, G. L., ET AL.: *Surgical treatment of muscular subaortic stenosis. Results from septectomy in twenty-six patients.* Circulation 35(Suppl. I):124, 1967.

44. FRYE, R. L., KINCAID, O. W., SWAN, H. J. C., ET AL.: *Results of surgical treatment of patients with diffuse subvalvular aortic stenosis.* Circulation 32:52, 1965.

45. KELLY, D. T., BARRATT-BOYES, B. G., AND LOWE, J. B.: *Results of surgery and hemodynamic observations in muscular subaortic stenosis.* J. Thorac. Cardiovasc. Surg. 51:353, 1966.

46. COOLEY, D. A., LEACHMAN, R. D., AND WUKASCH, D. C.: *Diffuse muscular subaortic stenosis and surgical treatment.* Am. J. Cardiol. 31:1, 1973.

47. REIS, R. L., HANNAH, H., CARLEY, J. E., ET AL.: *Surgical treatment of idiopathic hypertrophic subaortic stenosis: Postoperative results in 30 patients following ventricular septal myotomy and myectomy (Morrow procedure).* Circulation 53 and 54(Suppl. II):180, 1976.

48. MARON, B. J., MERRILL, W. H., FREIER, P. A., ET AL.: *Long-term clinical course and symptomatic status of patients after operation for hypertrophic subaortic stenosis.* Circulation 57:1205,1978.

49. WATSON, D. C., HENRY, W. L., EPSTEIN, S. E., ET AL.: *Effects of operation on left atrial size and the occurrence of atrial fibrillation in patients with hypertrophic subaortic stenosis.* Circulation 55:178, 1977.

50. REDWOOD, D. R., GOLDSTEIN, R. E., HIRSHFELD, J., ET AL.: *Exercise performance following septal myotomy and myectomy in patients with obstructive ASH.* Submitted for publication.

Atrial Septal Defect Secundum:
Clinical Profile with Physiologic Correlates
in Children and Adults

Wade T. Hamilton, M.D., Charles I. Haffajee, M.D.,
James E. Dalen, M.D., Lewis Dexter, M.D.,
and Alexander S. Nadas, M.D.

Over the past quarter of a century surgical closure of secundum atrial defect has become a safe procedure, with minimal risk of mortality or serious morbidity.[1-7] Currently, most authorities recommend routine closure of the defect as soon as the diagnosis is made. However, a number of questions still remain in the minds of some cardiologists.[8,9] First, what is the difference between the clinical and physiologic profiles of younger patients and those of patients over 20 years of age? Second, is there an appreciable difference between those operated on within the first two decades and those treated surgically at a later age with regard to surgical mortality, morbidity, and effectiveness? Finally, is there a physiologic profile which is diagnostic of smaller defects that may not require operation? We have attempted to answer some of these questions by a 30-year chart review of two Boston hospitals, Peter Bent Brigham and Children's Hospital Medical Center. A long-term followup of the survivors in this study group is underway.

MATERIALS

The records reviewed were from 412 patients with a secundum type atrial septal defect (ASD)[2] disclosed by catheterization or operation at the Peter Bent Brigham Hospital (PBBH) and the Children's Hospital Medical Center (CHMS). All patients were at least 16 years old (range 16 to 73) on July 1, 1977. To assess the role of age in clinical and physiologic profiles, symptoms, electrocardiogram (ECG), chest x-ray (CXR), and pertinent cardiac catheterization data obtained at the time of admission were evaluated. Details of operation, mortality, complications, and followup data of surgical survivors were also surveyed with respect to age. Patients were excluded from the study if they had ASD primum, concomitant rheumatic heart disease, or associated congenital heart disease, including pulmonary stenosis with peak systolic ejection gradient more than 30 mm. Hg and primary pulmonary hypertension with patent foramen ovale. Figure 1 shows the age distribution of the group which was 65 percent female and 35 percent male. Familial ASD was noted in four patients.

All PBBH patients (n=147) underwent cardiac catheterization upon admission, as did 60 percent (184) of the CHMC patients, resulting in a total of 331 catheterized patients (median age, 19.5 years). A total of 294 patients, 81 of whom did not undergo preoperative catheterization, underwent surgical repair at a median age of 16 years. The 118 remaining patients studied might have been operated upon later at another hospital, but we have no operative records.

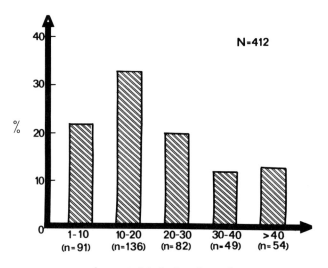

Figure 1. Admission age was defined as age at catheterization or, if there was no catheterization, the age at operation. One third of the 412 patients were teenagers when admitted to the study, with smaller percentages in the other age categories; one fourth were over age 30 years.

Of the 24 deaths in the group, 21 were operative deaths, and 3 occurred in older patients (ages 20, 40, and 55) who were unoperated and died during medical followup. These three patients had mean pulmonary artery pressures ($\bar{p}_{PA}$) greater than 55 mm. Hg, systemic arterial oxygen saturations less than 90 percent and pulmonary resistance (R_p) greater than 5 units/M².

Major noncardiac problems, congenital or acquired, were found in 14 percent (n = 60) of all patients. Neuropsychiatric disease (i.e. mental retardation, alcoholism) comprised 40 percent; orthopedic problems, 15 percent (including two patients with the Marfan syndrome); gastrointestinal problems, 10 percent (including liver disease and ulcer); genitourinary problems 12.5 percent; miscellaneous noncardiac disease, 25 percent (including systemic hypertension and diabetes mellitus).

Followup data were obtained from the hospital charts and included data from 149 of the 225 survivors (66 percent) of pump surgery who were last seen at least one year postoperatively. Mean followup time from surgery was 7.2 years. A long-term followup of all survivors is in progress.

RESULTS

Admission Profile

SYMPTOMS. Overall, almost one half (n=192) of the patients (ages 1 to 73 years) were asymptomatic at the time of initial catheterization or, if operated upon without catheterization, at time of surgery. One fifth (n=79) had severe symptoms (congestive heart failure requiring digitalis, chest pain, or cyanosis); one third had only mild symptoms (dyspnea on exertion, fatigue or palpitations). There were 11 patients with unusual symptoms such as severe headache, atypical chest pain, or syncope with effort. The percentage of asymptomatic patients declined as age increased: from 71 percent in the 1- to 10-year-olds to 4 percent in those over 40 years (Fig. 2). In a reciprocal fashion, the percentage of severe symptoms increased with age, from 8 percent in the 1- to 10-year-

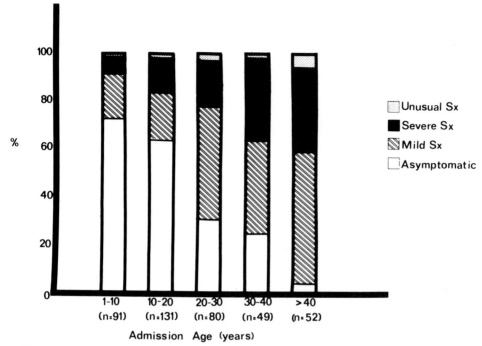

Figure 2. Symptoms increased with advancing age in unoperated patients with ASD.

old group to 36 percent among the few who were over 40 years when admitted to the study.

Of historical interest is the difference in symptoms with regard to decade of admission: 30 percent of the patients admitted between 1940 and 1960 were asymptomatic as compared to 56 percent of those seen in the 1970s.

CHEST X-RAY. Only 16 percent of patients with adequate chest radiograms (58/371) had normal-sized hearts at the time of admission to the study; 62 percent (230/371) had moderate cardiac enlargement and 22 percent (83/371) had severe cardiomegaly. The age distribution of patients with normal-sized hearts varied from a maximum of 26 percent (19/74) in the 20- to 30-year-olds to 2 percent (1/50) in those over 40.

Overall, 31 percent had greatly increased pulmonary markings on CXR, ranging from 5 percent (4/84) in the 1- to 10-year-old group to 79 percent (37/50) in those over 40.

ELECTROCARDIOGRAM. Electrocardiograms of 384 patients were available at admission to the study. Eighty-two percent (319/384) were in normal sinus rhythm (NSR), 8 percent (34/384) were in atrial fibrillation or flutter (AF/F), 1 percent (3/384) in complete heart block (CHB), and 8 percent (29/384) had miscellaneous disturbances, mostly complete right bundle branch block (CRBB). Figure 3 indicates that with advancing age, the percentage of those patients in NSR decreased and the incidence of severe rhythm disturbances increased. Similarly, the percentage of those with AF/F increased with increasing pulmonary resistance (R_p) from 7 percent (16/236) of those with $R_p \leq 2$ units/M² to 22 percent (13/60) among those with $R_p > 2$ units/M².

Of the 44 patients who complained of palpitations, 32 (73 percent) were in NSR, 8 (18 percent) showed AF/F and 4 (9 percent) showed CRBBB or other rhythm disturbance. Hence, a history of palpitations was not predictive of resting ECG abnormalities.

Overall, 88 percent (336/384) of the patients with electrocardiograms had right intraventricular conduction delay patterns in lead V_1 (RIVCD) at admission. Of the

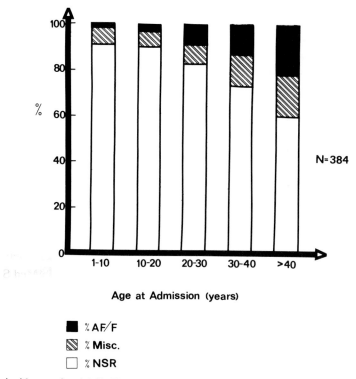

Figure 3. The incidence of atrial fibrillation or flutter (AF/F) increased with advancing age in patients with unoperated ASD. Miscellaneous disturbances, especially complete right bundle branch block and CHB, also were more common in older patients.

catheterized patients, 90 percent (187/207) had pulmonary to systemic flow ratios (Qp/Qs) of at least 2:1 and 76 percent (63/73) of those with calculated shunts of a lesser magnitude had right intraventricular conduction disturbance.

Complete heart block, classified under "miscellaneous" in Figure 3, was present in two patients over age 40 years and one in her twenties.

The height (mV) of r or R' in lead V_1 (RV_1) (whichever was taller) was correlated with R_p in Figure 4. It is noteworthy that 6 of 10 patients with RV_1 of 20 mV or more had marked elevation of R_p. By contrast, among those with the smallest RV_1 (≤ 5 mV) only 1 percent had severe elevation of R_p whereas the majority (79/86) had R_p less than 2 units/M^2.

HEART CATHETERIZATION. ASD secundum was discovered at cardiac catheterization in 331 patients who ranged in age from 1 to 72 years. Associated partial anomalous pulmonary venous return (PAPVR) was noted in 16 percent. Age distribution of the group at the time of catheterization was as follows: 1 to 10 years, 22 percent; 10 to 20 years, 28 percent; 20 to 30 years, 22 percent; 30 to 40 years, 14 percent; and 40 to 75 years, 14 percent. Five percent underwent catheterization in the 1940s, 45 percent in the 1950s, 39 percent in the 1960s, and 11 percent in the 1970s. Of the 18 patients catheterized in the 1940s, 12 were over 20 years of age; since then, in each decade, approximately 50 percent were over 20 years at catheterization.

Mean right atrial pressures ($\bar{p}_{RA}$), available for analysis in 306 patients, ranged from 1 to 25 mm. Hg with a mean of 5.2 ± 3.2 mm Hg (one standard deviation). Correlation between age at catheterization and mean right atrial pressures reveals the percentage of patients with $\bar{p}_{RA}$ greater than 10 mm. Hg increases with advancing age. Mean right

270

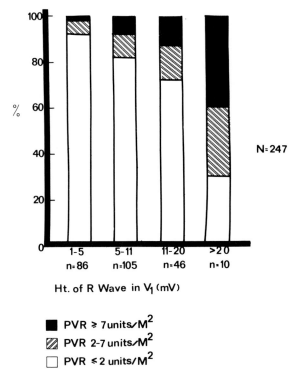

Figure 4. The height of the r or R′, whichever was taller, in ECG lead V₁ (RV₁) was a rough correlate of pulmonary resistance (R_p). However, in any given RV₁, a broad range of R_p is possible.

atrial pressure also was correlated with severe symptoms. Overall, 23 percent of catheterized patients exhibited severe symptoms: 18 percent (35/199) of those with $\bar{p}_{RA}$ between 1 and 5 mm. Hg, 68 percent (13/19) of those with $\bar{p}_{RA}$ >10 mm. Hg. Only one of 19 patients with $\bar{p}_{RA}$ greater than 10 mm. Hg was asymptomatic.

The pulmonary arterial mean pressures ($\bar{p}_{PA}$) of 311 patients averaged 24 (±18) mm. Hg; 31 percent of all patients had pulmonary arterial hypertension (PAH), with $\bar{p}_{PA}$ above 20 mm. Hg. A progressive increase in the percentage of patients with PAH was noted with age, from a low of 14 percent in the 1- to 20-year-old group to 53 percent in those catheterized when older than 30 years.

Pulmonary vascular resistance (R_p) (units/M²) was normal (less than 2 units/M²) in 79 percent, moderately elevated (2 to 7 units/M²) in 11 percent and severely raised (>7 units/M²) in 10 percent. A progressive decrease in percentage of patients with normal R_p was noted with age at the time of catheterization: 94 percent (138/147) of those catheterized before age 20 years had normal R_p as compared to 55 percent (49/88) of those catheterized after age 20 years (Fig. 5). Elevated R_p was rare under age 20.

Pulmonary systemic flow ratio (Qp/Qs) was measured in 317 patients; it was less than one in 5 percent, between 1 and 2 in 25 percent, between 2 and 3 in 34 percent and greater than 3 in 36 percent. In general, the patients with Qp/Qs < 2.0 were sicker; 36 percent (34/96) had severe symptoms compared to 18 percent (41/223) of those with Qp/Qs of 2 to 1 or greater. Qp/Qs is more useful when pulmonary vascular resistance is also known, as discussed in the sections on ECG and surgical mortality.

Arterial oxygen saturation, recorded in 307 patients, averaged 95 percent. The percentage of patients with oxygen saturation less than 90 percent increased with advancing age, ranging from 5 percent (7/144) in those catheterized before age 20 years to 15 percent (13/88) in those over age 30 years (Fig. 5).

Surgery

ALL OPERATED PATIENTS. Of the 412 patients, 294 (71 percent) —ranging in age from 3 to 69 years—underwent ASD closure (Fig. 6); five were later reoperated upon for residual defects. Overall, perioperative mortality was 7 percent (21/294). The mortality before 1960, when most of the nonpump operations were performed, was 19 percent (16/85); since 1960, 2 percent (5/205).

There were no major surgical complications (serious arrhythmias, paradoxical emboli, etc.) in 80 percent of all patients and in 93 percent of those with R_p less than 2 units/M² (Table 1). Complications became less common with advancing calendar time,

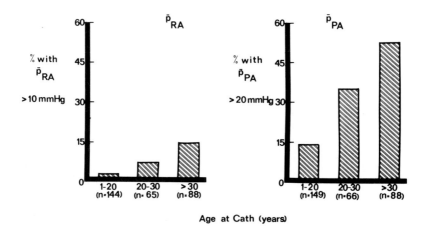

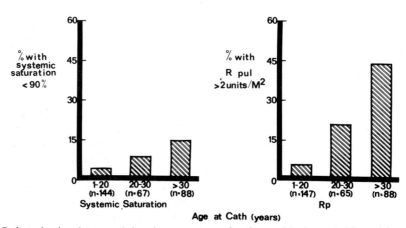

Figure 5. Catheterization data reveal that the percentage of patients with elevated right atrial pressure (p_{RA}), elevated pulmonary arterial pressure ($\bar{p}_{PA}$) systemic desaturation, and elevated pulmonary resistance (R_p) increased with advancing age, suggesting that these changes will eventually occur in some patients with unoperated ASD.

Table 1. Classification of surgical complications (59 complications/294 operations)

A. *Type of Complication*	*No.*
CNS: (including cerebral emboli and perioperative insults)	20
Cardiac Rhythm: (including postoperative admissions for AF/F and AV-dissociation)	9
Pulmonary: (including pneumonia, phrenic nerve paralysis, and pulmonary emboli)	9
Hematologic: (including clotting abnormalities, hemoglobinuria, and hepatitis)	9
Miscellaneous: (including postpump syndromes and non-CNS paradoxical emboli)	12

B. *Type of Surgery*	*Percentage of Complications*
Nonpump surgery	36% (21/59)
Pump surgery	17% (38/225)

and comprised 29 percent (25/85) in the 1950s, 19 percent (34/179) in the 1960s, and none in the 1970s.

NONPUMP SURGERY. Nonpump surgery (Bailey procedure, Sondergard procedure, "Well" technique) was performed in 59 patients (20 percent). Most of these were done before 1953 and all but four were done before 1960. Overall, mortality was 16/59 (27 percent); serious complications occurred in 21 (36 percent) (Fig. 6).

The generally older age of these patients, compared to those operated with cardiopulmonary bypass, may be a minor reason for the unfavorable outcome in terms of both mortality and morbidity; 50 percent of the nonpump patients were over 20 years of age at the time of surgery, but only 35 percent of those operated with cardiopulmonary bypass fell into this age group. Other obvious reasons for the poor results of surgery in this group are technical deficiencies, inadequacies of postoperative care, and—perhaps most importantly—unfamiliarity with proper indications for surgery, particularly as it relates to pulmonary resistance. No one survived nonpump surgery with a known $R_p >$ 2 units/M^2 and 12 of the 16 deaths occurred in this group: 8 with moderately elevated and 4 with severely elevated pulmonary resistance.

PUMP SURGERY. There were 5 deaths (2 percent) among the 225 patients who underwent atrial defect closure by means of cardiopulmonary bypass; only one of these deaths occurred among the 187 patients operated upon after 1961. The latter death occurred in a 33-year-old female with a pulmonary arterial pressure of 96/40 mm. Hg. Two of the other four deaths, all before 1961, occurred in patients, aged 32 and 38, with $\bar{p}_{PA}$ greater than 50 mm. Hg (84 and 57 mm. Hg, respectively). The other two deaths occurred in young patients; one 8-year-old girl (with $\bar{p}_{PA}$ = 19/10 mm. Hg) died after surgery of endotracheal and pulmonary hemorrhage. A 14-year-old boy with multiple congenital anomalies and mental retardation died of unclear causes on the first postoperative day.

To assess the effects of hemodynamic factors on surgical mortality, the 146 operated patients with adequate physiologic data were evaluated with regard to $\bar{p}_{RA}$, $\bar{p}_{PA}$, R_p, and systemic saturation (Fig. 7). Patients with $\bar{p}_{PA} >$ 50 mm. Hg, $R_p >$ 2 units/M^2 and systemic desaturation < 90 percent were at higher operative risk. Of 31 operated patients with $\bar{p}_{PA} >$ 20 mm. Hg, 21 had Qp/Qs > 2.0 with no deaths, whereas in the 10 whose flow ratio was less than 2, there were 2 deaths (22 percent). One woman, aged 48, survived operation with $\bar{p}_{PA}$ of 54 mm. Hg, Qp/Qs of 1.7:1 and R_p of 11 units/M^2. At a six-month postoperative recatheterization her pulmonary arterial mean pressure had dropped to 35 mm. Hg, but R_p was unchanged and she was still severely symptomatic.

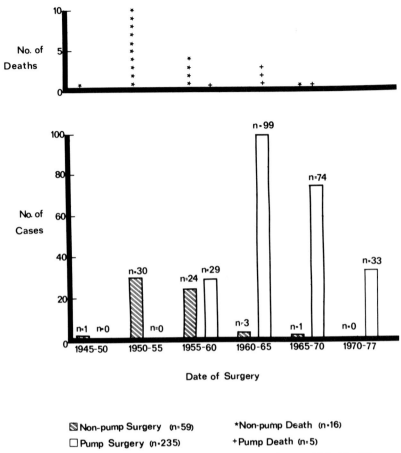

Figure 6. History of ASD surgery at CHMC and PBBH (total operations = 294). The 27 percent mortality associated with nonpump surgery, during the learning phase of ASD management, is attributable to both medical and surgical shortcomings. With the advent of pump surgery the mortality dropped to 2 percent.

The operative notes were reviewed relative to the size of the defect as measured by the surgeon in the operating room. The size was judged to be small (<2 cm.^{2}) in 22 percent, medium (2 to 10 cm.^{2}) in 44 percent and large (>10 cm.^{2}) in 34 percent. There was no correlation with body surface area or presence of noncardiac problems (i.e., Marfan syndrome, familial ASD, etc.). The correlation between defect size and shunt was not linear, but among the patients with small defects only 22 percent (4/18) had Qp/Qs greater than 3 compared to 44 percent (72/162) in the group with medium or large defects.

Follow-up

UNOPERATED PATIENTS. Since most of the unoperated patients were not followed up, we made the assumption that the previously presented admission profile of older patients may be a better representation of the results of medical management than the relatively small number of patients followed for at least a year after catheterization.

NONPUMP SURGERY. Followup of data of patients operated upon before the advent of pump surgery is not presented because it is irrelevant today.

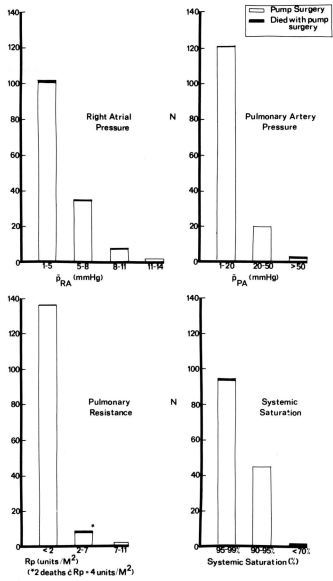

Figure 7. Hemodynamic deterioration is associated with an increased mortality in patients undergoing pump surgery. Perioperative deaths occurred in 2 of 3 patients with $p_{PA} > 50$ mm. Hg, 2 of 10 with $R_p > 2$ units/M^2, and in the only patient operated upon with significant systemic desaturation.

PUMP SURGERY. Of the 225 patients undergoing ASD closure utilizing cardiopulmonary bypass, 149 were seen again, at least one year after operation (mean followup = 7.2 years). Figure 8 illustrates the lack of change in cardiac rhythm and A-V conduction, the slight improvement in the degree of right ventricular hypertrophy (RVH), and the clearcut improvement in heart size and symptoms after surgery.

Almost 90 percent were asymptomatic at followup. Four of the five patients with dyspnea on exertion had been over age 20 years at operation. No one had severe symptoms at followup, compared to 9 percent preoperatively. Almost two thirds had normal heart size by CXR at followup. Mild to moderate residual cardiac enlargement

275

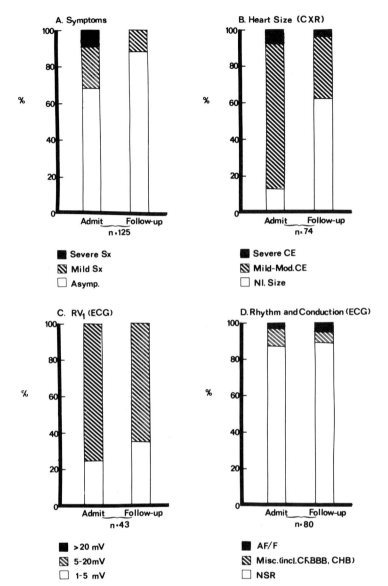

Figure 8. In patients seen at admission and again at followup at least one year after pump surgery, improvement was noted in symptoms and heart size, but little change in ECG.

was independent of age at operation. Severe residual cardiomegaly, however, was noted only in three patients, ages 29, 40, and 47 years, who were operated upon later in life.

CONCLUSIONS

A total of 412 patients with secundum type atrial septal defect (ASD) were evaluated on admission to an adult and a pediatric hospital. Symptoms, heart size, atrial arrhythmias, right ventricular hypertrophy, right atrial and pulmonary arterial pressure, and systemic desaturation increased progressively with advancing age. A concomitant increase in surgical morbidity and mortality also occurred in older patients and in those with pulmonary arterial hypertension and pulmonary vascular obstruction.

Survivors of successful ASD closure by means of cardiopulmonary bypass are almost invariably asymptomatic and seldom have residual cardiomegaly, unless the operation was performed after the second decade of life. Although most postoperative patients are in normal sinus rhythm, there is no evidence that pre-existing arrhythmias have been significantly ameliorated by surgery, nor can we state, on the basis of our data, whether early surgery prevents the late appearance of atrial arrhythmias. Right intraventricular conduction disturbance, with or without right ventricular hypertrophy, persists postoperatively, although the decrease in the height of R wave in V_1 suggests some involution of right ventricular hypertrophy.

This review of a large number of patients, ranging in age from childhood to late adulthood, documents spontaneous deterioration through the decades in terms of symptoms, heart size, electrocardiograms, and pulmonary vascular obstruction. Since surgical closure of the ASD within the first two decades carries a minimal mortality and since surgery at a later age is accompanied by much higher mortality and morbidity, as well as the danger of cardiovascular residua, routine early closure of all secundum atrial septal defects is strongly recommended.

REFERENCES

1. DEXTER, L.: *Atrial septal defect.* Br. Heart J. 18:209,1956.

2. DALEN, J. E., HAYNES, F. W., AND DEXTER, L.: *Life expectancy with atrial septal defect. Influence of complicating pulmonary vascular disease.* JAMA 200:442,1967.

3. ZAVER, A. G., AND NADAS, A. S.: *Atrial septal defect—secundum type.* Circulation 31–32(Suppl. III):24,1965.

4. KELLEY, J. J., AND LYONS, H. A.: *Atrial septal defect in the aged.* Ann. Intern. Med. 48:267,1958.

5. MARKMAN, P., HOWITT, G., AND WADE, E. G.: *Atrial septal defect in the middle-aged and elderly.* Q. J. Med. 34:409,1965.

6. RODSTEIN, M., ZEMAN, F. D., AND GERBER, I. E.: *Atrial septal defect in the aged.* Circulation 23:665,1961.

7. NASRALLAH, A. T., HALL, R. J., GARCIA, E., ET AL.: *Surgical repair of atrial septal defect in patients over 60 years of age.* Circulation 53:329,1976.

8. BIERMAN, F. Z., AND WILLIAMS, R. G.: *Subxiphoid two dimensional imaging of the atrial septum.* Am. J. Cardiol. 41:354,1978.

9. NADAS, A. S., AND FYLER, D.C.: *Pediatric Cardiology.* W.B. Saunders Co., Philadelphia, 1972.

Ventricular Septal Defect in the Adult

Mary Allen Engle, M.D., and Susan Anderson Kline, M.D.

CHANGING HISTORY

If pediatric cardiologists and cardiac surgeons have done their work well over the past 20 to 25 years, there should now be a higher percentage of adults who were born with a ventricular septal defect (VSD) than at any time in history. When Dr. Maude Abbott[1] in 1936 and Dr. Helen Taussig[2] in 1947 published their classic books on congenital heart disease, they recognized that the patients with a VSD who reached adulthood did so because they had small defects and no symptoms or else they had large defects with Eisenmenger syndrome. To that number are now added many patients who might in earlier times have died from cardiac failure in infancy[3-5] or from infective endocarditis and many more who have undergone cardiac surgery. How should the physician caring for adults evaluate and manage this mixed population that is far more varied than that which Drs. Abbott and Taussig had experienced 30 to 40 years ago? What is the magnitude of the problem?

PREVALENCE IN ADULTS

Ventricular septal defect is the most common congenital cardiac anomaly encountered at birth[6,7] and in necropsy series of cardiac anomalies.[1,8] It is equally divided among males and females. Though it occurs in 2/1000 live births,[9] its prevalence in school-aged children has been about 1/1000[7,9,10] and in adults approximately 0.5/1000.[7,9] In terms of its rank among congenital cardiac anomalies, VSD as the principal defect constituted 30 percent of the cardiac malformations at birth, 20 percent during childhood, and 10 percent in adult life.[11] Why this attrition?

In adults VSD was third in frequency in Mark and Young's 1965 report on 310 adults with congenital heart disease; patent ductus arteriosus and atrial septal defect were more common.[12] Their oldest patient with VSD was 73; but only 6 of the 38 adults were over 40. Perloff[13] and Walker[14] both commented that a patient with VSD seldom was seen after the fourth decade. Corone and coworkers from Paris, France, included 10 patients over the age of 40 in their study of 790 cases of VSD beyond the first year of life.[15] The oldest patient among Abbott's 50 necropsied cases was 49, and the oldest in Fontana and Edwards' series was 79.[8] In the recently completed cooperative study on the natural history of some common congenital anomalies were 1265 patients with VSD. Of these, 74 patients were over the age of 21 and the oldest was 58.

SURVIVORSHIP OF ADULTS

Campbell had an extensive personal experience with long-term followup for 20 or more years of patients diagnosed as having a VSD and to this he added series of cases he had carefully surveyed in the literature. His last publication on the natural history of VSD appeared in 1971.[17] Therein he computed that 27 percent of patients with VSD of all degrees had died by age 20, 53 percent by age 40, and 69 percent by age 60. However, if the defect was small, he stated that this group "now has an almost normal life expectation since treatment should eliminate the risk of dying from bacterial endocarditis."[17] Keith and associates shared this optimistic prognosis for those patients with small defects.[7]

If this be so, why should there be relatively so few adults recognized with VSD? Are they simply being overlooked or misdiagnosed? Is something happening to them? Some hurtful as well as some helpful events do occur in the natural history of this anomaly. Counteracting some of the harmful features is surgical intervention, which is meant only to be helpful but is itself sometimes harmful. In this "good news, bad news" blend, let us consider the bad news first.

HARMFUL EVENTS AFFECTING OUTCOME FOR ADULTS WITH VSD

Cardiac failure is the chief cause of death in infancy and in the first few months of life. While the condition is not limited to infancy, it is nonetheless peculiar to that early period of life. In adults cardiac failure due to VSD is rare.[15] In children the main cause of death is attempted cardiac surgery. After the age of three, death in patients born with VSD is apt to be related to other causes and not primarily to the heart.[9]

Before and early in the antibiotic era *infective endocarditis* took a heavy toll. It is now, for the most part, preventable[18] through physicians' attention to periods of risk of bloodstream infection. This risk is present most often following dental extraction, but also after cardiac catheterization or operation, genitourinary operations, or vaginal delivery.

The incidence of infective endocarditis now is low. It is reported to vary from 1:200 to 1:1200.[19] In 1971 Campbell estimated the risk to be 0.4 percent per year, from pooled data of 15 cases in 3886 patient years.[17] During the same year, Keith reported 1 percent incidence or 1 case in 787 patient-years among the 295 teenagers and young adults under long-term observation for an average of ten years.[7] Corone and coworkers studied 790 patients and emphasized that the risk is higher in adults than in children.[15] It did not occur in anyone under the age of two years, while in the 2- to 14-year-old group the rate was 1.2 per 1000 patient-years, and 7.1 per 1000 patient-years in the 15- to 20-year-old group. Five of the patients with infective endocarditis had undergone open heart surgery to close the VSD. Gersony and Hayes in the Natural History Study also demonstrated that the risk of infective endocarditis in the adult with VSD was higher than for children. They identified 16 cases in 10,403 patient-years, or 1.5/1000 patient-years. However, the complication was six times more common in those over 20 years of age than for those under 20.[19]

If infective endocarditis occurs, it should be promptly recognized because of the febrile illness without other obvious cause in an individual with the findings of a VSD. Proof by blood cultures and use of the appropriate antibiotic intravenously for a minimum treatment period of one month should permit recovery without sequelae. Although it seems that missed prophylaxis and missed diagnosis should not occur in the 1970s, apparently that can still happen, as illustrated by the report in 1976 by Wiegmann and associates.[20] They cited the case of a 40-year-old woman with diagnosis of VSD made at the age of 4 years, who had undergone three uneventful pregnancies. At the age of 33, cardiac catheterization documented a small VSD with normal pressures. Nonetheless, over the previous seven years she had undergone 21 dental procedures, all without antibiotic coverage. When she became ill with cough and fever, she was treated intermittently for one year with short courses of tetracycline or ampicillin. No blood cultures were taken during that whole period. Streptococcus viridans was then isolated; fortunately the patient responded to intravenous penicillin.

Pulmonary vascular obstructive disease may render the young child with large VSD less symptomatic, but at the price of seemingly inexorable progression to fixed, irreversible pulmonary hypertension with shunt reversal. Death generally results from a complication of cyanotic heart disease or of right-sided cardiac failure. If this course is interfered with by open-heart surgery before the age of two years, that young child has a chance of reversing the elevated pulmonary vascular resistance.[21] Among older children operated upon to close a large VSD when the pulmonary to systemic resistance ratios approach 0.7, the pulmonary pressure measured in the operating room drops only to the extent that the small left-to-right shunt is abolished. There usually is little decrease in pulmonary vascular resistance, and a late and progressive rise may even be observed postoperatively.[21,22] Table 1 is compiled from a child whose cardiac surgery was initially delayed because of discovery of a mediastinal tumor which upon excision was found to be a neuroblastoma. Though at first she appeared improved,[23] about 10 years later, signs of advancing pulmonary hypertension appeared[24] and thereafter, chronic right-sided cardiac failure ensued.

The Eisenmenger syndrome develops only in patients with a large VSD, not with small ones.[7,15] Although symptoms of exertional dyspnea and signs of shunt reversal usually appear in the late teens or early twenties, there may be no symptoms appreciated for many years. Once the evidence of worsening begins, however, the prognosis is poor for more than five or 10 more years of quiet life, on medication for right-sided cardiac failure and often with erythropheresis for excessive polycythemia. In Mark and Young's study of adults with VSD six of the nine with Eisenmenger syndrome died, three of cardiac failure, and one each from brain abscess, renal insufficiency, and sudden death.[12] Dysrhythmias and infective endocarditis are other lethal complications. In the 1977 Natural History Study, 6 of the 18 with Eisenmenger syndrome died.[27] Selzer reported one patient who survived to age 79.[25]

INCREASING SEVERITY OF PULMONIC STENOSIS. Since 1957 we have known about the natural transformation of ventricular septal defects into ventricular septal defects with pulmonic stenosis (PS).[26] Gasul's experience and that of most pediatric cardiologists would suggest that this initially helpful change occurs chiefly in infancy and childhood, but it may also begin or continue to progress during adult life.[15] Like the Eisenmenger

Table 1. Course of VSD in a patient with double outlet RV

	Age	RV	Pressures PA	SA	QP/ QS	Systemic O₂ Saturation
Preoperative Values	7	85/7	71/42	94/54	1.5	87%
	10	97/3	57/34	97/61	1.6	93%
Postoperative Values	11.5	55/3	43/13	112/70	1.0	96%
	21	120/5	112/60	70/42	1.0	88.5%

RV = right ventricle; PA = pulmonary artery; SA = systemic artery; QP = pulmonary flow; QS = systemic flow.

281

Table 2. Ventricular septal defect in a patient with pulmonic stenosis (valvular and infundibular)

Year:	1953	1959	1976
Age (Years):	6	13	30
Surgical Status:	Pre-Brock procedure	Post-Brock procedure	Pre-Open repair
Pressures (mm. Hg)			
RA ($\overline{X}$)	1	1	12
RV Inflow (S/D)	87/0	104/5	120/12
RV Outflow (S/D)	—	—	20/12
PA (S/D:$\overline{X}$)	27/0:11	24/7:15	20/11:18
P "C" ($\overline{X}$)	1	6	11
LV (S/D)	—	—	130/ 8
Flows (l./min.)			
QP/QS	0.7	1.9	1.5
QL→R	0	2.9	2.7
QL→R ÷ QP	0%	47%	31%
QR→L	1.5	0	0
QR→L ÷ QS	32%	0%	0%
Resistances (dynes-sec.-cm.$^{-5}$)			
PVR	248	118	64
Arterial Oxyhemoglobin Saturation			
	90%	97%	93%

Angiography
(1) RV hypertrophy and dilatation
(2) Moderately severe infundibular narrowing
(3) Moderate hypoplasia of pulmonary trunk and pulmonary anulus
(4) Thickened pulmonic valve leaflets
(5) L→R shunt at ventricular level; no R→L shunt at ventricular level
(6) Aortic and pulmonic valves side-by-side

Operative Findings
(1) Fibromuscular cristal hypertrophy
(2) Normal pulmonic valve
(3) Moderate-sized pulmonary trunk
(4) Large VSD (size of a quarter)

Procedure
(1) VSD patched
(2) Infundibulum resected (no patch); RV pressure ↓ to 35/5 (Ao = 95/5)

(X) = mean pressure; QP = pulmonary flow; QS = systemic flow; QL→R = left-to-right shunt; QR→L = right-to-left shunt; RA = right atrium; RV = right ventricle; PA = pulmonary artery; P "C" = pulmonary "capillary"; LV = left ventricle; S/D = systolic/diastolic pressure; PVR = pulmonary vascular resistance; SVR = systemic vascular resistance.

reaction, it develops in individuals with large VSD, not in those with small defects.[7,9,32] The infundibular hypertrophy decreases the size of the large left-to-right shunt and thus is helpful if the obstruction is just the right amount.

How often does this happen? In the newest U.S. Natural History Study[30] 3 percent of 828 medically managed children developed a systolic pressure gradient across the outflow tract of the right ventricle. This is a lower figure than the 5 to 10 percent estimate by Kaplan and coworkers[32] and the 6 to 11 percent found by Keith.[7] Corone's long-term study, reported in 1977,[15] stated that infundibular PS began in 7 percent of the 499 who had several examinations and was present in 13 percent at the initial examination. That group found that while PS in the childhood years was rare, it was far more common later on and was present in 21 percent of those over the age of 30. Perloff said that there were more adults like this with VSD and PS than with simple VSD alone.[33]

The harmful aspect of this natural transformation comes from continuation of the process to the point of severe obstruction to right ventricular outflow and shunt reversal. The condition is converted into a tetralogy of Fallot if the VSD remains large. This occurred in five of Corone's patients.[15] Longstanding infundibular hypertrophy becomes a dense fibromuscular barrier to pulmonary blood flow. Such a transformation from "pink tetralogy" to the symptomatic form is illustrated by the patient whose physiologic data is shown in Table 2.

ACQUISITION OF AORTIC REGURGITATION. Practically unheard of in babies under the age of two years, this development can take place in childhood but is even more apt to occur in adult life. Unlike simple VSD, there is a male preponderance.[28] Unlike the acquisition of pulmonary vascular obstructive disease (PVO) or PS, which occurs only with large defects, acquired aortic regurgitation (AR) is no respecter of size of the VSD. Shunt size may diminish as right ventricular outflow tract obstruction develops when the right aortic cusp prolapses and AR begins, so that a predominantly left-to-right shunt is converted into a left-to-left shunt. The AR is often the predominant feature,[28,29] and once present, it tends to progress (Fig. 1).

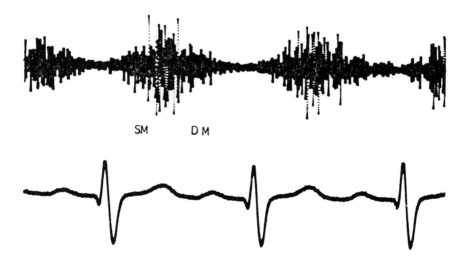

SM   D M

Figure 1. Phonocardiogram of an adolescent boy with marked aortic regurgitation superimposed on a large VSD. No history of infective endocarditis could be elicited. Note the late systolic crescendo and the diastolic decrescendo murmurs, maximal in the third left interspace.

AR is known to occur in patients with subpulmonic VSD, and both of these conditions are more prevalent in Orientals than in Occidentals.[28,29] In the U.S. Natural History Study[16,30] VSD was found at surgery to be subpulmonic in 13 and subaortic in 19 patients. In the study by Corone and coworkers of 790 medically treated patients with VSD, AR developed in 6.3 percent. This represents a rate of 4.3/1000 patient-years.[15] A history of infective endocarditis could be elicited in 5 of their 50 patients with VSD and AR, which is no surprise, but curiously, these patients tended to be more susceptible later to infective endocarditis than did those with competent aortic valves.[15] Somerville, Brandao, and Ross[31] summarized their experience with the clinical features and results of surgery and noted the variety of aortic abnormalities that were found when AR was superimposed on a VSD (Fig. 2).

Presence of other associated anomalies may adversely affect the adult with VSD. Extracardiac anomalies, such as the Down's, Turner, and Marfan syndromes, were recognized in 11 percent of Corone's group.[15] We found a 10 percent incidence of silent genitourinary anomalies in children with congenital heart disease undergoing cardiac catheterization with contrast visualization when we obtained a postangiographic film of the abdomen for visualization of kidneys, ureters, and bladder.[34]

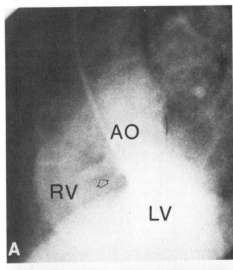

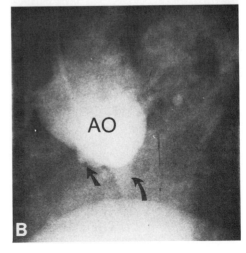

Figure 2. Cineangiocardiograms of an adult with VSD and aortic regurgitation. A, Left ventricular injection in the left anterior-oblique projection. Open arrow indicates the jet through the VSD. Note the dilatation of the aortic sinuses above the defect. B, Selective injection into the dilated aorta. Straight arrow points to the regurgitant jet into the right ventricle, a result of some prolapse of the aortic leaflet; the curved arrow points to the larger regurgitant stream into the left ventricle.

Other cardiac anomalies may also impair function and even survival of the patient. In the recent French study referred to earlier, Corone[15] found 649 of the subjects had VSD alone, while 140 had other cardiac lesions, the most frequent of which were atrial septal defect (in 49 patients) and patent ductus arteriosus (in 31). In addition to AR, which has already been considered, incompetence of one or more of the three other valves was also encountered. Figure 3 shows the pre- and postoperative films of a child with a large VSD with large left-to-right shunt. Closure of VSD abolished the left-to-right shunt, and as an adult she is asymptomatic but still has moderate mitral regurgitation and enlargement of the left ventricle and atrium. Figure 4 illustrates the findings in an adult with discrete membranous subaortic stenosis as well as a small VSD. Unlike the aforementioned cardiac anomalies which can be physiologically significant and make the prognosis worse, a clinically insignificant anomaly—a right aortic arch—was the third most frequent anomaly (found in 19 subjects).[15]

Uncommon, but of great significance medically and surgically to the person who has the condition, are three other associations with VSD: "corrected" *l*-transposition, double outlet right ventricle, and obstruction to pulmonary venous return.

"Corrected" transposition of the great arteries caught clinicians' attention when open heart surgery for VSD came into being.[35] In this condition venous return and atrial situs are appropriate, but the ventricles with their atrioventricular valves are inverted and the great arteries are in *l*-transposition, with the aorta located anterolaterally and the pulmonary trunk posteromedially. Systemic venous blood returns to the right atrium and passes through a bicuspid valve into the right-sided ventricle, an inverted anatomic left ventricle, which gives rise to the posteromedial great artery. Pulmonary veins drain into the left atrium, and then the oxygenated blood flows through a tricuspid valve into

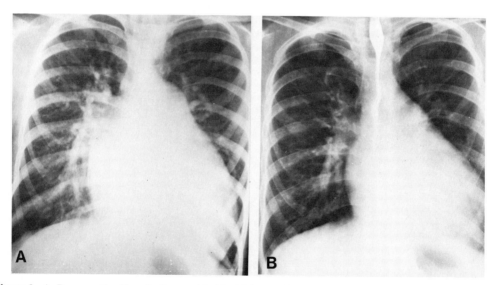

Figure 3. A, Preoperative film of a 7-year old girl with large VSD and with marked mitral regurgitation. Note gross cardiomegaly affecting all four cardiac chambers. The aortic knob is unusually slender, while the main pulmonary artery and both branches are quite distended from overfilling. Double density of enlarged left atrium is seen above the enlarged right atrium at lower right heart border. Not shown is the wide sweep of the barium-filled esophagus about the enlarged left atrium. B, Postoperative film after patch closure of large VSD, shows marked improvement with decrease in size of all cardiac chambers and the main pulmonary artery and branches. Barium column is no longer displaced by the left atrium. There is still some left ventricular enlargement persisting in the patient who is now an active, asymptomatic 25-year old woman; this is attributed to mild mitral regurgitation.

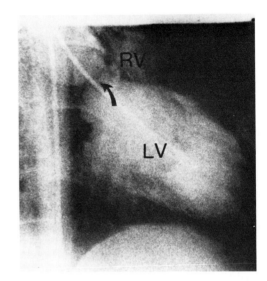

Figure 4. VSD and discrete membranous subaortic stenosis. Cineangiocardiogram in right anterior-oblique projection of adult with small VSD; selective left ventricular injection. Note faint opacification via the VSD of right ventricle superior to the left ventricle. Arrow points to the nonopacified discrete membrane beneath the aortic valve, producing discrete subaortic stenosis.

the left-sided ventricle, which is the mirror image of an anatomic right ventricle. The blood exits by way of an anterolateral aorta (Figs. 5 and 6). Blood flow is in the physiologic direction, and when there is a VSD (the most common condition when there is *l*-transposition) the effects are the same as with any other small, medium, or large defect, with one exception: the tendency to acquire high-grade heart block. If a large VSD in this setting is to be closed surgically,[36] the surgeon needs to be aware of the unusual location of the conduction system, which instead of coursing posteroinferiorly about the usual high defect, travels anterosuperiorly above the defect. There has been a higher incidence of surgically induced complete heart block when the

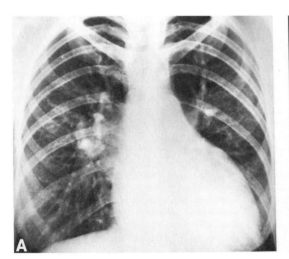
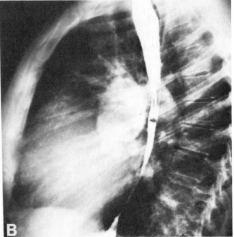

Figure 5. VSD and "corrected" transposition. Roentgenograms in frontal and lateral views of young woman with holosystolic murmur of VSD and loud second sound in second left interspace. A, Frontal view shows cardiomegaly with downward directed apex, increased pulmonary vascular markings in hilar regions, and slight convexity of pulmonary trunk, suggesting that it arises in the normal position. B, Lateral view, as well as the angiocardiogram in Figure 6, shows the pulmonary artery is a large posterior structure. It forms a border in the frontal view only because of its great size, not because of its point of origin.

286

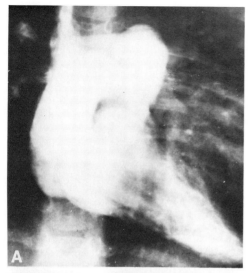

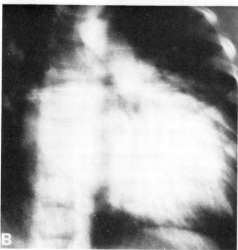

Figure 6. VSD and "corrected" transposition. See roentgenograms in Figure 5. Angiocardiogram with injection into superior vena cava showing: A, Flow of systemic venous blood through right atrium into an elongated, inverted left ventricle, and out the posteromedial but large pulmonary trunk forming a border. B, The pulmonary venous return to the left atrium, a globular ventricle on the left which is an inverted right ventricle, gives rise to the anterolaterally placed (*l*-position) aorta to the left of the pulmonary trunk. The shunt through the VSD is not seen in these two selected films.

vessels are in *l*-transposition than when a VSD with normally oriented aorta and pulmonary artery is closed.

Origin of both great arteries from the right ventricle (double outlet right ventricle) should be considered in any individual with a VSD when the systolic pressure measured in the right ventricle is identical with that in the left ventricle. Perhaps surprisingly, it may not be suspected before that time[37] because of the remarkable streaming of oxygenated blood from the left ventricle through a subaortic VSD (its only outlet) and into the aorta which arises above a conus, from the right ventricle. The patient may not appear cyanotic at all unless pulmonic stenosis[38,39] or pulmonary vascular obstructive disease decreases the left-to-right shunt and causes shunt reversal (Fig. 7).

We have spoken of the usual situation with VSD and double outlet right ventricle. It should be noted that in this spectrum VSD can be subaortic, subpulmonic, or uncommitted; the great arteries can be in normal external position; the aorta may be trans-

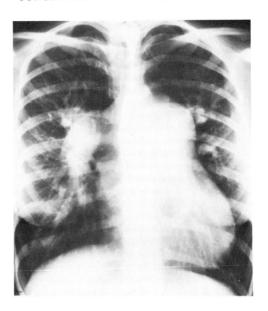

Figure 7. VSD, double outlet right ventricle, Eisenmenger syndrome in a 20-year-old woman. See angiocardiogram in Figure 8. Frontal roentgenogram shows great convexity of pulmonary trunk with enlargement of both hilar arteries but with clear lung fields beyond midpoint.

posed in front of the pulmonary artery in dextro- (Fig. 8) or levotransposition,[40-42] or the two may be side-by-side (Fig. 9). The VSD may decrease in size and thus become obstructive to left ventricular outflow (Fig. 10).[43] When the patient is a candidate for surgery, detailed preoperative delineation of the anatomy and skillful management at surgery can lead to successful repair;[44,45] Perloff cited an example, that of a 53-year-old patient who was successfully operated on by Morrow.[13]

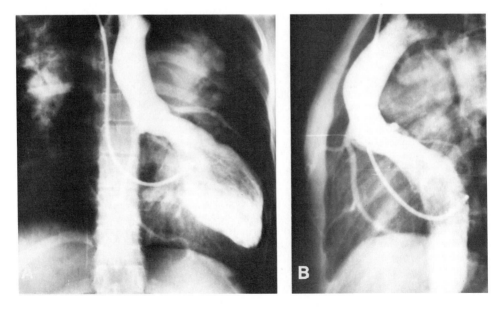

Figure 8. Angiocardiogram in frontal (A) and left lateral (B) views of an adult with pulmonary vascular obstructive disease and with origin of both the slender aorta (on the left and anteriorly) and the grossly enlarged pulmonary trunk from the right ventricle. The aorta stretches forward in a *d*-transposition.

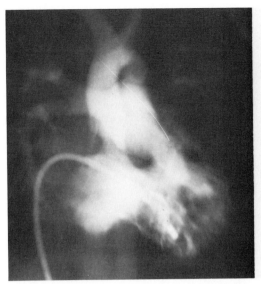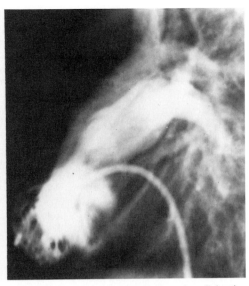

Figure 9. VSD with double outlet right ventricle and side-by-side arrangement of great arteries. Selective right ventricular injection in frontal (left) and simultaneous lateral (right) views. Both great arteries opacify simultaneously. The semilunar valves are at the same level; there is conal tissue beneath each one.

The third association to which we wish to call attention is *obstruction to pulmonary venous return* due to unusual conditions—cor triatriatum, supravalvular mitral stenosis,[46] congenital mitral stenosis,[47] and parachute mitral valve. Each of these conditions should be considered and ruled out in the patient with VSD and pulmonary hypertension before it is decided that he has fixed and irreversible pulmonary vascular obstructive disease due to precapillary vascular changes. Measurement at cardiac catheterization of a high pulmonary "wedge" pressure and angiocardiographic demonstration of delayed emptying and/or abnormality of the left atrium can confirm diagnosis. Echocardiography also contributes significant information concerning mitral valve and left atrial characteristics. Table 3 illustrates the physiologic data in a young

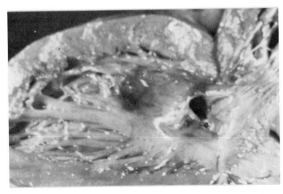

Figure 10. Postmortem specimen of double outlet right ventricle, with restrictive VSD just below the aortic leaflet of the mitral valve. The small size of the spontaneously closing VSD had the effect of contributing subaortic stenosis to left ventricular outflow.

Table 3. Ventricular septal defect in a 16-year-old patient with both arterial and pulmonary venous hypertension.

Pressures (mm. Hg)

RV (S/D):	105/5
PA (S/D:$\overline{X}$):	107/48; 73
P "C" ($\overline{X}$):	23
LA ($\overline{X}$):	23
LV (S/D):	107/6

Flows (l/min.)

QP/QS:	2.4
QL→R:	7.4
QL→R ÷ QP:	58%
QR→L:	0

Resistance (dynes-sec.-cm.$^{-5}$)

PVR:	314
SVR:	1223

Systemic Atrioventricular Valve

$\overline{X}$ Diastolic pressure gradient:	18 mm. Hg
Orifice area:	2.3 cm.^{2}

Angiography

(1) Large L→R shunt at ventricular level
(2) Thickening and limitation of motion of systemic A/V valve
(3) l-Transposition of the great arteries, "corrected"
(4) Ventricular inversion

(X) = mean pressure; QP = pulmonary flow; QS = systemic flow; QL→R = left-to-right shunt; QR→L = right-to-left shunt; RA = right atrium; RV = right ventricle; PA = pulmonary artery; P "C" = pulmonary "capillary"; LV = left ventricle; S/D = systolic/diastolic pressure; PVR = pulmonary vascular resistance; SVR = systemic vascular resistance.

adult who was rejected as a surgical candidate for VSD closure until it was demonstrated that the cause of his pulmonary hypertension was reparable: anatomic obstruction to pulmonary venous outflow.

Dysrhythmias are not a common problem for the adult with a VSD as they are in the adult with an atrial septal defect. However, they have been infrequently designated the cause of death in the natural history of the condition; in some details were not given,[15] but those with Eisenmenger syndrome seemed to be the group chiefly at risk for this problem.[12] It may be that in future years adults who have undergone surgery to close the VSD will be susceptible to dysrhythmias as a sequel to the operative intervention.[48]

Cardiomyopathy may or may not be part of the clinical picture for adults with large or small VSD. We have observed none in our personal experience at this medical center, but in 1961 Bloomfield reported nine cases of minor defects of the ventricular septum with evidence of cardiomyopathy of the left ventricle and death in cardiac failure. Three patients had small left-to-right shunts and the other six had imperforate defects. He speculated that VSD, even when closed, would interfere with systolic contraction and that it might compromise function if systemic hypertension or coronary artery disease were superimposed in adult life.[49] Graham and colleagues studied some children following surgical closure of VSD and found that myocardial function was sometimes impaired.[51,52] Jones and Ferrans[53] did electron microscopy on specimens from young and old patients with congenital heart disease associated with muscular obstruction to right ventricular outflow. Especially in the older subjects they found evidence of myocardial degeneration, and they speculated that this might affect cardiac performance and contribute to dysrhythmias. They believed that degenerative changes that occur in the late stage of hypertrophy are not reversible, and they urged that operative repair of congenital heart disease be undertaken at as early an age as is technically appropriate and that a maximal degree of intraoperative myocardial protection be provided, particularly in older patients who are likely to have some myocardial degeneration.

HELPFUL EVENTS AFFECTING THE OUTCOME OF ADULTS WITH VSD

The adult with VSD at birth has several favorable influences on his condition. The opportunity exists for spontaneous decrease in size or even complete closure, perhaps by formation of an aneurysm of the membranous septum. For those with large defects, there is the possibility of acquiring just the right amount of obstruction to right ventricular outflow to decrease the left-to-right shunt, as well as the chance to undergo surgery.

Spontaneous decrease in size of the defect which can lead to *complete, functional closure* is the best thing that could happen to a baby with VSD at birth. This fortunate event can occur in small muscular defects as well as large membranous defects. Although it was first described by two British physicians working independently of each other in 1918,[54,55] the phenomenon did not really command our attention until 1960 in the

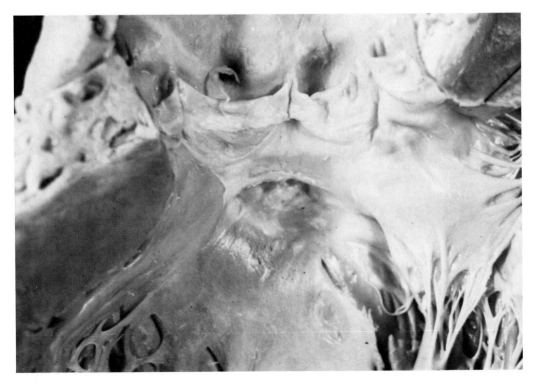

Figure 11. Postmortem specimen of an 81-year-old man who died a noncardiac death shows anatomic evidence of earlier spontaneous closure of a VSD. Note the crescentic fibrous rim arching over the depression where the VSD had been.

modern era of cardiac catheterization with contrast visualization for documentation on serial study.[56] This natural occurrence has been a topic of considerable interest, especially where it concerns the questions of "How?" and "How often?"

From pathologists' work[57–60] it appears that muscular defects most likely close by muscular encroachment and superimposed fibrosis. A fibrous plug or membrane formation in the center of the defect or near the endocardial surface of the right ventricle may begin the process.[59] For defects that involve the membranous septum, closure may be by diminution in size as the heart grows, by fibrosis about the circumference of the defect, by formation of an aneurysm of the membranous septum or by septal leaflet adhesion in the tricuspid valve which obliterates the shunt by formation of a pocket or by plastering down completely over the defect. Figure 11 shows a specimen from an elderly man who died from a noncardiac cause and who had undergone spontaneous closure of the defect.

How often does this occur? Keith estimated that 25 to 30 percent of defects present at birth would close spontaneously.[7] Campbell agreed, stating that spontaneous closure was common up to the fifth decade. He estimated that by age 30, 20 percent of those with VSD at birth were living with a closed defect and by age 60, 24 percent had a closed defect. He calculated a closing rate of 4.2 percent per year.[17] Hoffman was even more optimistic, suggesting that perhaps 50 percent of the defects closed in childhood, most frequently in the first year of life.[9] In the French study of 499 subjects with several examinations, 21 percent of the patients showed some degree of closing and 14 percent experienced complete closure. This occurred in 27 percent of the 215 with small VSD. In 28 percent of the 133 with medium-sized defect, closure was complete (in 10) or partial (in 27). In 10 percent of the 82 with a large defect, whose pulmonary arterial pressure elevated to 70 percent of systemic pressure, there was decrease in size and even closure. None of those with spontaneously closed defects had subsequent infective endocarditis.[15] The recent Natural History Study found that 7 percent of 828 patients had undergone definite spontaneous closure, mostly infants with small defects (17 percent) and rarely, children with large defects (1 percent).[16] Even a VSD acquired from trauma can close spontaneously.[14]

Although it is likely that most defects destined to close spontaneously do so early in childhood, instances of closure in adulthood have been reported. Schott documented the presence of a VSD with large left-to-right shunt (Qp/s = 2.5:1) and normal right heart pressures at the time of cardiac catheterization (age 23); a repeat study at age 40 revealed no evidence of a shunt except on left ventricular angiography, when a small amount of contrast medium was seen to jet across the membranous septum.[60] In the United States Natural History Study, closure was documented by serial cardiac catheterizations in one adult between the ages of 33 and 36.[25] Roberts and colleagues at the National Heart Institute reported the spontaneous closure of a ventricular septal defect in a 27-year-old adult for whom that defect had been advantageous—he had tricuspid atresia.[61] The defect had been in the basal portion of the muscular ventricular septum.

Aneurysm formation of the membranous septum (Fig. 12) is rated an advantage for the individual born with a VSD since it is one of the mechanisms for decreasing the shunt through the defect. The Natural History Study examined 119 patients with left ventricular cineangiocardiogram in the left anterior oblique position at serial cardiac catheterization.[62] An aneurysm of the membranous septum (AMS) developed in 26 patients who had had none at the first study; three were over the age of 12. Aneurysm formation was rare in infancy, the time when defects are most likely to close; therefore, these authors judged that aneurysm formation was not the chief method of closure during infancy. They found that AMS was present in only 12 percent of patients under age 2, in 45 to 50

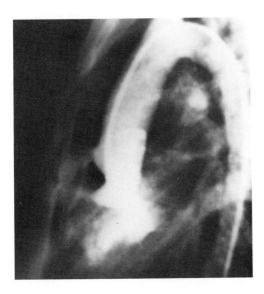

Figure 12. Aneurysm of membranous septum is the pyramidal structure extending from the left ventricle just beneath the aortic valve. A fine jet of contrast medium enters the right ventricle through this spontaneously closing defect.

percent of those aged 2 to 11 years, and in 62 percent of those over the age of 13. This certainly suggests an evolving process that begins early in childhood and continues into adult life. In 1969 Varghese and Rowe documented one case with aneurysm formation that went on to complete closure.[63] They collaborated with Freedom and colleagues in a study of the natural history of AMS over a four-year period, and while they found no evidence in these children of spontaneous closure, they did find that there were no serious complications attributable to the aneurysm. They suggested that the course in childhood was "usually stable and asymptomatic."[64]

Lambert and colleagues approached the question of ventricular septal aneurysms and their role in the natural history of VSD by reviewing 250 left ventricular cineangiograms of patients with VSD.[65] They found 44 with AMS. Thirty-six patients were followed up: 5 had no VSD; 4 had VSD plus a significant cardiac anomaly; and 27 had only VSD. The defect was small in everyone and in some the shunt was detected only by the hydrogen electrode. They confirmed the opinion that patients with VSD and aneurysm of the membranous septum have few physiologic consequences from AMS.

Steinberg first made the diagnosis of AMS in a living patient using angiocardiography.[66] Hoeffel and colleagues recently reviewed the radiologic patterns[67] and Tandon and Edwards the pathologic findings of the condition.[68] Sapire and Black described echocardiographic detection of AMS and advised that this noninvasive method be used in followup of patients.[69] In 1976 Vidne and associates reported their surgical experience in 29 patients. They recommended a change from their first plan of management, imbrication of the tissue in the suture line when closing the defect, because on postoperative study, five of their patients had a small residual VSD and three had a small residual AMS. They advocate excision of the aneurysm and closure of the VSD as the operation of choice.[70]

Acquisition of mild to moderate obstruction to right ventricular outflow offers an advantage to the individual with a persistent VSD, provided the infundibular muscular hypertrophy stops at just the right point. A desirable amount of hypertrophy is one that reduces the shunt so that the pulmonary blood flow is about 1.5 times the systemic flow, or less, and does not elevate the systolic pressure in the right ventricle beyond 40 to 50 mm. Hg. The process that initiates and terminates this development of infundibular

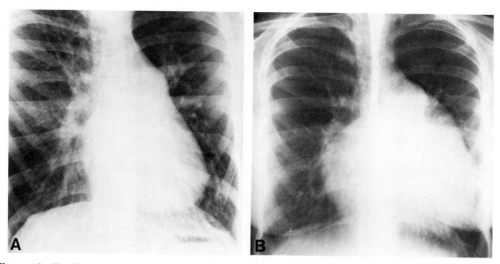

Figure 13. Ill effects of surgery to close a large VSD in a child with a borderline level of pulmonary hypertension and elevation of pulmonary vascular resistance to 70 percent of the systemic level. Left-to-right shunt was small. A, Preoperative film shows that the heart is only slightly enlarged, and that although the pulmonary trunk is abnormally convex, the pulmonary arterial markings are only slightly increased. B, Film taken five years postoperatively, just five years before her death in chronic, refractory right-sided cardiac failure. Although the defect was closed, the pulmonary vascular obstructive disease progressed, the right ventricle dilated and an aneurysmal dilatation appeared just beneath the convex pulmonary trunk. The right atrium enlarged. Pulmonary vascularity was average in the hilar regions, but decreased in the periphery.

pulmonic stenosis (PS) is not well understood and is beyond medical control. The ill effects of too much PS have been commented on earlier; the right ventricle acquires a pressure load, and the shunt may become right-to-left.

Cardiac surgery is the mechanism for helping the individual with a large VSD and a large left-to-right shunt that places a burden on the heart, lungs, and patient. By the time the patient reaches adulthood, the decision concerning suitability for surgery has usually been made. The operation has been carried out in childhood or, as has been done for the last five years if cardiac failure cannot be controlled or the baby fails to thrive, in early infancy.[11] Few adults with a simple, large VSD fulfill these criteria for operation. We do not believe that a simple, small VSD requires surgical closure and it is well known that the VSD associated with pulmonary vascular obstructive disease should not be closed (Fig. 13). The physician caring for adults will need to consider surgery for the few people who have acquired significant AR or PS. The surgeon may find defects in various locations of the ventricular septum.[75]

DIAGNOSTIC CONSIDERATIONS

The physician has in his diagnostic armamentarium the time-honored techniques of history-taking, physical examination, and electrocardiogram and cardiac roentgenograms; the now standard invasive techniques of cardiac catheterization with contrast visualization; and the newer modalities of echocardiography, radionuclide angiography, and the capability to stress the individual in a standardized fashion by dynamic and isometric exercise. Let us see how these measures apply, first to recognition of the unoperated adult with VSD, and then to the postoperative individual.

Unoperated VSD

For the person born with a condition, the way he feels is "normal" for him and he may not appreciate any symptoms until it is quite clear that he is unable to keep up with his peers. Children with VSD are usually totally asymptomatic, and so are adults with a small VSD. Those who have acquired the Eisenmenger syndrome or AR may acknowledge breathlessness or fatigue on exertion. More valuable than a careful history is the physical examination of the adult with VSD.

Roger's description of the findings with small VSD (Fig. 14) is still appropriate today. Freely translated from the French, his message was:

> There is a developmental defect of the heart from which cyanosis does not result despite a communication between the two ventricular cavities . . . It consists of an opening in the interventricular septum. It is revealed only on auscultation by a physical sign with a very definite character; this is a long loud murmur. . . It begins in systole and is prolonged to such an extent as to entirely cover the natural tic-tac of the heart sounds. It has its maximum intensity not at the apex nor at the base to the right or left, but over the upper third of the precordial region. It is chiefly medial in position like the septum itself, and from this central position it diminishes in intensity uniformly. It coincides with no other sign of heart disease except a harsh thrill which accompanies it. This murmur is the pathognomonic sign of an interventricular septal defect.

The electrocardiogram, the cardiac series of chest roentgenograms, and the echocardiogram in such a person would be normal, and if cardiac catheterization were carried out, only a small shunt or none at all would be detected by oxygen data. The hydrogen electrode would detect a small shunt, and the left ventricular angiocardiogram with the

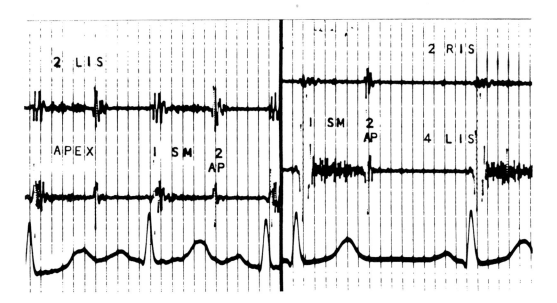

Figure 14. Phonocardiogram of small VSD, *maladie de Roger.* At the fourth interspace a smooth, high-pitched plateau-shaped holosystolic murmur radiates only a short distance. There is normal splitting of the second heart sound.

295

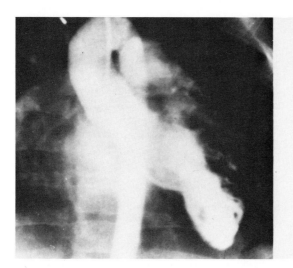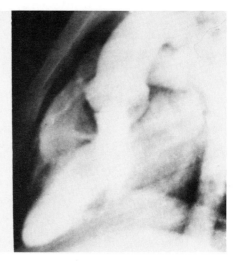

Figure 15. Small VSD demonstrated by selective left ventricular injection of contrast medium. Frontal view on left; simultaneous lateral view on right. Opacification of right ventricle and main pulmonary artery are seen on the frontal film as evidence of left-to-right shunt. In the lateral view the small jet of contrast medium passing through the high defect is easily seen.

patient in the left anterior oblique projection would show a "whiff" of contrast passing through the defect from left to right (Fig. 15). In this projection, the size, location, and number of defects can be identified: supracristal (subpulmonic)[72] or infracristal (membranous, muscular, or in the atrioventricular canal location).[73] Rosenquist and Sweeney's recent anatomic description of the membranous septum of the normal heart provides helpful information for interpretation of defects there.[74]

Eisenmenger's description of the syndrome that now bears his name is also appropriate today:[13,76] "The patient was a powerfully built man of 32 who gave a history of cyanosis and moderate breathlessness since infancy. He managed well enough . . . until January 1894 when dyspnea increased and edema set in . . . he improved with rest and digitalis, but collapsed and died more or less suddenly . . . following a large hemoptysis." At autopsy a 2 by 2.5 cm. defect was found in the region of the membranous septum.

On physical examination the striking diagnostic feature is the loudness and narrow splitting of the second heart sound in the second left interspace as the pressure in the pulmonary artery equals that in the aorta. As the left-to-right shunt diminishes, the systolic murmur shortens and appears diamond-shaped, ejection-type. A faint, high-pitched early diastolic decrescendo murmur is added when the pulmonary valve becomes incompetent (Fig. 16). Cyanosis appears as the shunt becomes right-to-left, and the plethora of polycythemia follows. The electrocardiogram reflects the systemic-pressure load of the right ventricle by showing right axis deviation and R/S reversal in precordial leads, indicative of right ventricular hypertrophy. The echocardiogram depicts the changes in ventricular wall and septum that are occurring as a result of hypertrophy and, later on, dilatation. The roentgenogram of the chest (Fig. 17) shows an average-sized heart (until cardiac failure occurs) with a prominently convex, dilated pulmonary trunk and branches that terminate abruptly in the hilar regions. Cardiac catheterization with contrast visualization documents the elevated pulmonary arterial

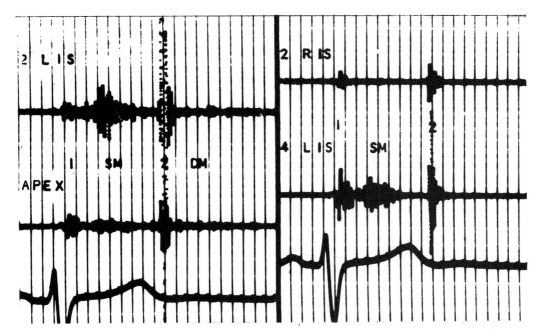

Figure 16. Auscultatory findings in Eisenmenger syndrome. Phonocardiogram shows mid-systolic ejection-type systolic murmur, more prominent at the second left interspace in the pulmonary area than in the fourth left interspace, where the usual holosystolic murmur of the ordinary VSD is maximal. The second sound is single and greatly exaggerated to auscultation due to superimposition of the sounds of aortic and pulmonic valves closing together at the same high pressure. Such an accentuated second heart sound is even palpable over the dilated pulmonary artery in the second left interspace. A faint decrescendo murmur in early and mid-diastole is caused by pulmonic regurgitation.

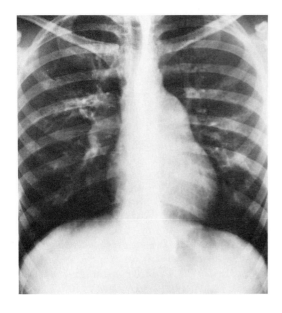

Figure 17. Eisenmenger syndrome, roentgenogram of the young man whose phonocardiogram is seen in Figure 16. The heart is average in size, but the pulmonary trunk is too prominent, as is the right pulmonary artery in the right hilus. Peripheral pulmonary arterial markings are "pruned." This 28-year-old man works daily and his condition is presently stable and free from symptoms during quiet activity.

297

pressure and resistance, which is equal to or in excess of the systemic vascular resistance, and the magnitude as well as direction of the shunt at ventricular level. Management of the patient is supportive by medical means, not by surgery. Some adults continue to function effectively at a quiet level of activity for many years.

The specific diagnostic features of associated cardiac anomalies referred to above (e.g., pulmonic stenosis and aortic regurgitation) are the auscultatory features of those abnormalities superimposed on the findings of VSD. Echocardiography and cardiac catheterization-angiocardiography provide precise analysis and diagnosis.

Postoperative VSD

It is unlikely that any adults will be encountered who underwent banding of the pulmonary trunk 10 or 20 years ago in an effort to decrease the left-to-right shunt through a large VSD that had caused refractory cardiac failure and failure to thrive. If there are any who have not already undergone surgery to deband the pulmonary trunk and close the VSD (if that is still patent), then those individuals as adults must have severe pulmonic stenosis (PS). The band on the pulmonary trunk does not increase in circumference as the child grows; so the effect is that of increasingly severe PS. If the defect is still patent, a right-to-left shunt occurs. Most adults who had this palliation in infancy as a life-saving measure have since undergone open heart surgery to repair the iatrogenic PS and to close the defect. They may therefore be considered the same as any other postoperative adult, with one exception: the possibility of some residual narrowing of the pulmonary trunk after the constricting band is removed or some abnormality of the pulmonic valves which had opened against the band.[77-79]

It has been more than 20 years since Lillehei and his colleagues reported the successful closure of VSD.[80] A whole generation of people with large VSDs have been operated upon, with success increasing at each five-year period: lower mortality rate (to about 2 percent for the usual simple VSD with large shunt) and with greater completeness of repair, minimal risk of heart block, and attention to preservation of myocardium. Many patients have had the defect closed with a patch after a right ventriculotomy permitted access to the defect; but some defects have been repaired via a transatrial[81] or transpulmonary arterial[82] approach, with the goal being the avoidance of a ventriculotomy.

How does one evaluate the postoperative adult? The history is important, with "before" and "after" comparisons and note of any recent trend. Symptoms may belie the true condition, however, and one must look beyond the presence or absence of symptoms to evaluate the cardiac status. It would be nice if all patients who underwent VSD closure were left with no murmur, and with normal heart size, electrocardiogram, and pressures. But this is not so.[24] Most still have a soft systolic murmur. That murmur accompanied by a thrill is highly suggestive of residual abnormality. Often there is wide, fixed splitting of the second heart sound because of surgically acquired complete right bundle branch block (CRBBB).[83] The intensity of the pulmonic (second) component of the second heart sound foretells the level of pulmonary artery pressure. There should be no diastolic murmur in the postoperative patient. The heart should not be enlarged on roentgenogram, although the pulmonary trunk may remain dilated for many years (Fig. 18). Overall pulmonary vascularity should be average. There should be normal sinus rhythm and often RBBB. We have made it a practice to perform cardiac catheterization postoperatively after a year has passed; in this manner we are able to define the pulmonary pressure and vascular resistance as well as the presence of a residual shunt or any previous or new abnormalities.[22,52,84-86] If any change occurs on followup, it may be necessary to repeat the cardiac catheterization. Maron and cowork-

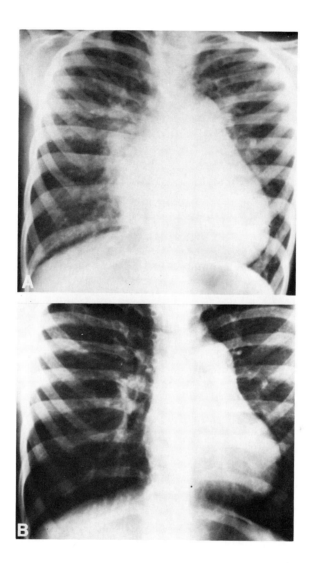

Figure 18. Pre- and postoperative films of six-year-old girl who was operated upon successfully to close a large VSD with large flow. A, Just prior to surgery there is marked cardiomegaly with prominence of the pulmonary trunk and overall pulmonary vascularity. B, Postoperative (one year) film; the findings are the same now, 21 years later. The decrease in cardiac size and overall pulmonary vascularity is striking and, in its way, as dramatic as her symptomatic improvement. The previously dilated pulmonary trunk remains dilated, however, as long, overstretched great arteries tend to do. The postoperative film of this patient with documentation by cardiac catheterization and contrast visualization of normality is not unlike Figure 17, taken from a man with Eisenmenger syndrome. (One must look beyond superficial appearance, history, and roentgenogram to obtain a valid clinical impression of the patient with VSD, unoperated or postoperative. When evidence is conflicting, painstaking physical examination augmented by electrocardiogram is apt to be more informative than the history or roentgenogram.)

ers have reported on the worth of intense upright exercise in evaluating postoperative pulmonary pressure and resistance.[87] Electrophysiologic studies can be performed at cardiac catheterization if a problem of dysrhythmia is detected on standard ECG or Holter monitoring.[83]

MANAGEMENT OF ADOLESCENTS AND ADULTS BORN WITH VSD

Management of adolescents and adults who had VSD at birth can be described as expectant, preventive, or therapeutic.[88] It can be summarized for convenience into six compartments:

1. Preoperative assessment in anticipation of surgery
2. Postoperative evaluation of results of surgery
3. Clarification of an obscure or complex condition
4. Followup of a specific problem, such as pulmonary hypertension
5. Documentation of the malformation in the adolescent or adult for such purposes as athletic competition, insurability, or job placement
6. Long-term evaluation of the effects of the defect

We have already commented on some of these. Let us consider some of the aspects of expectant management that are peculiar to adolescence.[88,89]

Expectant Management

The Adolescent with VSD

Typically the time of rebellion, these few years of adolescence pose a problem for physicians. The patient is apt to disappear from followup or to be lost in the transition from pediatric cardiologist to the physician who will be responsible for his care as an adult. The unwed teen-aged mother with congenital heart disease poses another problem. It has been suggested that some actually seek to become pregnant as proof to themselves that they are as "normal" and healthy as their friends. We have a separate afternoon session each week for adolescents with congenital heart disease so they "don't have to come with the babies." We schedule fewer patients for the doctors than usual so that there is ample time for communication. Suitability for sports, college, a job, or marriage are frequent topics of conversation. Suggested guidelines for utilization by people with the different categories of VSD, unoperated and postoperative, are given in Table 4; these have been taken from the Report of the Intersociety Commission on Heart Disease Resources whose objective was optimal long-term care of patients with congenital heart disease.[90] The teenagers are counselled as to the types of jobs appropriate for their physical condition. These youngsters usually attend clinic alone—not with their parents as in former years. We interpret to them their cardiac status and offer encouragement and reassurance when things are going well. Unless they have special problems, we extend the interval between visits to two or three years. They are reminded about dental care and penicillin prophylaxis for oral procedures and are given the recommendations in writing for their billfolds.

The Adult with VSD

Pediatric cardiologists try to have the individual with VSD in the best shape possible before he enters the adult world. Elective and indicated cardiac surgery has been

Table 4. Suggested guidelines for long-term care of patients with VSD

	Followup*	Activity Restriction†	Recreational Choice Restriction†	Occupational Choice Restriction†	Risk for Insurance
Not Operated					
—Spontaneous closure	4	None	None	None	None
—Small shunt with normal pulmonary arterial pressure	2	None	None	None	Slight
—Moderate or large shunt: a. normal pressure	1	None	None	None	Slight
b. PA < .50 aortic	1	None	None	Mild	Moderate
c. PA > .50 aortic	1	None/Mild	None/Mild	Moderate	Moderate
—With severe pulmonary vascular obstruction and little or no left-to-right shunt	2	Moderate	Moderate	Moderate	High
—With severe pulmonary vascular obstruction and predominant right-to-left shunt	1	Moderate	Moderate	Moderate	High
Operated					
—Defect closed with normal pulmonary arterial pressure	4	None	None	None	None
—Defect closed with pulmonary hypertension	3	None	Mild	Moderate/Severe	Moderate/High
—Residual defects—same as not operated					

*Code to recommendations for cooperative followup

Number	Center	Community
1	1–12 Months	P.R.N.
2	12 Months	3–6 Months
3	12–24 Months	12 Months
4	24–60 Months	6–24 Months

†Restriction categories:
Mild—Lift up to 50 lbs., carry up to 25 lbs.; team sports except for competition.
Moderate—Lift up to 20 lbs., carry up to 10 lbs.; modified physical education program, no team sports.
Severe—Mostly sitting, some walking.
Consider surgery to modify the restrictions indicated.

performed in childhood or adolescence to avoid the psychologic and medical handicaps of that undertaking after the adult has the responsibilities of a job and family.

Employability and *insurability* are status symbols of being able to function adequately as an adult. Attitudes of employers and insurers are now more favorable toward the adult born with VSD than they were 10 to 20 years ago.[96,97] Suggested guidelines for the different categories of VSD are given in Table 4.[90]

Marriage and a *family* are important considerations for the young person born with VSD, and their parents have usually asked long ago about these possibilities for their child. The young woman who has had remedial or palliative cardiac surgery or whose cardiac condition is so mild that surgery is not indicated has an excellent chance of an uneventful pregnancy and a healthy baby. The cyanotic woman with Eisenmenger syndrome has a better than average chance to miscarry or to have a baby with low birth weight,[91] and she is herself at risk of death during the pregnancy or soon after delivery.[17] Jones and Howitt reviewed the question of pregnancies in women with congenital heart disease. They added 188 personal cases to the 1284 that they reviewed. The maternal mortality was 27 percent in 37 women with Eisenmenger syndrome but only 1.8 percent in the 1247 women with all other malformations.[92]

Prospective parents sometimes ask if their baby will have congenital heart disease. No one can tell this in advance, but if there is no family history of congenital heart disease the risk of having a malformed child is somewhat greater than average; nonetheless, the chances of having healthy offspring are still excellent. If there is a family history of cardiac malformation, the risk is increased further.[93] If the anomaly is of a common type and occurs in one or more relatives, the chances of a malformation in the baby are increased about fourfold.[94,95]

Infective endocarditis occurs more often in adults than in children—perhaps because there are more years of adulthood than of childhood—so the adult patient is at risk for a longer time. Prophylaxis against this infection should continue to be stressed.

Preventive Management

Psychologic Considerations

The label "cardiac cripple" need rarely be applied in modern times because physicians can be optimistic in their expectant handling of the adult who was born with VSD. Knowledge is much more secure now than it was in earlier days and life expectancy is excellent for those with mild disorder, a small VSD, or one that has been reduced in size spontaneously or surgically. The informed physician does not overlay the majority of his patients with the blanket of worry that should be reserved for only a few. Psychologically as well as clinically, much has been gained these last 20 to 30 years in the management of the person with VSD. Emotional crippling can be prevented in patients with cardiac defects by the manner in which the physician handles the patient.

Infective Endocarditis

Infective endocarditis can almost always be prevented at times of predictable risk, e.g., patients undergoing dental extractions should be given penicillin in therapeutic doses immediately before and for three days after the procedure. Similar attention should be given at the time of vaginal delivery or genitourinary surgery. Infective endocarditis does still occur unpredictably and there is little one can do in the way of preventive medicine, except to encourage good dental hygiene at all times. The physician can, however, do the next best thing: recognize early any suggestion of infective endocarditis so that he can take several blood cultures and begin appropriate treatment. Patients can be asked to report promptly any febrile illness. Physicians should refrain from prescribing penicillin for the patient with VSD unless he knows he is treating a specific condition such as streptococcal sore throat or pneumococcal pneumonia. Treatment with penicillin for an unexplained fever will only temporarily suppress infective endocarditis and will prolong the period when cardiac damage and other complications can result from ongoing, inadequately treated, endocarditis.

Cerebral Abscess

The cyanotic individual with Eisenmenger syndrome is susceptible to two cerebral complications: brain abscess and cerebral thrombosis. The latter is apt to occur in the young adult who is polycythemic. Both of these complications are related to a pathway for venoarterial shunting, and obliteration of the shunt is not possible for these cyanotic individuals. Good dental hygiene should minimize the risk of brain abscess, and a periodic blood count to detect excessive polycythemia should minimize the risk of cerebral thrombosis. Erythropheresis may help keep the polycythemia of the older individual at a safe level.

Therapeutic Measures

At infrequent but crucial times in the life of the individual with congenital heart disease, certain situations may arise which call for specific treatment: cardiac failure, infective endocarditis, dysrhythmias and conduction disturbances, and cerebrovascular complications. The treatment for each of these is standard and not peculiar to the patient with VSD.

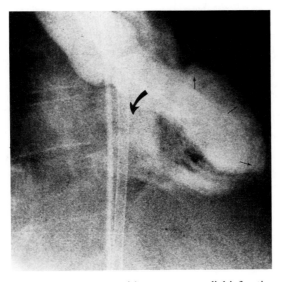

Figure 19. Acquired VSD in a middle-aged man with acute myocardial infarction. Left ventricular cineangiocardiogram shows retrograde catheterization of left ventricle; arrow indicates shunt of contrast medium from left to right ventricle.

303

To summarize the management that enables the patient with VSD to reach and progress through adulthood, we may say that the physician's goal is to enable these individuals to live as normal and full a life as is possible, not as invalids but as active, effective men and women. Many are accomplishing this now, and with each passing year still more will be able to do so.

THE ADULT WITH ACQUIRED VSD

A few adults acquire VSD as a result of trauma[98,99] or myocardial infarction. The latter is now the most common kind of VSD studied in our Adult Cardiac Catheterization Laboratory. Figures 19 and 20 are from cineangiocardiograms at cardiac catheteri-

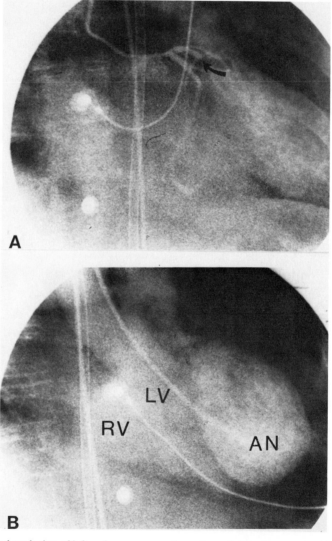

Figure 20. A, Total occlusion of left main coronary artery of an adult is demonstrated by coronary arteriography and indicated by arrow. B, The harmful effects of myocardial infarction have resulted in an acquired VSD, indicated by opacification of right ventricle (RV) at time of left ventricular injection, and an aneurysm (AN) of the left ventricle.

zation of two adults who had sustained a myocardial infarction that resulted in VSD. One of these patients (Fig. 20) had occlusion of the left main coronary artery and acquired not only the VSD but an aneurysm of the left ventricle as well, as is often the case. Because they have such large myocardial infarctions and often an aneurysm too, these patients tolerate the VSD poorly and require emergency surgery.[100]

CONCLUSIONS

The goals of long-term care of the individual born with VSD are to bring him to the peak of physical capability and to help him develop into a well adjusted and effective member of society.[90] Happily, these goals are increasingly being achieved, thanks to medical and surgical advances of the last three decades. So if you hear someone ask, "What happens to adults with VSD?" listen for them, and just look out, world; here they come.

REFERENCES

1. ABBOTT, M. E.: *Atlas of Congenital Cardiac Disease*. American Heart Association, New York, 1936, pp. 36–37, 60.

2. TAUSSIG, H. B.: *Congenital Malformations of the Heart*. Commonwealth Fund, New York, 1947, pp. 390–399.

3. ENGLE, M. A.: *Ventricular septal defect in infancy*. Pediatrics 14:16, 1954.

4. ENGLE, M. A.: *Editorial: The salvage of babies and children with congenital heart disease*. J. Pediatr. 81:203, 1972.

5. ENGLE, M. A.: *When the child's heart fails: Recognition, treatment, prognosis*. Prog. Cardiovasc. Dis. 12:601, 1970.

6. MITCHELL, S. C., KORONES, S. B., AND BERENDES, H. W.: *Congenital heart disease in 56,109 births. Incidence and natural history*. Circulation 43:323, 1971.

7. KEITH, J. D., ROSE, V., COLLINS, G., ET AL.: *Ventricular septal defect. Incidence, morbidity, and mortality in various age groups*. Br. Heart J. 33:81, 1971.

8. FONTANA, R. S., AND Edwards, J. E.: *Congenital Cardiac Disease: A Review of 357 Cases Studied Pathologically*. W. B. Saunders Co., Philadelphia, 1962, pp. 28–29, 72–75.

9. HOFFMAN, J. I. E.: *Natural history of congenital heart disease. Problems in its assessment with special reference to ventricular septal defects*. Circulation 37:97, 1968.

10. GROSSE-BROCKHOFF, F., AND LOOGEN, F.: *Ventricular septal defect*. Circulation 38:V13, 1968.

11. ENGLE, M. A.: *Ventricular septal defect: Status report for the seventies*. Cardiovasc. Clin. 4(3):281, 1972.

12. MARK, H., AND YOUNG, D.: *Congenital heart disease in the adult*. Am. J. Cardiol. 15:293, 1965.

13. PERLOFF, J. K., AND LINDGREN, K. M.: *Adult survival in congenital heart disease. Part 3. Common and uncommon defects with exceptional adult survival*. Geriatrics 29:93, 1974.

14. WALKER, W. J., GARCIA-GONZALEZ, E., CZARNECKI, S. W., ET AL.: *Interventricular septal defect. Analysis of 415 catheterized cases, ninety with serial hemodynamic studies*. Circulation 31:54, 1965.

15. CORONE, P., DOYON, F., GAUDEAU, S., ET AL.: *Natural history of ventricular septal defect. A study involving 790 cases*. Circulation 55:908, 1977.

16. WEIDMAN, W. H., BLOUNT, S. G., DuSHANE, J. W., ET AL.: *Clinical course in ventricular septal defect*. Circulation 56 (Suppl. I):156, 1977.

17. CAMPBELL, M.: *Natural history of ventricular septal defect*. Br. Heart J. 33:246, 1971.

18. *Prevention of Bacterial Endocarditis*. A statement prepared by the Committee on Rheumatic Fever and Bacterial Endocarditis of the Council on Cardiovascular Disease in the Young of the American Heart Association. Circulation 56:139A, 1977.

19. GERSONY, W. M., AND HAYES, C. J.: *Bacterial endocarditis in patients with pulmonary stenosis, aortic stenosis, or ventricular septal defect*. Circulation 56 (Suppl. I):184, 1977.

20. WIEGMANN, T., NAMEY, T. C., AND GODIN, M.: *Right-sided endocarditis and ventricular septal defect*. Can. Med. Assoc. 115:1110, 1974.

21. DuShane, J. W.: *Selection of cases of ventricular septal defect for surgery and late postoperative follow-up.* In Kidd, B. S. L., and Keith, J. D. (eds.): *The Natural History and Progress in Treatment of Congenital Heart Defects.* Charles C Thomas, Springfield, Ill., 1971, pp. 14–18.

22. DuShane, J. W., and Kirklin, J. W.: *Late results of the repair of ventricular septal defect on pulmonary vascular disease.* In Kirklin, J. W. (ed.). *Advances in Cardiovascular Surgery.* Grune and Stratton, Inc., New York, 1973, pp. 9–16.

23. Redo, S. F., Engle, M. A., Holswade, G. R., et al.: *Operative correction of ventricular septal defect with origin of both great vessels from the right ventricle,* J. Thorac. Surg. 45:526, 1963.

24. Engle, M. A., Garutti, R. J., Raptoulis, A. S., et al.: *Recent advances in the diagnosis and treatment of congenital heart disease,* South. Med. J. 70:597, 1977.

25. Selzer, A., and Laqueur, G. L.: *The Eisenmenger complex and its relation to the uncomplicated defect of the ventricular septum: Review of thirty-five autopsied cases of Eisenmenger's complex, including two new cases.* Arch. Intern. Med. 87:218, 1951.

26. Gasul, B. M., Dillon, R. J., and Vela, V.: *The natural transformation of ventricular septal defects into ventricular septal defects with pulmonary stenosis.* Am. J. Dis. Child. 94:424, 1957.

27. Weidman, W. H., DuShane, J. W., and Ellison, R. C.: *Clinical course in adults with ventricular septal defect.* Circulation 56 (Suppl. I):178, 1977.

28. Kawashima, Y., Danno, M., Shimuzu, Y., et al.: *Ventricular septal defect associated with aortic insufficiency: Anatomic classification and method of operation.* Circulation 47:1057, 1973.

29. Tatsuno, K., Konno, S., and Sakakibara, S.: *Ventricular septal defect with aortic insufficiency. Angiocardiographic aspects and a new classification.* Am. Heart J. 85:13, 1973.

30. Keane, J. F., Plauth, W. H., Jr., and Nadas, A.: *Ventricular septal defect with aortic regurgitation.* Circulation 56 (Suppl. I):172, 1977.

31. Somerville, J., Brandao, A., and Ross, D. N.: *Aortic regurgitation with ventricular septal defect: Surgical management and clinical features.* Circulation 41:317, 1970.

32. Kaplan, S., Daoud, G. I., Benzing, G., III, et al.: *Natural history of ventricular septal defect.* Am. J. Dis. Child. 105: 581, 1963.

33. Perloff, J. K. and Lindgren, K. M.: *Adult survival in congenital heart disease. Part 1. Common defects with expected adult survival.* Geriatrics 29:94, 1974.

34. Rao, S., Engle, M. A., and Levin, A. R.: *Silent anomalies of the urinary tract and congenital heart disease.* Chest 67:685, 1975.

35. Anderson, R. C., Lillehei, C. W., and Lester, R. G.: *Corrected transposition of the great vessels of the heart. A review of 17 cases.* Pediatrics 20: 626, 1957.

36. Olinger, G. N., and Maloney, J. V., Jr.: *Trans-pulmonary artery repair of ventricular septal defect associated with congenitally corrected transposition of the great arteries.* J. Thorac. Cardiovasc. Surg. 73:353, 1977.

37. Engle, M. A., Holswade, G. R., Campbell, W. G., et al.: *Ventricular septal defect with transposition of aorta masquerading as acyanotic ventricular septal defect.* Circulation 22:745, 1960.

38. Michaelsson, M., and Tuvemo, T.: *Double outlet right ventricle with spontaneously developing pulmonary outflow obstruction.* Br. Heart J. 36:937, 1974.

39. Van Praagh, R., Perez-Trevino, C., Reynolds, J. L., et al.: *Double outlet right ventricle (S, D, L,) with subaortic ventricular septal defect and pulmonary stenosis. Report of six cases.* Am. J. Cardiol 35:42, 1975.

40. Lev, M., Bharati, S., Meng, L., et al.: *A concept of double-outlet right ventricle.* J. Thorac. Cardiovasc. Surg. 64:271, 1972.

41. Zamora, R., Moller, J. H., and Edwards, J. E.: *Double-outlet right ventricle. Anatomic types and associated anaomalies.* Chest 68:672, 1975.

42. Lincoln, C., Anderson, R. H., Shinebourne, E. A., et al.: *Double outlet right ventricle with l-malposition of the aorta.* Br. Heart J. 37: 453, 1975.

43. Serratto, M., Arevalo, F., Goldman, E. J., et al.: *Obstructive ventricular septal defect in double outlet right ventricle.* Am. J. Cardiol. 19:457, 1967.

44. Kinsley, R. H., Ritter, D. G., and McGoon, D. C.: *The surgical repair of positional anomalies of the conotruncus.* J. Thorac. Cardiovasc. Surg. 67:395, 1974.

45. Kirklin, J. K., and Castaneda, A. R.: *Surgical correction of double-outlet right ventricle with noncommitted ventricular septal defect.* J. Thorac. Cardiovasc. Surg. 73:399, 1977.

46. LYNCH, M. F., RYAN, N. J., WILLIAMS, G. R., ET AL.: *Preoperative diagnosis and surgical correction of supravalvular mitral stenosis and ventricular septal defect.* Circulation 25:854, 1962.

47. HOLLMAN, A., AND HAMED, M.: *Mitral valve disease with ventricular septal defect.* Br. Heart J. 27:274, 1965.

48. GOODMAN, M. J., ROBERTS, N. K., AND IZUKAWA, T.: *Late postoperative conduction disturbances after repair of ventricular septal defect and tetralogy of Fallot. Analysis of His bundle recordings.* Circulation 49:214, 1974.

49. BLOOMFIELD, D. K.: *Association of left ventricular myopathy with minor congenital defects of the ventricular septum.* Circulation 24:889, 1961.

50. BLOOMFIELD, D. K.: *The natural history of ventricular septal defect in patients surviving infancy.* Circulation 29:914, 1964.

51. GRAHAM, T. P., JR.: *Myocardial performance after anatomic or physiologic corrective surgery.* Prog. Cardiovasc. Dis. 17:439, 1975.

52. JARMAKANI, J. M., GRAHAM, T. P., JR., AND CANENT, R. V., JR.: *Left ventricular contractile state in children with successfully corrected ventricular septal defect.* Circulation 45 (Suppl. I):102, 1972.

53. JONES, M., AND FERRANS, V. J.: *Myocardial degeneration in congenital heart disease. Comparison of morphologic findings in young and old patients with congenital heart disease associated with muscular obstruction to right ventricular outflow.* Am. J. Cardiol. 39:1051, 1977.

54. FRENCH., H.: *Spontaneous closure of a ventricular septal defect. A series of small points. Three clinical lectures, Lecture II.* Guy's Hosp. Gaz. 32:87, 1918.

55. WEBER, R. P.: *Can the clinical manifestations of congenital heart disease disappear with the general growth and development of the patient?* Br. J. Child. Dis. 15:113, 1918.

56. EVANS, J. R., ROWE, R. D., AND KEITH, J. D.: *Spontaneous closure of ventricular septal defects.* Circulation 22:1044, 1960.

57. SIMMONS, R. L., MOLLER, J. H., AND EDWARDS, J. E.: *Spontaneous closure of ventricular septal defect.* Mod. Med. December, 1966.

58. GLANCY, D. L., AND ROBERTS, W. C.: *Complete spontaneous closure of ventricular septal defect: Necropsy study of five subjects.* Am. J. Med. 43:846, 1967.

59. SUZUKI, H.: *Spontaneous closure of ventricular septal defects. Anatomic evidence in six adult patients.* Am. J. Clin. Pathol. 52:391, 1969.

60. SCHOTT, G. D.: *Documentation of spontaneous functional closure of a ventricular septal defect during adult life.* Br. Heart J. 35:1214, 1973.

61. ROBERTS, W. C., MORROW, A. G., MASON, D. T., ET AL.: *Spontaneous closure of ventricular septal defect. Anatomic proof in an adult with tricuspid atresia.* Circulation 27:90, 1963.

62. NUGENT, E. W., FREEDOM, R. M., ROWE, R. D., ET AL.: *Aneurysm of the membranous septum in ventricular septal defect.* Circulation 56:I–82, 1977.

63. VARGHESE, P. F., AND ROWE, R. D.: *Spontaneous closure of ventricular septal defects by aneurysmal formation of the membranous septum.* J. Pediatr. 75:700, 1969.

64. FREEDOM, R. M., WHITE, R. D., PIERONI, D. R., ET AL.: *The natural history of the so-called aneurysm of the membranous ventricular septum in childhood.* Circulation 49:375, 1974.

65. LAMBERT, M. E., WIDLANSKY, S., FRANKEN, E. A., ET AL.: *Natural history of ventricular-septal defects associated with ventricular-septal aneurysms.* Am. Heart J. 88:566, 1974.

66. STEINBERG, I.: *Diagnosis of congenital aneurysm of the ventricular septum during life.* Br. Heart J. 19:8, 1957.

67. HOEFFEL, J. C., HENRY, M., FLIZOT, M., ET AL.: *Radiologic patterns of aneurysms of the membranous septum.* Am. Heart J. 91:450, 1976.

68. TANDON, R., AND EDWARDS, J. E.: *Aneurysmlike formations in relation to membranous ventricular septum.* Circulation 47:1089, 1973.

69. SAPIRE, D. W., AND BLACK, I. F. S.:*Echocardiographic detection of aneurysms of the interventricular septum associated with ventricular septal defect. A method of noninvasive diagnosis and follow-up.* Am. J. Cardiol. 36:797, 1975.

70. VIDNE, B. A., CHIARIELLO, L., WAGNER, H., ET AL.: *Aneurysm of the membranous ventricular septum: Surgical consideration and experience in 29 cases.* J. Thorac. Cardiovasc. Surg. 71:402, 1976.

71. ROGER, H.: *Recherches cliniques sur la communication congenitale des deux coeurs, par inocclusion du septum interventriculaire.* Bull. Mem. Acad. R. Med. Belg. 8:1074, 1897.

72. STEINFELD, L., DIMICH, I., PARK, S. C., ET AL.: *Clinical diagnosis of isolated subpulmonic (supracristal) ventricular septal defect.* Am. J. Cardiol. 30:19, 1972.

73. TAYLOR, J. F. N., AND CHRISPIN, A. R.: *Interventricular septal defect shown by left ventricular cineangiocardiography.* Br. Heart J. 33:285, 1971.

74. ROSENQUIST, G. C.., AND SWEENEY, L. J.: *The membranous ventricular septum in the normal heart.* Johns Hopkins Med. J. 135:9, 1974.

75. GOOR, D. A., EDWARDS, J. E., AND LILLEHEI, C. W.: *The development of the interventricular septum of the heart: Correlative morphogenetic study.* Chest 58:468, 1970.

76. EISENMENGER, V.: *Die angeborenen Defecte der Kammerscheidwand des Herzens.* Z. Klin. Med. 32:1, 1897.

77. HUNT, C. E., FORMANEK, G., CASTANEDA, A., ET AL.: *Closure of ventricular septal defect and removal of pulmonary arterial band.* Am. J. Cardiol. 26:345, 1970.

78. STARK, J., TYNAN, M., ABERDEEN, E., ET AL.: *Repair of intracardiac defects after previous constriction (banding) of the pulmonary artery.* Surgery 67:536, 1970.

79. SEYBOLD-EPTING, W., REUL, G. J., JR., HALLMAN, G. L., ET AL.: *Repair of ventricular septal defect after pulmonary artery banding.* J. Thorac. Cardiovasc. Surg. 71:392, 1976.

80. LILLEHEI, C.W., COHEN, M., WARDEN, H. E., ET AL.: *The results of direct vision closure of ventricular septal defects in eight patients by means of controlled cross circulation.* Surg. Gynecol. Obstet. 101:446, 1955.

81. LINCOLN, C., JAMIESON, S., JOSEPH, M., ET AL.: *Transatrial repair of ventricular septal defects with reference to their anatomic classification.* J. Thorac. Cardiovasc. Surg. 74:183, 1977.

82. KAWASHIMA, Y., FUMITA, T., MORI, T., ET AL.: *Transpulmonary arterial closure of ventricular septal defect.* J. Thorac. Cariovasc. Surg. 74:191, 1977.

83. GODMAN, M. J., ROBERTS, N. K., AND IZUKAWA, T.: *Late postoperative conduction disturbances after repair of ventricular septal defect and tetralogy of Fallot—analysis of His bundle recordings.* Circulation 49:214, 1974.

84. HO, C. S., KROVETZ, L. J., STRIFE, J. L., ET AL.: *Postoperative assessment of residual defects following cardiac surgery in infants and children. II. Ventricular septal defects.* Johns Hopkins Med. J. 133:278, 1973.

85. ALLEN, H. D., ANDERSON, R. C., NOREN, G. R., ET AL.: *Postoperative follow-up of patients with ventricular septal defect.* Circulation 50:465, 1974.

86. FRIEDLI, B., KIDD, B. S. L., MUSTARD, W. R., ET AL.: *Ventricular septal defect with increased pulmonary vascular resistance: Late results of surgical closure.* Am. J. Cardiol. 33:403, 1974.

87. MARON, B. J., REDWOOD, D. R., HIRSHFELD, J. W., JR., ET AL.: *Postoperative assessment of patients with ventricular septal defect and pulmonary hypertension. Response to intense upright exercise.* Circulation 48:864, 1973.

88. ENGLE, M. A.: *Medical management of the patient with congenital heart disease.* Cardiovasc. Clin. 2(1):268, 1970.

89. STEINHERZ, L., AND ENGLE, M. A.: *Heart disease in the adolescent.* In Lopez, R. I. (ed.): *Adolescent Medicine.* Spectrum Publications, Inc., Holliswood, New York, 1976, pp. 109–147.

90. ENGLE, M. A., ADAMS, F. H., BETSON, R., ET AL.: *Resources for optimal long-term care of congenital heart disease. Report of Inter-Society Commission for Heart Disease Resources.* Circulation 44:A–205, 1971.

91. NEILL, C. A., AND SWANSON, S.: *Outcome of pregnancy in congenital heart disease.* Circulation 24:1003, 1961.

92. JONES, A. M., AND HOWITT, G.: *Eisenmenger syndrome in pregnancy.* Br. Med. J. 1:1627, 1965.

93. EHLERS, K. H., AND ENGLE, M. A.: *Familial congenital heart disease: 1. Genetic and environmental factors.* Circulation 34:503, 1966.

94. NORA, J. J.: *Multifactorial inheritance hypothesis for the etiology of congenital heart diseases.* Circulation 38:604, 1968.

95. NEILL, C. A.: *Etiology of congenital heart disease.* Cardiovasc. Clin. 4(3):137, 1972.

96. ENGLE, M. A.: *Editorial: Insurability and employability, congenital heart disease and innocent murmurs.* Circulation 56:143, 1977.

97. MANNING, J. A., AND HUTCHINSON, J. J.: *Insurability and employability of young cardiacs. Special report from the American Heart Association.* Circulation 56:335A, 1977.

98. HART, R. J., JR., AND GREGORATOS, G.: *Ventricular septal defects caused by stab wounds: Report of two cases.* Milit. Med. 139:289, 1974.

99. DEAL, C., DONNELLY, G. L., AND MONK, I.: *Ventricular septal defect caused by a penetrating wound of the heart.* Med. J. Aust. 1:29, 1971.

100. GRAHAM, A. F., STINSON, E. B., DAILY, P. O., ET AL.: *Ventricular septal defects after operative treatment.* JAMA 225:708, 1973.

Coarctation of the Aorta in the Adult

Barry J. Maron, M.D.

Coarctation of the aorta was one of the first congenital cardiovascular malformations for which operative repair became available.[1,2] Subsequently, a high degree of sophistication has been obtained with regard to both the clinical identification of coarctation of the aorta, the selection of patients for operation, and the surgical methods employed to repair this malformation.[3,4] Early studies emphasized that the vast majority of patients with coarctation of the aorta had improved symptomatically and had experienced substantial lowering of blood pressure shortly after operation.[3] These factors led to an initial euphoria among cardiologists and surgeons regarding the overall benefits of operative "correction" of this malformation. However, more recently it has become evident that a substantial number of patients with coarctation of the aorta may experience premature death or demonstrate residual cardiovascular abnormalities many years after apparently satisfactory operative repair.[5–7]

This review presents information currently available regarding both the natural and the unnatural history of isolated coarctation of the aorta ("adult-type"). In this regard the following two questions will be addressed: (1) What are the cardiovascular effects of coarctation of the aorta on the patient in adulthood if operation is not performed? (2) What are the cardiovascular effects on the patient in adulthood if apparently successful operative repair of coarctation of the aorta is performed earlier in life?

NATURAL HISTORY OF UNOPERATED PATIENTS WITH COARCTATION OF THE AORTA

Our knowledge of the natural history of coarctation of the aorta is derived principally from data obtained before the advent of operative repair of this malformation in 1945. This information emanates primarily from the large necropsy-based studies of Abbott[8] and of Reifenstein and coworkers[9] (a total of 304 patients) and a group of 161 patients identified clinically at three institutions and summarized by Campbell.[10,11] Drawing conclusions regarding the natural history of coarctation of the aorta from analysis of these 465 unoperated patients is fraught with a number of limitations (particularly bias in patient selection), but it is reasonable to derive the following conclusions:

1. In patients with coarctation of the aorta who did not undergo operation, life expectancy was probably severely shortened—e.g., the average age at death was about 35 years and nearly 90 percent of patients had died before 50 years of age (Fig. 1); the annual mortality rate increased from 2 percent in the first two decades to 7 percent in the sixth decade.

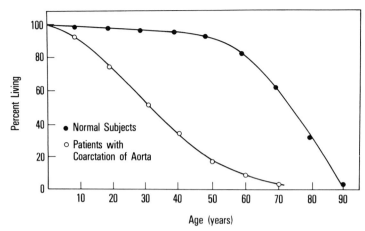

Figure 1. Survival plotted as a function of age for 465 unoperated patients with coarctation of the aorta who survived the first year of life and 1000 normal subjects who survived the first year. (Adapted from Campbell.[11])

2. The most common causes of death were congestive heart failure, aortic rupture, intracranial hemorrhage, or infective endocarditis or endarteritis (at the site of the coarctation or on a congenitally bicuspid aortic valve).

3. Systemic hypertension appeared to be the most deleterious component of this disease, since in most patients it was reasonable to consider death a consequence of the hypertension.

PROGNOSIS OF PATIENTS WITH REPAIRED COARCTATION OF THE AORTA

When repair of coarctation of the aorta was first introduced it was expected that this operation would be uniformly beneficial.[3] However, data are now available to suggest that satisfactory repair of coarctation of the aorta does not necessarily normalize systemic blood pressure or convey normal longevity.[5-7] In 1972 a retrospective analysis of 248 consecutive patients who had survived operation for coarctation of the aorta at Johns Hopkins Hospital between 1946 and 1960 revealed a surprisingly high prevalence of residual cardiovascular disease in these patients, often many years after operation.[5] In that study the average age at operation was 20 years and patients were followed for 11 to 25 years (average, 16 years) after operation. Only 12 of the 248 patients had associated cardiac malformations and all patients were over two years of age at operation. Fifty-five patients were either lost to followup or died of noncardiac causes.

Of particular interest was the finding that 12 percent of the patients in whom followup data were available had died of cardiovascular disease (average age, 35 years; average survival after operation, 9 years). Death was most commonly from a ruptured major artery (i.e., aorta or cerebral artery), associated aortic or mitral valvular disease with or without infective endocarditis, congestive heart failure, or coronary atherosclerosis with myocardial infarction, or else it was sudden and unexplained (presumably due to a ventricular arrythmia). The occurrence of premature cardiovascular death generally correlated with older age at the time of operation (and, therefore, longer duration of preoperative hypertension; Table 1), and was particularly high when repair was carried out after the age of 25 years (Fig. 2). In this regard, 14 of the 70 patients (or 20 percent) operated upon after 25 years of age had died, compared to only 8 (6 percent) of the 123 patients operated upon at or before 25 years of age (p < 0.01). A survival curve for the 193 patients who survived operation for coarctation of the aorta and in whom followup data were available is shown in Figure 3. The average annual mortality after operation

Table 1. Preoperative risk factors for patients with coarctation of the aorta

	Survivors	Deaths	
Age at Operation (years)	19	27	p < 0.005
Systolic Blood Pressure (mm. Hg)	165	169	
Diastolic Blood Pressure (mm. Hg)	92	92	p < 0.05
Arm-Leg Systolic Gradient (mm. Hg)	118	140	

for these patients was 1 percent; all patients died within the first 16 postoperative years. Systolic or diastolic blood pressure or the difference between arm and leg systolic blood pressure did not appear to be risk factors for late cardiovascular death (Table 1).

Fifty-nine of the patients in the study group underwent late postoperative inpatient evaluation. Almost 80 percent (46 of 59 patients) of this subgroup (average age, 40 years) had evidence of cardiovascular disease (Fig. 4). Cardiovascular abnormalities identified in these patients included aortic valvular disease (presumably on the basis of a congenitally bicuspid aortic valve which is present in a substantial number of patients with coarctation of the aorta), electrocardiographic conduction abnormalities, angina pectoris, or residual systemic hypertension (systolic, diastolic, or both).

It should be emphasized, however, that the patients studied at Johns Hopkins Hospital were operated upon later in life (mean age, 20 years) than those patients currently selected for operation. Nevertheless, there appears to be a substantial prevalence of postoperative cardiovascular problems in patients operated upon even at relatively young ages. Simon and Zloto[6] reviewed 241 patients at the University of Michigan Medical Center with coarctation of the aorta who underwent operation at an average age of about 12 years. These patients were followed for an average of only six years, and there was a 6 percent prevalence of premature cardiovascular death (mean age, 32

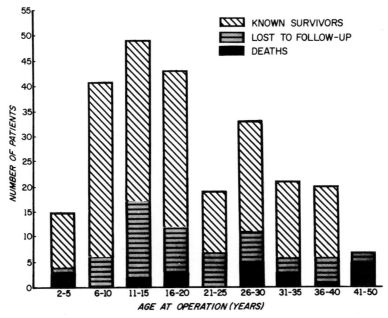

Figure 2. Age at operation and age at death for 248 patients with coarctation of the aorta. (From Maron et al.[5]; with permission of the American Heart Association, Inc.)

313

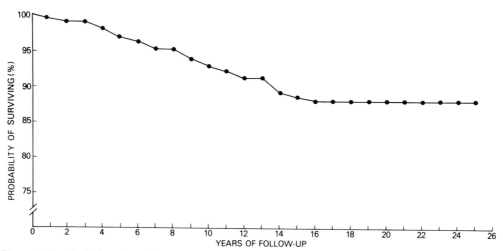

Figure 3. Survival plotted as a function of duration of followup after operative repair of coarctation of the aorta. This study group includes 193 patients in whom long-term followup data was available; excluded from this analysis were 19 deaths related to operation.

years). Such deaths were either sudden or the result of unexplained congestive heart failure, or they were attributed to associated congenital cardiac malformations (i.e., mitral regurgitation, hypoplastic aortic arch, aortic valve disease, atrial septal defect, or dissected aortic aneurysm). Indeed, other investigators have also emphasized the concomitant occurrence of a wide variety of congenital malformations of the mitral valve (including parachute deformity) that may result in either mitral regurgitation or stenosis.[12,13]

It is apparent that repair of coarctation of the aorta produces significant reduction in systemic blood pressure in the vast majority of patients.[14-19] However, in some patients the postoperative blood pressure (even when assessed many years after operation) does not return to normal. Persistent and unexplained systemic hypertension after repair of coarctation of the aorta has been noted to occur in 5 to 30 percent of patients,[5,6,14-19] and in the majority of these studies a sizeable prevalence of persistent hypertension (15

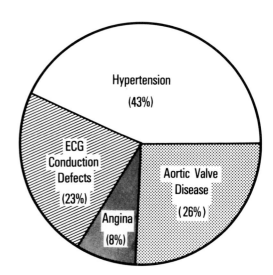

Figure 4. Cardiovascular disease present late postoperatively in 59 patients with coarctation of the aorta who were studied as inpatients.

314

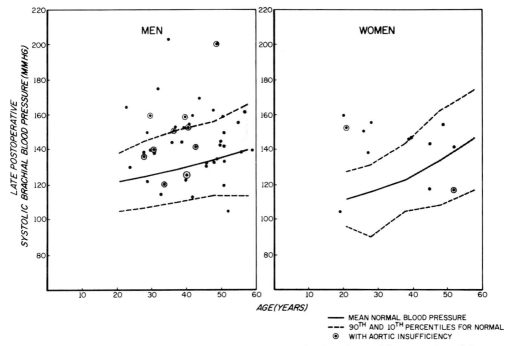

Figure 5. Late postoperative systolic brachial blood pressures in 59 patients with coarctation of the aorta. (From Maron et al.;[5] with permission of the American Heart Association, Inc.)

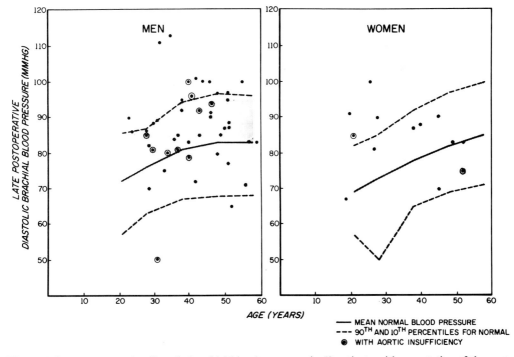

Figure 6. Late postoperative diastolic brachial blood pressures in 59 patients with coarctation of the aorta. (From Maron et al.;[5] with permission of the American Heart Association, Inc.)

315

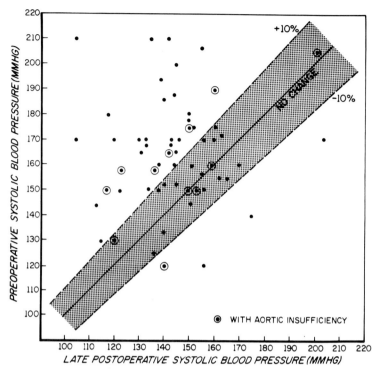

Figure 7. Comparison of preoperative and postoperative systolic brachial blood pressures in 59 patients with coarctation of the aorta. Symbols in the shaded area represent blood pressures unchanged by operation (21 of 59, or 35 percent). Blood pressures above the shaded area were lowered by operation (34 of 59, or 58 percent); those below the shaded area were elevated above the preoperative level (4 of 59, or 7 percent). (From Maron et al.;[5] with permission of the American Heart Association, Inc.)

percent or more) was reported. In the Johns Hopkins study,[5] about 40 percent of 59 patients demonstrated residual systemic hypertension (systolic, diastolic, or both) and showed unchanged or increased blood pressure as compared to preoperative pressures (Figs. 5–8). While the elevated blood pressure was caused by residual coarctation of the aorta or coexistent aortic regurgitation in a minority of these patients, the hypertension remained unexplained in about 30 percent of the 59 patients studied. Of interest, those patients with the highest systolic blood pressures at the most recent postoperative followup evaluation also had the highest blood pressures immediately after operation (p < 0.001) (Fig. 9). However, the magnitude of residual long-term postoperative hypertension does not appear to be related to the magnitude of preoperative hypertension (Fig. 10).

It is possible that the high prevalence of residual hypertension in the patients studied at Johns Hopkins Hospital[5] is related, in part, to the relatively advanced age at which operation was performed (and hence to the longer period of preoperative hypertension they experienced). Indeed, the age at which repair of coarctation of the aorta is undertaken may be an important determinant in the ultimate reduction of the postoperative blood pressure. This consideration is supported by the data of Nanton and Olley.[18] They studied patients operated upon between the ages of 4 and 15 years and found that the earlier the operation was performed the greater was the reduction in systemic blood pressure.

In addition, the relatively mild residual hypertension present under basal conditions in some patients after repair of coarctation of the aorta may be accentuated with

316

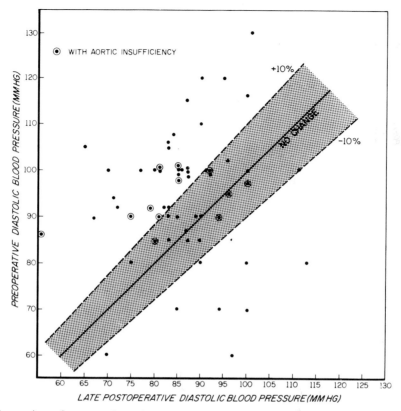

Figure 8. Comparison of preoperative and postoperative diastolic brachial blood pressures in 59 patients with coarctation of the aorta. Symbols in the shaded area represent blood pressures unchanged by operation (19 of 59, or 32 percent). Blood pressures above the shaded area were lowered by operation (32 of 59, or 55 percent); those below the shaded area were elevated above the preoperative level (8 of 59, or 13 percent).

exercise.[20,21] James and Kaplan[20] found that strenuous upright exercise (performed 6 to 15 months after operation) produced marked systolic hypertension (212 to 270 mm. Hg) in about two thirds of the patients, although the diastolic pressures usually decreased or were unchanged. Hence, it would seem prudent to identify and treat medically those patients who manifest residual hypertension after repair of coarctation of the aorta; furthermore, patients who demonstrate particularly marked elevations in blood pressure with exercise should be advised to avoid very strenuous or competitive physical activities.

The explanation for residual long-term postoperative hypertension (under basal conditions or with exercise) in patients with coarctation of the aorta is unclear. However, potential etiologic factors include residual limitation of the capacity and distensibility of the proximal aorta, disturbance of the renin-angiotensin system, or a disease process unrelated to the coarctation.

SUMMARY

It is generally accepted that repair of coarctation of the aorta ("adult-type") should be performed in childhood or adolescence in order to minimize the deleterious effects of systemic hypertension. However, while the vast majority of patients with coarctation of the aorta benefit from operative repair with subsequent substantial lowering of blood

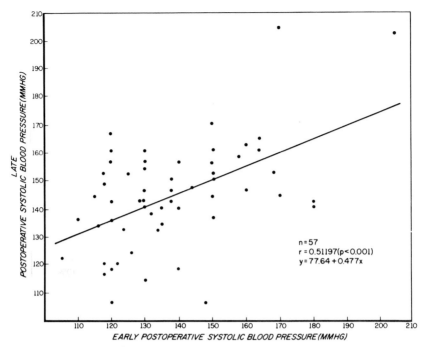

Figure 9. Relation of early and late postoperative systolic brachial blood pressures. Variance about the fitted line = 267.8. (From Maron et al.;[5] with permission of the American Heart Association, Inc.)

pressure, a significant number of patients may manifest persistent hypertension many years after operation. Furthermore, some patients experience premature cardiovascular death that may be sudden or the result of associated aortic or mitral valvular disease, infective endocarditis or endarteritis, unexplained congestive heart failure, or

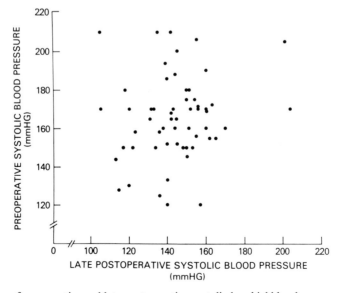

Figure 10. Relation of preoperative and late postoperative systolic brachial blood pressures.

318

rupture of a major artery (aorta or cerebral artery). Hence, continued close followup of patients after repair of coarctation of the aorta appears to be necessary in order to evaluate the potential long-term effects of these residual cardiovascular abnormalities.

REFERENCES

1. CRAFOORD, C., AND NYLIN, G.: *Congenital coarctation of the aorta and its surgical treatment*. J. Thorac. Surg. 14:347,1945.

2. GROSS, R. E., AND HUFNAGEL, C. A.: *Coarctation of the aorta: experimental studies regarding its surgical correction*. Surgery 18:673,1945.

3. SCHUSTER, S. R., AND GROSS, R. E.: *Surgery for coarctation of the aorta: review of 500 cases*. J. Thorac. Cardiovasc. Surg. 43:54,1962.

4. MORRIS, G. C., COOLEY, D. A., DEBAKEY, M. E., ET AL.: *Coarctation of the aorta with particular emphasis upon improved techniques of surgical repair*. J. Thorac. Cardiovasc. Surg. 40:705,1960.

5. MARON, B. J., HUMPHRIES, J. O., ROWE, R. D., ET AL.: *Prognosis of surgically corrected coarctation of the aorta: a 20-year postoperative appraisal*. Circulation 47:119,1973.

6. SIMON, A. G., AND ZLOTO, A. E.: *Coarctation of the aorta: longitudinal assessment of operated patients*. Circulation 50:456,1974.

7. FRASER, T. S., STOBEY, J., ROSSALL, R.E., ET AL.: *Coarctation of the aorta in adults*. Can. Med. Assoc. J. 115:415,1976.

8. ABBOTT, M. E.: *Coarctation of the aorta of the adult type II. Statistical study and historical retrospect of 200 recorded cases, with autopsy, of stenosis or obliteration of the descending arch*. Am. Heart J. 3:392,1928.

9. REIFENSTEIN, G. H., LEVINE, S. A., AND GROSS, R. E.: *Coarctation of the aorta: A review of 104 autopsied cases of the "adult type" 2 years of age or older*. Am. Heart J. 33:146,1947.

10. CAMPBELL, M., AND BAYLIS, J. H.: *The course and prognosis of coarctation of the aorta*. Br. Heart J. 18:475,1956.

11. CAMPBELL, J.: *Natural history of coarctation of the aorta*. Br. Heart J. 32:633,1970.

12. ROSENQUIST, G. C.: *Congenital mitral valve disease associated with coarctation of the aorta. A spectrum that includes parachute deformity of the mitral valve*. Circulation 49:985,1974.

13. FREED, M. D., KEANE, J. F., VAN PRAAGH, R., ET AL.: *Coarctation of the aorta with congenital mitral regurgitation*. Circulation 49:1175,1974.

14. RATHI, L., AND KEITH, J. D.: *Postoperative blood pressures in coarctation of the aorta*. Br. Heart J. 26:671,1964.

15. MARCH, H. W., HULTGREN, H. N., AND GERBODE, F.: *Immediate and remote effects of resection on the hypertension in coarctation of the aorta*. Br. Heart J. 22:361,1960.

16. SELLORS, T. H., AND HOBSLEY, M.: *Coarctation of the aorta: effect of operation on blood pressure*. Lancet 1:1387,1963.

17. CHIARIELLO, L., AGOSTI, J., AND SUBRAMANIAN, S.: *Coarctation of the aorta in children and adolescents*. Chest 70:621,1976.

18. NANTON, M. A., AND OLLEY, P.M.: *Residual hypertension after coarctectomy in children*. Am. J. Cardiol. 37:769,1976.

19. COUNIHAN, T. B.: *Changes in the blood pressure following resection of coarctation of the aortic arch*. Clin. Sci. 15:149,1956.

20. JAMES, F. W., AND KAPLAN, S.: *Systolic hypertension during submaximal exercise after correction of coarctation of the aorta*. Circulation 49 and 50(Suppl. II):27,1974.

21. TAYLOR, S. H., AND DONALD, K. W.: *Circulatory studies at rest and during exercise in coarctation of the aorta before and after operation*. Br. Heart J. 22:117,1960.

Patent Ductus Arteriosus in Adults

David T. Kelly, M.D.

HISTORY

In 181 A.D. Galen described the ductus arteriosus and its closure. This is possibly the first recorded description of a congenital cardiovascular malformation. Patent ductus arteriosus (PDA) has been known as the ductus Botallo since the 16th century but it is doubtful that Botallo described it; he rediscovered the foramen ovale, not the ductus.[1]

In 1628 Harvey described the direction of blood flow across the PDA, and in 1898, Gibson[2] described the "machinery murmur": "it begins softly and increases in intensity so as to reach its acme just about or immediately after the second sound and from that point gradually wanes till its termination. The second sound can be heard to be loud and clanging." This was a classic clinical observation documented many years later by phonocardiography. In 1938[3] Gross successfully ligated a PDA for the first time, and the procedure ushered in the era of modern cardiovascular surgery.

ANATOMY

The ductus arteriosus connects the left pulmonary artery to the aorta ventrolaterally distal to the origin of the left subclavian artery at an angle of about 30 degrees. The ductus is the embryological remnant of the distal sixth left aortic arch. During fetal life this vascular connection has a large lumen equal to both the aorta and pulmonary artery. When the ductus closes, the tissue forms a ligmentum arteriosus. In about one fourth of adult necropsies a small dimple is seen in the pulmonary artery on the aortic wall, but nothing unusual is ordinarily seen on the aortic side.[4]

The size and shape of PDA varies remarkably. It may be long and narrow or short and wide. The wall is usually thin. There is frequently a conical formation with the aortic end forming the mouth. The reverse also may occur. Ultrastructurally the ductus is different from the aorta. There is subendothelial vacuolization of medial smooth muscle cells, interruption of elastic lamina, and distended endoplasmic reticulum.[5]

INCIDENCE AND ETIOLOGY

The incidence of congenital thoracic cardiovascular malformations is 5 to 6 per 100 live births,[6] and about 10 percent of these (or 1 in 200 live births) result from PDA—one of the most common congenital cardiovascular anomalies.[7]

PDA may result from maternal rubella, often in association with other cardiac defects, primarily pulmonary arterial and systemic arterial stenoses.[8]

Frequently more than one member in a family has PDA, suggesting modified dominant or polygenetic inheritance. The children of a single parent with PDA have a 1 in 90 chance of having PDA, and this information is useful in genetic counseling.[9]

PDA is more frequent in females. In a study of 705 patients with PDA Keith[7] found a 68 percent female to 32 percent male prevalence. When PDA results from maternal rubella, prevalence is the same in both sexes.[10]

A fascinating study by Patterson showed that breeding poodles with PDA resulted in an 83 percent incidence of cardiovascular malformations with 80 percent concordance.[11] It was concluded that PDA was a polygenic threshold trait of high hereditability, and that normal ductal closure was impaired by extending aortic-like tissue differentiation into the ductal area. A proportion of offspring of poodles also showed incomplete closure, resulting in a ductus diverticulum at the aortic end.

Several conditions may modify the normal closing sequence of the PDA. Premature infants have a high incidence of PDA and respiratory distress in the newborn period is believed to delay normal ductal closure.[12] A ductus in the newborn may be closed by a high oxygen atmosphere, whereas anoxia will reopen the ductus or delay closure. Further effects of oxygen levels on ductal closure are seen in high altitude areas. Alzamora[13] showed that 30 percent of 110 infants with PDA were born at more than 4000 m. above sea level in Peru where only 2 percent of the population lived. Prostaglandin action on smooth muscle has been shown to maintain ductal patency in the newborn, and this therapy is used in the short-term management of cyanotic conditions such as transposition of the great vessels where ductal closure is deleterious.[14]

Aneurysm of the PDA is rare but reported in both young and old. Right-sided PDA, usually in association with a right-sided aortic arch, is uncommon.[6]

CLINICAL FEATURES

PDA is rare in adults and adolescents nowadays because a precordial murmur is usually identified early in life and appropriate surgery undertaken. Any patient with a typical Gibson continuous murmur, maximal in the second left interspace, must be suspected of having PDA. Adult patients with PDA are often asymptomatic. However, longstanding left-to-right shunt may cause dyspnea, often accompanied by sweating, as the result of left ventricular failure. Full-blown congestive heart failure may follow.

In addition to the characteristic murmur, the physical signs depend on the degree of left-to-right shunt. A small shunt will exhibit normal precordial activity and pulse; whereas a larger shunt will be accompanied by a wide pulse pressure and an enlarged and overactive left ventricle. The mid-diastolic flow murmur in the mitral area, often heard in the younger age groups, is rarely heard in adults. The echocardiogram shows enlargement of left ventricle and left atrium. The electrocardiogram is normal or may show increased voltage, i.e., the diastolic overload pattern. The chest radiograph in patients with significant left-to-right shunt may show enlarged main pulmonary arteries, particularly in older patients. Cardiomegaly with enlargement of the left ventricle, left atrium, and ascending aorta indicates a significant shunt. In older patients, fluoroscopy may show calcific deposits in the region of the ductus. This sign is common after the age of 30.[15] At cardiac catheterization the characteristic finding is a rise in oxygen saturation in the pulmonary artery. The catheter can usually be passed from the left main pulmonary artery through the ductus into the descending aorta. Figure 1 illustrates the typical hemodynamic findings and dye dilution curves. Except in patients with the Eisenmenger syndrome, significant pulmonary hypertension is uncommon. In a small PDA the left-to-right shunt may be minimal and therefore may go undetected in

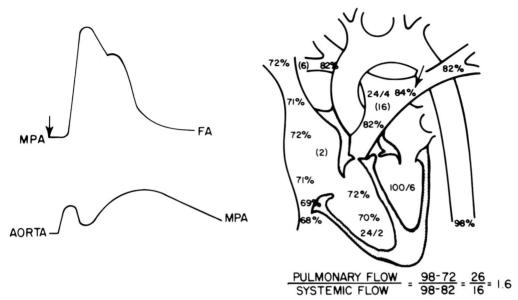

$$\frac{\text{PULMONARY FLOW}}{\text{SYSTEMIC FLOW}} = \frac{98-72}{98-82} = \frac{26}{16} = 1.6$$

Figure 1. Hemodynamic findings in PDA, with a rise in oxygen saturation at the pulmonary artery level. The right and left heart pressures are normal. Forward dye curve from main pulmonary artery (MPA) to femoral artery (FA) shows a left-to-right shunt. Reverse dye curve, i.e., from aorta to MPA, shows the shunt is at the great vessel level.

oxygen samples. More sensitive methods of shunt detection, such as hydrogen electrode or reversed dye techniques, may be needed. Aortography in the left lateral position usually will delineate the PDA and differentiate it from other causes of continuous precordial murmurs.

All adult patients with physical signs of PDA should have cardiac catheterization and angiography because there are other, less common, causes of continuous precordial murmurs in adults.

COMPLICATIONS

Eisenmenger's Syndrome

This disorder is the result of a large PDA in infancy. Cyanosis may not occur until adult life when it is more noticeable in the lower body. Cyanosis and clubbing of the toe nails, not the finger nails, are the characteristic features of PDA with reversal of flow. More generalized cyanosis occurs later. The physical signs are those of pulmonary hypertension with a right ventricular systolic impulse and a loud pulmonic second sound. The second sound often moves with respiration in the patient with an Eisenmenger ductus. A pulmonary ejection click is often present, but no continuous murmur is heard because the pressures in the aorta and pulmonary artery are equal.[16] The electrocardiogram reveals right ventricular hypertrophy and the chest radiograph, a normal-sized heart, large dilated central arteries and attenuated peripheral branches. An Eisenmenger ductus is often difficult to distinguish from a defect in the atrial or ventricular septum with associated severe pulmonary hypertension. Although no surgical treatment is possible, the exact diagnosis should be confirmed at cardiac catheterization because other rare and reversible conditions may resemble Eisenmenger's syndrome.

Congestive Heart Failure

The adult with PDA frequently develops congestive heart failure, which is often accompanied by atrial fibrillation. The irregular rhythm, the low cardiac output, and the moderate rise in pulmonary pressure all tend to attenuate the intensity of the continuous precordial murmur and may confuse the diagnosis. The wide pulse pressure, the "overactive" left ventricle, and the large central and peripheral pulmonary arteries help to confirm the proper diagnosis.

Infective Arteritis

This infection usually occurs and proliferates at the pulmonary end of the PDA. Vegetations tend to dislodge and embolize to the lungs, producing septic pneumonitis and infarcts. Infective arteritis is most common in the second and third decades of life.[6]

Of 1435 patients with infective endocarditis (or arteritis) studied by Espino-Vela,[15] 38 (3 percent) had PDA. Better recognition of cardiac defects and antibiotic prophylaxis have undoubtedly decreased the incidence of "endocarditis," which accounted for approximately one third of the deaths from PDA 40 years ago.[17] Although estimation is difficult, Campbell[18] has suggested that the incidence of arteritis is just under 1 percent per annum.

Aneurysm and Diverticulum of Ductus

Ductal aneurysm is uncommon and usually found in infants. It may occur in association with a patent ductus or with a ductus closed at only one end. It also may occur after operative closure of PDA. Rupture of the aneurysm has been reported.[19,20]

Ductal diverticulum is more rare than ductal aneurysm and is associated with incomplete closure of the ductus. Genetic studies in poodles with PDA have shown that a significant number of offspring have a ductus diverticulum.[11] The exact incidence in humans is unknown. Infection may occur in the diverticulum and cause distal embolization; rupture also may occur. Ductus diverticulum may be the cause of unexplained blood stream infections and of fever of unknown origin. This possibility can be ruled in or out by an aortogram in the left lateral position.

PROGNOSIS

Of 60 necropsied, unoperated patients with PDA studied by Keys and Shapiro,[17] the average age of death was 39 in males and 36 in females. These authors estimated that among patients over age 17 with PDA, life expectancy was half that of the general population. This data, however, was accumulated before operative therapy for PDA. Some adults with PDA have small left-to-right shunts and never develop symptoms of cardiac dysfunction. White described a 90-year-old man with PDA whom he had followed for 40 years.[21]

Good hemodynamic data in adults with PDA are not available. However, severe pulmonary hypertension does not appear to occur in later years if pulmonary resistance is not elevated by the second or third decades.

From earlier necropsy data, Campbell[18] suggested that by the age of 30, 20 percent of patients with PDA die; by age 40, the mortality rate rises from 2.5 to 4 percent per year. By age 60, 60 percent of patients with PDA have died, mainly from congestive cardiac failure, "endocarditis" (arteritis), or consequences of pulmonary hypertension.

Campbell[18] calculated that the rate of spontaneous closure of PDA is 0.6 percent per annum for the first four decades. Closure after one year is rare.[6,7]

DIFFERENTIAL DIAGNOSIS

In an adult with a continuous murmur maximal in the left precordium, other alternatives to a ductus should be considered, especially coronary artery anomalies, such as coronary artery fistula to right atrium or ventricle or coronary vein, anomalous origin of the left coronary artery from the pulmonary trunk, rupture of sinus of Valsalva aneurysm, and VSD associated with aortic regurgitation. Other lesions to be ruled out include aorticopulmonary defect (window), severe coarctation of the pulmonary arteries, arteriovenous fistula (both pulmonary and systemic), and anomalous arterial lesions. Aorticopulmonary defect is often quoted in the differential diagnosis, but it is usually a large defect and in adults is nearly always associated with Eisenmenger's syndrome. Although clinical nuances may help to distinguish all these lesions from PDA, cardiac catheterization and angiography are essential to confirm the diagnosis.

TREATMENT

The asymptomatic adult with a proven PDA and a normal-sized heart may be treated conservatively.[22] Antibiotic prophylaxis is indicated for minor operative procedures. The incidence of "endocarditis" in these patients appears lower now than in earlier years.[6] Although some risk is present from "endocarditis," division or suture obliteration of a PDA is not an easy operation in an adult; the risk is much higher than in infants and children. In a patient with PDA who has had "endocarditis" or who has cardiomegaly, operative closure of the PDA is indicated.[23]

Calcific deposits in the PDA are common in persons over age 30 with this condition. When calcified, however, operative repair is difficult and may require cardiopulmonary bypass or other special techniques, such as bypass from left subclavian artery to distal descending aorta.[24,25]

Reported long-term results of surgery for PDA are surprisingly sparse.[26,27] When the ductus is ligated or divided in children under two years of age who have no other major cardiovascular defects, late sequelae are exceptionally rare. If an adult with significant pulmonary hypertension has operative closure of PDA, the pulmonary hypertension may persist and progress nonetheless. If pulmonary resistance is not significantly elevated, however, long-term results are excellent. Even patients with PDA in their fifties and sixties with congestive heart failure and cardiomegaly may have excellent long-term results after operative closure of the PDA.

Recanalization of the PDA after operative closure has been reported frequently in the past, but currently is rare. If a continuous precordial murmur is still heard after operative "closure" of a PDA, alternative causes of a continuous murmur in addition to recanalization must be considered. Ductal aneurysm following operative closure of a PDA is rare.[28]

PDA is now rarely encountered in adults. If clinically suspected because of a classic continuous precordial murmur, PDA must be confirmed and the left-to-right shunt quantitated by cardiac catheterization, because other anomalies may simulate PDA. Surgery is usually beneficial and not contraindicated because of age per se. However, if the left-to-right shunt is small, the risk of complications is low and the patient may never require operative closure.

REFERENCES

1. BOYER, N.H.: *Patent ductus arteriosus*. Ann. Thorac. Surg. 4: 570,1967.
2. GIBSON, G.A.: *Disease of the Heart and Aorta*. Pentland, London, 1898.
3. GROSS, R.E., AND HUBBARD, J.P.: *Surgical ligation of a patent ductus arteriosus*. JAMA 112: 729,1939.

4. QUIROGA, C.: *Partial persistence of the ductus arteriosus.* Acta Radiol. 55:103,1961.
5. CASSELS, D.E.: *The Ductus Arteriosus.* Charles C Thomas, Springfield, Ill., 1973.
6. KEITH, J.D., ROWE, R.D., AND VLAD, P.: *Patent ductus arteriosus.* In *Heart Disease in Infancy and Childhood,* ed. 2. Macmillan, New York, 1967.
7. COGGIN, C.J., PARKER, K.R., AND KEITH, J.D.: *Natural history of isolated patent ductus arteriosus and the effect of surgical correction: Twenty years' experience at The Hospital for Sick Children, Toronto.* Canad. Med. Assoc. J. 102:718,1970.
8. CAMPBELL, M.: *Place of maternal rubella in the aetiology of congenital heart disease.* Br. Med. J. 1:691,1961.
9. RENWICK, D.H.G.: *The combined use of a central registry and vital records for incidence studies of congenital defects.* Br. J. Prev. Soc. Med., 22:61,1968.
10. CAMPBELL, D.C., HOOD, R.H., AND DOOLEY, B.N.: *Patent ductus arteriosus. Review of literature and experience with surgical corrections.* Lancet, 87:415,1967.
11. PATTERSON, D.F., PILE, R.L., BUCHANAN, J.W., ET AL.: *Hereditary patent ductus arteriosus and its sequelae in the dog.* Circ. Res. 29:1,1971.
12. KITTERMAN, J.A., EDMUNDS, L.H., JR., GREGORY, G.A., ET AL.: *Patent ductus arteriosus in premature infants: incidence, relation to pulmonary disease and management.* N. Engl. J. Med. 287:473,1972.
13. ALZAMORA-CASTRO, V., BATTILANA, G., ABUGATTAS, R., ET AL.: *Patent ductus arteriosus and high altitude.* Am. J. Cardiol. 5:761,1960.
14. OLLEY, P.M.: *Nonsurgical palliation of congenital heart malformations.* N. Engl. J. Med. 292:1292,1975.
15. ESPINO-VELA, J., AND ZAMORA, C.: *Patent ductus arteriosus—the natural history after the first year of life.* In Keith, J.D., and Kidd, B.S.L. (eds.): *Congenital Heart Defects,* Charles C Thomas, Springfield, Ill., 1971.
16. WOOD, P.: *The Eisenmenger syndrome or pulmonary hypertension with reversed central shunt.* Br. Med. J. 2:701,755,1958.
17. KEYS, A., AND SHAPIRO, M.J.: *Patency of the ductus arteriosus in adults.* Am. Heart J. 25:158,1943.
18. CAMPBELL, M.: *Natural history of persistent ductus arteriosus.* Br. Heart J. 30:40,1968.
19. WAGENER, O.: Deutsch Arch. Klin. Med. 79:90,1920.
20. DAS, J.B., AND CHESTERMAN, J.T.: *Aneurysus of the patent ductus arteriosus.* Thorax 11:295,1956.
21. WHITE, P.D., MAZURKIE, S.J., AND BOSCHETTI, A.E.: *Patency of the ductus arteriosus at 90.* N. Engl. J. Med. 280:146,1969.
22. NADAS, A.S., AND FYLER, D.C.: *Congenital heart disease—patent ductus arteriosus.* In *Pediatric Cardiology,* ed. 3. W. B. Saunders Co., Philadelphia, 1972.
23. BLACK, L.L., AND GOLDMAN, B.S.: *Surgical treatment of the patent ductus arteriosus in the adult.* Ann. Surg. 175:290,1972.
24. MORROW, A.G., AND CLARK, W.D.: *Closure of the calcified patent ductus.* J. Thorac. Cardiovasc. Surg. 51:534,1966.
25. PIFARRE, R., RICE, P.L., AND NEMICKAS, R.: *Surgical treatment of calcified patent ductus arteriosus.* J. Thorac. Cardiovasc. Surg. 65:635,1973.
26. LUCHT, U., AND SONDERGAARD, T.: *Late results of operation for patent ductus arteriosus.* Scand. J. Thorac. Cardiovasc. Surg. 5:223,1971.
27. CAMPBELL, M.: *Patent ductus arteriosus: some notes on prognosis and on pulmonary hypertension.* Br. Heart J. 17:511,1955.
28. MUSTARD, W.T.: *Surgery for patent ductus arteriosus.* In Keith, J.D., and Kidd, B.S.L. (eds.): *Congenital Heart Defects.* Charles C Thomas, Springfield, Ill., 1971.

Pulmonic Valve Stenosis in Adults

Samuel Kaplan, M.D., and Robert J. Adolph, M.D.

ETIOLOGY

Although the etiology of pulmonic stenosis is unknown, several factors have been reported which may help in counseling families in which one or several members have this malformation. All forms of congenital heart disease can be considered to be associated with genetic factors, chromosomal abnormalities, or exogenous factors. Examples of these three teratogenic categories have been reported in association with pulmonic stenosis, but the causation of this anomaly is still unexplained in the great majority of instances.

Repeated occurrences of pulmonic stenosis in *siblings* is more frequent than transmission through several generations.[1-5] Also, siblings of patients with pulmonic stenosis may be affected by various other forms of congenital heart disease. However, Warkany[1] points out that the occurrence of familial cases in the same generation is not convincing evidence of a genetic etiology since repetitive or persistent environmental or maternal factors could be responsible for cardiac malformations in several children born to the same mother. The studies of McKeown and coworkers[6] indicate that the prevalence of congenital heart disease is increased in siblings but not in parents or cousins of affected individuals. On the other hand, the data of Lamy and coworkers[3] suggest that genetic factors may be important since they found a high incidence of pulmonic stenosis in offspring of consanguineous marriages. Nevertheless, pulmonic stenosis has been recognized in mothers and some of their offspring and, in some patients, has been associated with deaf-mutism.[7,8] In families where atrial septal defect occurs as a dominant hereditary trait, pulmonic stenosis has also been diagnosed in some members.[9]

A variety of congenital cardiac defects, including pulmonic stenosis, has been described in general disorders known to be inherited recessively. Thus, pulmonic stenosis has been diagnosed as one of the many cardiovascular anomalies occurring in patients with the Laurence-Moon-Biedl syndrome.[10] Congenital heart disease is known to occur frequently in patients with chromosomal abnormalities (especially trisomy 21, 18, and 13–15). Isolated pulmonic valve stenosis is rare in trisomy 21, but right ventricular outflow obstruction has been reported in trisomy 18 and 13–15. Although maternal rubella is most frequently associated with patent ductus arteriosus and pulmonary arterial branch stenosis, pulmonic valve stenosis also may be present.

Noonan's Syndrome

A syndrome of pulmonic valve stenosis and other associated noncardiac abnormalities was described by Noonan and Emke.[11] Although some features of the Turner's syndrome are present, both males and females are affected and the karyotypes are normal.[12] This syndrome has been variously designated as male Turner syndrome, male Ullrich syndrome, Turner phenotype and the XX or XY Turner phenotype.[13] However, the features of Noonan's syndrome are sufficiently distinctive that a separate eponym is now used frequently.[14]

The noncardiac abnormalities described in Noonan's syndrome include small stature, mild mental retardation, hypertelorism, low-set ears, triangular-shaped face, ptosis, webbed neck, dental malocclusion, prominent pectus carinatum with distal pectus excavatum, and undescended testes (Fig. 1). The syndrome may be familial[13] and in some families the parents may show minor stigmata of Noonan's syndrome. Although pulmonic stenosis is the commonest associated cardiac abnormality, many other forms of congenital heart disease also may occur.[15]

The appearance of the stenotic pulmonic valve may be similar to classic dome stenosis, but in many instances the valve is dysplastic and similar to that described by Koretzky and coworkers.[16] The dysplastic valve has greatly thickened, shortened, and rigid cusps without significant commissural fusion. The valve opening may be further impeded by prominent fibrous masses in the depth of the sinuses. The obstruction results in significant right ventricular hypertrophy with or without infundibular stenosis. Associated anomalies may be present, including supravalvar or pulmonary arterial branch stenosis, atrial septal defect, and dysplasia of other valves—especially the aortic.

Although a loud pulmonic systolic ejection murmur is audible in patients with dysplastic valves, other clinical findings are different from those produced by classic pulmonic valve stenosis. These include absence of a pulmonic ejection click, left axis or marked right axis deviation ranging from +170 to +270 degrees and a QRS vector which is either posterior, superior, and rightward; or anterior, inferior, and rightward. In severe cases the peak right ventricular pressure may exceed 200 mm. Hg. Right ventriculography does not demonstrate classic doming of the pulmonic valve; a systolic

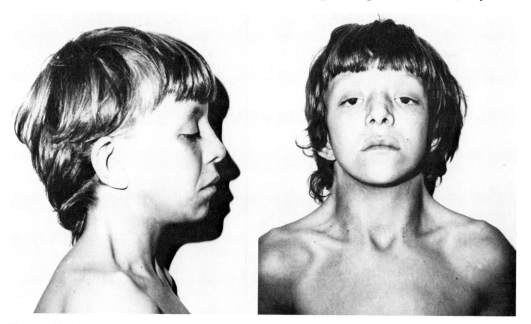

Figure 1. Facial features of Noonan's syndrome in a 16-year-old boy. Ptosis, hypertelorism, webbed neck, and low-set ears are evident. He had a normal male karyotype.

jet of contrast is unusual; the thickened cusps are visualized especially in diastole; and poststenotic dilatation is frequent.

Classic pulmonary valvotomy is not the surgical procedure of choice if the valves are dysplastic since the obstruction is not produced by commissural fusion. The various surgical procedures used include excision of one or all valve leaflets with or without valve replacement (usually with a porcine heterograft), incision of the pulmonary anulus with insertion of a right ventricular outflow patch, and resection of subvalvar hypertrophied myocardium.

CLINICAL ESTIMATION OF SEVERITY OF OBSTRUCTION

The majority of patients, even those with significant obstruction, deny symptoms.[17] Fatigue and dyspnea are the commonest complaints, and they tend to occur more frequently with higher grades of obstruction, though some adults may have these symptoms even with mild gradients. Angina pectoris and syncope with or without hypoxic spells usually denote severe obstruction. Momentary stabbing, nonradiating chest pain unrelated to exercise occurs frequently and is probably psychogenic in origin.

The physical findings depend in part on whether the stenosis is mild, moderate, or severe. To the extent that the obstruction is not progressive, severe stenosis, i.e., right ventricular systolic pressure (RVSP) greater than 120 mm. Hg is uncommon in the older adult, whereas mild stenosis (RVSP < 65 mm. Hg) and sometimes moderate (RVSP 65 to 120 mm. Hg) stenosis is compatible with the absence of symptoms and the ability to live a normal life.[18] Infective endocarditis, however, may interrupt this otherwise uncomplicated life pattern. Patients with moderately severe to severe pulmonic valvular stenosis may develop right heart failure and/or cyanosis in early adult life. Cyanosis occurs when right atrial pressure exceeds left atrial pressure and there is a right-to-left shunt at the atrial level. Right atrial pressure is elevated because of decreased right ventricular compliance or right heart failure. When the interatrial septum is embryologically intact, the right-to-left shunt develops in response to a patent foramen ovale made incompetent by the high right atrial pressure. The cyanosis is accentuated by exercise, which lowers systemic vascular resistance and thereby increases the right-to-left shunt.

Jugular Venous Pulse

The clue to diagnosis may be a giant A wave in the deep and external jugular venous system. With right ventricular outlet obstruction the wall hypertrophy results in decreased compliance or distensibility which, in turn, increases the impedance to right atrial emptying during atrial systole. A giant A wave in the jugular venous pulse and a right ventricular fourth (presystolic) heart sound are reflections of this pathologic state. In the presence of an atrial or ventricular septal defect and pulmonic stenosis, the A wave may be the predominant venous wave in the neck but a giant wave is never present. A giant A wave indicates that the right atrium in presystole is contracting against an increased resistance to emptying and that the septa are intact. The differential diagnosis of a giant A wave is limited. The likely causes are junctional rhythm, tricuspid valve stenosis, pulmonic valve stenosis, or pulmonary arterial hypertension. Junctional rhythm is easily ruled in or out by an electrocardiogram. Tricuspid valvular stenosis is associated with slowed right ventricular filling, causing a slow "y" descent in the jugular pulse; it is also almost always associated with evidence of mitral and aortic valve disease. Pulmonary hypertension can usually be differentiated easily from pulmonic stenosis at the bedside. In the former, the second heart sound is single or closely split and loud, and the systolic ejection murmur is short, soft and localized to the left upper parasternal edge. In the latter, the second heart sound is widely split with a soft second component and the systolic ejection murmur is long, loud and transmits to the neck.

An abnormal lower left parasternal movement is common and more easily appreciated in younger patients with thin chests. There has been some disagreement as to whether the movement is sustained through systole, as reported by Schmidt and Craige,[19] or exaggerated but not sustained in the majority of patients, as reported by Holt and Eddleman.[20] The difference is probably related to the method of measurement, an apexcardiogram in the former study and a kinetocardiogram in the latter. An abnormal presystolic movement corresponding to the giant right atrial A wave and presystolic gallop also is recorded by apexcardiography.

Auscultatory Findings

Typically, the murmur of pulmonic stenosis is a long and loud systolic ejection murmur. With pulmonic valvular stenosis the murmur is loudest in the second left intercostal space parasternally and it transmits to the clavicle, the suprasternal area, and left neck. Radiation down the left sternal border is less intense. Typically, it is at least grade 3 to 4 intensity (on a scale of 6) and when grade 4 or louder it may be associated with a thrill in the second and third intercostal spaces and, occasionally, in the suprasternal notch. The duration of the murmur gives a rough indication of the severity of the stenosis. As the severity increases, right ventricular ejection is prolonged and the murmur tends to peak later (the kite-shaped murmur) and to encompass and mask the first component of the second heart sound (S_2), namely, aortic closure (A_2). A soft murmur, symmetrical in shape, that peaks in midsystole and ends before the first component of S_2 typifies mild stenosis. Murmurs recorded from patients with valvular stenosis of progressive severity are illustrated in Figures 2, 3, and 4. The murmur is louder and longer during the tachycardiac phase following inhalation of amyl nitrite,

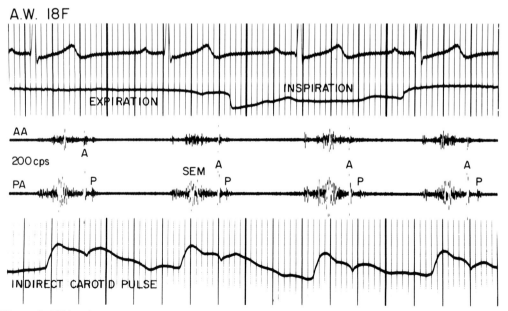

Figure 2. Mild pulmonic valvular stenosis (28 mm. Hg) in an 18-year-old girl. The long systolic ejection murmur peaks in midsystole. Aortic (A_2) and pulmonic (P_2) closures are sharp and easily heard. Respiratory variation in the splitting of S_2 is minimal. No definite systolic ejection click is recorded.

330

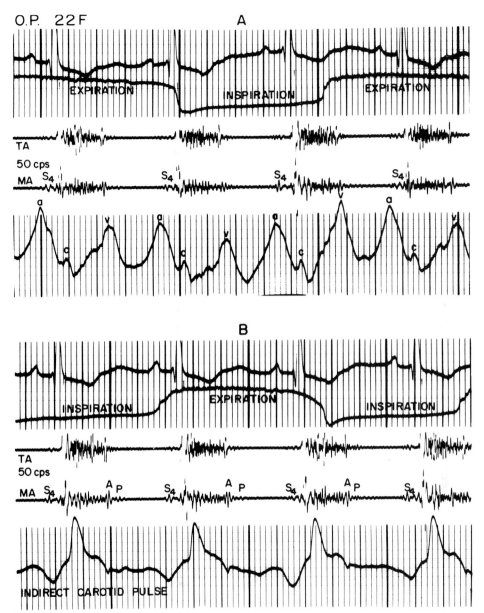

Figure 3. Moderately severe pulmonic valvular stenosis is a 22-year-old woman. The long systolic ejection murmur peaks in midsystole. P_2 is delayed and decreased in intensity. A loud, right-sided S_4 gallop which increases in intensity during late inspiration is best recorded at the apex and corresponds in time to a prominent jugular venous A wave.

presumably a consequence of increased venous return.[21] This change in the loudness and duration of the murmur following amyl nitrite inhalation is indicative of an intact ventricular septum. In tetralogy of Fallot, for example, the decrease in systemic vascular resistance exceeds the decrease in pulmonary vascular resistance, so that left-to-right shunting decreases and right-to-left shunting increases. This results in a softer and shorter pulmonary flow murmur. Amyl nitrite helps differentiate the murmur of pulmonic stenosis from that of a ventricular septal defect but not from aortic or subaortic stenosis. The use of the Valsalva maneuver, isometric handgrip exercise, and pressor agents are not sufficiently discriminating to warrant their routine application in differential diagnosis. Although it usually is unaffected, the murmur may sometimes increase in intensity during normal inspiration.

The *second heart sound* is abnormal in pulmonic valvular stenosis. The second component of the second heart sound, pulmonic closure (P_2), is progressively delayed and softer with more severe degrees of stenosis. Leatham[22] plotted a linear relationship between the delay in P_2 during expiration and right ventricular systolic pressure. In mild stenosis the splitting of S_2 may be 0.03 to 0.06 sec. in expiration and P_2 is only slightly diminished in intensity. Respiratory variation in the splitting can usually be appreciated. The murmur ends before P_2, and A_2 is easily heard in the pulmonic area. When the stenosis is moderate the splitting of S_2 is wider, perhaps 0.06 to 0.10 sec., and P_2 is diminished in loudness. Inspiratory widening of the splitting is difficult to discern on auscultation but can be seen on phonocardiography. A_2 may be masked by the later peaking murmur. With severe stenosis the splitting of S_2 may approach 0.14 sec. and P_2 may be inaudible although it can usually be recorded. A_2 may be inaudible because the murmur overlaps the sound and extends through it. The resultant auscultatory illusion is that of a pansystolic murmur at the upper left sternal edge since neither A_2 nor P_2 is heard following the long murmur. A small ventricular septal defect, tricuspid valve regurgitation, or mitral valve regurgitation with unusual transmission may be incorrectly suspected. The steps to unraveling the illusion are as follows: inching downward along the left sternal edge with the stethoscope, a point is reached where the murmur is less intense and A_2 is uncovered; the murmur obviously extends through A_2. The high location of the thrill makes ventricular septal defect unlikely. The absence of C-V or regurgitant waves in the neck excludes tricuspid valve regurgitation. Indeed, the normal A_2 tends to exclude significant aortic valvular stenosis as well.

On auscultation another characteristic feature of mild or moderate pulmonic valvular stenosis is a *pulmonary systolic ejection sound or click*. It is heard at the base of the heart and at the upper left sternal edge but not at the apex, unlike the ejection click of aortic valvular stenosis. The ejection click closely follows the first heart sound (S_1) and in mild to moderate stenosis may be confused with audible splitting of S_1 or S_1 itself. Characteristically, it is louder during expiration and diminishes in intensity or disappears with inspiration (Fig. 2). The mechanism responsible for expiratory augmentation of the ejection click was investigated by Hultgren and coworkers.[23] In pulmonic valvular stenosis the ejection click is valvular in origin. The high-pitched transient is produced by sudden doming or checking of the stenotic membrane when it reaches its maximum excursion shortly after the onset of ejection. Forward excursion of the valve is normally initiated by systolic contraction during the isovolumic period. In patients with pulmonic valvular stenosis during expiration, pressure in the right ventricle at end-diastole is lower than the pressure in the pulmonary artery. This allows ventricular systole to produce an opening motion of the closed, slack leaflets. During inspiration, however, right ventricular end-diastolic pressure exceeds the diastolic pressure in the pulmonary artery. Increased venous return augments right atrial systole and moves the valve forward to its ejection position by end-diastole. Hence, the sudden deceleration of the valve that occurs with ejection is absent and the ejection sound moves closer to the first heart sound. In severe stenosis, it may be absent entirely during both phases of respiration (Fig. 4).

Right atrial (S_4) gallops are common in pulmonic stenosis, but right ventricular (S_3) gallops are uncommon in the absence of right heart failure. We have been interested in the finding of a right-sided atrial gallop in patients with noncompliant hypertrophied right ventricles and strong right atrial contractions. It is better heard over the right

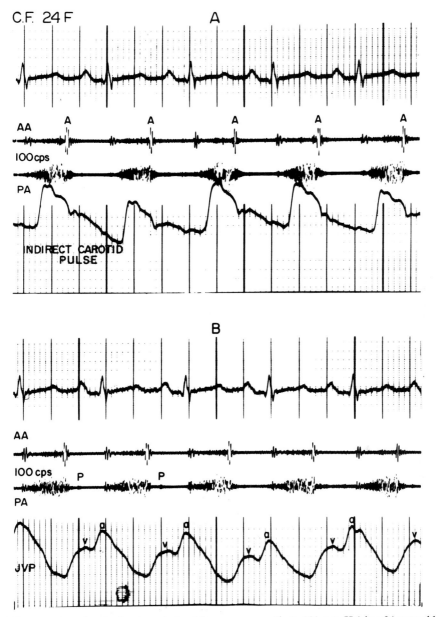

Figure 4. Severe pulmonic valvular stenosis (systolic pressure gradient, 166 mm. Hg) in a 24-year-old woman. In the upper panel a long, loud and late-peaking systolic ejection murmur that obscures aortic closure was recorded in the pulmonic area. P_2 was neither heard nor recorded. In the lower panel a late, miniscule P_2 was recorded. A prominent jugular venous A wave was present.

jugular vein than along the left sternal border.[24] At the left sternal border it is a reflection of presystolic ventricular filling. In the neck it is a reflection of the giant A wave which rapidly distends and sets into vibration the jugular venous wall. Both right-sided atrial and ventricular gallops tend to be accentuated by inspiration (Fig. 3).

Electrocardiogram

Ellison and coworkers[17] correlated the peak systolic pressure gradient across the right ventricular outflow tract with various combinations of the R and T waves in lead V_1. In patients with small gradients a small R wave (< 10 mm.) is followed by an inverted T wave; the latter is explained by persistence of the juvenile T wave pattern. With higher gradients the T wave tends to become isoelectric or upright before the R wave increases in voltage; and with still further increase in gradient the R wave in V_1 exceeds 10 mm. and the T wave again becomes inverted because of right ventricular "strain."

Chest Roentgenogram

Varying degrees of prominence of the right heart are present on the chest roentgenograms in patients with moderate or severe obstruction, and in the latter the cardiac silhouette can be greatly enlarged because of dilatation of the right atrium and ventricle. In the adult the pulmonic valve may become calcified.[26] The pulmonic valve is located more anteriorly and cephalad than the aortic valve. Recognition of a right aortic arch with clinical findings of pulmonic stenosis has generally been considered to be sound evidence for the presence of an associated ventricular septal defect. However, isolated pulmonic stenosis is occasionally associated with a right aortic arch (Fig. 5)[26] so that preoperative angiocardiography is essential in these patients to evaluate the integrity of the ventricular septum. The degree of poststenotic dilatation of the pulmonary trunk bears no relationship to severity of obstruction and persists after valvotomy.

CLINICAL COURSE

There is no unanimity about the course of pulmonic valvular stenosis. Johnson and coworkers[18] followed 21 catheterized patients for an average of 15 years. There were no cardiac deaths or clinical deterioration in this group of patients. This study contrasts with that of Campbell[27] who observed only a 12 percent probability of survival to the sixth decade, even with moderate obstruction (peak right ventricular pressure of ≤ 70 mm. Hg). Survival to beyond the sixth decade has been reported.[28-30] Favorable

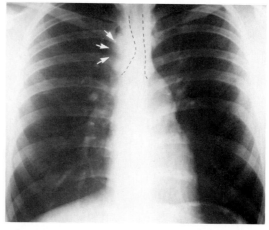

Figure 5. Postero-anterior chest roentgenogram in 22-year-old man with pulmonic valvular stenosis, intact ventricular septum and right aortic arch. The right border of the right aortic arch is indicated by the arrows. The right arch also indents the trachea (dotted lines).

prognostic features in patients beyond middle age include absence of symptoms, a normal resting cardiac output, peak right ventricular pressures of less than 100 mm. Hg, and a normal pulmonary arterial pressure.

The generally held optimistic view concerning the clinical course[31-34] was confirmed by the study of Nugent and coworkers[35] which included 120 patients between 12 and 21 years of age. Medical therapy alone was employed in 68 of these patients who had right ventricular outflow gradients of less than 80 mm. Hg (and in 64 the gradient was less than 50 mm. Hg). There were no cardiac deaths in this group of 68 patients. When two cardiac catheterizations were undertaken 4 to 8 years apart, the pressure gradient remained stable in the majority. A meaningful increase in gradients did not occur in patients over the age of 12 if the initial gradient was less than 50 mm. Hg. Infective endocarditis is also rare in isolated pulmonic valvular stenosis[36] although Engle and coworkers[32] reported an incidence of 7 percent.

The clinical course in 304 patients after surgical treatment for pulmonic valvular stenosis was described by Nugent and coworkers.[35] Of the 304 patients, 52 were between the ages of 12 and 21 at the time of surgery; 30 had preoperative gradients exceeding 80 mm. Hg and in 14 the gradient was between 50 and 79 mm. Hg. Stenosis did not recur in any of these patients. Although some decrease of gradient did occur in the late postoperative period, it was seldom dramatic. Thus, the decrease in right ventricular pressure after pulmonary valvotomy is immediate and lasting. There are occasional anecdotes about stenosis recurring many years after surgery, and we have seen one patient where a gradient of 85 mm. Hg was relieved but recurred 15 years later with a right ventricular peak systolic pressure of 190 mm. Hg. Most observers agree that patients with gradients exceeding 80 mm. Hg should undergo surgical treatment, preferably in childhood or adolescence. Although there is some disagreement about the management of patients whose gradient is between 50 and 79 mm. Hg, long-term evaluation indicates that the results with surgery are better than those without surgery.[36] Occasionally, surgery is advisable in patients with gradients of about 40 mm. Hg to relieve the myocardium of long-term pressure overload. It is clear that the prognosis is excellent in patients with trivial pulmonic stenosis (i.e., gradients less than 25 mm. Hg).

Children with isolated pulmonic stenosis generally do extremely well for many years after valvotomy. However, in adults the results may not be uniformly good.[37] Right ventricular dysfunction may persist despite a technically excellent pulmonic valvotomy.[38] This dysfunction has been attributed to a stiff, poorly filling right ventricle due to persistent hypertrophy and fibrosis. The clinical picture in these patients is dominated by elevated systemic venous pressure and reduced cardiac output with resultant fatigue and exertional dyspnea.

Jonsson and Lee[39] studied the hemodynamic response to muscular exercise in 17 adults after pulmonic valvotomy. They found that during exercise a persistent low cardiac output in relation to oxygen uptake remained after operation. They did not attribute this postoperative abnormality to right ventricular myocardial disease since the right ventricular end-diastolic pressure and duration of systole became normal after operation. These authors suggested that the persistent low cardiac output after pulmonic valvotomy was related to the ability of the peripheral circulation to extract and utilize oxygen to a greater degree, and that this ability developed during early childhood.

Significant preoperative infundibular hypertrophy may result in persistence of right ventricular hypertension even after an adequate pulmonic valvotomy.[40] This may contribute to the low cardiac output syndrome seen occasionally after pulmonic valvotomy so that infundibular resection is sometimes required, especially in patients with severe right ventricular hypertension which persists intraoperatively. Although spontaneous regression of infundibular stenosis is normal in the years following valvotomy, its persistence also may contribute to the compromised diastolic function which results from myocardial hypertrophy and fibrosis.

POSTOPERATIVE PULMONIC VALVE REGURGITATION

Trivial pulmonic valve regurgitation is common after valvotomy and is manifest as an early diastolic murmur along the left sternal edge. Generally, the benign postoperative course described above is unaffected by the regurgitation. However, in patients with severe pulmonic regurgitation (comprising about 3 percent of patients having pulmonic valvotomy), significant cardiomegaly persists with electrocardiographic signs of right atrial and ventricular enlargement (Figs. 6 and 7) and echocardiographic evidence of right volume overload. With persistence of right volume overload, tricuspid valve regur-

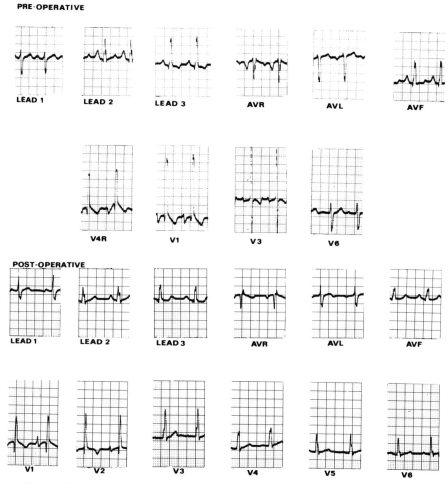

Figure 6. Preoperative and postoperative electrocardiograms in a patient with severe pulmonary stenosis (preoperative gradient, 180 mm. Hg). Pulmonic valvotomy was done at age 9. Postoperative cardiac catheterization showed a right ventricular pressure of 38/3 mm. Hg, virtual abolition of the gradient and gross pulmonic valve regurgitation. The postoperative electrocardiogram at age 30 shows persistence of right atrial and right ventricular hypertrophy.

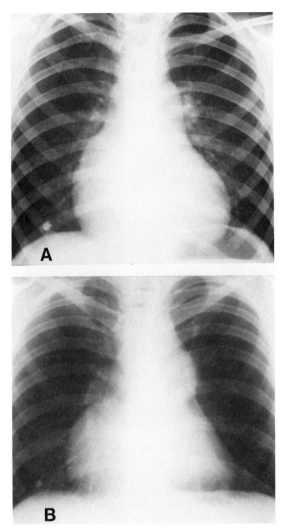

Figure 7. Preoperative (A) and postoperative (B) postero-anterior roentgenograms of patient in Figure 6 show persistence of cardiomegaly 21 years after operation. The persistent cardiomegaly is attributed to pulmonic valve regurgitation.

gitation may develop. Although these patients are frequently asymptomatic, the ultimate prognosis is guarded.

SUMMARY

The prognosis is excellent in patients with trivial pulmonic stenosis (peak right ventricular systolic outflow pressure gradients of less than 25 mm. Hg). Although there is no unanimity concerning the course of pulmonic valvular stenosis in adults, generally an optimistic view is justifiable based on long-term followup studies. A meaningful increase in gradient in adult life does not occur if cardiac catheterization beyond the age of 12 years shows a resting gradient of less than 50 mm. Hg. Generally, the clinical course after surgery for moderate or severe pulmonic stenosis in childhood is excellent. Recurrence of stenosis in adult life is rare and the decrease of right ventricular systolic pressure after valvotomy is immediate and lasting. The results of surgery for moderate or severe pulmonic stenosis in adults may not be uniformly good because of persistent right ventricular dysfunction. Furthermore, persistence of a low cardiac output during exercise in adults after pulmonic valvotomy is frequent.

REFERENCES

1. WARKANY, J.: *Congenital Malformations.* Year Book Medical Publishers, Inc., Chicago, 1971, pp. 459–470.

2. EHLERS, K.H., AND ENGLE, M.A.: *Familial congenital heart disease. 1. Genetic and environmental factors.* Circulation 34:503,1966.

3. LAMY, M., DeGROUCHY, J., AND SCHWEISGUTH, O.: *Genetic and non-genetic factors in the etiology of congenital heart disease: A study of 1188 cases.* Am. J. Hum. Genet. 9:17,1957.

4. WATSON, G.H.: *Pulmonary stenosis, cafe-au-lait spots and dull intelligence.* Arch. Dis. Child. 42:303,1967.

5. COBLENTZ, B., AND MATHIVAT, A.: *Stenose pulmonaire congenitale chez duex soeurs.* Arch. Mal. Coeur 45:490,1952.

6. McKEOWN, T., MacMAHON, B., AND PARSONS, C. G.: *The familial incidence of congenital malformations of the heart.* Br. Heart J. 15:273,1953.

7. LEWIS, S. M., SONNENBLICK, B. P., GILBERT, L., ET AL.: *Familial pulmonary stenosis and deaf mutism: Clinical and genetic considerations.* Am. Heart J. 55:458,1958.

8. KOROXENIDES, G., WEBB, N. C., JR., MOSCHOS, C. B., ET AL.: *Congenital heart disease, deaf mutism and associated somatic malformations occurring in several members of one family.* Am. J. Med. 40:149,1966.

9. WEIL, M. H., AND ALLENSTEIN, B. J.: *A report of congenital heart disease in five members of one family.* N. Engl. J. Med. 265:661,1961.

10. McLOUGHLIN, T. G., KROVITZ, L. J., AND SCHIEBLER, G. L.: *Heart diseases in the Laurence-Moon-Biedl-Bardet syndrome.* J. Pediatr. 65:388,1964.

11. NOONAN, J. A., AND EMKE, D. A.: *Associated noncardiac malformations in children with congenital heart disease.* J. Pediatr. 63:468,1963.

12. NOONAN, J. A.: *Hypertelorism with Turner phenotype.* Am. J. Dis. Child. 116:373,1968.

13. BOLTON, M. R., PUGH, D. M., MATTIOLI, L. F., ET AL.: *The Noonan syndrome: A family study.* Ann. Intern. Med. 80:626,1974.

14. SUMMITT, B. L.: *Turner syndrome and Noonan's syndrome.* J. Pediatr. 74:155,1969.

15. PHORNPHUTKUL, C., ROSENTHAL, A., AND NADAS, A. S.: *Cardiomyopathy in Noonan's syndrome. Report of three cases.* Br. Heart J. 35:99,1973.

16. KORETZKY, E. M., MOELLER, J. H., KORNS, M. E., ET AL.: *Congenital pulmonary stenosis resulting from dysplasia of valve.* Circulation 40:43,1969.

17. ELLISON, R. C., FREEDOM, R. M., KEANE, J. F., ET AL.: *Indirect assessment of severity in pulmonary stenosis.* Circulation 56 (Suppl. I):14,1977.

18. JOHNSON, L. W., GROSSMAN, W., DALEN, J. E., ET AL.: *Pulmonic stenosis in the adult: Long term followup results.* N. Engl. J. Med. 287:1159,1972.

19. SCHMIDT, R. E., AND CRAIGE, E.: *Precordial movements over the right ventricle in children with pulmonary stenosis.* Circulation 32:241,1965.

20. HOLT, J. H., JR., AND EDDLEMAN, E. E., JR.: *The precordial movements in adults with pulmonic stenosis.* Circulation 35:492,1967.

21. PERLOFF, J. K.: *The Clinical Recognition of Congenital Heart Disease.* W. B. Saunders Co., Philadelphia, 1970.

22. LEATHAM, A., AND WEITZMAN, D. W.: *Auscultatory and phonocardiographic signs of pulmonary stenosis.* Br. Heart J. 19:303,1957.

23. HULTGREN, H. N., REEVE, R., COHN, K., ET AL.: *The ejection click of valvular pulmonic stenosis.* Circulation 40:631,1969.

24. ADOLPH, R. J.: *Diagnosis and significance of gallop rhythm.* Cardiovasc. Clin. 6(3):1,1975.

25. ROBERTS, W. C., MASON, D. T., MORROW, A. G., ET AL.: *Calcific pulmonic stenosis.* Circulation 37:973,1968.

26. GAMBLE, W. J., AND NADAS, A. S.: *Severe pulmonic stenosis with intact ventricular septum and right aortic arch.* Circulation 32:114,1965.

27. CAMPBELL, M.: *The natural history of congenital pulmonic stenosis.* Br. Heart J. 31:394,1969.

28. WILD, J. B., ECKSTEIN, S. W., VANEPPS, E. F., ET AL.: *Three patients with congenital pulmonic valvular stenosis surviving for more than 57 years. Medical histories and physiologic data.* Am. Heart J. 53:393,1957.

29. CAMPBELL, M., AND MISIEN, G. A. K.: *Survival in good health until 65 years with pulmonary valvar stenosis.* Guy's Hosp. Rep. 108:390,1959.

30. WHITE, P. D., HURST, J. W., AND FENNELL, R. H.: *Survival to the age of 75 years with pulmonary stenosis and patent foramen ovale.* Circulation 2:558,1950.

31. BARRITT, D. W.: *Simple pulmonary stenosis with normal aortic root.* Br. Heart J. 16:381,1954.

32. ENGLE, M. A., TOMIKO, I., AND GOLDBERG, H. P.: *The fate of the patient with pulmonic stenosis.* Circulation 30:554,1964.

33. TINKER, S., HOWITT, G., MARKMAN, P., ET AL.: *The natural history of isolated pulmonary stenosis.* Br. Heart J. 27:151,1965.

34. SNELLEN, H. A., HARTMAN, H., BOIS-LIEM, T. N., ET AL.: *Pulmonary stenosis.* Circulation 37, 38(Suppl. V):93,1968.

35. NUGENT, E. W., FREEDOM, R. M., NORA, J. J., ET AL.: *Clinical course in pulmonary stenosis.* Circulation 56 (Suppl. I):38,1977.

36. NADAS, A. S.: *Clinical course. Summary and conclusions.* Circulation 56 (Suppl. I):70,1977.

37. MARON, B. J., ROSING, D. R., GOLDSTEIN, R.E., ET AL.: *Long-term postoperative prognosis of patients with congenital heart disease.* Chest 72:499,1977.

38. MCINTOSH, H. D., AND COHEN, A. I.: *Pulmonary stenosis: The importance of the myocardial factor in determining clinical course and surgical results.* Am. Heart J. 65:715, 1963.

39. JONSSON, B., AND LEE, S. J. K.: *Haemodynamic effects of exercise in isolated pulmonary stenosis before and after surgery.* Br. Heart J. 30:60,1968.

40. NADAS, A. D.: *Pulmonic stenosis: indications for surgery in children and adults.* N. Engl. J. Med. 287:1196,1972.

Tetralogy of Fallot in Adults

*Arthur Garson, Jr., M.D., Dan G. McNamara, M.D.,
and Denton A. Cooley, M.D.*

According to Fallot in 1888,

> . . . cyanosis is the result of a small number of malformations. One of these is
> much more frequent than the others since we have found it in about 74 percent of
> our cases; this is what the clinician should diagnose, and in doing so, his chances of
> error are relatively slight. This malformation consists of a true anatomopathologic
> type represented by a tetralogy. . .[1]

It is still true today that the child with cyanotic congenital heart disease has a 75
percent chance of having tetralogy of Fallot (TOF).[2] However, the activity in cardiac
centers all over the world virtually assures that practically all patients with TOF will
henceforth receive total correction during infancy and childhood, and large numbers of
these patients will reach adult life and no longer be cyanotic.

The clinical and hemodynamic features of the patient with surgically repaired TOF
are unlike those of any of the naturally occurring types of heart disease. The medical
problems of these patients are unique and their long-term futures are still uncertain.
The purpose of this chapter is to present to the cardiologist and internist the characteristics of this group of adult patients, many of whom still require regular examinations
and medical or surgical management, despite surgical treatment and symptomatic improvement.

INCIDENCE AND DEFINITION OF TETRALOGY OF FALLOT

About 24,500 children are born each year with congenital heart disease;[2,3] about 2700
(11 percent) of these have TOF.[4-6] Based on our current data regarding surgical treatment, we estimate that 87 percent of those patients, or 2260 per year, will survive to
adulthood.

For the purpose of this chapter, patients were excluded if they had any of the
anatomic variations of TOF that would have altered either the natural clinical course or
the result of surgical repair: variations such as right ventricular (RV) outflow or pulmonary artery atresia (pseudotruncus), associated aortic origin of a pulmonary artery or a
restrictive ventricular septal defect (VSD). Concern is directed toward the patient with
TOF who has lived longer than 15 years.

PATIENT POPULATION

In addition to reviewing the literature, we have included the clinical and hemodynamic data of 253 of our own patients with TOF, all born more than 15 years before January 1, 1977. The median age of 123 patients on whom we could obtain recent information, was 22.5 years (range 15.2 to 44.5). Of the entire group, 154 were male and 99 were female (1.56:1 ratio). All patients but one have been operated upon: 19 had palliation only and 233 had intracardiac repair (ICR) following a variety of anastomotic procedures (Fig. 1). There were 27 surgical deaths (11.6 percent) during ICR. Of the survivors, 120 underwent cardiac catheterization from three months to 15 years postoperatively (median 1.1 years). The followup period ranged from one month to 15.6 years (mean 5.2 years). The incidence of late death is difficult to estimate since many patients from foreign countries have been lost to followup. Therefore, the late cardiac-related mortality is a minimum figure (Table 1). The total cardiac-related mortality of patients who underwent ICR was 16.3 percent (38/233).

It is likely that these data will differ in the next five to ten years since the adult patients in the future will not have had the same management during childhood as the current adult patient. There is an ever-increasing trend toward ICR in younger children. We expect this will allow for a higher percentage of survival beyond childhood. Today, the adult who has had surgical treatment of TOF has a life expectancy ten times greater than the patient who lived before 1944, when the first palliative Blalock-Taussig operation was performed.

The following three sections correspond to the types of treatment which have been performed. The first section refers to nonsurgically treated patients; the second to

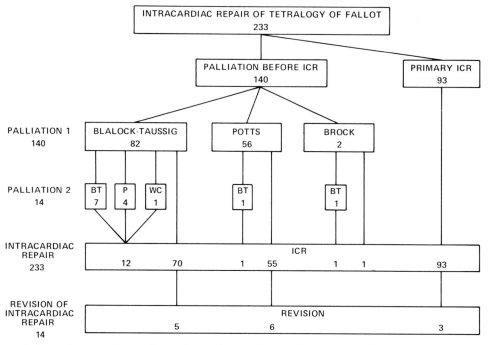

Figure 1. Surgical course of our patients who had intracardiac repair of tetralogy of Fallot. Not included in the figure are 19 patients who had surgical palliation only and one patient who has not had surgery. BT = Blalock-Taussig; ICR = intracardiac repair; P = Potts; WC = Waterston-Cooley; Revision = reclosure of VSD and/or removal of residual obstruction to right ventricular outflow.

Table 1: Cardiac-related mortality following intracardiac repair of tetralogy of Fallot

Operative Group	EARLY[1]				LATE[2]				TOTAL	
	N*	%	Cause of Death	Age (Years) at Death Mean (Range)	N	%	Cause of Death	Age (Years) at Death Mean (Range)	N	%
Blalock-Taussig, prior to repair[3]	10/74	13.5	3 hemorrhage 6 low CO 1 CAVB	16.4(7.0–28.0)	2/61	3.3	1 BE 1 PAH	9.3(13.1–18.5)	12/74	16.2
Potts, prior to repair[3]	6/54	11.1	1 PAH 5 low CO	11.5(4.5–18.4)	4/48	8.3	1 PAH 1 CHF 2 sudden	13.8(3.0–19.9)	10/54	18.5
Palliation prior to repair[4]	16/129	12.4		14.0(4.5–28.0)	6/110	5.5		12.3(3.0–19.9)	22/129	17.1
Primary repair	10/90	11.1	3 hemorrhage 7 low CO	8.9(3.0–19.0)	2/80	2.5	2 sudden	24.0(15.0–33.0)	12/90	13.3
Revision of repair[5]	1/14	7.1	1 PAH	12.0	3/13	23.1	3 sudden	17.0(16.0–17.9)	4/14	28.6
All repair	27/233	11.6		13.9(3.0–28.0)	11/203	5.4		17.1(3.0–33.0)	38/233	16.3

*N refers to number of patients, not number of operations.

[1] Early mortality = within 30 days of operation.

[2] Late mortality—this figure excludes three patients who died in accidents.

[3] Excludes those who had revision of intracardiac repair.

[4] This row is made up of summation of two rows above it, plus one patient with prior Brock procedure.

[5] Revision = reclosure of VSD, revision of residual infundibular or valvular or branch pulmonary stenosis.

BE = bacterial endocarditis; CAVB = complete atrioventricular block; CHF = congestive heart failure; CO = cardiac output; PAH = pulmonary arterial hypertension.

patients who have had surgical palliation; and the third to patients who have had intracardiac repair.

THE UNOPERATED PATIENT

In our series of 253 patients, all but one 32-year-old man required surgical treatment. Since the unoperated adult patient is a relative rarity, it is necessary to provide data on the natural history only for comparison with the improved status brought about by operative intervention.

Natural History

Most investigators[7-9] report approximately 50 percent of patients with untreated TOF die by the age of five years (Fig. 2). By the age of 10 years, an additional 25 percent are dead; and between the ages of 10 and 20 years (during puberty) most have died, so that by the age of 25 years, only 3 to 5 percent are alive.[7-13] Survival into adulthood has been reported.[9,14,15] The oldest known survivor died at age 69 of a cerebrovascular accident, but coexistent adenocarcinoma of the prostate could have been the cause. The predominant nonsurgical causes of death which have been reported are approximately evenly distributed between (1) paroxysmal hypoxemic spells, (2) cerebrovascular accident and brain abscess, (3) bacterial endocarditis, and (4) pneumonia and congestive cardiac failure.[9,12,13] It is surprising that pneumonia and congestive cardiac fail-

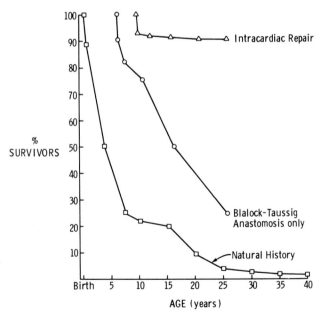

Figure 2. Natural and surgically modified survival in patients with tetralogy of Fallot. The percentage of survivors at the end of each interval is graphed for each of three courses. The natural history data were combined from six authors,[7-12] while the estimated survival following a single Blalock-Taussig anastomosis combined two studies,[29-30] and the data following ICR (with or without prior operation) are ours combined with one other study.[26] The curves representing survival following operation are constructed with the following assumptions: (1) the beginning point is the mean age at operation; (2) the initial vertical decrease corresponds to 30-day mortality; and (3) no patient died before operation.

ure are listed as major causes of death. In our experience pneumonia is a rare complication of TOF. Furthermore, we have never encountered congestive cardiac failure in unoperated patients. Adults with TOF only rarely have paroxysmal hypoxemic spells, and their deaths result from the other causes listed. In one series[13] 40 percent of the patients died suddenly and unexpectedly, and it may be that cardiac dysrhythmia was the cause of death in these patients. Adults with chronic lung disease superimposed upon TOF seem to be in special danger. Systemic blood shunted from right to left through an intracardiac defect not only has a decreased concentration of oxygen but also an increased concentration of carbon dioxide. Therefore, patients with relatively mild lung disease may manifest arterial hypercarbia if a portion of the systemic venous blood bypasses the lungs.[15]

The clinical, laboratory, and cardiac catheterization findings are much the same in untreated adults as in children with TOF.[16] Oakley[15] has provided an excellent review on the untreated adult patient with TOF. With respect to pregnancy, Neill and Swanson[17] found a high incidence of spontaneous abortion when the hematocrit value in the mother was 65 percent or more. Fifty-five pregnancies have been reported in 46 women with unoperated TOF. Of these, 10 to 20 percent of the mothers died during pregnancy. Maternal difficulties with pregnancy have been reported to include congestive cardiac failure, paroxysmal hypoxemic spells, pulmonary hemorrhage, and paradoxical emboli.[18]

Management Question: Whether or Not to Perform Phlebotomy?

While blood hyperviscosity related to polycythemia may be detrimental to some patients, an appropriate degree of polycythemia protects the patient with arterial hypoxemia. Ideally, arterial blood has an oxygen content of 15 volumes percent. This is the level attained in a healthy individual with a 95 percent arterial blood oxygen saturation and a hemoglobin level of 12 gm./dl. In the patient with an arterial blood oxygen saturation reduced to 80 percent, the ideal level of oxygen content of 15 volumes percent is achieved with a hemoglobin level of 14 gm./dl. Furthermore, a hemoglobin level of 18 gm./dl. is necessary for ideal oxygen content if the arterial blood oxygen saturation is 60 percent. In fact, if the patient who has an arterial blood oxygen saturation of 60 percent has less than 18 gm./dl. of hemoglobin, he may require iron therapy. Therefore, a balance must be maintained between increased tissue oxygenation with more red blood cells and increasing viscosity. The maximum beneficial hematocrit value is approximately 65 percent.[19] Above this value, symptoms appear that are related to cerebral ischemia, and clotting abnormalities are manifest: prolonged bleeding time, increased capillary fragility and abnormal platelet survival. Somewhat less frequently encountered are thrombocytopenia, prolonged prothrombin time, and decreased fibrinogen level.[19,20] These abnormalities can be corrected transiently with phlebotomy and a resultant hematocrit level of 60 to 65 percent.[12,20]

Phlebotomy can be dangerous, however, particularly in patients with TOF. If the systemic blood pressure drops during phlebotomy, a hypoxemic spell may be precipitated. We have observed cerebrovascular accidents in this situation, possibly from a decreased oxygen-carrying capacity. For these reasons, in patients who are not being considered for surgery, we recommend phlebotomy only to relieve symptoms or to correct a manifest bleeding disorder. When intracardiac repair is considered, an abnormality of any of the clotting studies, including platelet aggregation tests, indicates the need for phlebotomy. Without benefit of platelet function studies, it is customary in some centers to perform phlebotomy before operation to lower the hematocrit level to between 60 and 65 percent. In patients with TOF we replace the volume of blood removed with a 5 percent solution of albumin in Ringer's lactate.

Management Question: When to Operate on the Adult with Tetralogy of Fallot Who Has Had No Prior Procedure?

To answer this question one must examine the risks with and without operation to the unoperated patient. We have seen from the natural history data that by the age of 15, 80 percent of patients with TOF have died. The results of primary ICR in adults seem to be no different than those in children.[16,21-24] Early mortality in adults with primary ICR varies from 0[23] to 11 percent.[22] Probably the only adults who should not have intracardiac repair are those with extremely hypoplastic pulmonary arteries.

THE PATIENT WHO HAS HAD PALLIATIVE SURGERY

In our series of 253 adults with TOF, 158 (63 percent) had surgical palliation. The figures from other centers on the number of patients with palliation before ICR range from 50 to 89 percent.[22,24] Since we are following only two patients over the age of 15 who have had surgical palliation alone, we will briefly review the data from the literature on the longevity and special problems associated with each of the major types of aorticopulmonary anastomosis, as well as the Brock transpulmonary valvotomy operation.

Blalock-Taussig Anastomosis

Before 1944 there was no specific treatment for TOF. When Blalock and Taussig[25] introduced the anastomosis between the subclavian artery and pulmonary artery, surgery for TOF was initiated. This is the most common type of procedure encountered in adults who have had palliative operation during childhood.[24,26-28]

Clinical Course

In series where patients have had the anastomosis alone and have not had corrective surgery, approximately 20 percent die postoperatively every five years (Fig. 2).[29,30] Thus, approximately 60 percent of the children who have had anastomoses between the ages of 3 and 5 years will live to be adults.[31] One half of the nonsurgical deaths following the Blalock-Taussig procedure are from brain abscess.[4] The other causes of death are similar in type and frequency to those in the unoperated patient.

Morbidity Associated with Blalock-Taussig Anastomosis

Following this procedure, 4 to 6 percent of the patients had brain abscess and 2 to 5 percent had cerebrovascular accidents.[28,29] This figure is higher than for patients who have had ICR. A possible association is the subclavian steal syndrome in which collateral flow to the arm on the side of the anastomosis is supplied by the ipsilateral vertebral artery and may cause blood to be shunted away from the brain.[32]

Bacterial endocarditis occurred in one third of Deuchar's patients before ICR. In our 88 patients with a subclavian anastomosis, bacterial endocarditis occurred in five (5.8 percent), whereas only one of our 253 patients had bacterial endocarditis before an operation. Horner's syndrome of ptosis, miosis, enophthalmos, and anhydrosis is caused by injury of the cervical sympathetic chain at operation. It is frequent in the immediate postoperative period but resolves in most cases.[33]

Because the anastomosis may not grow with the patient, palliation often will decrease in effectiveness with increasing age.[34] Following the Blalock-Taussig anastomosis, between 35 and 50 percent of the patients will experience a return of symptoms within five years.[29,34] Pulmonary vascular obstructive disease (PVOD) is rare following Blalock-Taussig anastomosis but does occur in 1 to 5 percent of cases.[35,36]

Clinical Findings

The findings in adults basically do not differ from those in children.[16] By the time the patient reaches adulthood, the arm on the side of the anastomosis may be smaller than the other arm.[16] The pulse is usually absent, and the blood pressure is difficult to obtain because of the narrow pulse pressure in the arm being supplied by collateral vessels. Only one case of ischemic gangrene of the arm following Blalock-Taussig anastomosis has been reported.[36]

Effect of Prior Blalock-Taussig Anastomosis on Intracardiac Repair

The morbidity and mortality associated with prior Blalock-Taussig is the same as for primary repair. The most recent surgical mortality figures for patients undergoing ICR following Blalock-Taussig anastomosis vary from 4.2 to 8 percent.[16,27,28]

Potts Anastomosis

In 1946 Potts, Smith, and Gibson[38] reported a procedure in which the descending thoracic aorta was anastomosed side-to-side to the left pulmonary artery. In reports on older patients the Potts anastomosis was as common as the Blalock-Taussig procedure,[24] but in recent years it has become less popular for reasons described later.

Clinical Course

Among patients who did not have ICR, 15 percent died within the first ten years after operation, with approximately 85 percent surviving to adulthood.[39,40] The major causes of late death are congestive cardiac failure from a shunt which is too large (38 percent), followed by complications of PVOD in 15 percent. Another 15 percent die from bacterial endocarditis and 4 percent from cerebrovascular accident.

Morbidity Associated with Potts Anastomosis

Pulmonary over-circulation, commonly seen in children, is less often observed in the adult. PVOD after Potts anastomosis is observed much more often in the adult, since this complication is related to duration of the anastomosis.[41] Newfeld[36] reported no instances of PVOD among patients observed for five years following Potts anastomosis, but after five years 50 percent of the patients had histologic changes of PVOD evident on lung biopsy (Heath and Edwards[42] grade III or higher).

Clinical Findings

Two clinical features suggest that PVOD is likely to develop in the patient with a large Potts anastomosis: severe cardiac enlargement on chest roentgenogram (cardiothoracic ratio greater than 0.58) and electrocardiographic evidence of left ventricular hypertrophy. In the patient with these findings disappearance of the Potts continuous murmur and return of right ventricular hypertrophy suggest that PVOD has developed.

Cardiac Catheterization

It is essential to calculate the pulmonary/systemic resistance ratio (Rp/Rs). This is best done by averaging the main, right, and left pulmonary artery saturation.[41] An Rp/Rs ratio greater than or equal to 0.7 almost assuredly is associated with PVOD. Newfeld[36] found that all patients with a main pulmonary artery (MPA) *mean* pressure greater than or equal to 40 mm. Hg (without distal obstruction) had changes of PVOD evident on lung biopsy.

Effect of Prior Potts Anastomosis on Intracardiac Repair

The surgical mortality for patients with ICR after Potts anastomosis is higher than for all other types of palliation and higher than for primary ICR. Reports of mortality range from 15 to 60 percent.[16,27,28] The most common reason for the increase in mortality is PVOD. In addition to the increased risk of PVOD following Potts anastomosis, ICR takes more time and causes more risk when closure of the anastomosis is required;[16] for these reasons few surgeons currently use the Potts procedure for palliation of TOF.

Waterston-Cooley Anastomosis

Waterston[43] first described the extrapericardial approach to the ascending aorta-to-right pulmonary artery anastomosis in 1962. This was modified by Cooley and Hallman[44] in 1966. In the more recent series[27] and in our own experience, this operation is taking the place of the Potts anastomosis and is considered an effective means of palliation for infants. Therefore, more adults eventually will appear who have had this procedure.

Clinical Course

The late death rate ten years following the Waterston-Cooley anastomosis has been reported to be between 4 and 10 percent.[45,46] Death was caused by either excessive or inadequate flow through the anastomosis.

Morbidity Associated with a Waterston-Cooley Anastomosis

Theoretically, the Waterston-Cooley procedure could have the same associated sequelae as the Potts anastomosis.[46] Indeed, in one series there was a 26 percent incidence of late congestive cardiac failure following this procedure. PVOD occurred in six percent of the patients followed by Greenwood and coworkers;[46] two of these four patients exhibited elevated pulmonary resistance within four years of anastomosis.

Clinical Findings

Patients have findings similar to those with Potts anastomosis (see previous section), except the continuous murmur is heard best in the third intercostal space, to the right of the sternum.

Cardiac Catheterization

The major complication of Waterston-Cooley anastomosis is kinking and distortion of the right pulmonary artery.[45] Obstruction of blood flow can occur either to the left lung[47] or to the right lung,[48] depending upon which side of the right pulmonary artery is obstructed. In this situation it is important to ascertain if there is PVOD in the lung receiving the majority of the blood flow. This can be assessed by pulmonary arterial wedge angiography.[49,50]

Effect of Prior Waterston-Cooley Anastomosis on Intracardiac Repair

In a recent study by Greenwood and associates[46] there was a significantly higher surgical mortality associated with ICR following the Waterston-Cooley anastomosis (29.5 percent) than there was following primary ICR (6 percent). Clayman[28] found a 25 percent mortality for ICR following the Waterston-Cooley procedure. The reasons attributed to the increased mortality were similar to those given for the Potts anastomosis: immediate postoperative pulmonary hypertension with low cardiac output, hemorrhage, or residual obstruction of the distal right pulmonary artery.

Brock Procedure

Brock[51] first described his procedure—intrapericardial transventricular valvotomy for palliation of TOF—in 1948. Unfortunately, the results have been poor: either there was inadequate relief of obstruction, or congestive cardiac failure resulted from increased left-to-right flow through an unrestricted VSD. In addition, the intrapericardial approach rendered subsequent total correction more difficult.[16] For these reasons there are few adults in the U.S. with prior Brock procedures for palliation of TOF.

Management Question: When Should Intracardiac Repair Be Performed on the Patient with Previous Surgical Palliation?

In our experience, there is a slightly increased mortality rate for ICR in older patients who have had prior surgical anastomosis. Nonetheless, in most cases we believe the risk is acceptable and the patient should have ICR.

However, there are several relative-to-absolute contraindications in this situation. The first is PVOD. If the Rp/Rs is greater than 0.4, or if the MPA mean pressure is greater than 40 mm. Hg, we do not recommend repair. If an anastomosis has resulted in significantly reduced or absent flow to one lung, the presence of PVOD in the shunted lung is a contraindication to repair. Finally, the distortion of the pulmonary arterial architecture may be a relative contraindication. Kirklin[16] cautions against repair if anastomosis has resulted in clotting of either the right or left main branch of the pulmonary artery.

THE PATIENT WHO HAS HAD INTRACARDIAC REPAIR

In our series of 253 adult patients, 233 had ICR (92 percent). Today's adult has had ICR at an older age than will future adults, since ICR is currently being performed in younger infants and children. Our series of adults had ICR at a mean age of 10.9 years (range, 11 months to 36 years); 43 of our patients had repair done when they were over the age of 15 years.

Clinical Course

Estimates of late mortality are similar in all series and range from 1.7[23] to 7.1 percent[28] in patients followed for 10 to 15 years after operation. Our figure of 5.4 percent was in the middle range (Table 1). There are four reasons for the late deaths. In most series the majority of deaths were sudden and thought to be caused by cardiac dysrhythmias.[23,26,52,55] Of our patients sudden death occurred in eight (4 percent), three months to eight years after operation. Premature ventricular contractions or supraventricular tachycardia were reported in most patients who later died suddenly.[23,54] All eight patients in our series who died suddenly had premature ventricular contractions before their death. Of our patients who experienced sudden death, half died during strenuous exercise. A second reason for postoperative death was congestive cardiac failure associated with a residual left-to-right shunt at the ventricular level.[27,28] Some investigators[16,26] report a high surgical mortality associated with reoperation for residual defects—either VSD or pulmonary outflow obstruction. We have not established this correlation since we have had only one surgical death in 14 cases of reoperation. Finally, those patients with PVOD and resultant pulmonary arterial hypertension have a high late mortality.[56] In our experience five of these eight patients died between one and eight years postoperatively. At least 75 percent of our adult patients who had ICR are believed to be alive.

Morbidity Following Intracardiac Repair

Bacterial endocarditis occurred in only one of our patients following intracardiac repair and it was responsible for his death. Nine other patients had had bacterial endocarditis (total 5 percent) before ICR. There was no difference in exercise tolerance or hemodynamic parameters when those patients who had had bacterial endocarditis previously (mean 9.8 years) were compared with those who had not.

None of our patients had a cerebrovascular accident beyond the immediate postoperative period following ICR. Of the six patients (3 percent) who had cerebrovascular accidents either before or immediately after ICR, five were alive for a mean of ten years following their cerebrovascular accident (one died of bacterial endocarditis). Of the five, two had residual hemiparesis, two had seizure disorders, and one was lost to followup.

Symptoms

Eighty-one percent of our patients had unlimited exercise tolerance (N.Y.H.A. class I) and 14 percent were in class II. Ten of 203 patients (5 percent) were in class III and one patient was in class IV. Poor exercise tolerance generally implied either a residual VSD or RV hypertension.[28,57,58] Eighty-six percent of Rocchini's patients with symptoms of congestive cardiac failure had a residual VSD.[58] In our patients with decreased exercise tolerance, 9/11 had residual hemodynamic abnormality. In patients with PVOD a high MPA pressure has correlated with decreased exercise tolerance.[57] Several investigators have found no direct relationship between presence or severity of pulmonary valvular incompetence (PI) and exercise tolerance.[59-61]

Unfortunately, the normal exercise tolerance displayed by 80 to 95 percent of patients following ICR does not necessarily imply a good hemodynamic result.[16,28,57,62] Of our 54 patients with a RV systolic pressure equal to or greater than 40 mm. Hg, only 6 were symptomatic; of 10 with a hemodynamically significant VSD, only 3 were symptomatic.

Patient Questionnaire: Psychosocial and Medical Followup

We sent questionnaires to 203 patients believed to be alive and 95 (47 percent) responded. Ninety-one percent reported they were not limited by their disease in any way. Fifteen had undergone noncardiac surgical procedures without difficulty, varying from a Harrington rod procedure for scoliosis to pyloroplasty and vagotomy for peptic ulcer disease.

Forty-two percent of those who responded are currently students; 37 of the 51 who are no longer students have attended college. Twenty of these patients graduated from college and six had advanced professional degrees. Occupations held by more than two patients each included banker, construction worker, computer programmer, music instructor, and truck driver.

Eighteen men and ten women have married. Two marriages have ended in divorce. No patient has reported infertility, and there were no reported miscarriages in either the female patients or wives of the male patients. Nine men and six women have had children, none of whom has congenital heart disease.

In a previous study, there was evidence for a neurotic tendency, despite normal intelligence, in adults following ICR of TOF.[63] We have found that some young adults need encouragement to a normal life, but others have had tremendous success. One 23-year-old man who had ICR at the age of 11 recently graduated from college where he was commanding officer of his cadet company and responsible for leading the exercise routine, frequently running two to six miles per day.

Physical Examination

At followup, an average of five years after operation, the height and weight of our patients were normal. All patients had a crescendo-decrescendo murmur at the third left intercostal space. This murmur became louder and harsher as the right ventricular-to-pulmonary artery gradient increased. Seven (4 percent) of those with a short, low-pitched murmur had a gradient greater than 25 mm. Hg, while 42 percent of those with a harsh, long murmur had a gradient greater than 25 mm. Hg. Eight patients were believed to have a separate pansystolic plateau murmur of a residual VSD. These 8 patients had VSD according to results of cardiac catheterization, as did 11 other patients, including 5 with a Qp/Qs greater than 1.5:1 in whom the diagnosis was missed clinically. It seems that the physical examination is an inadequate means of assessing postoperative result.

One hundred twelve patients (55 percent) had a low-pitched diastolic decrescendo murmur which was separated from the aortic component of the second heart sound and was believed to represent pulmonary valvular incompetence. One patient had a high-pitched diastolic decrescendo murmur immediately following the aortic component of the second heart sound and was believed to have aortic valvular incompetence. This was the only case of aortic valvular incompetence observed at cardiac catheterization.

Chest Roentgenogram

Forty-one percent of our patients had a normal chest roentgenogram following ICR. In 42 percent the film was interpreted as showing generalized cardiomegaly. This was generally associated with the degree of pulmonary valvular incompetence (Fig. 3). We have been unable to predict the residual outflow gradient or left-to-right shunt from the chest roentgenogram. Abnormalities frequently interpreted included isolated right ventricular hypertrophy, increased pulmonary arterial vascular markings, and undue prominence of the MPA segment. Less frequently encountered were isolated left ventricular hypertrophy, prominent aortic arch, concave MPA segment, asymmetrical pulmonary vascular markings, and pulmonary edema.

Electrocardiogram

CONDUCTION DISTURBANCES. Complete right bundle-branch block (RBBB) occurs in 80 to 95 percent of these patients postoperatively.[55] It is impossible to determine from surface electrocardiograms whether (1) the RBBB has occurred because the peripheral ramifications of the right bundle were severed by the ventriculotomy or (2) the central right bundle-branch was injured during sewing of the interventricular patch (Fig. 4).

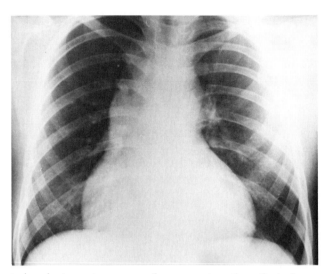

Figure 3. Posteroanterior chest roentgenogram of an asymptomatic patient nine years after intracardiac repair. At cardiac catheterization this patient had normal right heart pressures and no shunt; the cardiomegaly is presumably caused by pulmonary valvular incompetence.

Regardless of its origin, RBBB pattern alone has not been associated with any known complication. However, since Wolff's[64] original report quoting a 12.5 percent incidence of sudden death associated with the RBBB–left anterior hemiblock pattern (RBBB–LAH), controversy has appeared in the literature concerning the morbidity and mortality of this entity. The incidence of this pattern following ICR varies from 7 to 25 percent.[65] Gillette,[53] from this center, was unable to find consistent intracardiac conduction abnormalities in patients with this pattern. Most authors[53,55,66] now agree that

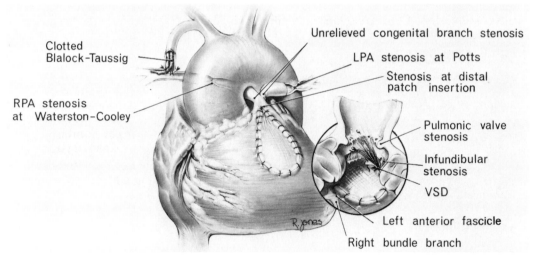

Figure 4. Composite drawing of the most common technical causes of a poor result after ICR. Obstruction to right ventricular outflow can occur at the infundibulum, at the valve, or within the pulmonary arteries. The residual VSD is usually at the upper margin of the patch; the right bundle-branch and left anterior fascicle are shown in close proximity to the patch in an area prone to injury. LPA = left pulmonary artery; RPA = right pulmonary artery; VSD = ventricular septal defect.

RBBB–LAH is not associated with sudden death or increased morbidity. In our series 8.4 percent of patients had RBBB–LAH and none died.

On the other hand, true trifascicular block indicated by RBBB–LAH and a long H-V interval may lead to sudden death. Gillette[53] found no correlation between this pattern and late postoperative mortality. However, 80 percent of Narula's elderly patients with coronary artery disease and trifascicular block died.[67] Presumably, such patients develop complete AV block.

Late development of complete AV block is said to be rare following ICR of TOF, with only single cases being reported in the literature.[28,56] We have identified none. However, this complication has been reported to occur up to 14 years after operation,[65] with only complete RBBB evident on the surface electrocardiogram.[68] No positive association has been made between transient postoperative complete AV block and late permanent AV block.

We believe patients with (1) transient postoperative complete AV block, (2) first degree AV block with RBBB–LAH (which is associated with trifascicular block),[54] (3) late development of second or third degree AV block, and (4) those with Stokes-Adams attacks should all be studied with intracardiac electrocardiography. Any suspicion of complete AV block with a wide QRS complex is an indication for a pacemaker, as is Mobitz II second degree AV block.

RHYTHM DISTURBANCES. The incidence of supraventricular tachycardia has been reported at between 8 and 11 percent.[19,57] Patients with PVOD seem to be particularly prone to this disorder which may be the result of right atrial enlargement.

Premature ventricular contractions (PVCs) are the most ominous findings in a patient after ICR. The incidence of this dysrhythmia on routine electrocardiogram varies from 5 to 18 percent during the postoperative period.[53,54,69] With exercise, especially in the postexercise recovery period, the incidence of PVCs is increased, and in one study 23 percent of postoperative patients had this dysrhythmia.[53] In our group of 203 patients 21 (10.4 percent) had PVCs on the resting electrocardiograms. The PVCs first appeared from two months to ten years after ICR. Twelve of sixty patients (from another series in our hospital) who had a treadmill exercise test following ICR had PVCs during or after exercise. Half of these had no PVCs on resting electrocardiograms.

The most important association with PVCs on the resting electrocardiogram was an elevated RV systolic or end-diastolic pressure. Of the 18 patients with PVCs who had cardiac catheterization, 16 had RV systolic pressures equal to or greater than 60 mm. Hg and end-diastolic pressures greater than 7 mm. Hg. Each of the other two patients with a normal RV systolic pressure had an end-diastolic pressure elevated to 8 mm. Hg. PVCs were found in 12 of the 32 (38 percent) patients who had pulmonary stenosis causing an RV systolic pressure greater than 60 mm. Hg, while 6 of the 8 patients (75 percent) with distal pulmonary arterial hypertension (distal pressure greater than 40 mm. Hg) had PVCs. There was no association between PVCs and the presence or severity of pulmonary valvular incompetence, or with cardiomegaly on chest roentgenogram in those patients whose RV systolic pressure was less than 60 mm. Hg. Therefore, it seems to be systolic pressure overload, rather than cardiac dilation, which is the major determinant of PVCs in this clinical setting.

Of the 21 patients in our series who had PVCs on the resting electrocardiogram, 8 died suddenly (38 percent). No other patient has died suddenly. All of the patients who died suddenly had an RV systolic pressure greater than 70 mm. Hg and an RV end-diastolic pressure greater than 7 mm. Hg. Five of the eight patients who died with PVCs were receiving digitalis at the time of their deaths, and one was additionally receiving quinidine. From our data we conclude:

1. PVCs are dangerous in patients following ICR and should be treated. If the heart is normal sized on chest roentgenogram, we would begin treatment with propranolol. If

the heart size is large, we would use quinidine which has been shown to be effective in reducing the number of PVCs following ICR of TOF.[69,70] Phenytoin may be used if there are contraindications to propranolol or quinidine.

2. All patients should undergo exercise testing following ICR, and if there are any PVCs during or after the test, the patient should be started on antidysrhythmic therapy.

3. If the RV systolic pressure is less than 60 mm. Hg, the likelihood of PVCs is reduced. If surgically accessible outflow obstruction is the cause of RV hypertension, operation is indicated. We speculate that PVCs may decrease following such surgery.

4. Patients with PVOD are likely to have PVCs and the combination of these two problems is likely to be responsible for the death of the patient.

Echocardiogram

In our laboratory we have noted certain common features in patients who have had ICR: (1) an enlarged RV, (2) an enlarged aortic root that may appear to override the ventricular septum, (3) paradoxical septal motion associated with pulmonary valvular incompetence, or (4) anterior septal motion in early systole, presumably the result of RBBB. These features may be present whether or not the patient has had an excellent hemodynamic result.

Response to Exercise

The data on exercise provide us with a measure of the functional adequacy of anatomic repair of TOF. Following ICR, patients have been reported to respond normally to *submaximal* exercise.[67,71] In another series from our hospital 40 of 53 patients (75 percent) had normal physical work capacity. Other studies have revealed an abnormal response to *maximal* exercise in these patients, with a 30 to 40 percent reduction in maximal oxygen uptake and a 20 percent lower cardiac index than expected for age and weight.[71] The deficit appears to be related to an inadequate stroke volume since the maximal heart rate is normal in most studies. It has been postulated that decreased contractility is the cause of the decreased stroke volume.[72,73] The decrease in maximal work capacity seems to occur more frequently in patients who had ICR after the age of 10 years.[69] Children operated upon earlier than this would be expected to have not only less fibrosis of the RV,[74] but also earlier relief of symptoms and increased exercise tolerance during the growth period.[63] James and associates[69] have suggested an exercise program for patients following repair of TOF in an effort to counteract the years of inactivity and possibly improve myocardial function.

Cardiac Catheterization

We have seen that evidence of a poor hemodynamic result can be missed from the history, physical examination, and noninvasive assessment. For this reason we recommend that cardiac catheterization be performed on all patients within one year or so of ICR for TOF.

A problem in interpreting the published results of followup catheterization data is that the criteria for operative results differ; using a variety of definitions, between 8 and 34 percent of patients have a "poor" result[24,28,52] (Fig. 4).

Because of the noted association between sudden death and an RV systolic pressure equal to or greater than 60 mm. Hg, and the association between symptoms, residual VSD, and a Qp/Qs greater than 1.5:1, we designated the term "poor" to cardiac catheterization results which indicated the presence of either of these factors, or the presence of pulmonary arterial hypertension (distal pulmonary artery pressure greater

Table 2. Cardiac catheterization pressure data after repair of tetralogy of Fallot

Pressure	N*	Mean†	SEM†	Range†	Median†	n>Normal‡(mm. Hg)
RV systolic	120	45.5	2.5	20–115	35	58>40
MPA	120	29.0	1.7	10–115	25	20>40
RPA systolic	83	24.8	2.3	10–115	17	8>40
LPA systolic	72	24.3	2.5	1–14	17	8>40
RV end-diastolic	120	7.2	0.26	1–14	6	37> 8
Aorta	120	114.0	3.0	95–150	110	—
LA (wedge)	81	8.8	0.34	2–15	7	13>12
Proximal gradient§	120	13.0	1.9	0–85	0	47>10
Distal gradient§	83	5.3	1.6	0–85	0	22>10
Total gradient	83	18.3	2.2	0–50	10	50>20

*N = number of patients with this parameter recorded
†values in mm. Hg
‡n = number of patients who exceed the normal value for our laboratory.
§Proximal gradient: infundibulum, pulmonary valve, proximal outflow patch insertion; distal gradient: distal outflow patch insertion, distal MPA, RPA, LPA.
LA = left atrium; LPA = left pulmonary artery; MPA = main pulmonary artery; RPA = right pulmonary artery; RV = right ventricle.

than or equal to 40 mm. Hg). Using these criteria 31 percent of our patients had a poor result. There was no relationship between the result and the age at operation or prior anastomosis.

It is generally accepted that if the RV pressure is less than 40 mm. Hg and there is no residual VSD, the result is excellent. Between 40 and 60 percent (51 percent in our series) have received an excellent result from ICR.[24,28,56] Results of the pressure data from our 120 postoperative cardiac catheterizations are given in Table 2 and Figures 5 and 6.

RESIDUAL RV OUTFLOW GRADIENT. There are a number of possible sites for residual anatomic obstruction to RV outflow (compare Figures 7 through 9). In our series 40 percent of the patients had RV pressure equal to or greater than 40 mm. Hg with an outflow gradient such that the distal MPA pressure was normal. Forty-seven of our fifty patients with gradients had a gradient proximal to the mid-MPA (at the infundibulum,

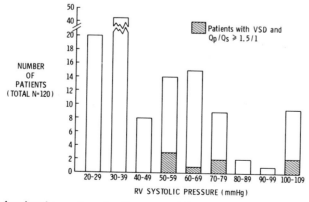

Figure 5. Histogram showing the number of patients at each level of right ventricular systolic pressure of our 120 patients who underwent ICR for TOF. In only two of the eight patients with VSD was the elevated RV pressure caused by the VSD, and not by RV outflow obstruction. Qp/Qs = pulmonary to systemic flow ratio; RV = right ventricle; VSD = ventricular septal defect.

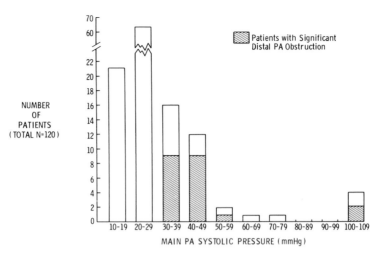

Figure 6. Histogram showing the number of patients at each level of main pulmonary artery systolic pressure. Eight patients had increased pulmonary artery pressure (greater than 40 mm. Hg) without demonstrable obstruction. PA = pulmonary artery.

valve, or proximal patch insertion) (Fig. 8). In our experience[27] the proximal gradient has occurred with equal frequency among patients with a pulmonary outflow patch as in those without such a patch. Of the 50 patients, 22 had gradients distal to the mid-MPA. It was not always possible to ascertain if the gradient was caused by unrelieved congenital proximal pulmonary branch stenosis or by obstruction at the site of distal patch insertion (Fig. 9).

Of our nine patients with prior Potts anastomosis, only one had a residual kink causing obstruction to the left pulmonary artery. Ruzyllo and associates,[24] from this center, found a 4.8 percent incidence of kinked left pulmonary artery following Potts anastomosis and 3.3 percent incidence of blocked left pulmonary artery from clotted Blalock-Taussig anastomosis. From our experience we would expect a high incidence

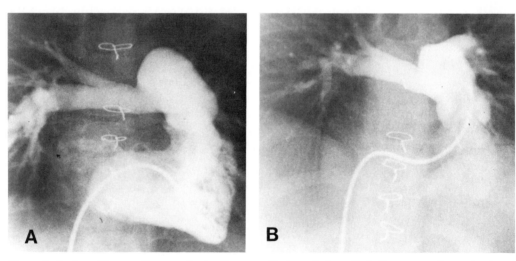

Figure 7. Angiocardiograms from a patient with an excellent surgical result. A, Posteroanterior projection of a right ventricular angiocardiogram. The left pulmonary artery frequently cannot be visualized in this projection. B, With the patient in a 45-degree sitting position the left pulmonary artery is clearly seen.

356

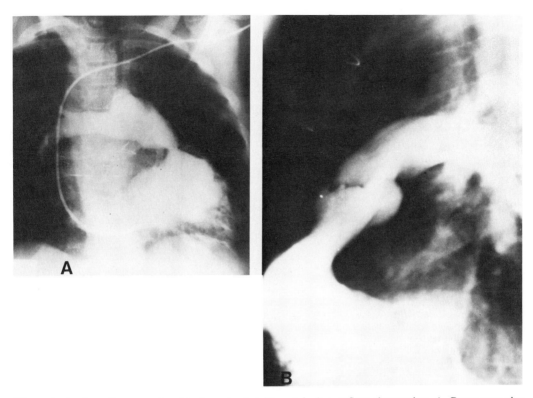

Figure 8. Angiocardiograms of residual *proximal* right ventricular outflow obstruction. A, Posteroanterior projection of a right ventricular angiocardiogram shows persistent infundibular obstruction. B, In another patient lateral projection of a right ventricular angiocardiogram shows valvular stenosis.

of distortion of the right pulmonary artery anatomy from Waterston-Cooley anastomosis.

From long-term serial cardiac catheterization data we infer that if the RV systolic pressure is below 60 mm. Hg at the first cardiac catheterization, it is likely to remain stable or decrease. However, if the pressure is above 60 mm. Hg, it is unlikely to decrease and it may increase.[24,57,62,75]

RESIDUAL LEFT-TO-RIGHT SHUNT. In our group 19 of 120 (16 percent) had a residual VSD; in eight (5.9 percent) the Qp/Qs was equal to or greater than 1.5:1 (Fig. 10). This is similar to the incidence of hemodynamically significant VSDs found by others (between 3 and 7 percent).[24,26,28] In all of our patients with a hemodynamically significant VSD, the RV systolic pressure was equal to or greater than 40 mm. Hg, but in only two patients was the distal pulmonary artery pressure elevated (the remaining seven patients had coexistent obstruction to RV outflow) (Figs. 5 and 6).

A residual insignificant left-to-right shunt (Qp/Qs less than 1.5:1) was present in 5 of 37 patients (13.5 percent) through a patent Potts anastomosis, and 3 of 40 patients (7.5 percent) with a Blalock-Taussig anastomosis.

DISTAL PULMONARY ARTERIAL HYPERTENSION. In our study 8 of the 120 patients (6.7 percent) had pulmonary arterial hypertension (Fig. 5). Two of these patients had VSD with a large residual left-to-right shunt; the remaining six had no left-to-right shunt and PVOD. Of these six, four had had a prior Potts anastomosis, one a prior Blalock-Taussig procedure, and one patient had had left ventricular failure following primary ICR. Kinsley[57] found that all of his patients with PVOD following ICR had had prior Potts

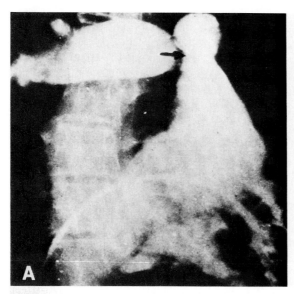
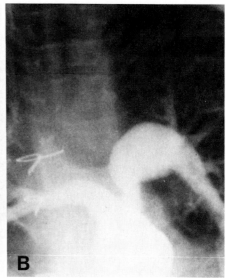

Figure 9. Angiocardiograms of residual *distal* right ventricular outflow obstruction. A, Posteroanterior projection of a right ventricular angiocardiogram shows narrowing of main pulmonary artery at the site of distal patch insertion (arrow). B, In another patient posteroanterior projection of a main pulmonary artery angiocardiogram with the patient in the sitting position (inclined 45 degrees) shows unrelieved congenital bilateral pulmonary arterial branch stenosis.

anastomosis. The theoretical incidence of development of PVOD following a Waterston-Cooley anastomosis is approximately the same as that of a Potts anastomosis.

Nihill,[76] in our center, is currently studying the effect of treating patients who have increased pulmonary arterial resistance with a combination of either acetylsalicylic acid with cyproheptadine, acetylsalicylic acid with dipyridamole, or dipyridamole and cyproheptadine, in an effort to decrease the occurrence of thrombi in the small pulmonary arteries.

PULMONARY VALVULAR INCOMPETENCE (PI). The incidence of postoperative PI is 60 to 70 percent.[24] It is suggested either by the presence of a low pulmonary artery diastolic pressure (less than 10 mm. Hg), or by the regurgitant stream seen following the injection of contrast into the MPA. Severe PI is associated with an elevated RV end-diastolic pressure.[52] Severity is more marked in the presence of distal obstruction either in the large pulmonary arteries or from PVOD in the small muscular arteries.[26,27]

In our patients there was no association between the presence or degree of PI and decreased exercise tolerance, PVCs, or mortality. Epstein[60] found no relationship between maximal work capacity and the presence or degree of PI. Most authors believe PI is well tolerated for long periods of time.[26,59,75] However, patients with isolated PI have developed congestive cardiac failure beyond the age of 25, especially during pregnancy.[78]

We agree with Kirklin's[16] caution that a longer period of followup is required to determine the ultimate hemodynamic significance of PI.

VENTRICULAR FUNCTION. The right ventricle appears to function normally in the patient following ICR. Graham and associates[79] found a normal end-diastolic volume and RV ejection fraction in patients, unless an outflow patch had been used, in which case both parameters were abnormal. Shah[80] also found a normal RV systolic ejection rate in patients at rest and during exercise.

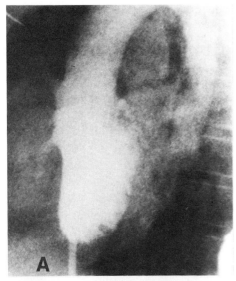

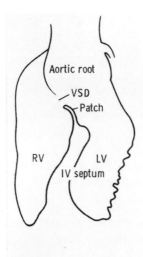

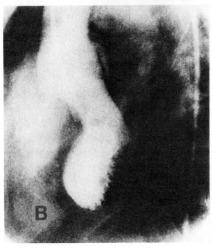

Figure 10. Residual VSD. Both views are lateral projections of left ventricular angiocardiograms. A, A small VSD. B, A larger defect. The diagram (top right) indicates the position of the defect. IV = interventricular; LV = left ventricle; RV = right ventricle; VSD = ventricular septal defect.

Graham found that the left ventricle was dilated with mild to moderate functional impairment. The average ejection fraction was 50 percent.[81,82]

There was no correlation found between indices of ventricular function and morbidity or mortality. Such studies of ventricular function should be performed during cardiac catheterization to determine clinical correlation and long-term implications.

Management Question: When Should Revision of Unsatisfactory Intracardiac Repair Be Undertaken?

There are three basic reasons for performing a revision of ICR: residual VSD, residual proximal RV outflow obstruction, and residual distal RV outflow obstruction. Most authors agree that repair is indicated if any VSD results in a pulmonary-to-systemic flow ratio in excess of 1.5:1.[24,26] Poirier and associates,[26] at the Mayo Clinic, recommended reoperation if the total outflow gradient is greater than 70 mm. Hg or if the gradient is 50 mm. Hg in a symptomatic patient. We believe that if the RV systolic

359

pressure is greater than 60 mm. Hg at postoperative cardiac catheterization, surgery should be performed. In our patients, RV pressure of this magnitude was associated with a high incidence of sudden death. In addition, we found that such a high pressure is not likely to decrease.[13,47]

Recommendations for the Practical Management of the Patient

Pregnancy

Despite the fact that we have found no increased incidence of problems associated with pregnancy in patients who had successful ICR, an expectant mother should be followed closely by a cardiologist, especially through the third trimester. Patients with severe PI or residual VSD should be watched carefully for development of congestive cardiac failure. If revision of ICR is required, it should be done before pregnancy is contemplated. Antibiotic prophylaxis should be given for bacterial endocarditis at the beginning of labor and for at least three days postpartum.

Risk of Congenital Heart Disease in the Offspring of TOF Patients

The risk of congenital heart disease in any first degree relative (sibling or child) of a patient with TOF is 3.2 percent.[83] If the parent with TOF already has one child with congenital heart disease, the risk for each subsequent child is estimated to be 6.4 percent.

Precautions for Noncardiac Surgery

If the result of repair is good, there is little increased risk from anesthesia for other surgical procedures. Antibiotics should be prescribed for prophylaxis against bacterial endocarditis. The electrocardiogram of all patients should be monitored during and immediately following anesthesia. Patients with increased distal pulmonary artery pressure have an increased risk of anesthesia, and cardiac dysrhythmias—especially supraventricular tachycardia and PVCs—are common. The anesthesiologist should administer a high concentration of oxygen during and immediately following operation for protection against hypoxia.

Exercise

If a treadmill or bicycle stress test reveals no abnormalities, exercise should be encouraged. We believe that if a patient has an excellent hemodynamic result and no abnormalities on periodic exercise testing, competitive sports may be allowed. In patients with less than an excellent result competitive sports should be restricted.

Patients with cardiac dysrhythmias should not exercise until drug therapy has been instituted and a subsequent exercise test proves that the medication is protective. In that case, light exercise may be permitted.

Life Expectancy

Using our actuarial estimates, there is an 85 percent probability that a patient with TOF born 15 years ago is alive today. The probability is 75 percent that this patient will live to be 40 years old (Fig. 11). We have not followed patients for a sufficient period of time to predict survival beyond the age of 40. It is unknown if the ventricle subjected to open heart surgery can function adequately for a full life span. In patients who have had

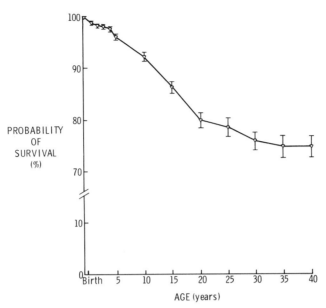

PROBABILITY OF SURVIVAL (%)

AGE (years)

Figure 11. Life table of 253 patients with tetralogy of Fallot. All patients were born more than 15 years before the study. The mean probability of survival to each age is indicated ($\pm$ 1 SEM). Of the 253 patients, 51 were known to have died (all causes, including accidental death) at a median age of 12.5 years (range 1.5 to 26.5 years); 123 were known to be alive at median age of 22.5 years (range 15.2 to 45.5 years). Using this method we predict that approximately 75 percent of our patients will reach 40 years of age.

earlier primary repair it is possible that the right ventricle will have undergone less stress, and survival is thus improved further. Patients with an excellent hemodynamic result do not seem to exhibit changes during annual examinations; some have remained stable for as long as 15 years after surgery. We believe they will continue to lead normal and active lives.

REFERENCES

1. FALLOT, A.: *Contribution à l'anatomie pathologique de la maladie bleue (cyanose cardiaque)*. Marseille Médical 25:418, 1888.

2. NADAS, A. S., AND FYLER, D. C.: *Pediatric Cardiology*, ed. 3. W. B. Saunders, Philadelphia, 1972.

3. *Current Population Reports (U.S. Census 1970) Population Estimates and Projections*. Series P-25, No. 481, U.S. Dept of Commerce, U.S. Government Printing Office, Washington, D.C., 1972.

4. CAMPBELL, M.: *Late results of operations for Fallot's tetralogy*. Br. Med. J. 2:1175,1958.

5. THOMPSON, W. M., CARTAYA, A. L., VANHOUTTE, J. J., ET AL.: *Tetralogy of Fallot*. J. Okla. State Med. Assoc. 69:434,1976.

6. BOESEN, I.: *Tetralogy of Fallot in Denmark. Incidence in newborns and prognosis up to the age of three years*. Dan. Med. Bull. 18(Suppl. 2):22,1971.

7. RYGG, I. H., OLESEN, K., AND BOESEN, I.: *The life history of tetralogy of Fallot*. Dan. Med. Bull. 18(Suppl. 2):25,1971.

8. CAMPBELL, M.: *Natural history of cyanotic malformations and comparison of all common cardiac malformations*. Br. Heart J. 34:31,1972.

9. IKEDA, M., AND HIROSAWA, K.: *Tetralogy of Fallot*. Circulation 37 (Suppl. V):21, 1968.

10. HIRSCHFELD, A. D.: *Diseases of the Heart and Aorta*. J.B. Lippincott, Philadelphia, 1910.

11. DONZELOT, E., HEIM DE BALZAC, R., EMAM-ZADE, A. M., ET AL.: *Étude de 200 cas de tétrade de Fallot*. Arch. Mal. Coeur 42:98,1948.

12. BOWIE, E. A.: *Longevity in tetralogy and trilogy of Fallot. Discussion of patients and presentation of two further cases*. Am. Heart J. 62:125,1961.

13. ABBOTT, M.: *Atlas of Congenital Cardiac Disease.* American Heart Association, New York, 1936.

14. BAIN, G. O.: *Tetralogy of Fallot: Survival to seventieth year.* Arch. Pathol. 58:176,1954.

15. OAKLEY, C., OLSEN, E., HUDSON, R. E. B., ET AL.: *A case of long survival with Fallot's tetralogy.* Br. Med. J. 2:748, 1966.

16. KIRKLIN, J. W., AND KARP, R. B.: *The Tetralogy of Fallot from a Surgical Viewpoint.* W.B. Saunders Company, Philadelphia, 1970.

17. NEILL, C. A., AND SWANSON, S.: *Outcome of pregnancy in congenital heart disease.* Circulation 24:1003,1961.

18. JACOBY, W. J.: *Pregnancy with tetralogy and pentalogy of Fallot.* Am. J. Cardiol. 14:886,1964.

19. JEPSON, J. H.: *Polycythemia: pathophysiology, hematological and cardiological consequences.* In Jepson, J. H., and Frankl, W. S. (eds): *Hematological Complications in Cardiac Practice.* W. B. Saunders Company, Philadelphia, 1975.

20. EKERT, H., GILCHRIST, G. S., STANTON, R., ET AL.: *Hemostasis in cyanotic congenital heart disease.* J. Pediatr. 76:221,1970.

21. TRIMBLE, A. S., MORCE, J. E., FROGGATT, M. B., ET AL.: *Total intracardiac repair of the adult cyanotic tetralogy of Fallot.* Can. Med. Assoc. J. 103:911,1970.

22. BENDER, H. W., HALLER, J. A., BRAWLEY, R. K., ET AL.: *Experience in repair of tetralogy of Fallot malformations in adults.* Ann. Thorac. Surg. II:508,1971.

23. BEACH, P. M., BOWMAN, F. O., KAISER, G. A., ET AL.: *Total correction of tetralogy of Fallot in adolescents and adults.* Circulation 43(Suppl. I):37,1971.

24. RUZYLLO, W., NIHILL, M. R., MULLINS, C. E., ET AL.: *Hemodynamic evaluation of 221 patients after intracardiac repair of tetralogy of Fallot.* Am. J. Cardiol. 34:565,1974.

25. BLALOCK, A., AND TAUSSIG, H. B.: *The surgical treatment of malformations of the heart in which there is pulmonic stenosis or patent ductus arteriosus.* JAMA 128:189,1945.

26. POIRIER, R. A., McGOON, D. C., DANIELSON, G. K., ET AL.: *Late results after repair of tetralogy of Fallot.* J. Thorac. Cardiovasc. Surg. 73:900,1977.

27. CHIARIELLO, L., MEYER, J., WUKASCH, D. C., ET AL.: *Intracardiac repair of tetralogy of Fallot.* J. Thorac. Cardiovasc. Surg. 70:529,1975.

28. CLAYMAN, J. A., ANKENEY, J. L., AND LIEBMAN, J.: *Results of complete repair of tetralogy of Fallot in 156 consecutive patients.* Am. J. Surg. 130:601,1975.

29. REID, J. M., COLEMAN, E. N., BARCLAY, R. S., ET AL.: *Blalock-Taussig anastomosis in 126 patients with Fallot's tetralogy.* Thorax 28:269,1973.

30. DEUCHAR, D., BESLOS, L. L., AND CHAKORN, S.: *Fallot's tetralogy: A 20 year surgical follow-up.* Br. Heart J. 34:12,1972.

31. TAUSSIG, H. B., KALLMAN, C. H., NAGEL, D., ET AL.: *Long-time observations on the Blalock-Taussig Operation. VIII. 20–28 year follow-up on patients with a tetralogy of Fallot.* Johns Hopkins Med. J. 139:13,1975.

32. MORRISS, J. H., AND McNAMARA, D. G.: *Residuae, sequelae and complications of surgery for congenital heart disease.* Prog. Cardiovasc. Dis. 18:1,1975.

33. ENGLE, M. A.: *Postoperative syndromes.* In Moss, A. J., and Adams, F. H. (eds.): *Heart Disease in Infants, Children and Adolescents.* Williams and Wilkins, Baltimore, 1968.

34. KAPLAN, S., HELMSWORTH, J. A., AHEARN, E. N., ET AL.: *Results of palliative procedures for tetralogy of Fallot in infants and young children.* Ann. Thorac. Surg. 5:489,1968.

35. TAUSSIG, H. B., CROCETTI, A., ESAGHPOUR, E., ET AL.: *Long-time observations on the Blalock-Taussig operation, III. Common complications.* John Hopkins Med. J. 129:274,1971.

36. NEWFELD, E. A., WALDMAN, J. D., PAUL, M. H., ET AL.: *Pulmonary vascular disease after systemic-pulmonary shunt operations.* Am. J. Cardiol. 39:715,1977.

37. WEBB, W. R., AND BURFORD, T. H.: *Gangrene of the arm following use of the subclavian artery in pulmonary-systemic (Blalock) anastomosis.* J. Thorac. Surg. 23:199,1952.

38. POTTS, W. J., SMITH, S., AND GIBSON, S.: *Anastomosis of the aorta to a pulmonary artery.* JAMA 132:627,1946.

39. COLE, R. B., MUSTER, A. J., FIXLER, D. E., ET AL.: *Long-term results of aorticopulmonary anastomosis for tetralogy of Fallot.* Circulation 48:263,1971.

40. POTTS, W. J., GIBSON, S., BERMAN, E., ET AL.: *Surgical correction of tetralogy of Fallot.* JAMA 159:95,1955.

41. VON BERNUTH, G., RITTER, D. G., FRYE, R. L., ET AL.: *Evaluation of patients with tetralogy of Fallot and Potts anastomosis.* Am. J. Cardiol. 27:259,1971.

42. HEATH, D., AND EDWARDS, J. E.: *The pathology of hypertensive pulmonary vascular disease: A description of six grades of structural changes in the pulmonary arteries with special reference to congenital cardiac septal defects.* Circulation 18:533, 1958.

43. WATERSTON, D. J.: *Fallot's tetralogy in children under one year of age.* Rozhl. Chir. 41:181,1962.

44. COOLEY, D. A., AND HALLMAN, G. L.: *Intrapericardial aortic-right pulmonary arterial anastomosis.* Surg. Gynecol. Obstet. 122:1084,1966.

45. ALVAREZ-DIAZ, F., BORITO, J. M., CORDOVILLA, G., ET AL.: *Ascending aorta-right pulmonary artery anastomosis: Waterston's operation.* Thorax 28:152,1973.

46. GREENWOOD, R. D., NADAS, A. S., ROSENTHAL, A., ET AL.: *Ascending aorta-to-pulmonary artery anastomosis for cyanotic congenital heart disease.* Am. Heart J. 94:14,1977.

47. WALDHAUSEN, J. A., FRIEDMAN, S., TYERS, G. F. O., ET AL.: *Ascending aorta-to-right pulmonary artery anastomosis: Clinical experience with 35 patients with cyanotic congenital heart disease.* Circulation 38:463,1968.

48. HALLMAN, G. L., YASHER, J. J., BLOODWELL, R. D., ET AL.: *Intrapericardial aorta-pulmonary artery anastomosis for tetralogy of Fallot: Clinical experience.* Arch. Surg. 95:709,1967.

49. HIRSCHHUT, E., PUIGBO, J. J., APARICIO, J. M., ET AL.: *Algunas applicationes de la angiografia selectiva del pulmon.* Memorias del IV Congreso Mundiae de Cardiologia (Mexico) Vol. IB:28,1962.

50. CASTELLANOS, A., HERNANDEZ, F. A., AND MERCADO, H. G.: *Wedge pulmonary arteriography in congenital heart disease.* Radiology 85:838,1965.

51. BROCK, R. C.: *Pulmonary valvulotomy for relief of congenital pulmonary stenosis: Report of three cases.* Br. Med. J. 1:1121,1948.

52. SOULÍE, P., FOUCHARD, J., BOUCHARD, F., ET AL.: *Résultats de la réparation complète de la tétralogie de Fallot.* Arch. Mal. Coeur 64:1751,1971.

53. GILLETTE, P. C., YEOMAN, M. A., MULLINS, C. E., ET AL.: *Sudden death after repair of tetralogy of Fallot: Electrocardiographic and electrophysiologic abnormalities.* Circulation (in press).

54. QUATTLEBAUM, T. G., VARGHESE, P. J., NEILL, C. A., ET AL.: *Sudden death among postoperative patients with tetralogy of Fallot.* Circulation 54:289,1976.

55. JAMES, F. W., KAPLAN, S., AND CHOU, T. C.: *Unexpected cardiac arrest in patients after surgical correction of tetralogy of Fallot.* Circulation 52:691,1975.

56. GERSONY, W. M., BATTHANY, S., BOWMAN, F. O., ET AL.: *Late follow-up of patients evaluated hemodynamically following total correction of tetralogy of Fallot.* J. Thorac. Cardiovasc. Surg. 66:209,1973.

57. KINSLEY, R. H., McGOON, D. C., DANIELSON, G. C., ET AL.: *Pulmonary arterial hypertension after repair of tetralogy of Fallot.* J. Thorac. Cardiovasc. Surg. 67:110,1974.

58. ROCCHINI, A. P., ROSENTHAL, A., FREED, M., ET AL.: *Chronic congestive heart failure after repair of tetralogy of Fallot.* Circulation 56:305,1977.

59. FISH, R. G., TAKARO, T., AND CRYMES, T.: *Prognostic considerations in primary isolated insufficiency of the pulmonic valve.* N. Engl. J. Med. 261:739,1959.

60. EPSTEIN, S. E., BEISER, G. D., GOLDSTEIN, R. E., ET AL.: *Hemodynamic abnormalities in response to mild and intense upright exercise following operative correction of an atrial septal defect or tetralogy of Fallot.* Circulation 47:1065,1973.

61. JONES, E. L., CONTI, C. R., NEILL, C. A., ET AL.: *Long-term evaluation of tetralogy patients with pulmonary valvular insufficiency resulting from outflow patch correction across the pulmonic annulus.* Circulation 47(Suppl. III):11,1973.

62. FINNEGAN, P., HARDER, R., PATEL, R. G., ET AL.: *Results of total correction of the tetralogy of Fallot. Long-term hemodynamic evaluation at rest and during exercise.* Br. Heart J. 38:934,1976.

63. GARSON, A., Jr., WILLIAMS, R. B., Jr., AND RECKLESS, J.: *Long-term follow-up of patients with tetralogy of Fallot: Physical health and psychopathology.* J. Pediatr. 85:429,1974.

64. WOLFF, G. S., ROWLAND, T. W., AND ELLISON, R. C.: *Surgically induced right bundle-branch block with left anterior hemiblock.* Circulation 45:587,1972.

65. YABEK, J. M., JARMAKANI, J. M., AND ROBERTS, N. K.: *Diagnosis of trifascicular damage following tetralogy of Fallot and ventricular septal defect repair.* Circulation 55:23,1977.

66. CAIRNS, J. A., DOBELL, A. R. C., GIBBONS, J. E., ET AL.: *Prognosis of right bundle-branch block and left anterior hemiblock after intracardiac repair of tetralogy of Fallot.* Am. Heart J. 90:549,1975.

67. NARULA, O. S., GANN, D., AND SAMET, P.: *Prognostic value of H-V intervals.* In *His Bundle Electrocardiography and Clinical Electrophysiology.* F.A. Davis Company, Philadelphia, 1975.

68. MOSS, A. J., KLYMAN, G., AND EMMANOULIDES, G. C.: *Late onset of complete heart block.* Am. J. Cardiol. 30:884,1972.

363

69. JAMES, F. W., KAPLAN, S., SCHWARTZ, D. C., ET AL.: *Response to exercise in patients following total surgical correction of tetralogy of Fallot.* Circulation 54:671,1976.

70. GEY, G. O., LEVY, R. H., PETTET, G., ET AL.: *Quinidine plasma concentration and exertional arrhythmias.* Am. Heart J. 90:19,1975.

71. GOTSMAN, M. S.: *Hemodynamics and cine-angiographic findings after one-stage repair of Fallot's tetralogy.* Br. Heart J. 28:448,1966.

72. BJARKE, B.: *Oxygen uptake and cardiac output during submaximal and maximal exercise in adult subjects with totally corrected tetralogy of Fallot.* Acta Med. Scand. 197:177,1975.

73. MOCELLIN, R., BASTANIER, C., HOFACKER, W., ET AL.: *Exercise performance in children and adolescents after surgical repair of tetralogy of Fallot.* Eur. J. Cardiol. 4:367,1976.

74. JONES, M., AND FERRANS, V. J.: *Myocardial degeneration in congenital heart disease: Comparison of morphologic findings in young and old patients with congenital heart disease associated with muscular obstruction to right ventricular outflow.* Circulation 55:1051,1977.

75. BRISTOW, J. D., KLOSTER, F. E., LEES, M. H., ET AL.: *Serial cardiac catheterizations and exercise hemodynamics following correction of tetralogy of Fallot.* Circulation 41:1057,1970.

76. NIHILL, M. R.: Personal communication, 1977.

77. ELLISON, R. G., BROWN, W. J., YEH, T. S., ET AL.: *Surgical significance of acute and chronic pulmonary valvar insufficiency.* J. Thorac. Cardiovasc. Surg. 60:549,1970.

78. PRICE, B. O.: *Isolated incompetence of the pulmonic valve.* Circulation 23:596,1961.

79. GRAHAM, T. P., CORDELL, D., ATWOOD, G. F., ET AL.: *Right ventricular volume characteristics before and after palliative operation in tetralogy of Fallot.* Circulation 54:417,1976.

80. SHAH, P., AND KIDD, L.: *Hemodynamic response to exercise and to isoproterenol following total correction of Fallot's tetralogy.* J. Thorac. Cardiovasc. Surg. 52:138,1966.

81. GRAHAM, T. P.: *Ventricular performance in patients following corrective surgery for congenital heart disease.* Adv. Cardiol. 11:81,1974.

82. JARMAKANI, J., GRAHAM, T. P., CANENT, R. V., ET AL.: *Left heart function in children with tetralogy of Fallot, before and after palliative or corrective surgery.* Circulation 46:478,1972.

83. NORA, J. J., McGILL, C. W., AND McNAMARA, D. G.: *Empiric recurrence risks in common and uncommon congenital heart lesions.* Teratology 3:325,1970.

Transposition of the Great Arteries in the Adult

Langford Kidd, M.D., F.R.C.P., and
J. O'Neal Humphries, M.D.

Transposition of the great arteries (TGA) can be complete or corrected. At birth complete transposition is five times more common than corrected transposition, but until recently patients with corrected transposition survived into adult life more often than those with complete transposition.

DEFINITIONS AND TERMINOLOGY

Complete and corrected transposition are part of a group of congenital heart malformations, the cono-truncal malpositions, in which the relationship between the great arteries and the heart is abnormal. The term "transposition" means that the aorta and pulmonary trunk are placed across the ventricular septum so that the aorta arises anteriorly from the right ventricle and the pulmonary trunk from the left.

In complete transposition the atria and the ventricles are normally related, but the aorta arises anteriorly, high and to the right from the right ventricle. The pulmonary trunk arises posteriorly, low and to the left from the left ventricle. This produces two separate circulations in parallel rather than in series (Fig. 1). The course of blood flow is as follows: right atrium to right ventricle to aorta to body to systemic veins to right atrium on one side, and left atrium to left ventricle to pulmonary artery to lungs to pulmonary veins to left atrium on the other side.

This dichotomous arrangement is obviously incompatible with life unless there is some communication between the two circuits; thus, it was very rare for a patient to survive beyond infancy with this condition. Recently, however, procedural intervention has improved survival and a group of patients with isolated complete transposition, salvaged by a variety of techniques developed over the past 30 years, is now approaching adulthood. A second group of patients survive naturally into adult life because of the congenital presence of adequate communication between the two circuits, either by a ventricular septal defect (VSD) or single ventricle (SV). These adults have either pulmonic stenosis or severe pulmonary vascular disease. Most patients are cyanotic and considerably limited physically.

Corrected transposition is so called because although the great arteries are transposed—the aorta arising from the right ventricle and the pulmonary trunk from the left—the transposition is "corrected" by the fact that the ventricles are inverted, with the right ventricle on the left and the left ventricle on the right. The course of the circulation then is as follows: right atrium to left ventricle to pulmonary artery to lungs to pulmonary veins to left atrium to right ventricle to aorta to body to systemic veins to

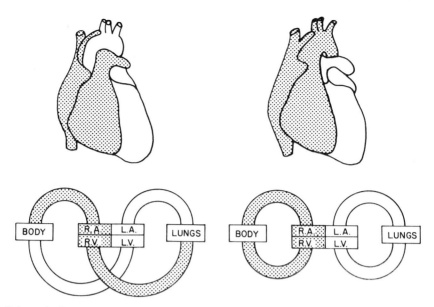

Figure 1. Schematic diagram of blood flow in complete transposition of the great arteries (TGA) as contrasted with normal.

right atrium; this is a physiologically "correct" circuit (Fig. 2). The aorta arises anteriorly, high and to the left, in corrected transposition and the pulmonary trunk arises posteriorly, low and to the right. The side-to-side inversion of the ventricles occurs during the ventricular looping stage of cardiac development, when the ventricular part of the cardiac tube loops to the left (an *l*-loop) instead of the more usual direction, to the right (a *d*-loop). This accounts for the alternative names for the transpositions: *l*-transposition (corrected) and *d*-transposition (complete).

Patients with corrected transposition have an essentially normal circulation and might therefore be expected to lead normal lives. However, associated anomalies such as SV or VSD, pulmonic stenosis, left atrioventricular (AV) valve regurgitation, and heart block are frequent, and truly normal hearts are rare.

DIAGNOSTIC APPROACH

In the vast majority of patients with transposition of the great arteries the diagnostic problem is one of chronic central cyanosis, the features of which are well known and

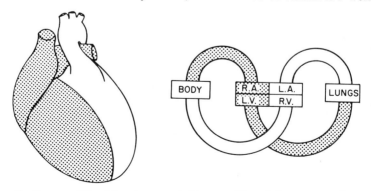

Figure 2. Schematic diagram of blood flow in corrected transposition of the great arteries.

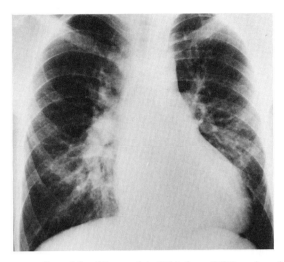

Figure 3. Chest roentgenogram of an adult with complete TGA, large VSD, and markedly elevated pulmonary vascular resistance. The shape of the heart is similar to the shadow of a large summer squash. The pulmonary conus is not prominent, but the central and peripheral branches of the pulmonary arteries are conspicuous.

easily recognized. The clinical examination may yield some helpful information, as described below, and the ancillary noninvasive tests will be of value. The definitive and anatomically accurate diagnosis, however, depends on cardiac catheterization and selective angiocardiography.

Chest X-ray

There is nothing specific on the chest roentgenogram to establish the diagnosis of TGA. However, the presence of an elongated, moderately enlarged heart with a narrow waist (similar to the shadow of a large summer squash) is highly suggestive of TGA. The pulmonary vasculature will vary according to the associated lesions.

In the patient with either *d* or *l* TGA and a large VSD without pulmonic stenosis, the pulmonary trunk is not clearly detected despite great prominence of the proximal portions of both the right and left main pulmonary arteries (Fig. 3). Prominence of the pulmonary vasculature is present all the way to the periphery of the lung fields despite markedly elevated pulmonary vascular resistance. "Pruning" of the peripheral vasculature, so often present in adult patients with isolated VSD and elevated pulmonary vascular resistance, is not seen with TGA and VSD.

In the patient with pulmonic stenosis (PS) in addition to VSD or SV and TGA, the x-ray shows normal or diminished pulmonary vasculature (Fig. 4). The aortic arch may be to the right as in this patient.

In the acyanotic patient with corrected TGA, intact ventricular septum, and atrioventricular valve regurgitation the area of the pulmonary conus is remarkably small when compared to other signs of pulmonary congestion and pulmonary hypertension; also, the ascending aorta may be identified at the left upper heart border in some of these patients (Fig. 5).

Electrocardiogram

The electrocardiogram usually shows right ventricular hypertrophy, right or left axis deviation in the frontal plane, abnormal P waves, and various degrees of AV heart

367

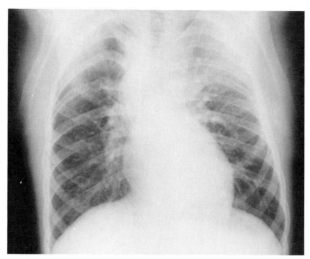

Figure 4. Chest roentgenogram of an adult with complete TGA, large VSD, and PS. There is a right-sided aortic arch.

block. The presence of a QS wave in V_1 and the absence of a Q wave in V_6 in a patient with cyanotic heart disease suggests, but is not diagnostic of, corrected TGA.

Echocardiography

With new echocardiographic techniques it is possible to establish the relationship of the great vessels to each other, to the ventricles, and to the ventricular septum. These studies performed prior to catheterization and angiography are of great value to the angiographer who can complete the studies more quickly and thoroughly. An example of a two-dimensional echocardiogram in a patient with *d*-TGA and a VSD is shown in Figure 6.

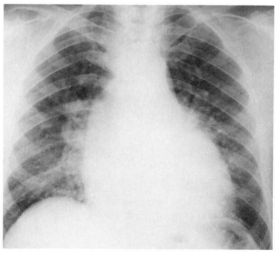

Figure 5. Chest roentgenogram of an adult with corrected TGA, intact ventricular septum, and left-sided atrioventricular valvular regurgitation. There is marked pulmonary congestion but the pulmonary conus is not prominent. The ascending aorta is in the left hilar shadows.

368

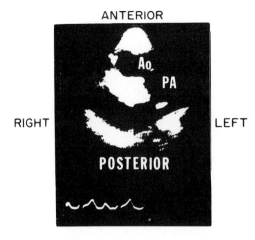

Figure 6. Two-dimensional echocardiogram of an adult with complete TGA and a large VSD. The aorta (Ao.) is to the left of the pulmonary artery (PA) and overrides the ventricular septal defect.

Angiography and Cardiac Catheterization

The angiographic demonstration of the aorta arising anteriorly over the right ventricular outflow tract establishes the diagnosis of TGA. However, it is also important to establish the following: whether the aorta is to the right or to the left of the pulmonary trunk; whether either of the great arteries overrides the ventricular septum; whether there is a single ventricle or a large VSD; whether there is pulmonic stenosis; the level of pulmonary vascular resistance; the anatomical position of the atria, and the competence of the atrioventricular valves. Associated lesions such as persistent ductus arteriosus and coarctation of the aorta must be sought.

COMPLETE TRANSPOSITION OF THE GREAT ARTERIES

Survival in Infancy

The basic feature of the circulation in complete transposition is the presence of two separate circuits (Fig. 1). With limited mixing between them, the immediate consequence following birth is severe hypoxemia and ensuing metabolic acidosis. About one half of the patients have an intact ventricular septum and in these infants death ensues rapidly. Of the other half, approximately 80 percent have a large VSD and 20 percent have SV; these defects allow bidirectional shunting and mixing of the two blood streams. Naturally occurring atrial septal defects are rare in this condition; the ductus arteriosus is persistent for the first few days in nearly all patients and then it usually closes spontaneously.

Thus, in the presence of VSD or SV, mixing of the pulmonary and systemic circulations results in less severe hypoxia and distress. However, those without pulmonic stenosis develop congestive heart failure early, a result of pulmonary overperfusion and hypoxemia; they also die early.[2] The total mortality figures for all types of complete transposition for the years up to 1965 at the Hospital for Sick Children, Toronto, showed that 50 percent of the infants were dead in one month, 66 percent in three months, and 90 percent in 12 months: only 5 percent survived two years. The survivors are likely to be those who have VSD or single ventricle[3] allowing for mixing, and who have either had pulmonic stenosis of moderate degree from birth, or have rapidly developed progressive pulmonary vascular obstructive disease (the Eisenmenger syndrome).[4] Rarely, an atrial septal defect is the only mixing site; paradoxically, these children with the poorest immediate prognosis have the best long-term outlook if they survive the newborn period.[5]

Survival into Adult Life

The Johns Hopkins Hospital records of patients with complete transposition who survived to 15 years of age without procedural intervention (and are presently being followed in the Adolescent Cardiac Clinic) show that all patients had either a large VSD or SV; approximately one third had pulmonic stenosis and two thirds had high pulmonary vascular resistance.

Shaher[5] found 43 cases in his Hospital for Sick Children series and in the literature who had survived for more than 10 years without surgery. The majority of these had VSD, but 26 percent (the oldest at age 47) had communications at the atrial level only. Complications due to high hematocrit and pulmonary hypertension were frequent, and a common cause of death was severe pulmonary or gastrointestinal bleeding. Cerebrovascular accidents were fairly frequent and there was one case of brain abscess and one of gout. Other late complications include infective endocarditis, atrial and ventricular arrhythmias, paradoxical emboli, and epistaxis. These patients experience the abnormal bleeding,[6] proteinuria,[7] scoliosis,[8] acne, and other skin infections of all patients with cyanosis and polycythemia.

Survival statistics in this condition improved rapidly in the mid-1960s. The low-risk balloon atrial septostomy procedure introduced by William Rashkind[9] superseded Blalock-Hanlon[10] and other surgical septostomy techniques. This greatly improved the outlook for the crucial first month or so of life in patients with an intact ventricular septum. Secondly, a "corrective" surgical procedure was introduced by William Mustard[11] which, by transposing the venous streams with an intra-atrial baffle of pericardium, resulted in "normalization" of the circulation (Fig. 7).

Banding of the pulmonary trunk in the infant with TGA and an associated VSD or SV but no PS may be life saving and retard the rate of development of pulmonary vascular damage. Later, internal repair can be considered after careful laboratory delineation of the anatomy. In the infants with PS and VSD or SV considerable reduction in cyanosis and increase in exercise tolerance can be expected if a systemic to pulmonary artery anatomosis is created, but the operative risk is higher and long-term results are not as good as they are in patients with typical tetralogy of Fallot.[12] Later, "corrective" surgery for this complex combination of heart abnormalities can be successful.[13]

Thus, there are three groups of patients with complete transposition now surviving into adult life: one with a "natural" history—the unoperated patient who has had reasonable mixing and either pulmonic stenosis or an Eisenmenger reaction; a second group with an "unnatural history, i.e., palliative surgery; and a third group, the survivors of "corrective" surgery. Each group will present with its own distinctive set of problems.

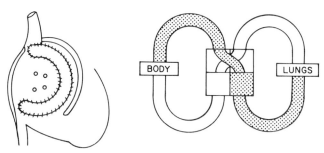

Figure 7. Artist's conception of the Mustard surgical procedure to correct the blood flow in a patient with complete TGA.

Natural History of Complete Transposition:
Clinical Picture and Patient Management

Transposition of the Great Arteries with Intact Ventricular Septum

For the reasons outlined above, survival to adult life of patients with this isolated situation is rare. There are no adult patients in this clinic with this isolated disorder, nor were there any in the review by Shaher.[5]

Occasionally a patient will be seen who has survived naturally with an atrial septal defect. These patients are usually deeply cyanosed with marked clubbing and limitation on exertion. Heart failure is not frequent. On examination there is usually a parasternal heave, a loud S_1 and single S_2. A soft ejection systolic murmur is frequent. The chest roentgenogram shows an enlarged heart with a narrow pedicle and increased pulmonary vascular markings. The electrocardiogram will show right ventricular hypertrophy; the echocardiogram usually shows a large right ventricle and an anterior great vessel which is to the right of the posterior one. At cardiac catheterization the usual diagnostic features of complete transposition are present; a left-to-right and right-to-left shunt is demonstrated at the atrial level and the catheter passes easily from the right atrium to the left atrium. In the majority of these rare cases the pulmonary vascular resistance has remained low so that such patients are ideal candidates for correction using the Mustard procedure.

Transposition of the Great Arteries with VSD or SV Without PS

Some patients with this combination will survive to adulthood, though pulmonary vascular changes develop more rapidly and are more severe than those seen in patients with large VSD and normally positioned great vessels. Adult patients with TGA and a large VSD are severely limited with little exercise ability; both weakness and breathlessness result from exertion and there is marked cyanosis and clubbing. The hematocrit is usually about 60 percent and may rise as high as 90 percent if excessive fluid loss occurs, as with febrile or diarrheal illnesses. Skin complications include acne, petechiae, purpura, and ulcerations. Spontaneous thrombosis in the venous system may cause serious and fatal complications. Prominent A waves are commonly seen in the jugular pulse and peripheral edema does occur. The precordium is active with heaves parasternally and at the apex; a presystolic heave is often present. The fourth sound is audible and the second sound loud and single. A systolic murmur may be present but is not impressive. A murmur of pulmonic valve regurgitation may develop; this murmur may be decrescendo but is likely to be plateau-shaped, harsh, and easily mistaken for a systolic murmur. The course is slowly progressive with decreasing exercise tolerance and more and more complications, i.e., hemoptysis, vascular thrombosis, infections, arrhythmias, and eventually systemic congestion. The oldest patient in this clinic with this disorder is now 35 years old. His hematocrit has been as high as 85 percent but has been maintained at about 60 percent by repeated phlebotomies. He feels considerably better when the hematocrit is between 55 and 60 percent than when it is between 65 and 70 percent, and presumably this also reduces the risk of systemic and pulmonary intravascular thrombosis. He has had episodes of acute gout involving the great toe and elbow joints with uric acid levels as high as 17 mg. percent; the uric acid has been maintained at normal levels with the use of allopurinol. He has been hospitalized on several occasions because of bloody diarrhea. Hemoptysis occurs frequently, but has never been of large quantities. His chest X-ray and ECG are shown in Figures 3 and 8, respectively.

It is most unusual for patients with this disorder to survive to age 40. Treatment is

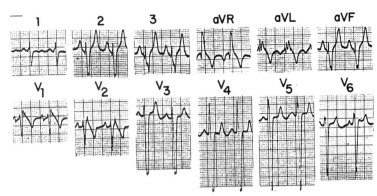

Figure 8. The ECG of an adult with complete TGA, large VSD, and markedly elevated pulmonary vascular resistance.

largely limited to management of complications. In patients in whom the hematocrit rises to about 60 percent, improvement in exercise tolerance and sense of well-being is observed following phlebotomy. Hemoptysis, common in older patients with pulmonary hypertension, can be suppressed by phlebotomy if the hematocrit is elevated. Phlebotomy may have to be repeated periodically to maintain a hematocrit below 60 percent. Iron medication should not be given; an iron-depleted state is purposefully maintained.

Paradoxically, if the hematocrit drops too low—into the low 40s—from excessive phlebotomies or other blood loss, the patient's symptoms may be severely worsened because of the relative anemia. It will then be necessary to give these patients iron temporarily.

Total surgical repair of these defects is extremely hazardous in the adult, although palliation may be helpful. Lindesmith and colleagues[14] have proposed a "palliative Mustard procedure" for these patients. In this procedure the intra-atrial baffle is placed to redirect the venous returns to the opposite ventricles, but the VSD is untouched. Results so far[15] are encouraging, with reported improvement in oxygen saturation, hemoglobin, and hematocrit. The Mayo Clinic group[16] has reported that the improvement seems to be more than would be expected from mere switching of the aortic and pulmonary artery oxygen saturations and conversion of the patient from a transposition Eisenmenger into a straightforward Eisenmenger situation. It is hoped that the advance of progressive pulmonary vascular disease might be slower in these postoperative cases.

Transposition of the Great Arteries with VSD and PS

The degree of anatomical obstruction to pulmonary blood flow determines the hemodynamic and, thus, the clinical patterns in this combination.

Mild Pulmonic Stenosis. Patients with this disorder behave similarly to those with transposition and VSD without pulmonic stenosis. The systolic murmur may be loud, but it is usually not long.

Moderate Pulmonic Stenosis. These patients are slightly cyanotic and clubbed, but function well during childhood without symptoms. Clinical examination reveals a loud, long systolic murmur, loudest along the sternal border but very widely transmitted. The second sound may be single or split and a loud ejection click is common. There is arterial desaturation but the hematocrit is usually in the 50s. The ECG shows signs of right ventricular hypertrophy. On the chest roentgenogram the pulmonary vessels appear normal or slightly increased. At catheterization there is a pressure gradient between the ventricles and the pulmonary trunk and the pulmonary blood flow exceeds the systemic flow.

Unfortunately, the pulmonary vascular resistance may increase slowly in these patients. This is accompanied by the development of easy fatigue and decreased exercise tolerance. There are no marked changes in the ECG, but left ventricular forces may appear.[17] As this process continues the patient may develop all of the complications of longstanding pulmonary hypertension. An 18-year-old patient in our clinic has exhibited this course; the results of cardiac catheterizations in 1963 and 1971 are shown in Table 1. Internal repair of the VSD and relief of the pulmonic sternosis before the development of elevated pulmonary vascular resistence would have provided improvement in symptoms and life expectancy.

SEVERE PULMONIC STENOSIS. These patients have severe cyanosis and clubbing and are small in stature; they often exhibit kyphoscoliosis and usually have symptoms of easy fatigue and dyspnea on exertion. The systolic murmur is loud and long and the second sound is usually single and loud. On chest x-ray there is usually a concavity in the area of the proximal pulmonary artery and normal or diminished peripheral pulmonary vasculature.

The hematocrit is usually in the 60s. Normal or low pulmonary artery pressure is found beyond valvular and/or subvalvular stenosis. Most patients with this combination of disorders have undergone some type of operative procedure before reaching adulthood. The occasional adult without previous cardiovascular surgery is usually disabled enough to mandate the consideration of operative intervention. An operation to totally "correct" the hemodynamics is preferable, but benefit is obtained from operations designed to increase the pulmonary blood flow by the creation of a shunt from the systemic to the pulmonary circulation. The Blalock-Taussig operation is much preferred to the Waterston or Potts operations.[18]

Correction is probably best obtained by the Rastelli procedure.[13] In this technique the VSD is baffled to the aorta, and the pulmonary trunk is ligated and divided. The distal pulmonary trunk is then connected to the anterior aspect of the right ventricle via a valved conduit.

PULMONIC ATRESIA. Patients with this combination of defects are severely disabled and rarely survive to adulthood. Those who do survive have evidence of significant anatomical communications between the aorta and the pulmonary arteries—either a persistent ductus arteriosus or prominent bronchial collateral arteries. Cyanosis, acne, retarded growth, and skeletal abnormalities are present. One or more continuous murmurs are present depending on the location of the aortic-pulmonic connections. The second sound is loud and single and there may be an ejection click. Precordial activity is usually quiet, though a parasternal heave may be present. The chest x-ray shows a small heart, absence of proximal pulmonary artery prominence, and, not uncommonly, a distinct reticular pattern indicative of bronchial vasculature.[19] The pulmonary artery

Table 1. Progressive pulmonary vascular resistance in an 18 year-old patient with TGA and PS

		RA	RV	AO	LV	PA	Hematocrit (%)
1963	Pressure (mm.Hg)		98/0	96/72	104/0-10	36/22 (32)	57
	Oxygen Saturation (%)	64	84	82	98	93	
1971	Pressure (mm.Hg)	11*	115/0-12	115/75 (93)	115/0-12	75/45 (56)	57
	Oxygen Saturation (%)	46	76	77	80	84	

*Mean pressure

RA = right atrium; RV = right ventricle; AO = aorta; LV = left ventricle; PA = pulmonary artery pressure cannot ordinarily be measured unless a ductus arteriosus is present, in which case the pressure is usually low. Angiography may demonstrate the pulmonary vasculature; the pulmonary arteries are usually very small. "Corrective" operative repair is hazardous if the pulmonary arteries are small; a systemic to pulmonary shunt may result in enlargement of the pulmonary arteries and allow "corrective" surgery at a later date.[20]

"Unnatural" History of Complete Transposition: Clinical Picture and Patient Management

Palliative Procedures

ATRIAL SEPTOSTOMY. For a child with TGA and an intact ventricular septum to survive, adequate mixing at the atrial level is essential. Prior to 1967 the surgical procedures used most frequently to achieve this were the Blalock-Hanlon technique,[10] in which a large portion of the atrial septum is excised from behind, and the Edwards procedure,[21,22] in which the atrial septum is shifted leftward so that the right pulmonary veins drain into the right atrium. Since 1967 transvenous balloon atrial septostomy has virtually replaced the operative procedures for the emergency management of these patients. Patients who have undergone these procedures frequently have good mixing, resulting in systemic arterial oxygen saturations between 70 and 80 percent. They show few physical signs apart from the chronic cyanosis, a soft ejection systolic murmur, and a single second heart sound. The chest x-ray shows the mild cardiomegaly and the narrow pedicle, with moderately increased pulmonary vascularity. These patients usually remain markedly limited and are liable to all of the complications of a chronic right-to-left shunt. Management of these patients is by a Mustard repair.

PULMONARY ARTERY BANDING. If the patient had TGA with VSD, as well as atrial septostomy, pulmonary artery banding was commonly added.[23] If the band is tight enough, pulmonary blood flow will fall and the clinical picture is that of TGA with VSD and pulmonic stenosis. Cyanosis is prominent, and a long, harsh ejection murmur is heard with a single second sound. The chest x-ray shows an enlarged heart with diminished lung vascularity and the electrocardiogram often shows combined ventricular hypertrophy. These patients are also candidates for surgical correction, though at considerable risk.

PARTIAL REPAIR. The most commonly used partial repair palliation for TGA was that described by Baffes.[24] In this procedure the right pulmonary veins were transferred to the right atrium, and the inferior vena cava was routed to the left atrium. These patients have improved mixing and better arterial oxygen saturation. The physical signs will depend on whether they have an additional VSD or not. If there is no VSD, then surgical management is by completion of the intra-atrial correction. If there is VSD, the Eisenmenger reaction will have developed[25] and a palliative Mustard procedure might be of value.

SYSTEMIC-PULMONARY ANASTOMOSES. As mentioned above, some of the patients with TGA, VSD, and PS may in fact be limited by their pulmonary oligemia if the PS is severe. In these cases systemic-pulmonary anastomoses have been valuable, the most commonly used being the Blalock-Taussig shunt. These patients will feature the continuous murmur of their shunt and may do well for many years.

A recent review by Taussig[12] showed that a high percentage of patients (85 percent) lived into their second decade of life after being palliated by this shunt; one third of them were still alive 20 years after the operation and some of these were in their 30s and 40s. Some died at repeat surgery, and other, sometimes fatal, complications included heart failure, infective endocarditis, brain abscess, renal failure, arrhythmias, and pulmonary vascular disease. Medical management of these patients will be dictated by the depth of cyanosis, the presence or absence of heart failure, and other complications. Consideration of corrective surgery should be based on anatomical considerations and the presence or absence of pulmonary vascular disease.

Corrective Procedures

THE MUSTARD REPAIR. In 1964 Mustard[11] introduced his technique of intra-atrial repair using a pericardial baffle; it has been widely and successfully used ever since. Both the early and long-term results have been encouraging.[11,26] The most immediate observation is the return of oxygen saturation to normal. There are occasionally residual baffle leaks but these have generally been small.[27] Other more serious complications include arrhythmias, baffle obstruction, pulmonary vascular disease, and decreased right ventricular contractility. The incidence of these problems may increase as these patients reach adulthood.

Arrhythmias. Considering the extent of the intra-atrial surgery, it is not surprising that supraventricular arrhythmias are fairly common. The excision of the atrial septum destroys two of the internodal tracts[28] and the stitching of the intra-atrial baffle comes perilously close to not only to the atrioventricular node but the sinoatrial node and the sinus node artery as well. Damage to these structures may result in AV block and/or the "sick sinus" syndrome.[29] In the Toronto series,[23] 26 percent of 102 long-term survivors had major dysrhythmias, mostly of the supraventricular tachy-brady dysrhythmia type. The incidence varies, however, and in the Auckland series[30] 40 of 46 patients had sinus rhythm at late followup. In the series from Houston[31] the frequency of late dysrhythmias was about 98 percent and increased with time. Major arrhythmias are probably the most common cause of both sudden death and late morbidity. Evidence from Baltimore and elsewhere[29,30,32,33] has implicated structural damage to the sinus node as the chief cause of these tachy-brady dysrhythmias. Only time will tell whether further modification of the surgical placement of the cannulae and sutures for the baffle will reduce the incidence, or whether these arrhythmias are inevitable long-term consequences of late changes in the baffle.

Episodes of paroxysmal junctional and atrial tachycardia can best be treated with propranolol. If atrial flutter or fibrillation has been established, digoxin with or without the addition of propranolol will best control the ventricular rate. Bradycardia at an inadequate rate, either transient or persistent, will require a permanent pacemaker.

Baffle Obstruction. Either primary misplacement of the baffle or secondary changes in it can result in obstruction of either the systemic or pulmonary veins. Caval obstruction is usually mild, but can be severe. Superior vena caval obstruction may present with facial swelling, edema, and distension of the upper extremity veins. These signs may improve as collateral channels in the azygos and other venous systems develop and expand. Inferior caval obstruction is rarer, and will present as ascites, liver distension, and lower limb edema. Caval obstruction has been linked in some centers to the knitted Dacron used to construct the baffle;[34,35] in severe cases operative refashioning of the baffle may be required.[36]

Pulmonary venous obstruction has been attributed by Mustard[35] to redundancy of the baffle in its mid-portion so that it adheres to itself and creates a narrow opening between the pulmonary vein area and the tricuspid valve area. In the early postoperative period this causes pulmonary edema and is clearly identifiable. Later on, however, its onset is slow and insidious and pulmonary artery hypertension will ensue. This can be suspected when the patient becomes breathless on exertion, or goes into heart failure with pulmonary and systemic venous congestion. The chest x-ray may show large distended pulmonary arteries and veins, and the electrocardiogram, increased left ventricular forces. Again, the treatment of this is surgical and requires removal of the baffle and its replacement.

Pulmonary Vascular Disease. As previously mentioned, pulmonary vascular disease (Eisenmenger reaction) occurs early in patients with complete transposition, and is almost universally present in patients with VSD. However, it has also been reported in patients with an intact septum,[37] and it has been known to progress following successful Mustard repair.[38-40] Again, the signs and symptoms are those of pulmonary hypertension. Congestive heart failure will develop, at which time digitalis and diuretics may help. There is no long-term solution to this problem, and the patient will continue on a downhill course.

Right Ventricular Dysfunction. There is reason for continuing concern for the function of the systemic right ventricle in patients who have had a surgical correction of complete transposition with an intra-atrial baffle. One worry has been whether tricuspid regurgitation would be a problem.[41] However, it has been shown recently that this is most often related to instances where the valve has been damaged at the time of VSD repair.[42,43]

As Rushmer[44] has pointed out, the right ventricle is, by virtue of its design and bellows-like action, suited to low-pressure, large-volume work, while the design of the left ventricle is more suited to a "pressure-pump" function. The question then is whether this bellows-like right ventricle can function as the systemic ventricle over a prolonged period of time.

Initially the good clinical results were encouraging with regard to ventricular function, and contractility indices suggested that in a good proportion of cases the right ventricle of transposition patients was functioning like a normal left ventricle.[42] However, volume data have consistently shown larger right ventricular end-diastolic volumes and smaller ejection functions in transposition patients.[45,46]

Graham[47] recently carried out volume and contractility index studies on the same patients and confirmed that the contractility indices were normal despite poor volume data. Therefore, the conclusion is uncertain and the concern remains. Only the passage of time will tell how these right ventricles will stand up to the continued systemic load as the patients advance into adult life.

ARTERY-SWITCHING TECHNIQUE. The concern with the long-term results of the Mustard procedure[11] has prompted a new look at the previously abandoned artery-switching technique. Using new aortocoronary bypass graft techniques, it has been possible to overcome the difficulties with myocardial perfusion that were previously encountered, and a small number of patients with both TGA and VSD have been operated on with success.[48-50] The patients are too few, too recent, and too young to establish this as a long-term solution to the problem yet.

RASTELLI PROCEDURE. Surgery for repair of transposition of the great arteries, VSD, and pulmonic stenosis or pulmonary atresia has been the most complicated. In 1969 a new procedure for these patients was described by both Cooley[51] and Rastelli.[13] This procedure involved removing the pulmonary trunk from the left ventricle and placing a baffle from the VSD to the aorta so that the left ventricle ejected exclusively into the aorta. The last step is the placement of a valved conduit from the anterior surface of the right ventricle back to the distal pulmonary arteries. Early experience by the Mayo group[13] using aortic homografts indicated that the immediate results were good, but calcification of the conduit increased with the passage of time in many patients, eventually leading to significant obstructions in the conduit.[52,53] More recently, Dacron conduits with porcine valves have been used with excellent results.[20,54] But again, substantiated followup is still scarce, and it is likely that these tissue valves also will deteriorate with time and have to be replaced as the patients approach adulthood.

376

CORRECTED TRANSPOSITION OF THE GREAT ARTERIES

In contradistinction to complete transposition, survival to adulthood of patients with corrected transposition is likely, and many adults with this condition are asymptomartic. These patients should theoretically be entirely normal, but they have three groups of problems which render them at high risk for disability and premature death.

First, in a series of 101 cases seen at the Hospital for Sick Children, Toronto,[55] a high percentage of patients had either VSD (44 percent) or SV (40 percent). For an unoperated survivor of this group to reach adulthood he would have to have either pulmonic stenosis (53 percent of this same group) or pulmonary vascular disease (Eisenmenger syndrome).

The second problem involves the left-sided atrioventricular valve, which anatomically is the tricuspid valve. This valve is frequently incompetent and often has an Ebstein-type configuration.[56] This produces signs and symptoms of "mitral" regurgitation.

The third difficulty involves atrioventricular conduction. Because of the ventricular inversion the course of the His bundle is abnormal and prolonged in these patients; thus, varying degrees of heart block which often progress to complete heart block are common.

Corrected Transposition with an Intact Ventricular Septum

About half of these patients are recognized during childhood because of the presence of a systolic murmur at the apex of the heart. They are often thought to have mitral regurgitation of other etiologies. These patients and those unrecognized during childhood generally present with symptoms and signs of pulmonary congestion between the third and sixth decades of life. The clinical presentation is so like that of mitral regurgitation that the correct diagnosis is often not identified until angiography, surgery, or necropsy.[57] The simulating features may include heart failure, cardiomegaly, an apical pansystolic murmur, atrial fibrillation, and a history of heart murmur. Angiography usually clarifies the clinical problem if the anterior and leftward position of the aorta is observed. Clues on the routine chest x-ray include an ascending aorta which lies along the left hilum and the absence of a prominent pulmonary conus despite pulmonary congestion. Management aims toward control of the atrial fibrillation, digitalis, and diuretic therapy.

If the patient is significantly symptomatic, surgical repair or replacement of the left atrioventricular valve should be considered, i.e., plastic surgery to the valve or replacement with a prosthetic valve. The latter has proved more successful in our hands because of the frequency of severe valvular malformation and the Ebstein-type displacement of its attachments. Even with successful valve surgery, however, the prognosis is not excellent. The left-sided anatomical right ventricle is pumping against systemic resistance and usually dilates and fails prematurely, despite correction of the valvular regurgitation.

Patients with corrected transposition are also prone to atrioventricular block. This block may begin with prolongation of the P-R interval and progress through second degree block to complete block. These conduction disturbances may play a significant role in the presentation of these patients as adults and may necessitate the insertion of a permanent pacemaker.

The reports of Cumming[38] and Rotem and Hultgren[59] reviewing corrected transposition without associated anomalies, suggest that these patients may have a normal life span with minor impairment of cardiac function. Heart block may occur suddenly after the age of 20, and can be life-threatening; however, pacemakers and valve replacement may improve this outlook. Nagle and coworkers,[60] Dodek,[61] and Selden[62] have reported cases of middle-aged men with angina and congestive heart failure due to this lesion. Benchimol and coworkers[63] suggest that although the oldest known patient was 73 years old,[64] a normal life span is unlikely.

Corrected Transposition with VSD or SV

Here the clinical picture is one of a large left-to-right shunt with pulmonary hyperperfusion present from infancy. These children present in infancy with a murmur indistinguishable from that seen in children with normally positioned great vessels and a large VSD or SV. The abnormal ventricular and great artery relationships become apparent only through catheterization and angiography; then the pulmonary trunk can be noticed in a much more medial location and the ascending aorta is recognized as forming the upper left anterior cardiac border. Treatment of this combination is either pulmonary artery banding, as palliation, or repair of the defect. The latter is a difficult procedure as the access is limited from the right-sided left ventricle, and repair is often associated with the development of complete heart block which requires a permanent pacemaker. The operative mortality rate is probably around 40 percent.[55] When SV is present, palliation by pulmonary artery banding is advisable; at a later date, surgical repair by the insertion of a Dacron ventricular septum is feasible. McGoon and his colleagues[65] report moderately good short-term results in such patients.

Some of these patients will survive "naturally" into adult life and will develop an Eisenmenger reaction. Clinically they will be indistinguishable from patients with Eisenmenger VSD or SV with complete transposition, except for a high incidence of conduction abnormalities and "mitral" incompetence.

Corrected Transposition with VSD or SV and Pulmonic Stenosis

Here the presentation is very similar to patients with normally positioned great vessels or with complete transposition, VSD, and pulmonic stenosis. If the pulmonic stenosis is mild, then the picture is that of a large left-to-right shunt. If it is moderate, the patient may be asymptomatic for many years and not require operative intervention. When the obstruction is severe, cyanosis may be a major problem and may be alleviated by systemic-pulmonary anastomoses. "Corrective" surgery is possible, but would certainly be a high-risk undertaking because of the difficult access to the pulmonic valve and subvalvular region.[55]

SUMMARY

Transposition of the great arteries may be defined as complete or corrected, according to the rotation or looping of the ventricle beneath the transposed great arteries. The clinical presentation, clinical course, and management are, to a large extent, determined by the presence or absence of associated congenital cardiac defects. Complete TGA with an intact ventricular septum is exceedingly rare in adults. Corrected TGA with an intact ventricular septum is compatible with long-term survival, and its clinical course is determined by the presence or absence of left-side atrioventricular valve regurgitation and/or severity of atrioventricular heart block.

Adults with either complete or corrected TGA commonly have a large VSD or SV and develop all of the complications of longstanding pulmonary arterial hypertension. Other adults with TGA and VSD or SV also will have PS and the course will be somewhat like the course of a patient with tetralogy of Fallot.

A wide variety of operative interventions have been used in infants and children with TGA. They fall into two major categories: palliation and "total correction." The palliative procedures are designed to increase mixing of the systemic and pulmonary circulations; pulmonary artery banding, also palliative, is designed to reduce pulmonary artery blood flow. Corrective procedures alter the anatomy so that the flow of blood through the heart is physiologically "correct" and mixing of the two circulations is eliminated. Many of these patients are surviving to adulthood and present a host of new and difficult clinical problems such as arrhythmias and deterioration of graft material.

REFERENCES

1. HENRY, W. L., MARON, B. J., AND GRIFFITH, J. M.: *Cross-sectional echocardiography in the diagnosis of congenital heart disease: identification of the relation of the ventricles and great arteries.* Circulation 56:267,1977.

2. KIDD, B. S. L., TYRELL, M. J., AND PICKERING, D.: *Transposition 1969.* In Kidd, B. S. L., and Keith, J. D. (eds.): *The Natural History and Progress in Treatment of Congenital Heart Defects.* Charles C Thomas, Springfield, Ill., 1971.

3. KIDD, B. S. L.: *The fate of children with transposition of the great arteries following balloon atrial septostomy.* In Kidd, B. S. L., and Rowe, R. D. (eds.): *The Child with Congenital Heart Disease After Surgery.* Futura, New York, 1976.

4. WOOD, P.: *The Eisenmenger syndrome.* Br. Med. J. 2:701,755,1958.

5. SHAHER, R. M.: *Complete Transposition of the Great Arteries.* Academic Press, New York and London, 1973.

6. HARTMANN, R. C.,: *A hemorrhagic disorder occurring in patients with cyanotic congenital heart disease.* Johns Hopkins Med. J. 91:49,1952.

7. SPEAR, G. S.: *Implications of the glomerular lesions of cyanotic congenital heart disease.* J. Chronic Dis. 19:1083,1966.

8. JORDAN, C. W., WHITE, R. I., FISHER, K. C., ET AL.: *Scoliosis of congenital heart disease.* Am. Heart J. 84:463,1972.

9. RASHKIND, W. J., AND MILLER, W. M.: *Creation of an atrial septal defect without thoracotomy. A palliative approach to complete transposition of the great arteries.* JAMA 196:992,1966.

10. BLALOCK, A., AND HANLON, C. R.: *The surgical treatment of complete transposition of the aorta and pulmonary artery.* Surg. Gynecol. Obstet. 90:1,1950.

11. MUSTARD, W. T., KEITH, J. D., TRUSLER, G. A., ET AL.: *The surgical management of transposition of the great vessels.* J. Thorac. Cardiovasc. Surg. 48:953,1964.

12. TAUSSIG, H. B., KEINONEN, R., MOMBERGER, N., ET AL.: *Long-time observations on the Blalock-Taussig operation. VII. Transposition of the great vessels and pulmonary stenosis.* Johns Hopkins Med. J. 135:161,1974.

13. RASTELLI, G. C., McGOON, D. C., AND WALLACE, R. B.: *Anatomic correction of the great arteries with ventricular septal defect and subpulmonary stenosis.* J. Thorac. Cardiovasc. Surg. 58:545,1969.

14. LINDESMITH, G. C., STILES, W. R., TUCKER, B. L., ET AL.: *The Mustard operation as a palliative procedure.* J. Thorac. Cardiovasc. Surg. 63:75,1972.

15. LINDESMITH, G. G., STANTON, R. E., LURIE, P. R., ET AL.: *An assessment of Mustard's operation as a palliative procedure for transposition of the great vessels.* Ann. Thorac. Surg. 19:514,1975.

16. MAIR, D. D., RITTER, D. G., DANIELSON, G. K., ET AL.: *The palliative Mustard operation: rationale and results.* Am. J. Cardiol. 37:762,1976.

17. ELLISON, C., AND RESTIEAUX, N.: *Vectorcardiography in Congenital Heart Disease.* W. B. Saunders, Philadelphia, 1972.

18. SHUMWAY, N. E., GRIEPP, R. B., AND STINSON, E. B.: *Surgical management of transposition of the great arteries.* Am. J. Surg. 130:233,1975.

19. HAROUTUNIAN, L. M., AND NEILL, C. A.: *Pulmonary pseudofibrosis in cyanotic heart disease. A clinical syndrome mimicking tuberculosis in patients with extreme pulmonic stenosis.* Chest 62:587,1972.

20. MARCELLETTI, C., MAIR, D. D., McGOON, D. C., ET AL.: *Complete repair of transposition of the great arteries with pulmonary atresia.* J. Thorac. Cardiovasc. Surg. 72:215,1976.

21. EDWARDS, W. S., BARGERON, L. M., AND LYONS, C.: *Repositioning of right pulmonary veins in transposition of great vessels.* JAMA 188:522,1964.

22. TRUSLER, G., AND KIDD, B. S. L.: *Surgical palliation in complete transposition of the great vessels—experience with the Edwards procedure.* Am. J. Surg. 12:83,1969.

23. TRUSLER, G. A., MULHOLLAND, H. C., TAKEUCHI, Y., ET AL.: *Long term results of intra-arterial repair of transposition of the great arteries.* In Davila, J. C. (ed.): *Second Henry Ford Hospital International Symposium on Cardiac Surgery.* Appleton-Century-Crofts, New York, 1977, p. 368.

24. BAFFES, T. G.: *New method for surgical correction of transposition of aorta and pulmonary artery.* Surg. Gynecol. Obstet. 102:227,1956.

25. PAUL, M. H.: *Transposition of the great arteries: Physiologic data.* In Kidd, B. S. L., and Keith, J. D., (eds.): *The Natural History and Progress in Treatment of Congenital Heart Defects.* Charles C Thomas, Springfield, Ill., 1971.

26. CHAMPSAUR, G. L., SOKOL, D. M., TRUSLER, G. A., ET AL.: *Repair of transposition of the great arteries in 123 pediatric patients.* Circulation 48:1032,1973.

27. KIDD, L., AND MUSTARD, W. T.: *Hemodynamic effects of a totally corrective procedure in transposition of the great vessels.* Circulation 33(Suppl. I):28,1966.

28. JAMES, T. N.: *The connecting pathways between the sinus node and A-V node and the right and left atrium in the human heart.* Am. Heart J. 66:498,1963.

29. VARGHESE, P. J., AND ROLAND, J. M. A.: *Sick sinus syndrome in post-operative children.* In Kidd, B. S. L., and Rowe, R. D. (eds.): *The Child with Congenital Heart Disease After Surgery.* Futura, New York, 1976, p. 233.

30. CLARKSON, P. M., BARRATT-BOYES, B. G., AND NEUTZE, J. M.: *Late dysrhythmias and disturbances of conduction following Mustard operation for complete transposition of the great arteries.* Circulation 53:519,1976.

31. EL-SAID, G., ROSENBERG, H. S., MULLINS, C. S., ET AL.: *Dysrhythmias after Mustard's operation for transposition of the great arteries.* Am. J. Cardiol. 30:526,1972.

32. RODRIQUEZ-FERNANDEZ, H. L., KELLY, D. T., COLLADO, A., ET AL.: *Hemodynamic data and angiographic findings after Mustard repair for complete transposition of the great arteries.* Circulation 46:799,1972.

33. GILLETTE, P. C., EL-SAID, G. M., SIVARAJAN, N., ET AL.: *Electrophysiological abnormalities after Mustard's operation for transposition of the great arteries.* Br. Heart J. 36:186,1974.

34. STARK, J., SINGH, A., LEVAL, M., ET AL.: *Early versus late Mustard operation for "simple" transposition of the great arteries.* In Kidd, B. S. L., and Rowe, R. D. (eds.): *The Child with Congenital Heart Disease After Surgery.* Futura, New York, 1976, p. 187.

35. MUSTARD, W. T.: *Baffle problems in transposition of the great arteries.* In Kidd, B. S. L., and Rowe, R. D. (eds.): *The Child with Congenital Heart Disease After Surgery.* Futura, New York, 1976, p. 195.

36. VENABLES, A. W., EDIS, B., AND CLARKE, C. P.: *Vena caval obstruction complicating the Mustard operation for complete transposition of the great arteries.* Eur. J. Cardiol. 1(4):401,1974.

37. LAKIER, J. B., STANGER, P., HEYMANN, M. A., ET AL.: *Early onset of pulmonary vascular obstruction in patients with aortopulmonary transposition and intact ventricular septum.* Circulation 51:875,1975.

38. MAIR, D. D., DANIELSON, G. K., WALLACE, R. B., ET AL.: *Long term follow-up of Mustard operation survivors.* Circulation 50(Suppl. II):11,1974.

39. ROSENGART, R., FISHBEIN, M., AND EMMANOULILIDES, G. C.: *Progressive pulmonary vascular disease after surgical correction (Mustard procedure) of transposition of great arteries with intact ventricular septum.* Am. J. Cardiol. 35:107,1975.

40. NEWFELD, E. A., PAUL, M. H., MUSTER, A. J., ET AL.: *Pulmonary vascular disease in complete transposition of the great arteries: A study of 200 patients.* Am. J. Cardiol. 34:75,1974.

41. TYNAN, M., ABERDEEN, E., AND STARK.: *Tricuspid incompetence after the Mustard operation for transposition of the great arteries.* Circulation 45:13,1972.

42. GODMAN, M. J., FRIEDLI, B., PASTERNAC, A., ET AL.: *Hemodynamic studies in children four to ten years after the Mustard operation for transposition of the great arteries.* Circulation 53:532,1976.

43. CLARKSON, P. M., NEUTZE, J. M., BARRATT-BOYES, B. G., ET AL.: *Late postoperative hemodynamic results and cine-angiocardiographic findings after Mustard atrial baffle repair for transposition of the great arteries.* Circulation 53:525,1976.

44. RUSHMER, R. F.: *Cardiovascular Dynamics.* W. B. Saunders, Philadelphia, 1970.

45. JARMAKANI, J. M. M., AND CANENT, R. W.: *Pre- and post-operative right ventricular function in children with transposition of the great vessels.* Circulation 48 (Suppl. IV):23,1973.

46. GRAHAM, T. P., JR., ATWOOD, G. P., BOUCEK, R. J., ET AL.: *Right heart volume characteristics in transposition of the great arteries.* Circulation 51:881,1975.

47. GRAHAM, T. P., ATWOOD, G. F., BOUCEK, R. J., ET AL.: *Transposition of the great arteries—right and left*

ventricular function problems. In Kidd, B. S. L., and Rowe, R. D. (eds.): *The Child with Congenital Heart Disease After Surgery.* Futura, New York, 1976, p. 207.

48. JATENE, A. D., FONTES, V. F., PAULISTA, P. P., ET AL.: *Successful anatomic correction of transposition of the great vessels. A preliminary report.* Arq. Bras. Cardiol. 28:461,1975.

49. ROSS, D., RICKARDS, A., AND SOMMERVILLE, J.: *Transposition of the great arteries: logical anatomical arterial correction.* Br. Med. J. 1:1109,1976.

50. YACOUB, M. H., RADLEY-SMITH, R., AND HILTON, C. J.: *Anatomical correction of complete transposition of the great arteries and ventricular septal defect in infancy.* Br. Med. J. 1:1112,1976.

51. COOLEY, D. A., AND HALLMAN, G. L.: *Surgical Treatment of Congenital Heart Disease.* Lea & Febiger, Philadelphia, 1966.

52. McGOON, D. C., WALLACE, R. B., AND DANIELSON, G. K.: *The Rastelli operation. Its indications and results.* J. Thorac. Cardiovasc. Surg. 65:65,1973.

53. SOMERVILLE, J.: *Homograft reconstruction of the right ventricular outflow tract–pulmonary atresia extreme tetralogy of Fallot–Late results.* In Davila, J. C. (ed.): *2nd Henry Ford Hospital International Symposium on Cardiac Surgery.* Appleton-Century-Crofts, New York, 1977.

54. SAKAKIBARA, S., IMAI, Y., IMAMURA, E., ET AL.: *Rastelli operation employing composite graft of porcine pulmonary valve and vascular prosthesis.* In Davila, J. C. (ed.): *2nd Henry Ford International Symposium on Cardiac Surgery.* Appleton-Century-Crofts, New York, 1977.

55. BJARKE, B. B., AND KIDD, B. S. L.: *Congenitally corrected transposition of the great arteries. A clinical study of 101 cases.* Acta Paediatr. Scand. 65:153,1976.

56. SCHIEBLER, G. L., EDWARDS, J. E., BURCHELL, H. B., ET AL.: *Congenital corrected transposition of the great vessels.* Pediatrics 27:851,1961.

57. ROBERTS, W. C., ROSS, R. S., AND DAVIS, F. W., JR.: *Congenital corrected transposition of the great vessels in adulthood simulating rheumatic valvular disease.* Johns Hopkins Med. J. 114:157,1964.

58. CUMMING, G. R.: *Congenital corrected transposition of the great vessels without associated intracardiac anomalies. A clinical hemodynamic and angiographic study.* Am. J. Cardiol. 10:605,1962.

59. ROTEM, C. E., AND HULTGREN, H. N.: *Corrected transposition of the great vessels without associated defects.* Am. Heart J. 70:305,1965.

60. NAGLE, J. P., CHEITLIN, M. D., AND McCARTY, R. J.: *Corrected transposition of the great vessels without associated anomalies: report of a case with congestive failure at 45.* Chest 60:367,1971.

61. DODEK, T. P. AND NEILL, W. A.: *Corrected transposition of the great arteries masquerading as coronary artery disease.* Am. J. Cardiol. 30:910,1972.

62. SELDEN, R., SCHAEFER, R. A., KENNEDY, B. J., ET AL.: *Corrected transposition of the great arteries simulating coronary heart disease in adults.* Chest 69:188,1976.

63. BENCHIMOL, A., TIO, S., AND SUNDARARAJAN, V.: *Congenital corrected transposition of the great vessels in a 58-year-old man.* Chest 59:634,1971.

64. LIEBERSON, A. D., SCHUMACKER, R., AND CHILDRESS, D.: *Corrected transposition of the great vessels in a 73 year old man.* Circulation 39:96,1969.

65. McGOON, D. C., MARCELLATTI, C., DANIELSON, G. K., ET AL.: *The problem of correcting single and common ventricle.* Circulation 54, 54 Suppl. II):101,1976.

Complex Cyanotic Congenital Heart Disease in Adults

Thomas P. Graham, Jr., M.D. and
Gottlieb C. Friesinger, M.D.

Cyanotic congenital heart disease in adults is rare. Table 1 lists the large number of cyanotic congenital lesions which may be encountered in adults and divides lesions into those associated with decreased pulmonary blood flow (a consequence of pulmonary stenosis or pulmonary atresia) and those having increased pulmonary vascular resistance. The more common causes of cyanotic congenital heart disease in the adult have been discussed in the chapters on the Eisenmenger complex and tetralogy of Fallot. Transposition of the great vessels, a rare cause of cyanosis in the adult, has also been

Table 1. Cyanotic congenital heart disease encountered in adults

I. Lesions Relatively Frequently Encountered
    A.   Reduced pulmonary blood flow
           1. Tetralogy of Fallot (PS with VSD)
           2. Pulmonary atresia with VSD
           3. Pulmonary stenosis with atrial right-to-left shunt
    B.   Increased pulmonary vascular resistance
           1. VSD with Eisenmenger reaction
           2. Patent ductus arteriosus with Eisenmenger reaction
           3. ASD with Eisenmenger reaction
II. Lesions Less Frequently Encountered
    A.   Reduced pulmonary blood flow
           1. Single ventricle with pulmonary stenosis or atresia
           2. Tricuspid atresia with pulmonary stenosis, atresia, or small VSD
           3. Transposition with pulmonary stenosis or atresia
    B.   Increased pulmonary vascular resistance
           1. Single ventricle with Eisenmenger reaction
           2. Transposition with Eisenmenger reaction
           3. Truncus arteriosus
    C.   Ebstein's anomaly with atrial right-to-left shunt
III. Lesions Rarely Encountered
    A.   Double outlet right ventricle with or without pulmonary stenosis
    B.   Congenital pulmonary arteriovenous fistula
    C.   Congenital vena caval to left atrial communication
    D.   Mitral atresia
    E.   Double outlet left ventricle
    F.   Asplenia or polysplenia syndromes
    G.   Total anomalous pulmonary venous return

discussed elsewhere in this monograph. It should be emphasized that the lesions being considered in this chapter are so rare that they may never be seen by a cardiologist; they are included to indicate the range of possibilities which should be considered in the adult who presents with cyanotic congenital heart disease. Because of their rarity and the fact that pathognomonic signs are not apt to be present, an elaborate differential diagnosis is not presented here.

We shall consider *single ventricle, tricuspid atresia, Ebstein's anomaly,* and *truncus arteriosus* in some detail and comment briefly on several other entities. All lesions considered in this chapter are extremely rare at birth and the severity of each malformation makes survival to adult life unlikely unless some operative procedure is undertaken. The increasing use of operative procedures in patients with these malformations, however, means that occasionally such patients will be seen as adults in a cardiologic practice.

SINGLE OR COMMON VENTRICLE

For purposes of this review, the terms single and common ventricle will be used interchangeably and are indicative of the condition in which one ventricular chamber receives both the tricuspid and mitral valves. The majority of patients with single ventricle die in infancy or early childhood unless palliative surgery is performed, but at least 33 patients over age 15 with this condition have been reported.[1-3] The increasing success with palliation and repair of this abnormality has increased the probability that the physician dealing with heart disease may encounter such a patient.

Patients with single ventricle can be divided into two basic anatomic types: those with an outlet chamber giving rise to one great vessel and those with no outlet chamber.

The absence of pulmonic stenosis leads to excessive pulmonary blood flow with resulting congestive heart failure, poor weight gain, and (frequently) death in infancy or early childhood, unless vigorous anticongestive measures are effective. Some patients develop elevated pulmonary vascular resistance, experience an improvement in the symptoms of congestive heart failure, and show only moderate limitation of physical activity until pulmonary blood flow is diminished to the degree that cyanosis, polycythemia, and other complications associated with the Eisenmenger reaction appear. Figure 1 is a schematic illustration of a single ventricle with an outlet chamber. This is the most common type of single ventricle—approximately 80 percent of patients with single ventricle will have an outlet chamber.[4,5] This outlet chamber probably represents embryologically the conus cordis which normally forms the infundibulum or outflow tract of the right ventricle. This condition has been called *double inlet left ventricle,* indicating that both mitral and tricuspid valves enter the "left ventricle" and there is failure of formation of the body of the right ventricle. Among patients with single ventricle, approximately 85 percent have transposed great vessels, half being *d*-transposition (aorta anterior and to the right of the pulmonary artery) and half being *l*-transposition[4] (Fig. 1). The small number of patients without transposition (15 percent of those with an outlet chamber) have a "Holmes heart," a malformation described by W. F. Holmes in 1824.[6]

In our review of 33 reported patients who reached the age of 15 or older, the oldest was 56 years old. Of those in whom the information was available, 67 percent had transposition of the great arteries and a differentiation between a *d*- or *l*-transposition was not possible from the majority of reports. Of these adult patients, 42 percent had pulmonic stenosis and 80 percent of them had an outlet chamber. These findings are similar to data reported previously in patients of all ages with single ventricle.[4,5]

384

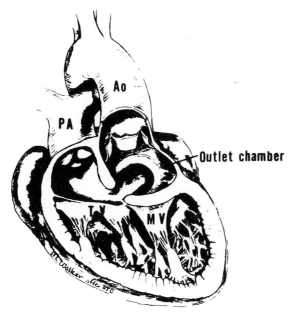

Figure 1. Schematic representation of single ventricle associated with an outlet chamber and *l*-transposition of the great arteries.

Clinical Presentation

The clinical presentation in a patient with single ventricle is primarily dependent on the presence or absence of pulmonic stenosis. Patients with pulmonic stenosis will have a prominent systolic murmur from early infancy with obvious cyanosis. With severe pulmonic stenosis, cyanosis is marked and the patient may succumb in infancy to problems associated with hypoxemia. With a moderate degree of pulmonic stenosis patients may have only moderate limitation of physical activity.

Physical Examination

All adults with single (common) ventricle will show varying degrees of cyanosis, although in a rare patient with a moderate degree of pulmonic stenosis systemic desaturation can be inconspicuous. In patients with significant pulmonic stenosis, a parasternal life will be present. The first heart sound is usually normal and the second sound is single and sometimes obscured by the murmur. The majority of patients will have transposition of the great vessels and when the aorta is in the *l* position, a palpable loud single sound will be felt and heard at the upper left sternal border. The murmur of pulmonic stenosis will usually be maximal in the second and third left interspace. In patients with *l*-transposition, the murmur may be present maximally at the upper right sternal border.

It is rare to have a pulmonary ejection click because the pulmonic stenosis is most frequently subvalvular. With increasing severity of pulmonic stenosis, the murmur can become softer because less blood is ejected through the valve to the lungs. The bronchial collateral circulation in these instances will increase and, rarely, continuous murmurs will be heard posteriorly over the chest.

In patients without pulmonic stenosis the first heart sound is usually normal or accentuated, and the second heart sound is markedly increased and usually single. A

385

pulmonary ejection sound may be heard at the upper left sternal border and, occasionally, at the upper right sternal border in patients with *l*-transposition of the great arteries. The murmur of pulmonic regurgitation may be present in patients with severe elevation of pulmonary vascular resistance. A prominent systolic murmur over the pulmonic valve area is rare.

These patients also can have subaortic stenosis. The subaortic gradient is usually at the site where the common ventricle enters the rudimentary outflow chamber. These murmurs are heard best along the left sternal border and may radiate to the lower left sternal border. With excessive pulmonary blood flow, a short, rumbling, mid-diastolic mitral murmur may be present, often introduced by a loud third heart sound.

Chest X-ray

The chest x-ray will usually show moderate-to-severe cardiac enlargement when pulmonic stenosis is absent. With severe pulmonic stenosis cardiac enlargement is only mild-to-moderate. The vascular pedicle often is quite narrow as a result of transposed great vessels. The upper left border may show a prominent convexity in patients with an outlet chamber in the inverted position and *l*-transposition of the great arteries.

Figure 2 is the chest x-ray of a 35-year-old man with single ventricle, *d*-transposition of the great vessels, and pulmonary hypertension. There was no gradient across the pulmonic valve, and he had profound polycythemia, cyanosis, and clubbing. At age 25 typical gout appeared, but it has been well controlled by allopurinol. In adult patients with extreme polycythemia, gout is common since increased bone-marrow activity results in high uric acid.

Figure 3 is the chest x-ray of a 27-year-old man with single ventricle, *d*-transposition of the great vessels, and pulmonic stenosis. Note the difference in the heart size and shape and the pulmonary vasculature as compared to Figure 2. Polycythemia, cyanosis, and clubbing were marked and transient cerebral ischemic attacks had occurred. Phlebotomy with volume replacement by plasma or plasmanate has been used for several years to reduce blood viscosity.

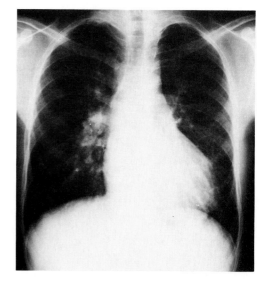

Figure 2. Chest x-ray of a 35-year-old man with single ventricle, *d*-transposition of the great vessels, pulmonary hypertension and increased pulmonary vascular resistance. At catheterization, no gradient was present across the pulmonic valve. The heart is enlarged (C/T ratio, 0.57), the central vessels are prominent, and the distal pulmonary arteries are small.

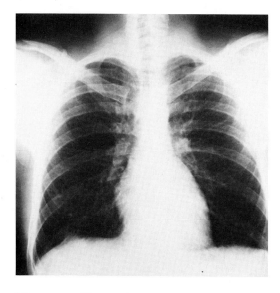

Figure 3. Chest x-ray of a 27-year-old man with single ventricle, *d*-transposition of the great vessels and pulmonary stenosis. Note the difference in the heart size and shape and the pulmonary vasculature as compared to Figure 2. The heart is normal in size (C/T ratio, 0.43), the main pulmonary artery segment is inconspicuous, and the peripheral pulmonary arteries are not enlarged. The pulmonary artery pressure was moderately elevated (systolic, 50 mm. Hg) possibly because of vascular disease resulting from longstanding polycythemia.

Electrocardiography

Sinus rhythm ordinarily is present, and in patients with longstanding pulmonic stenosis or elevated pulmonary vascular resistance right atrial enlargement is a common electrocardiographic finding.[3,7-9] The presence of first-degree heart block should indicate that ventricular inversion of the outlet chamber with *l*-transposition of the great arteries is likely. These patients can progress to complete heart block. In patients with ventricular inversion and *l*-transposition, there is usually an abnormal initial QRS vector producing abnormal Q waves in the right precordial leads with a qR pattern frequently present in V_4R and V_1. These patients may have a superior axis in the frontal plane. The electrocardiogram will frequently mimic the findings of patients with congenitally corrected transposition of the great vessels. Patients with *d*-transposition of the great vessels will frequently have a normal axis or superior axis in the frontal plane and absence of Q waves in the precordial electrocardiographic leads. Similarly, patients with single ventricle and normally related vessels frequently have a normal QRS axis in the frontal plane and stereotype Rs or rS across the precordial leads, again without Q waves. It is apparent that the electrocardiographic findings are extremely variable in the single ventricle with "left" ventricular hypertrophy, "right" ventricular hypertrophy, absent right heart forces, and the precordial stereotype Rs or rS patterns seen in various anatomic types.

Figure 4 is the electrocardiogram from a 35-year-old patient whose chest x-ray is shown in Figure 2. The stereotype rS pattern across the precordium is most striking.

Figure 5 is the electrocardiogram from the 25-year-old patient whose chest x-ray is shown in Figure 3. Despite severe right axis deviation, the r/s ratio in V_1 is not increased, indicating a discordance between the rightward frontal plane axis and the lack of signs of severe right ventricular hypertrophy in V_1. Such discordance should lead one to consider the diagnosis of single ventricle.

Echocardiography

Standard M mode echocardiography has been used to aid in the diagnosis of single ventricle.[10,11] The simultaneous recording of both mitral and tricuspid valves without an intervening septal echo is excellent presumptive evidence of single ventricle. In patients

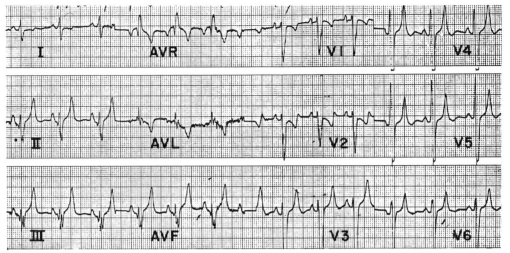

Figure 4. Electrocardiogram from the 35-year-old patient whose chest x-ray is shown in Figure 2. The tracing shows right atrial hypertrophy, small right heart forces, and an rS pattern across the precordium without q waves.

with an outlet chamber, a small ridge of "septum" may be visualized together with a small anterior chamber which does not contain an atrioventricular valve. Patients with a common AV valve and single ventricle are quite difficult to distinguish from patients with mitral or tricuspid atresia and a large ventricular chamber. In addition, patients with congenitally corrected transposition and ventricular septal defect are difficult to distinguish by echocardiography from patients with single ventricle because the ventricular septum may be virtually perpendicular to the standard echo beam positions in corrected transposition making delineation difficult. Contrast echocardiography can improve the diagnostic accuracy for single ventricle.[12]

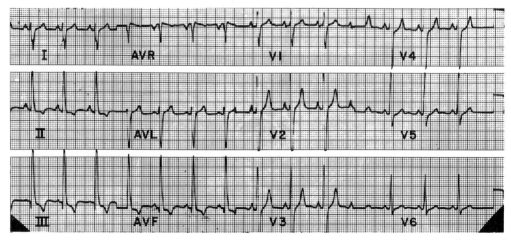

Figure 5. Standard 12-lead electrocardiogram from the 27-year-old patient whose chest x-ray is shown in Figure 3. Right atrial hypertrophy and profound right axis deviation are seen. There is a 7.5 mm. R wave in V_1 with a 15 mm. S wave.

Therapeutic Principles

Medical care consists of anticongestive therapy for patients with increased pulmonary blood flow causing high output failure. This problem exists primarily in infants and young children in whom banding of the pulmonary trunk may be required for control of heart failure. Patients with the Eisenmenger reaction should have regular followup care, with attention given to the complications of polycythemia and elevated pulmonary resistance as outlined elsewhere in this monograph.

Patients with pulmonic stenosis and severe limitation of pulmonary blood flow usually can benefit from systemic-to-pulmonary shunt procedures. Indications for operation include effort intolerance and severe polycythemia (usually with a hematocrit > 65 percent). The procedure of choice is a Blalock-Taussig (subclavian-to-pulmonary artery) shunt. The risk of operation is probably less than 5 percent in most centers which perform the procedure regularly. Complete catheterization information is required before the shunt is performed, i.e., angiographic and/or pressure data substantiating pulmonic stenosis, pressure data regarding the presence or absence of subaortic stenosis, angiographic definition of the pulmonary arteries, and exclusion by angiography (or echocardiography) of any left-sided obstructive lesion such as mitral stenosis, mitral atresia, pulmonary-vein stenosis, or cor triatriatum. Such lesions can be clinically occult when pulmonary flow is low, but will cause intractable pulmonary edema immediately following a shunt procedure. Finally, the aortic arch and vessels should be visualized angiographically and an aberrant, retroesophageal subclavian artery must be ruled out before operation since this vessel is difficult to use for the shunt. Details of the shunt construction are of great importance in these patients and operations should be performed only by surgeons and centers with extensive experience in the operative treatment of congenital heart disease.

In contrast to the shunting (palliative) operations, successful reparative operations employing septation of the univentricular heart have been reported by a number of groups and recently summarized by McGoon and coworkers.[13] These surgeons reported on 35 patients with single ventricle. The average age of their patients was 13, but several adults (including one 36-year-old patient) were included. The operative mortality was high (approximately 50 percent) with additional small numbers of patients having severe chronic heart failure postoperatively. Improvements in patient selection and operative technique will undoubtedly result in an improved outcome for a larger number of patients in the future. Currently many important questions remain unanswered about reparative operations for this complex congenital abnormality, but the data reported thus far encourages development of improved surgical approaches.

TRICUSPID ATRESIA

Most patients with tricuspid atresia will die in infancy or childhood unless operative intervention is successful, but unoperated adults have been reported, including one 57-year-old patient.[14] The increasing success of operative palliation or "repair" of tricuspid atresia ensures that the management of the adult patient with this condition will soon be an important problem.

Tricuspid atresia has been classified into eight basic categories by Keith, Rowe, and Vlad[15] based on the associated lesions shown in Table 2. Patients with associated pulmonic atresia (Types IA and IIA) do not survive infancy unless they have an operative shunt or a persistent patent ductus. Patients with pulmonic stenosis (Types IB, IIB, IIIA) account for approximately 70 percent of all patients with tricuspid atresia and virtually all adults with this condition.[14] Patients with Type IC usually have congestive heart failure early in infancy but develop cyanosis which increases as the VSD (fre-

Table 2. Tricuspid atresia classification (percentages refer to all cases, the majority of whom are first seen in childhood and infancy)

Type I.	Normally Related Great Arteries (69%)
	A. Pulmonary atresia*
	B. Pulmonary stenosis and VSD*
	C. Large VSD; no pulmonary stenosis*
Type II.	*D*-Transposition of the Great Arteries (27%)
	A. Pulmonary atresia*
	B. Pulmonary stenosis and VSD*
	C. Large VSD; no pulmonary stenosis
Type III.	*L*-Transposition of the Great Arteries (3%)
	A. Pulmonary stenosis
	B. Subaortic stenosis

*These types are most frequently encountered. Virtually all adults with tricuspid atresia who have not had palliative operations have types IB, IIB, or IIIA.

quently located in the muscular septum) gets smaller, sometimes closing spontaneously. These patients then require operative intervention in order to reach adult life.

Clinical Presentation

Adults with unoperated tricuspid atresia give a history of cyanosis since early infancy. The degree of cyanosis is variable and depends on the adequacy of pulmonary blood flow. Growth and development may be mildly retarded if cyanosis is severe. Impaired effort tolerance is the most prominent symptom and, again, usually is directly related to the degree of cyanosis. Sudden deterioration may follow the onset of an atrial dysrhythmia, usually atrial fibrillation.

Physical Examination

Central cyanosis and digital clubbing are prominent features. Peripheral pulses usually are normal. Precordial palpation reveals an increased left ventricular apical impulse without a significant parasternal right ventricular impulse. The left ventricular impulse is directly related to pulmonary flow and can be normal with markedly decreased pulmonary perfusion.

The first heart sound is single and frequently loud. The second sound usually is single also because of the frequent occurrence of significant pulmonic stenosis with an inaudible or very soft pulmonary component. A systolic murmur of pulmonic stenosis usually is present. The intensity and duration of this murmur varies directly with the degree of pulmonary flow: the louder the murmur, the more blood is being ejected into the lungs. The pulmonic stenosis is usually subvalvular and a pulmonary ejection sound is rare.

When the great arteries are not transposed, a long, harsh, systolic murmur can be generated at the site of accompanying VSD which is generally in the muscular septum and small to moderate in size. With transposition of the great arteries the VSD usually is large, and ejection from left ventricle through VSD and out the aorta is associated with a variable systolic murmur—harsh and pansystolic if the defect is significantly less than aortic orifice size; short and of medium frequency when the VSD is equal to or larger than the aortic valve orifice. Rarely, a murmur of mitral regurgitation can develop with the onset of left heart failure.[3]

Chest X-ray

The most frequently occurring type of tricuspid atresia seen in adults is associated with pulmonic stenosis and normally related great arteries. The contour of the heart in the posteroanterior view reveals a concavity of the pulmonary trunk and slight prominence of the right atrium. The overall heart size and pulmonary vascularity vary with the degree of pulmonic stenosis; with markedly decreased pulmonary flow the heart is small and the lung fields oligemic. The left anterior oblique view frequently has a distinctive "humped" appearance (prominent superior margin with flat receding inferior margin) because of right atrial enlargement in the absence of a right ventricle.[3] Left atrial enlargement is almost always present; the degree of enlargement varies directly with the amount of pulmonary blood flow. With transposition of the great arteries the pulmonary trunk is usually quite concave with a narrow vascular pedicle.

Figure 6 is the chest x-ray of a 22-year-old man with tricuspid atresia who had a Potts procedure done at age 5 which resulted in an excessive increase in pulmonary blood flow and volume overload of the left ventricle. The left ventricular configuration of the heart and markedly increased pulmonary blood flow is easily appreciated in this x-ray. A second operative procedure was performed at age 22 and reduction of the size of the Potts anastomosis was accomplished.

Electrocardiography

The ECG frequently provides the diagnosis in patients with tricuspid atresia. Right atrial enlargement is nearly always present, with P waves $\geq$ 2.5 mm. and peaked in leads 2 and V_1 through V_3. Left atrial enlargement can also be apparent, with broad, notched P waves in 1, 2, aVF, V_2 through V_4 and a prominent negative component in V_4R and V_1. The PR interval is normal or short. The frontal QRS axis is virtually always superior and to the left. Rarely, an adult patient with a more adequate right ventricle will have an axis between 0 and 90 degrees or, occasionally, to the right. The right precordial leads usually show small r and deep S waves with the left precordial leads showing tall R waves indicative of left ventricular hypertrophy. Leads V_5 and V_6 frequently show flat or inverted T waves, suggesting a left ventricular strain pattern.

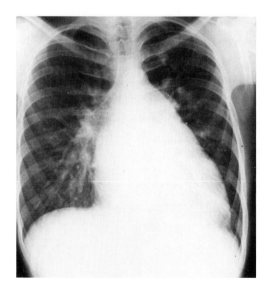

Figure 6. Chest x-ray of a 22-year-old man with tricuspid atresia who had a Potts procedure done at age 5 which resulted in excessively increased pulmonary blood flow and volume overload to the left ventricle. Heart size is markedly increased (C/T ratio, 0.61), and the pulmonary vascularity is exceedingly prominent.

391

Echocardiography

The M mode echo can be useful in patients with suspected tricuspid atresia since a tricuspid valve echo cannot be obtained. This "negative" information is most helpful in children in whom the tricuspid valve echo can virtually always be obtained when this valve is present. Obtaining a reliable echo from the tricuspid valve in adults is far more difficult. The echo is also useful for quantitation of left atrial size and left ventricular size and function. Cross-sectional echo should provide useful information in diagnosis of this condition as well as in delineating the size of the right ventricle and the presence and severity of pulmonic stenosis, but these applications have not been substantiated to date.

Cardiac Catheterization

Cardiac catheterization is indicated to diagnose the condition correctly, determine the presence of associated defects, assess the severity of pulmonic stenosis if present, evaluate pulmonary vascular resistance, evaluate the size of the atrial septal defect, and evaluate left ventricular function.

The catheter will usually pass readily across the atrial defect into the left atrium and left ventricle. A pullback pressure tracing from left to right atrium provides data regarding size of the atrial defect. In some patients the VSD can be crossed with a floating balloon catheter to obtain right ventricular and pulmonary artery pressures. In patients with surgical shunts (aorta-to-pulmonary artery) a retrograde study with pulmonary artery pressure, obtained by passing the catheter from the aorta, may be possible. Ideally, pressures and oxygen data in pulmonary artery, aorta, pulmonary vein, both atria, and both cava should be obtained for pressure and resistance calculations. This is frequently impossible and angiographic data must be used to provide inferential information regarding pulmonary flow and resistance.

A right atrial angiogram is necessary to establish the diagnosis. Contrast material flows readily from right atrium to left atrium to left ventricle. In patients with severe tricuspid stenosis or pulmonary atresia with intact ventricular septum and very small right ventricle, a similar right atrial angiogram can be seen but these conditions seldom are encountered in adults.

The most useful angiogram is obtained by a left ventricular injection with the patient in a tilted left anterior oblique position as described by Bargeron.[16] This will delineate VSD size, right ventricular size, and degree of pulmonic stenosis. Figure 7 is a cineangiographic frame from a patient with tricuspid atresia, VSD, pulmonic stenosis, and normally related great vessels. A left ventricular angiogram also can be used for volume calculations to provide data on left ventricular size, function, and output. La Corte and coworkers[17] reported left ventricular volume data which indicated a significant incidence of left ventricular dysfunction in patients with tricuspid atresia and longstanding volume overload. We have similar data from our laboratory[18] and believe that the cyanosis contributes to the hemodynamic alterations. Myocardial hypoxia and resultant altered function might result from periods of high myocardial oxygen demand (increased wall tension, tachycardia) and limited supply (decreased arterial oxygen content, tachycardia, increased wall tension) during periods of stress.

Clinical Course and Operative Treatment

The clinical course of older patients with tricuspid atresia is determined primarily by the adequacy of pulmonary blood flow. Unoperated adults virtually never have excessive pulmonary flow and resultant high output congestive failure as can be seen in

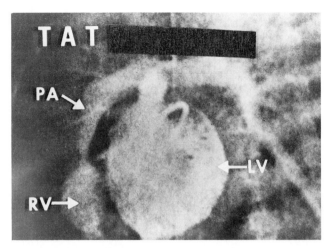

Figure 7. Cineangiogram frame from a patient with tricuspid atresia and normally related great vessels. The injection was into the left ventricle which is large. There is filling of a small right ventricle through multiple ventricular defects. Subvalvular pulmonic stenosis is present.

infants. Patients with adequate pulmonary flow often have minimal symptoms or none at all while at rest. Dick and coworkers[19] reported the clinical courses of 101 patients with tricuspid atresia who were followed at Boston Children's Hospital. Survival was manifested by three distinct phases. Phase I included a mortality of 40 percent during the first year of life. This figure could probably be lowered considerably with current improvements in operative management. Phase II was a prolonged stable phase lasting for approximately 15 years experienced by 50 percent of all patients. Phase III, which began around the middle of the second decade, was a gradual attrition attributed to congestive heart failure. The three oldest patients in this series (which included patients seen at Children's Hospital from 1941 to 1973) were in their thirties.

In 1975 Kyger and coworkers[20] reported on surgical palliation of 105 patients with tricuspid atresia and decreased pulmonary flow who were seen at the Texas Heart Institute between 1953 and 1973. Operative shunts included the Potts anastomosis, Blalock-Taussig shunt, aorta-to-right-pulmonary-artery shunt, and Glenn procedure. Overall, early operative mortality was 9 percent. Patients undergoing operations more than 15 years before the report had a 45 percent (9/20) survival. Taussig and coworkers[21] reported a similar 20-year survival of 42 percent (18/43) in patients with a Blalock-Taussig shunt.

Williams and coworkers[22] reported their management of 160 patients with tricuspid atresia who were seen at the Hospital for Sick Children in Toronto between 1947 and 1974. Mortality from a shunt procedure in 52 patients older than 6 months of age at the time of the procedure was 13 percent. Seven years after a shunt procedure, 91 percent of the patients were alive with 25 percent asymptomatic and 65 percent having only mild limitation of exercise tolerance. Seven years postoperatively, 25 percent of patients with a Potts shunt, 19 percent of patients with a Glenn shunt, and 50 percent of patients with a Blalock-Taussig shunt required an additional procedure because the shunt no longer provided adequate pulmonary flow. Of 31 repeat shunt procedures there was only 1 death (3 percent mortality).

In 1971 Fontan and Baudet[23] presented data on an entirely new approach to the operative treatment of tricuspid atresia. The superior vena cava was anastomosed to the distal end of the transected right main pulmonary artery, the right atrium was anastomosed to the proximal end of the right main pulmonary artery with an interposed aortic homograft, the atrial septal defect was closed, a homograft valve was inserted into the inferior vena cava, and the pulmonary trunk was ligated. This operation was performed in three patients and resulted in perfusion of the right lung by the superior vena cava with left lung blood flow pumped by the right atrium. The patients' ages were 12, 36, and 23 years. Two patients survived with no postoperative resting cyanosis.

Subsequent experience with this operation by six different groups was recently summarized by Kreutzer.[24] At the time of his report (June 1975), 35 operations of the Fontan type had been performed with 10 hospital deaths and 2 late deaths (34 percent mortality). Henry and coworkers[25] reported an important modification of the technique in which the homograft or valved conduit is anastomosed to the right ventricular outflow tract and the atrial and ventricular defects are closed as depicted (Fig. 8). Many centers have adopted this modification when the right ventricular and pulmonary artery anatomy are favorable and have reported improved results, particularly in terms of a decreased incidence of postoperative right heart failure. Whether or not a superior-vena-cava-to-right-main-pulmonary-artery anastomosis should be combined with this operation for optimal results is still unclear. In addition, the question of the need for homograft or prosthetic inferior vena caval valve insertion remains unanswered. Many patients have a fairly well developed Eustachian or inferior vena caval valve of their own and clearly do not need a valve inserted.

From the aforementioned data, it is clear that operative management of tricuspid atresia is in a state of change. Infants who require an operation for cyanosis need a shunt procedure since the Fontan operation does not appear to be a reasonable alternative until about 5 years of age. Unfortunately, some patients with a shunt procedure will develop an elevated pulmonary vascular resistance which makes them poor candidates for any additional surgery, including the Fontan operation. The older patient who requires an operation and has a fair-sized right ventricle, a relatively normal pulmonic valve, normal pulmonary vascular resistance, reasonably-sized pulmonary arteries, and sinus rhythm is a good candidate for the Fontan-type procedure with the atrium anastomosed to the right ventricular outflow tract (Fig. 8). But only occasionally will an adult fall into this category. Proponents of the shunt operation for the older patient would argue that very good results are obtained with shunts in older patients, and it is

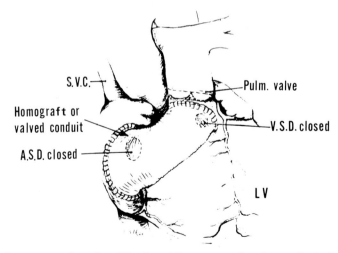

Figure 8. Schematic representation of modification of Fontan procedure for repair of tricuspid atresia. Right atrium is anastomosed to right ventricular outflow tract using a homograft or valved conduit. Ventricular and atrial defects are closed. Right atrium and small right ventricle "in series" pump blood to the lungs.

still unclear whether patients with the Fontan operation will either outlive or have less morbidity than shunted patients. It will require a number of years and careful followup studies to determine the "best" operation for an individual patient.

It is important to recognize, however, that these patients can lead active, productive lives, and medical as well as surgical management should be pursued vigorously. The outlook for the patient with tricuspid atresia has improved greatly over the last 10 years as a result of shunt procedures, and it is hoped that the Fontan-type operation will add a new dimension to the long-term outlook for patients with this malformation.

EBSTEIN'S ANOMALY

Ebstein's anomaly, like the other entities discussed in this chapter, is rarely seen in adults, but Wilhelm Ebstein's first clinical and anatomical description[26] was of a 19-year-old boy with pulmonary tuberculosis who had shortness of breath and palpitations since childhood. He had the ausculatory findings regularly associated with Ebstein's anomaly as well as advanced right heart failure. At necropsy the tricuspid valve was markedly abnormal with valvular tissue attached partially to the tricuspid anulus and adherent to the right ventricular myocardium; thus, the attachment was displaced distally down into the cavity of the right ventricle. The foramen ovale was patent and the right heart chambers were dilated. This is the basic malformation in Ebstein's anomaly—a downward displacement of the origin of the tricuspid valve into the right ventricle. The anterior cusp is the least affected and usually is quite large. The downward displacement of the valve origin results in a division of the right ventricle into a proximal "atrialized" portion which has an atrial pressure and, usually, a thinned-out wall, and a distal portion which in severe cases is only the outflow tract of the right ventricle. Netter's drawing[27] of this anomaly is extremely useful for visualizing the actual anatomical abnormalities.

The hemodynamic abnormalities which can result are tricuspid regurgitation, akinesis or dyskinesis of the atrialized part of the right ventricle, and a decrease in filling of the small distal right ventricular chamber. A patent foramen ovale or a true atrial septal defect is present in approximately 50 percent of patients, with right-to-left atrial shunting occurring in most patients.[28–30]

The severity of the anatomic and the resultant hemodynamic abnormalities is extremely variable and ranges from a normal-sized heart and minimal tricuspid regurgitation to severe cardiomegaly, massive tricuspid regurgitation, and large right-to-left atrial shunt. Survival to age 79 as well as death in infancy have been reported; these variations are summarized by Perloff.[3]

Clinical Presentation

Patients with relatively severe abnormalities of the tricuspid valve usually have significant cyanosis as neonates: high pulmonary vascular resistance increases the severity of tricuspid regurgitation, right atrial dilatation and increased pressure occur, and atrial right-to-left shunting ensues. With the normal fall in pulmonary resistance the forward output of the right ventricle increases and tricuspid regurgitation and cyanosis decrease. Clinical improvement in this situation is marked, and these patients can then be relatively asymptomatic for many years.

Adults with symptoms generally report effort intolerance and dyspnea. Palpitations and definite episodes of tachycardia are common and may be associated with Type B Wolff-Parkinson-White pre-excitation. Chest pain has been reported[31,32] and is usually related to effort or exposure to cold. It can resemble pericardial pain or be "anginal-like," but the cause has not been determined.

Physical Examination

Patients with a mild anomaly usually are acyanotic and have abnormalities of the first heart sound, audible third and/or fourth heart sounds, and a systolic murmur of mild tricuspid regurgitation.[33] Because this review is concerned mainly with cyanotic adults, physical findings in the mild cases will not be discussed in detail. However, adults with mild degrees of Ebstein's anomaly will not be cyanotic and only come to the physician's attention because of abnormal physical findings, electrocardiographic abnormalities, or palpitations and arrhythmias.

The frequency of cyanosis in adults with Ebstein's anomaly has been estimated to be as high as 80 percent[3] and as low as 15 percent.[34] This variation undoubtedly is attributable to differences in the severity of the abnormality among different series. All degrees of cyanosis exist, with more severe cyanosis usually occurring with the more severe degrees of tricuspid regurgitation.

The peripheral pulses are usually normal or slightly diminished in patients with low output heart failure. Despite significant tricuspid regurgitation, jugular venous pulsations are rarely strikingly abnormal, probably because of the damping effect of a large right atrium.[3,35]

Precordial activity is usually inconspicuous, but a rippling or undulating motion occasionally seen over the mid to left lower sternal border during held expiration can be quite helpful in diagnosis.[3,32,35] It probably represents abnormal systolic motion of the "atrialized" portion of the right ventricle. A systolic thrill is occasionally palpated between the left sternal border and apex.

Auscultation is most helpful. The first heart sound is abnormal with a loud second component of S_1 which is delayed and can resemble a pulmonary ejection sound.[3,31-33,34-37] It is probably caused by the abrupt cessation of motion of the large sail-like anterior tricuspid leaflet as it reaches the limit of its systolic excursion, and has been designated the sail sound.[37] The second sound may be prominently split, but in cases with severely decreased pulmonary flow the pulmonary component may be inaudible and S_2 will be single. Both S_3 and S_4 are frequently present and can produce triple or quadruple rhythms.

The systolic murmur of tricuspid regurgitation varies from a soft, scratchy, short, and superficial-sounding murmur to a pansystolic murmur with a thrill. The murmur is frequently heard best toward the apex over the displaced tricuspid valve and can be mistaken for mitral regurgitation. The murmur has often been mistaken for a pericardial rub. An inspiratory increase in the intensity of the murmur can help to differentiate the source, but this sign is not always present and is apt to be absent in more severe cases in which the small distal right ventricular chamber cannot increase its stroke volume with inspiration.[3]

Chest X-ray

The typical chest x-ray in a symptomatic patient consists of a "balloon-shaped," enlarged heart with a narrow vascular pedicle suggesting pericardial effusion. The right atrium is usually quite prominent and can be massively enlarged, virtually filling the major part of the right chest. The pulmonary vascularity correlates with atrial right-to-left shunting; in cyanotic patients pulmonary flow is diminished and the lung fields are oligemic.

Figure 9 is the chest x-ray of a 28-year-old woman. The cardiac silhouette is typical of Ebstein's anomaly. Fatigue was a prominent symptom and diabetes mellitus was present. The electrocardiogram showed right bundle branch block and left axis deviation and typical auscultatory findings of Ebstein's anomaly were present. At catheterization

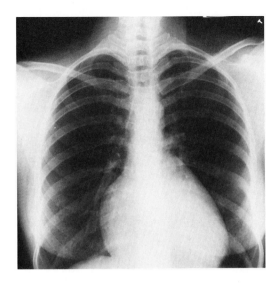

Figure 9. Chest x-ray of a 28-year-old woman. The cardiac silhouette is typical for that seen in Ebstein's anomaly. The heart is enlarged (C/T ratio, 0.61) with the right atrium quite prominent. The pulmonary vascularity is normal.

pressures were normal and no shunts were present. The displacement of the tricuspid valve was demonstrated by simultaneous pressure and intracardiac electrocardiographic studies as well as angiography.

Electrocardiography

The rhythm is usually sinus. The PR interval frequently is prolonged in patients without the Wolff-Parkinson-White (WPW) syndrome.[29] The P waves usually demonstrate right atrial enlargement: peaked, amplitude $\geq$ 2.5 mm. in 2, aVF, V_1 through V_3. The QRS usually is also distinctive with a right bundle branch pattern of a "splintered" V_4R and V_1 consisting of rsR' or rsR'S' complexes with the R' voltage usually relatively low. Prolongation of the QRS to a mild degree is frequently present, probably as a result of depolarization over the abnormal atrialized portion of the right ventricle.

Type B WPW pre-excitation of the right ventricle occurs in as many as 25 percent of patients.[29] The pattern has been described as intermittent. The anatomic correlate of this pattern undoubtedly is myocardial tissue "bridging" the atrioventricular ring in the region of the atrialized portion of the right ventricle. These patients are most prone to paroxysmal supraventricular tachycardias—a rhythm disorder that occurred in 30 of 65 (46 percent) patients reported by Bialostozky and coworkers.[29]

Echocardiography

M mode echocardiography usually shows a prominent, easily recorded, tricuspid valve echo with increased amplitude of excursion which can be recorded further to the left than normal. Tricuspid valve closure is usually delayed, with the difference between q wave to mitral valve closure and q wave to tricuspid valve closure being greater than 65 msec. in most patients with Ebstein's anomaly; it is virtually never this high in any other known condition. Type B WPW pre-excitation does not appear to influence this delayed closure significantly.[38,39] Septal motion can be normal, flat or paradoxical. Thus, the echocardiogram can be extremely useful in substantiating the diagnosis of Ebstein's anomaly.

Cardiac Catheterization

Cardiac catheterization will frequently be needed to firmly establish the diagnosis. The clinical, electrocardiographic, radiographic, and echocardiographic findings are often so characteristic, however, that the diagnosis is virtually certain before catheterization. An increased risk of catheterization has been suggested from early reports of intracardiac investigation. Watson[30] reported 13 deaths (3.6 percent) and 6 cardiac arrests (1.7 percent) successfully resuscitated in a retrospective cooperative study of 363 cardiac catheterizations from 57 centers around the world. Paroxysmal dysrhythmias were reported during 100 (28 percent) of these 363 studies. The only predisposing factor to distinguish patients at greatest risk for dysrhythmia was a large heart since the incidence of pre-excitation and history of previous dysrhythmias were similar in patients with and without this complication.

It is our opinion that the current risk of cardiac arrest and/or death during cardiac catheterization is considerably less than 5 percent for patients with Ebstein's anomaly. There were no deaths among 49 patients with Ebstein's anomaly catheterized as part of the cooperative study published in 1968,[40] and Nadas and Fyler[41] report no deaths in 33 patients studied at their institution since 1955. It is imperative, however, that preparations be made to treat promptly any dysrhythmia which occurs during catheterization. These studies should be undertaken only at institutions which deal with significant numbers of patients with congenital heart problems.

The principal reasons for catheterization are to substantiate the diagnosis, quantify right-to-left shunting, estimate the degree of tricuspid regurgitation, estimate the size of the atrialized and distal right ventricular cavities, measure cardiac output, and identify any associated anomalies.

The methods for substantiating the diagnosis are the intracardiac electrogram and angiography. In most patients a simultaneous intracardiac electrogram and pressure recording obtained from the atrialized portion of the right ventricle will show an atrial pressure and a ventricular electrogram. This combination theoretically is diagnostic of Ebstein's anomaly and should be sought by a careful, slow pullback of the electrode catheter from right ventricle to right atrium. Lowe and Watson[35] have emphasized that this finding should be considered only as confirmatory of the diagnosis since false-negatives and positives have been reported.

Angiocardiography will substantiate the diagnosis in virtually all patients with Ebstein's anomaly. Frequently, a single injection into the distal right ventricular chamber will reveal the following characteristic findings in the frontal view: tricuspid regurgitation and two notches on the diaphragmatic border of the right heart—one representing the displaced or false anulus and the other the true anulus. The "atrialized" portion of the right ventricle lies between these two notches (Fig. 10). The size of the distal and proximal right ventricular cavities, the degree of paradoxical motion of the "atrialized" chamber, and the degree of tricuspid regurgitation usually can be determined best with cineangiocardiography. The position of the right coronary artery when visualized in the frontal view can be used to locate the right atrioventricular groove and thus the approximate position of the true tricuspid valve ring.

Clinical Course and Operative Treatment

As might be expected from the anatomic variations of this lesion, there are considerable differences in clinical course. Bialostozky and coworkers[29] reported on all 65 patients followed at the National Cardiology Institute in Mexico and reported only 5 patients (7.7 percent) over 30 years of age. In an international cooperative study of 505 cases of Ebstein's anomaly, Watson[30] found only 67 patients (13 percent) over 25 years of

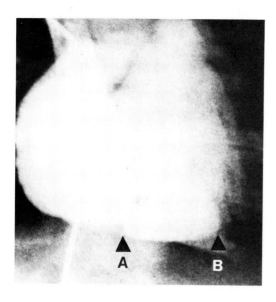

Figure 10. Right atrial angiocardiogram of a patient with Ebstein's anomaly. A, The site of the true tricuspid anulus. B, The displaced false anulus. Simultaneous electrocardiographic and pressure recording from a catheter positioned between A and B showed an atrial pressure curve and a ventricular electrogram.

age. Thus, the majority of patients do not live to adulthood. Known causes of death other than operative include congestive heart failure and sudden death, presumably from a dysrhythmia. A previous history of dysrhythmia or a pre-excitation pattern do not necessarily predispose to sudden death.[30] Extreme cardiomegaly can be an unfavorable prognostic sign but exceptions to this correlation are common. The onset of progressive clinical symptoms of exercise intolerance, heart failure, and cyanosis are indications that operative intervention should be considered.

Two basic operative approaches have been used recently in this condition: replacement of the tricuspid valve[42] and annuloplasty associated with plication of the atrialized segment to obliterate the akinetic or dyskinetic abnormality of this chamber.[43] Tricuspid valve replacement alone has not been satisfactory in most centers.[30] McFaul and coworkers[44] recently reported a 100 percent survival rate in 8 patients with plication, annuloplasty, and resection of redundant right atrial free wall. These same authors had only 1 of 5 patients survive valve replacement. Thus, optimal operative therapy for these patients is still evolving at present and may have to be individualized for each patient because of the anatomic variability of the lesion.

Patients with uncontrolled dysrhythmia and type B WPW pre-excitation are candidates for intracardiac mapping and division of the anomalous pathway,[44,45] but these procedures rarely will be required.

TRUNCUS ARTERIOSUS

Truncus arteriosus is a condition in which one great artery arises from the heart above a large ventricular septal defect. Both the coronary arteries and the pulmonary arteries arise from this great vessel. The 1949 classification of truncus by Collett and Edwards[46] remains useful, but minor changes in it seem appropriate because of the large surgical experience with this lesion since its original classification. Type I truncus remains as originally described—a single pulmonary trunk arises from the ascending aorta and it branches into right and left main pulmonary arteries. The length of the pulmonary trunk is usually short and can be virtually an aorticopulmonary window. Types II and III have been classified together now as Type II and consist of the pulmonary arteries arising separately from the posterolateral aspect of the ascending aortic trunk.[47] Type IV of Collett and Edwards now is considered to be a form of pulmonary atresia with no pulmonary arteries arising from the aorta. Associated anomalies or variations include hemitruncus (one pulmonary artery arising from the ascending aorta and one from the right ventricle), interrupted aortic arch, truncal valve regurgitation, atrial septal defect, single ventricle, common atrioventricular valve, and right aortic arch.

The majority of patients with this lesion die in infancy or early childhood. Survival to adulthood is rare and, when encountered, is virtually always associated with severe elevation of pulmonary vascular resistance or some type of surgical intervention.

Clinical Presentation

Patients have a history of cyanosis and dyspnea on exertion from infancy or early childhood. If pulmonary vascular resistance falls to normal or near normal levels in the first few weeks of life, severe congestive heart failure develops. Those patients who survive infancy usually do so because of increased pulmonary vascular resistance. These patients can have a relatively stable condition with only cyanosis and dyspnea on exertion for a number of years. Their clinical course will be similar to that described in the chapter on Eisenmenger's syndrome.

Physical Examination

Adolescents and adults show cyanosis of varying degrees, digital clubbing, and, usually, prominence of the anterior left chest. Pulses can be accentuated from the pulmonary "runoff" in patients without severe pulmonary vascular disease or the frequently associated truncal valve regurgitation.

In older patients precordial activity is dominated by the right ventricle with a parasternal life, but an accentuated left ventricular apical impulse also can be present. S_1 is normal or slightly accentuated. A truncal ejection click is frequently present; it is usually constant and heard well at the apex and left sternal border. S_2 is usually palpable, loud, and single. A split S_2 is rare but has been recorded,[48,49] and is probably a result of asynchronous closure of abnormal truncal valve leaflets of which there may be from two to six. Prominent, harsh systolic murmurs which are crescendo-decrescendo and end before S_2 are common. These murmurs are probably caused by turbulence from the truncal orifice (due to the abnormal truncal valves), from the pulmonary artery origins, or from tricuspid regurgitation. The systolic murmur frequently transmits well to the upper right sternal border.[3]

A diastolic decrescendo murmur beginning shortly after S_2 usually indicates truncal valve regurgitation in the adolescent or adult. When pulmonary flow is markedly increased—as occurs in younger children—a virtually continuous murmur with its origin in the pulmonary arteries can be heard and the diagnosis of truncal regurgitation is difficult on clinical grounds.

Chest X-ray

The chest x-ray usually shows cardiac enlargement, a concave pulmonary trunk, and an uplifted apex. The pulmonary vessels are prominent and the right main pulmonary artery is located more superiorly than normal. A right aortic arch is present in approximately 25 percent of patients.

Electrocardiography

The ECG usually shows sinus rhythm, right atrial enlargement, and right ventricular hypertrophy. Left ventricular hypertrophy is also present in younger patients with increased pulmonary flow and in patients with truncal regurgitation.

Echocardiography

M mode echocardiography is useful in showing that the aorta overrides the ventricular septum. The only other condition which consistently is associated with this finding is tetralogy of Fallot. Enlargement of the right ventricle, the aortic root, and, frequently, the left ventricle can be quantitated. Truncal valve regurgitation will usually be associated with mitral valve flutter.

Cardiac Catheterization

To substantiate the diagnosis, right ventricular and aortic angiocardiography are necessary. Aorticopulmonary window can usually be differentiated by the absence of VSD and clear delineation of pulmonary and aortic valves.

Pulmonary vascular resistance must be estimated if an operation is to be considered. Both pressure and oxygen saturations must be obtained in both pulmonary arteries, truncus, pulmonary veins (or wedge), as well as mixed venous samples. The main pulmonary arteries frequently can be entered with balloon-tipped catheters from the venous side. If this approach is not successful, retrograde catheterization of the pulmonary arteries should be attempted. Flows are estimated using the Fick principle and Rp estimated in units M^2 by dividing (PAP-LAP or pulmonary wedge) by (Qp/B.S.A.) where PAP = pulmonary artery pressure, LAP = left atrial pressure, Qp = pulmonary flow from a Fick determination, and B.S.A. = body surface area. Two articles by the Mayo Clinic group are especially helpful regarding these calculations in patients with truncus arteriosus and including those patients with only one pulmonary artery or previous pulmonary artery banding.[50,51] Since systemic oxygen saturation is directly related to Qp, patients with two pulmonary arteries, no pulmonary stenosis, and an oxygen saturation < 85 percent are probably inoperable because of pulmonary vascular obstructive disease. This finding usually correlates with an Rp value > 12 units M^2.

Truncal regurgitation is assessed by a truncal root angiogram. Patients with severe truncal regurgitation, if operated upon, will require valve replacement; this has been associated with an increased mortality.[50]

Clinical Course and Operative Treatment

A successful operation to repair truncus arteriosus by McGoon, Rastelli, and Ongley in 1968[52] radically changed the outlook for many patients with this disease. The operation usually is referred to as the Rastelli procedure and consists of detachment of the pulmonary artery or arteries from the truncus, making an "aortic" closure of the VSD so that the left ventricle pumps blood into the aorta, and establishing continuity from right ventricle to pulmonary arteries with an aortic homograft or valved conduit (Fig. 11). Griepp and coworkers[53] recently reviewed the overall mortality rate for this operation in patients reported since 1968 and found it to be 30 percent. The Mayo Clinic group reported only a 9 percent mortality for older children operated on since 1972.[51]

The natural history of this lesion indicates that unless operation is undertaken in infancy or childhood, the majority of patients will die from congestive heart failure or will have such severe pulmonary vascular disease as to be inoperable.[54] In 1976 Marcel-

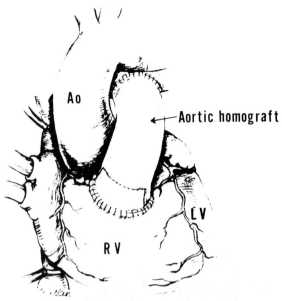

Figure 11. Schematic representation of Rastelli repair of truncus arteriosus. The ventricular septal defect is closed so that the left ventricular output is out the aorta (truncus). The pulmonary arteries are detached from the truncus and continuity with the right ventricle established using a homograft or valved conduit.

letti and coworkers[54] reported the followup status of 23 unoperated patients originally referred to Mayo Clinic between 1957 and 1967. All 10 patients referred as infants with congestive heart failure have died. Of the remaining 13 patients, referred originally at ages 2 to 16 years, 4 died—2 in congestive heart failure at ages 11 and 18 years and 2 suddenly at ages 15 and 24 years. The remaining 9 patients ranged in age from 11 to 26 years at the time of the report and all but one were symptomatic (Class II or III). The oldest surviving patients reported died at ages 35,[55] 36,[56] and 43.[57] All died with signs of chronic passive congestion, undoubtedly a result of right heart failure. Lung pathology was available in only one case and was consistent with pulmonary vascular obstructive disease.[57] Right and left ventricular hypertrophy were present in all three patients, and scattered myocardial fibrosis was commented upon in two of the three patients.[56,57]

It is clear, therefore, that the majority of patients presenting to the adult cardiologist will be those who have had previous operative procedures. The following case report illustrates the type of patient who will be seen and some of the possible problems which may be encountered.

Case Report

This 18-year-old boy has been followed at Vanderbilt University since infancy with initial symptoms of congestive heart failure. Initial cardiac catheterization revealed Type I truncus arteriosus, and he underwent bilateral pulmonary artery banding. At age 14 he underwent repair with a Hancock conduit used to establish continuity between the right ventricle and pulmonary artery. Because of severe truncal regurgitation, this valve was replaced with a Björk-Shiley prosthesis. His postoperative course was complicated by bleeding (requiring multiple blood transfusion), cytomegalovirus infection, congestive heart failure, and thoracotomy wound infection. Despite these problems, he was able to return to school and resume normal activities in six months. At age 17 he underwent postoperative cardiac catheterization which revealed a systolic gradient

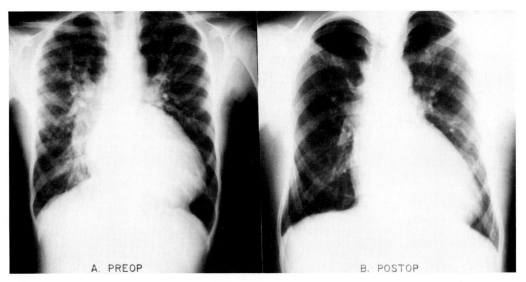

Figure 12. A, Preoperative chest x-ray of a 14-year-old boy with truncus arteriosus and bilateral pulmonary artery banding. The heart is enlarged (C/T ratio, 0.67), the pulmonary trunk is absent, and the pulmonary vascularity appears increased despite the banding. B, Postoperative film at age 17. The heart remains enlarged (C/T ratio, 0.68), the pulmonary vascularity is normal, and a porcine xenograft valve ring and a prosthetic aortic (truncal) valve are in place.

from right ventricle to pulmonary artery of 82 mm. Hg, right ventricular pressure 105/5 mm. Hg, and pulmonary artery pressure 23/7 mm. Hg. The gradient appeared to be largely across the porcine valve. There were no residual shunts or truncal regurgitation. Cardiac output was 5.8 l/min./M² by indicator dilution curve. The pulmonary vascular resistance was 2 units M².

Because of his good exercise tolerance and lack of symptoms, it was elected not to replace his conduit. At the present time he is able to work and plays basketball with his brothers. His chest x-ray (Fig. 12B) continues to show severe cardiomegaly. His current medications are digoxin, warfarin, and folic acid. On a recent visit his resting ECG showed bigeminy with two different foci. The rhythm reverted to sinus with mild exercise for one minute.

This patient's course and current findings illustrate some of the problems which will face the cardiologist who cares for these patients. When should a stenotic conduit or homograft be replaced? What exercise limitations should these patients have? How will the right ventricle continue to function under the handicap of a large ventriculotomy (possibly multiple ventriculotomies with the need for conduit replacements) associated usually with some degree of right ventricular hypertension? Despite these problems, patients with truncus arteriosus now enjoy a greatly improved prognosis in comparison with the almost hopeless situation before the introduction of the Rastelli procedure.

SUMMARY

This chapter deals with four relatively uncommon congenital heart defects that until the last 10 years presented only diagnostic problems rather than therapeutic dilemmas. Operative intervention for these lesions has dramatically changed the outlook for these patients. We are beginning an exciting new phase in the care of patients with complex congenital heart disease in which careful study of the long-term results of new operative approaches will be required to determine optimal therapeutic management.

REFERENCES

1. FONTANA, R. S., AND EDWARDS, J. E.: *Congenital Cardiac Disease: A Review of 357 Cases Studied Pathologically.* W. B. Saunders, Philadelphia, 1962.

2. PENMAN, H. G., AND WHITTIG, R. H.: *Cor triolculare biatriatum.* Br. Heart J. 25:141,1963.

3. PERLOFF, J. K.: *The Clinical Recognition of Congenital Heart Disease.* W. B. Saunders, Philadelphia, 1970.

4. VAN PRAAGH, R., ONGLEY, P. A., AND SWAN, H. J. C.: *Anatomic types of single or common ventricle in man. Morphologic and geometric aspects of 60 necropsied cases.* Am. J. Cardiol. 13:367,1964.

5. EDWARDS, J. E., CAREY, L. S., NEUFELD, H. N., ET AL.: *Congenital Heart Disease.* W. B. Saunders, Philadelphia, 1965.

6. HOLMES, W. F.: *Case of malformation of the heart.* Trans. Med. Chir. Soc. Edin. 1:252,1824.

7. SHAHER, R. M.: *The electrocardiogram in single ventricle.* Br. Heart J. 25:465,1963.

8. VAN PRAAGH, R., VAN PRAAGH, S., VLAD, P., ET AL.: *Diagnosis of the anatomic types of single or common ventricle.* Am. J. Cardiol. 15:345,1965.

9. DAVICHI, F., AND MOLLER, J. H.: *Electrocardiogram and vectorcardiogram in single ventricle.* Am. J. Cardiol. 23:19,1969.

10. CHESLER, E., JOFFE, H. S., VECHT, R., ET AL.: *Ultrasound cardiography in single ventricle and the hypoplastic left and right heart syndromes.* Circulation 42:123,1970.

11. ASSAD-MORELL, J. L., TAJIK, A. J., AND GIULIANI, E. R.: *Echocardiographic analysis of the ventricular septum.* Prog. Cardiovasc. Dis. 17:219,1974.

12. SEWARD, J. B., TAJIK, A. J., HAGLER, D. J., ET AL.: *Contrast echocardiography in single or common ventricle.* Circulation 55:513,1977.

13. McGOON, D. C., DANIELSON, G. K., RITTER, D. G., ET AL.: *Correction of the univentricular heart having two atrioventricular valves.* J. Thorac. Cardiovasc. Surg. 74:218,1977.

14. JORDAN, J. C., AND SANDERS, C. A.: *Tricuspid atresia with prolonged survival.* Am. J. Cardiol. 18:112,1966.

15. KEITH, J. D., ROWE, R. D., AND VLAD, P.: *Heart Disease in Infancy and Childhood,* ed. 2. Macmillan Co., New York, 1967.

16. BARGERON, L. M., JR., ELLIOTT, L. P., SOTO, B., ET AL.: *Axial cineangiography in congenital heart disease.* Circulation 56(6):1075,1977.

17. LA CORTE, M. A., DICK, M., SCHEER, G., ET AL.: *Left ventricular function in tricuspid atresia.* Circulation 52:996,1975.

18. GRAHAM, T. P., JR., ATWOOD, G. F., AND BOUCEK, R. J.: *Left ventricular function in cyanotic congenital heart disease.* Circulation 56(Suppl. III):172,1977.

19. DICK, M., FYLER, D. C., AND NADAS, A. S.: *Tricuspid atresia: clinical course in 101 patients.* Am. J. Cardiol. 36:327,1975.

20. KYGER, E. R., III, REUL, G. J., JR., SANDIFORD, F. M., ET AL.: *Surgical palliation of tricuspid atresia.* Circulation 52:685,1975.

21. TAUSSIG, H. G., KEINONEN, R., MOMBERGER, N., ET AL.: *Long-term observations on the Blalock-Taussig operation. IV. Tricuspid atresia.* Johns Hopkins Med. J. 132:135,1973.

22. WILLIAMS, W. G., RUBIS, L., FOWLER, R. S., ET AL.: *Tricuspid atresia: results of treatment in 160 children.* Am. J. Cardiol. 38:235,1976.

23. FONTAN, F., AND BAUDET, E.: *Surgical repair of tricuspid atresia.* Thorax 26:240,1971.

24. KREUTZER, G.: *Recent surgical approaches to tricuspid atresia.* In Langford Kidd, B. S., and Rowe, R. D. (eds.): *The Child with Congenital Heart Disease After Surgery.* Futura, Mount Kisco, N.Y.,1976.

25. HENRY, J. N., DEVLOO, R. A., RITTER, D. G., ET AL.: *Tricuspid atresia. Successful surgical "correction" in two patients using porcine xenograft valves.* Mayo Clinic Proc. 49:803,1974.

26. EBSTEIN, W.: *On a very rare case of insufficiency of the tricuspid valve caused by a severe malformation of the same.* Arch. Anat. Physiol. Wissensch. Med., Leipz. 238, 1866. Translated by Schiebler, G. L., Gravenstein, J. S., and Van Mierop, L. H. S. Am. J. Cardiol. 22:867,1968.

27. NETTER, F. H., ALLEY, R. D., AND VAN MIEROP, L. H. S.: *Diseases—Congenital Anomalies.* In Yonkman, F. F. (ed.): *Ciba Collection of Medical Illustrations. Vol. 5. Heart.* Prepared by F. H. Netter. Ciba, New York, 1969.

28. KUMAR, A. E., FYLER, D. C., MIETTINEN, O. S., ET AL.: *Ebstein's anomaly.* Am. J. Cardiol. 28:84,1974.

29. BIALOSTOZKY, D., HORIVITZ, S., AND ESPINO-VELA, J.: *Ebstein's malformation of the tricuspid valve.* Am. J. Cardiol. 29:826,1972.

30. WATSON, H.: *Natural history of Ebstein's anomaly of tricuspid valve in childhood and adolescence.* Br. Heart J. 36:417,1974.

31. VACCA, J. B., BASSMAN, D. W., AND MUDD, J. G.: *Ebstein's anomaly. Complete review of 108 cases*. Am. J. Cardiol. 2:210,1958.

32. GENTON, E., AND BLOUNT, S. G., JR.: *The spectrum of Ebstein's anomaly*. Am. Heart J. 73:395,1967.

33. POCOCK, W. A., TUCKER, W. A., AND BARLOW, J. B.: *Mild Ebstein's anomaly*. Br. Heart J. 31:327,1969.

34. WOOD, P.: *Diseases of the Heart and Circulation,* ed. 2. Eyre and Spottiswoode, London, 1956.

35. LOWE, K. G., AND WATSON, H.: *Ebstein's anomaly of the tricuspid valve*. In Watson, H. (ed.): *Paediatric Cardiology.* C. V. Mosley, St. Louis, 1968.

36. CREWS, T. L., PRIDIE, R. B., BENHAM, R., ET AL.: *Auscultatory and phonocardiographic findings in Ebstein's anomaly. Correlation of first heart sound with ultrasonic records of tricuspid valve movement.* Br. Heart J. 34:681,1972.

37. FONTANA, M. E., AND WOOLEY, C. F.: *Sail sound in Ebstein's anomaly of the tricuspid valve.* Circulation 46:155,1972.

38. LUNDSTRÖM, N-R.: *Echocardiography in the diagnosis of Ebstein's anomaly of the tricuspid valve.* Circulation 47:597,1973.

39. MILNER, S., MEYER, R. A., VENABLES, A. W., ET AL.: *Mitral and tricuspid valve closure in congenital heart disease.* Circulation 53:513,1976.

40. BRAUNWALD, E., AND SWAN, H. J. C.: *Cooperative study on cardiac catheterization.* Circulation 37(Suppl. III):1,1968.

41. NADAS, A. S., AND FYLER, D. C.: *Pediatric Cardiology,* ed. 3. W. B. Saunders, Philadelphia, 1972.

42. BARNARD, C. N., AND SCHRIRE, V.: *Surgical correction of Ebstein's malformation with prosthetic tricuspid valve.* Surgery 54:302,1963.

43. HARDY, K. L., MAY, I. A., WEBSTER, C. A., ET AL.: *Ebstein's anomaly: A functional concept and successful definitive repair.* J. Thorac. Cardiovasc. Surg. 48:927,1964.

44. MCFAUL, R. C., DAVIS, Z., GIULIANA, E. R., ET AL.: *Ebstein's malformation.* J. Thorac. Cardiovasc. Surg. 72:910,1976.

45. COBB, F. F., BLUMENSCHEIN, S. D., SEALY, W. C., ET AL.: *Successful surgical interruption of the bundle of Kent in a patient with Wolff-Parkinson-White syndrome.* Circulation 38:1018,1968.

46. COLLETT, R. W., AND EDWARDS, J. E.: *Persistent truncus arteriosus: A classification according to anatomic types.* Surg. Clin. North Am. 29:1245,1949.

47. VAN PRAAGH, R.: *Classification of truncus arteriosus communis.* Am. Heart J. 92:129,1976.

48. GOLDBERG, M. J., AND MCGREGOR, M.: *Persistent truncus arteriosus. Report of a case with atypical radiologic features.* Am. Heart J. 55:360,1958.

49. VICTORICA, B. E., GESSNER, I. H., AND SCHIEBLER, G. L.: *Phonocardiographic findings in persistent truncus arteriosus.* Br. Heart J. 30:812,1968.

50. MAIR, D. D., RITTER, D. G., DAVIS, G. D., ET AL.: *Selection of patients with truncus arteriosus for surgical correction.* Circulation 49:144,1974.

51. MCFAUL, R. C., MAIR, D. D., FELDT, R. H., ET AL.: *Truncus arteriosus and previous pulmonary artery banding: Clinical and hemodynamic assessment.* Am. J. Cardiol. 38:626,1976.

52. MCGOON, D. C., RASTELLI, G. C., AND ONGLEY, P. A.: *An operation for the correction of truncus arteriosus.* JAMA 205:59,1968.

53. GRIEPP, R. B., STINSON, E. B., AND SHUMWAY, N. E.: *Surgical correction of types II and III truncus arteriosus.* J. Thorac. Cardiovasc. Surg. 73:345,1977.

54. MARCELLETTI, C., MCGOON, D. C., AND MAIR, D. D.: *The natural history of truncus arteriosus.* Circulation 54:108,1976.

55. MACGILPIN, H. H.: *Truncus arteriosus communis persistens.* Am. Heart J. 39:615,1950.

56. CARR, F. B., GOODALE, R. H., AND ROCKWELL, A. E. P.: *Persistent truncus arteriosus in a man aged thirty-six years.* Arch. Pathol. 19:833,1935.

57. SILVERMAN, J. J., AND SCHIENESSON, G. P.: *Persistent truncus arteriosus in a 43-year-old man.* Am. J. Cardiol. 17:94,1966.

Congenital Cardiovascular Abnormalities Usually "Silent" until Adulthood: Morphologic Features of the Floppy Mitral Valve, Valvular Aortic Stenosis, Discrete Subvalvular Aortic Stenosis, Hypertrophic Cardiomyopathy, Sinus of Valsalva Aneurysm, and the Marfan Syndrome

William C. Roberts, M.D.

Congenital heart disease most commonly consists of *defects* (absent tissue) in cardiac septa causing shunts, *obstructions* (excess tissue) at or near valvular levels, *anomalous connections* between arteries and veins or between arteries or veins and cardiac chambers, and *combinations* of these three malformations. Less commonly, a congenital cardiovascular malformation consists of an improperly formed tissue which functions normally or almost normally at birth and during the early decades of life, but later causes cardiac dysfunction. This chapter describes certain morphologic features in six of these conditions.

FLOPPY ATRIOVENTRICULAR VALVE

Delineation of the click-late systolic murmur syndrome was a major addition to cardiologic knowledge in the 1960s.[1-5] It is now apparent that the click-late systolic murmur is common, probably occurring in 5 percent or more of persons older than 15 years.[6,7] Although generally not considered as such, the click-systolic murmur syndrome, probably in the majority of persons, is a form of congenital heart disease and, therefore, is the most common congenital heart disease. The auscultatory manifestations, however, are usually not manifest until adulthood.

The click-murmur syndrome may be viewed from both auscultatory and morphologic standpoints as manifesting three stages (Fig. 1): (1) systolic click(s) only, (2) click(s) plus a mid-to-late systolic murmur, and (3) pansystolic murmur only. Although progression from stage one to stage three has been documented in relatively few patients, it appears likely that this is the natural sequence of events in some patients. In others, there may be no progression from stage 1; patients in stage 2 may revert to stage 1; patients in stage 1 may lose their click(s) altogether; and patients appearing in stage 3 (pansystolic murmur) may have had no documentation of stages 1 and 2. This condition in stages 1 and 2 is usually unassociated with symptomatic evidence of cardiac dysfunction; the rare exceptions are patients with arrhythmias and/or chest pain. Patients in stage 3 may have congestive heart failure because of the associated severe mitral regurgitation. The stage 3 floppy mitral valve appears to be a major cause, possibly the most common, of severe *pure* mitral regurgitation requiring valve replacement. As a consequence, there is considerable anatomic information available on the floppy mitral valve which produces a pansystolic murmur (stage 3) and causes severe mitral regurgitation.[8-18] In contrast, there is relatively little anatomic information available in patients with systolic click(s) only (stage 1) or those with both click(s) and late systolic murmur (stage 2).

407

THE SPECTRUM OF MITRAL VALVE PROLAPSE

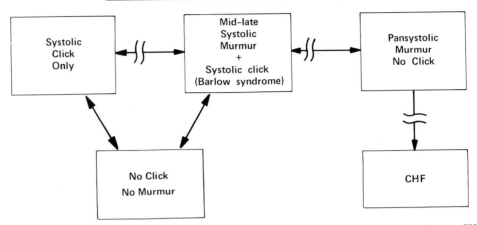

Figure 1. Diagram showing likely auscultatory progression in the prolapsing mitral valve syndrome. CHF = congestive heart failure.

Several names applied to this syndrome describe to some extent what the valve looks like anatomically; "prolapsing posterior mitral leaflet," "prolapsing mitral valve," "billowing or ballooning mitral leaflet syndrome," "overshooting or hooded mitral valve," "floppy mitral valve," and "myxomatous" or "mucinous degeneration of the mitral valve." The common anatomic denominator of the floppy mitral valve is either *excessive leaflet tissue* or *excessive length of chordae tendineae,* or both. Of these, the most common is excessive leaflet tissue. The excess most commonly results from an increase in the transverse or commissure-to-commissure dimension of the leaflet (width). This excess may be focal, involving only a portion of one or both leaflets, or it may be diffuse, involving both leaflets but not necessarily uniformly. The increase in transverse dimension causes the circumferences of the leaflets, measured on a line corresponding to the distal margin of the posterior leaflet, to be much larger than the circumference of the mitral valve anulus; in the normal valve the two are equal. The result is analogous to an accordian not fully extended, or better, a skirt gathered at the waist. The leaflets or the opened normal mitral valve are flat or smooth (like the mucosa of the ileum) whereas those of the opened floppy mitral valve are undulating (like the mucosa of the duodenum or jejunum).

Excessive leaflet tissue also results when there is an increase in the longitudinal or base-to-distal margin dimension of the leaflet (length). Again, this increase may be focal, involving portions of one or both leaflets, or diffuse when both leaflets are involved throughout, though not necessarily uniformly. In some patients there may be an increase in both the transverse and longitudinal dimensions of the leaflets.

Excessive length of chordae tendineae may be an additional cause of mitral valve prolapse. Again, all chordae may be elongated (diffuse) or just a few of them (focal). Elongation of chordae by itself is probably the least frequent mechanism of prolapse. In some patients there appears to be both excessive leaflet tissue and excessive length of chordae tendineae.

Opportunities for structural study of a mitral valve associated with click(s) only have been extremely rare. Figure 2 depicts such a valve. This child was examined while alive by Dr. John Barlow of Johannesburg, South Africa, who by auscultation heard three systolic clicks and no precordial murmur. The child had no symptoms of cardiac dysfunction and died of leukemia; necropsy revealed a perfectly competent mitral valve but three distinct foci where leaflet overlapped adjacent leaflet. The leaflets otherwise were

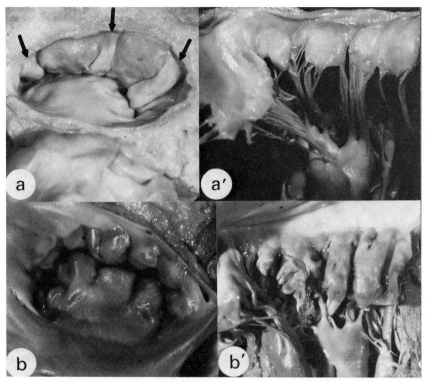

Figure 2. Mitral valves of two children, aged 9 and 13, who died of leukemia. Neither had symptoms of cardiac dysfunction. *a* and *a'*, Mitral valve as viewed from left atrium (a) and after opening (a'). Three areas of leaflet overlap (arrows) are present with the valve intact and the orifice is competent. The leaflets are devoid of scallops and relatively smooth (a'). This child had three systolic clicks during life but no precordial murmur. *b* and *b'*, Mitral valve as viewed from left atrium (b) and after opening (b'). Both leaflets of this valve, in contrast to the valve above, are highly scalloped causing the orifice to be incompetent. This child had a systolic click and a late systolic murmur. (The children whose valves are shown here were examined by Dr. John Barlow in Johannesburg, South Africa, and the auscultatory findings described above were those of Dr. Barlow. I am indebted to him for allowing me to photograph each of these hearts.)

smooth and notably devoid of so-called scallops. There are no reported anatomic descriptions, to my knowledge, of mitral valves producing one or more systolic clicks without an associated precordial systolic murmur. I recently learned, however, of a young woman in her 20s who had, on different occasions, one or more systolic clicks without murmur, associated with recurring arrhythmias. She died during an arrhythmia and a competent pathologist described the mitral valve at necropsy as "entirely normal."

The opportunity to examine the mitral valves (at necropsy) of patients who had systolic click(s) plus a mid-to-late systolic murmur (Barlow syndrome) also is infrequent since this stage is usually asymptomatic. Death in stage 2—as in stage 1—is usually from a noncardiac cause. The mitral valves of three such patients are illustrated in Figures 2 to 4. In this stage the most characteristic feature is leaflet scalloping, which represents excessive leaflet due to an increase in the transverse or commissure-to-commissure dimension of the leaflet. The mitral anulus, as in stage 1, is not dilated. The chordae tendineae may or may not be elongated and they may even be shorter than normal.

The major anatomic characteristic of stage 3 "floppiness" is dilatation of the mitral anulus.[19] Normally, the mitral anulus in adults measures about 9 cm. in circumference.

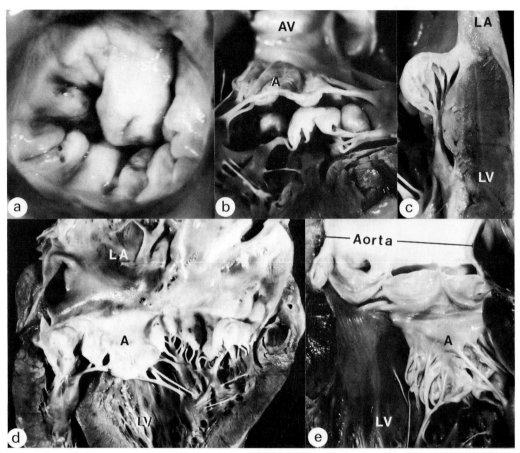

Figure 3. *Floppy mitral valve* in an 18-year-old girl who died of Ewing's sarcoma. She never had symptoms of cardiac dysfunction despite an active life. She had a mid-systolic click and a grade 3/6, ejection-type systolic murmur over the precordium, loudest over the apex. Necropsy revealed Ebstein's anomaly of the tricuspid valve. The mitral valve leaflets shown are elongated transversely, but the chordae are not elongated. *a,* Mitral valve as viewed from left atrium showing marked scalloping. *b,* Same valve as viewed from left ventricle. (A = anterior mitral leaflet; AV = aortic valve) *c,* Longitudinal section of left atrium (LA), billowing posterior mitral leaflet and left ventricle (LV). *d,* Opened mitral valve. *e,* View of anterior mitral leaflet (A) from the left ventricular (LV) aspect. The mitral leaflets and chordae tendineae contained excessive amounts of acid mucopolysaccharide material.

In patients with left ventricular dilatation from any cause with or without mitral regurgitation, the circumference of the mitral anulus usually dilates slightly, to about 11 cm. or less than 25 percent.[19] Among patients with floppy mitral valves associated with severe mitral regurgitation, the circumference of the mitral anulus generally increases by well over 50 percent of normal dimensions (15 to 18 cm.).[19] When the anulus dilates to this extent, the leaflets may "stretch" or flatten transversely, and this stretching diminishes the amount of scalloping. In addition, the left ventricular dilatation may cause longitudinal stretching of the leaflets. The amount of scalloping in the stage 3 valves, therefore, appears to be less than that observed in the stage 2 valves.

Microscopically, the floppy mitral valve leaflets contain an excessive amount of acid mucopolysaccharide material. Both the normal and the floppy mitral leaflet consists of two elements, the fibrosa and the spongiosa. The fibrosa consists of fibrous tissue (collagen), and the spongiosa, of mucoid or myxomatous material high in acid

410

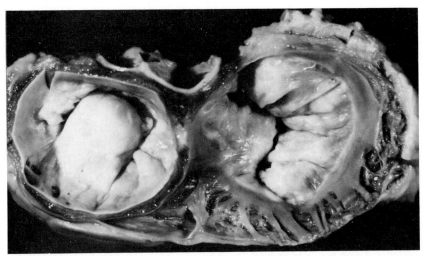

Figure 4. *Floppy mitral valve* (left) and *floppy tricuspid valve* (right) in a 51-year-old man who died suddenly at a dance. Although always asymptomatic, he was found to have a precordial systolic murmur when he was 36 years old. When evaluated about one year before death, he had a systolic murmur; echocardiogram disclosed the classic "hammocking" of the mitral leaflets during ventricular systole, and left ventricular angiography also showed "classic" mitral leaflet prolapse during ventricular systole.

At necropsy, at least one third of the posterior mitral leaflet had prolapsed toward left atrium; several chordae tendineae to this prolapsed segment were thickened and a few were absent, indicating that rupture had occurred. The anterior mitral leaflet appeared normal from the left ventricular aspect, but from the left atrial aspect it was thickened as a result of abnormal contact by the large prolapsed segment of posterior leaflet. All chordae tendineae from the anterior leaflet were elongated, whereas those from the posterior leaflet were thickened. The tricuspid-valve leaflets also were elongated but only mildly thickened compared to the mitral leaflets. There was no clinical evidence of dysfunction of the tricuspid valve. Both atria were mildly dilated. The coronary arteries were normal in course and size and free of significant luminal narrowing. The myocardial walls were free of foci of necrosis or fibrosis.

This case is an example of sudden death in a previously asymptomatic patient with classical auscultatory, echocardiographic and left ventricular angiographic features of the systolic click–late systolic murmur syndrome.

mucopolysaccharide material. In most valve diseases the fibrosa element proliferates and may entirely replace the spongiosa element. In the floppy mitral valve the spongiosa element comprises the more central portion of the leaflet, and appears to proliferate with a far less proportional increase in the fibrosa element. The resulting proliferated myxoid or myxomatous stroma, however, does not appear abnormal, i.e., degenerated, simply increased in amount. Thus, the term myxoid or myxomatous "degeneration" for this condition is not appropriate. The fibrosa element makes up the periphery of the leaflet, and is also increased focally in this condition. The fibrosa element may be subdivided into two components, the *auricularis,* which normally is a thin layer forming the atrial or contact aspect of the leaflet, and the *ventricularis,* which normally is a relatively thick layer which covers the ventricular aspect of the leaflet. The atrial aspect of the floppy mitral leaflet often is focally thickened. This change is considered secondary to abnormal friction from contact between the prolapsed segment of the leaflet and its "opposite number," i.e., the other leaflet, or between two prolapsed segments of the same leaflet.[17,18] The changes on the ventricular surface of the leaflet consist of connective tissue "pads" forming primarily in the interchordal segments. This proliferation of fibrous tissue may extend into adjacent chordae tendineae and onto ventricular endocardium behind the posterior mitral leaflet.[18] The interchordal collections of fibrous tissue are considered responses to the tension and stretching that occurs at the undersurface of prolapsed leaflet or segment of leaflet.[18] This increase in fibrous tissue,

411

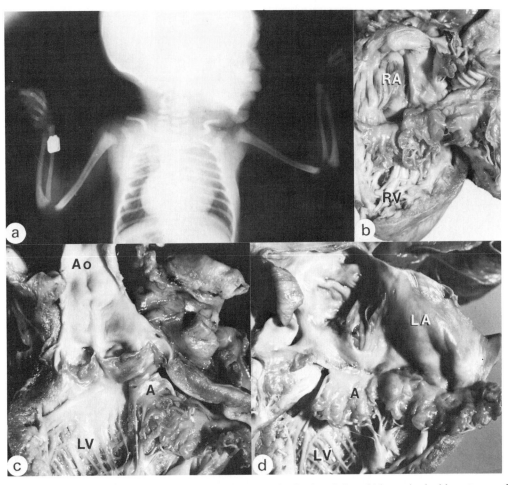

Figure 5. Congenital *floppy mitral valve* and *floppy tricuspid valve* in a 2-day-old boy who had long toes and fingers, a high-arched palate, and a grade 3/6 precordial systolic murmur typical of mitral regurgitation. The heart was enlarged *(a)* and he died of congestive cardiac failure. At necropsy, the intima of the ascending aorta (Ao) was wrinkled *(c)* suggesting that the underlying media was abnormal at this early stage. Shown here is the opened aorta, aortic valve, and left ventricle (LV) (A = anterior mitral leaflet). *(d)* Opened left atrium (LA), mitral valve, and left ventricle (LV). The mitral leaflets are considerably elongated in both longitudinal and transverse dimensions. The left atrium (LA) is dilated. *b,* The tricuspid valve leaflets also are elongated in both transverse and longitudinal dimensions (RA = right atrium; RV = right ventricle).

particularly on the ventricular surface of the valve, has, on occasion, caused this type of valve to be considered as rheumatic in origin rather than floppy.[17]

Ultrastructural studies of floppy mitral valves[20] have disclosed alterations of the collagen fibers in the leaflets and in the chordae tendineae. These changes have included fragmentation, splitting, swelling and coarse granularity of the individual collagen fibers, as well as spiraling and twisting of the fibers.[20] Also, some elastic fibers are fragmented and contain cystic spaces. These alterations in the structure of the collagen may be more important than the accumulation of the acid mucopolysaccharide material in that they lead to focal weaknesses in the leaflets. The left ventricular systolic pressure exerted against these weakened areas may lead to prolapse or focal interchordal hooding. Although the actual prolapse of the mitral valve may be acquired and a consequence of the left ventricular systolic (closing) pressure, the focally weak areas of

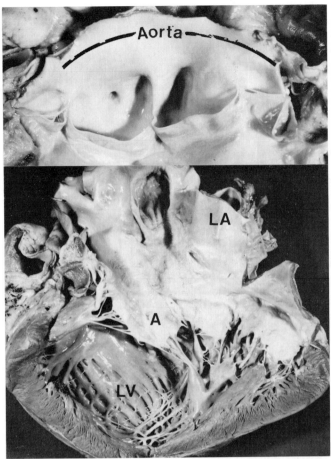

Figure 6. *Floppy mitral valve*—pure mitral regurgitation without aortic disease—in the *Marfan syndrome* in a 28-year-old man who died from severe mitral regurgitation. He had been well until age 24 when he developed exertional dyspnea and hemoptysis and was found to have cardiomegaly. Catheterization was performed at age 25 and the pressures (in mm. Hg) were: pulmonary artery, 19/10; right ventricle, 19/5; right atrial mean, 5; pulmonary arterial wedge mean, 10; and systemic artery 130/80. The cardiac output was 2.3 L./min. He remained functionally class II for the next three years but during his last year of life the congestive heart failure worsened and he became class IV. When examined seven days before his death he was quite ill. A grade 5/6 pansystolic precordial murmur, loudest over the apex, was audible. No diastolic murmur was present. The chest radiograph showed a big heart and severe kyphoscoliosis. Electrocardiogram showed sinus rhythm and left ventricular hypertrophy. He died of progressive heart failure.

At necropsy, the heart was huge (850 gm.). Although the sinuses were dilated, the aorta was entirely normal histologically (top). The mitral leaflets (bottom) were mildly thickened and elongated and the mitral anulus was severely dilated (15 cm.). Calcific deposits were present in the anulus behind the posterior mitral leaflet. The left atrium (LA) was quite dilated as was the left ventricle (LV) (A = anterior mitral leaflet).

the leaflets are probably most often congenital in origin. This focal leaflet weakness may be analogous to the berry aneurysm of the cerebral artery—the weakness in the arterial wall is almost certainly congenital in origin and the later bulging, with or without rupture, is acquired as a consequence of a high intra-arterial pressure. Mitral valve prolapse also may be higher in persons with elevated left ventricular systolic pressures than in persons with normal levels of this pressure. Certainly, calcification of the mitral anulus is more common in hypertensive than in normotensive individuals,[21] and mitral anular calcification is more common in persons with floppy mitral valves

413

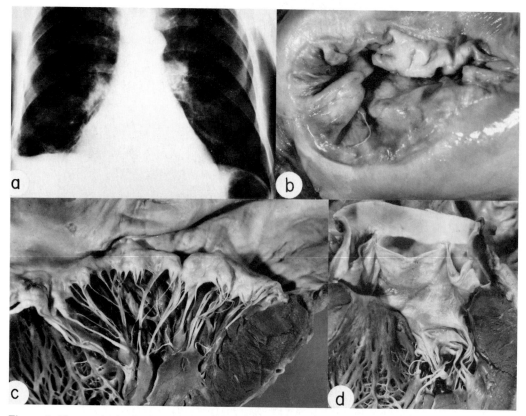

Figure 7. *Floppy mitral valve* in a 70-year-old man who died of gastric carcinoma. During life a grade 3/6 pansystolic blowing murmur was heard, loudest over the apex with radiation to the left axilla. The rhythm was atrial fibrillation. He never had symptoms of cardiac dysfunction. The heart was enlarged by radiograph (*a*), but at necropsy it weighed only 310 gm. Both atria were quite dilated. The mitral leaflets protruded toward the left atrium (*b*) because the chordae tendineae were too long. A portion of opened mitral valve showing the elongated chordae is shown in *c*. *d*, The opened left ventricle and aortic valve show excessively long chordae. Focal calcific deposits also were present in the mitral anulus.

than it is in individuals of similar age and sex without floppy mitral valves.[21,22] Another factor supporting the concept that the underlying fault of mitral floppiness is congenital is its high frequency in patients with other congenital defects (atrial septal defect)[23–26] or deficiencies (the Marfan syndrome)[14,21,27–34] (Figs. 5–7).

Recognized complications of the floppy mitral valve are listed in Table 1. Because a valve may be floppy or prolapsed without mitral regurgitation, it appears reasonable to consider mitral regurgitation as a complication of floppiness rather than a necessary component of this syndrome. Calcification of the mitral anulus almost surely is the second most frequent complication of mitral floppiness (Fig. 8). Rupture of mitral chordae tendineae may be the consequence of infective endocarditis, or rupture may occur without evidence of infection ("spontaneous" rupture)[35-37] (Figs. 9 and 10). Chordal rupture is probably noninfective more often than infective in origin.[38] Nevertheless, because patients with systolic murmurs are at increased risk to develop infective endocarditis and because infection superimposed on a floppy valve is usually highly destructive, antibiotic prophylaxis against this valvular infection appears warranted.

The cause of the arrhythmias is unclear.[39] There is no anatomic evidence in these patients of "a myocardial factor" or abnormality in course or size of any of the major

Table 1. Complications of prolapsing mitral valve.

1. Mitral regurgitation
2. Calcification, mitral "anulus"
3. Rupture of chordae tendineae
   A. Infective endocarditis
   B. Non-infective ("spontaneous")
4. Infective endocarditis
5. Arrhythmias
6. Chest pain
7. Stroke (transient ischemic attacks)
8. Sudden death

coronary arteries. An attractive but unproven explanation is the considerable friction between chordae tendineae and the underlying left ventricular mural endocardium.[18] The cause of the chest pain which occurs occasionally in these patients is also unknown. Associated coronary arterial disease is clearly not the explanation for the chest pain in the majority of these patients. Acute nonprogressive strokes or transient cereb-

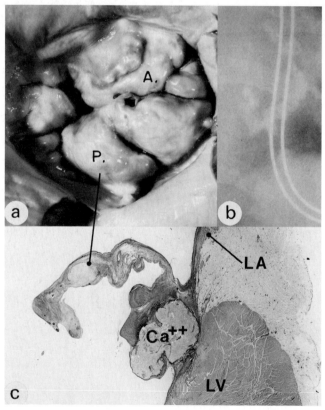

Figure 8. *Floppy mitral valve* and *calcium in the mitral anulus* of a 70-year-old woman who had a grade 3/6 murmur of mitral regurgitation, atrial fibrillation and complete heart block. *a,* Mitral valve from left atrial aspect (A., P. = anterior and posterior mitral leaflets, respectively). *b,* Radiograph taken while the patient was alive shows a C-shaped deposit of calcium in the mitral anular area. Pacing wires also are visible. *c,* Photomicrograph through wall of left atrium (LA), prolapsed posterior leaflet, and left ventricle (LV). The calcium (CA++) in the anular area is apparent.

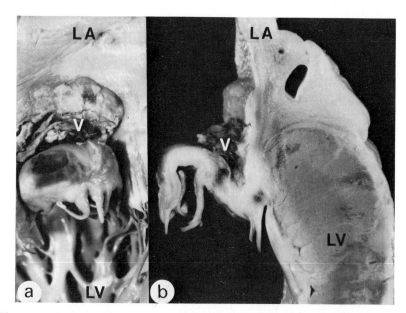

Figure 9. *Floppy mitral valve* with superimposed *Staphylococcus aureus endocarditis* in a 52-year-old man who was known to have a murmur of mitral regurgitation for 10 years. He was asymptomatic, however, until he developed typical clinical features of active infective endocarditis which caused a fatal septic cerebral embolus. Necropsy revealed a portion of posterior mitral leaflet prolapsed toward left atrium (LA) and vegetative (V) material at the acute angle formed by the hooded posterior leaflet and mural endocardium of left atrium. (This junction is a common location of fibrin-platelet deposits in patients with prolapsed posterior mitral leaflets.) *a*, Closeup of hooded segment of posterior leaflet with the superimposed vegetation. *b*, Longitudinal section through left atrium, prolapsed and thickened posterior leaflet and left ventricle (LV).

ral ischemic attacks recently have been noted to occur with increased frequency in these patients.[40] In some patients, small fibrin-platelet thrombi have been observed on the atrial aspects of the prolapsed segments of mitral leaflet at junctions with the left atrial mural endocardium.[18] It has been suggested that dislodgement of these small fibrin-platelet thrombi and their migration to the cerebral arteries is the explanation for the transient cerebral ischemia. It is also possible that these minute thrombi dislodge and embolize to the coronary arteries, triggering an arrhythmia or chest pain or both.[41]

AORTIC VALVE STENOSIS AND THE CONGENITALLY MALFORMED AORTIC VALVE

If papillary muscle dysfunction is excluded, valvular aortic stenosis (AS) is the most common fatal cardiac valve lesion; it was found in 50 percent of patients older than 15 years with valvular heart disease whom I have studied at necropsy.[42-44] Of the patients with AS (with or without aortic regurgitation), the lesion was isolated in 66 percent; in the other 34 percent the mitral valve was stenotic or incompetent or both. The evidence is substantial that the cause of AS, when associated with mitral valve disease, is rheumatic.[44] In contrast, the evidence is substantial that isolated AS (anatomically normal mitral valve) is nonrheumatic in origin.[42-44] This section focuses on patients with isolated AS.[42-50]

In contrast to what was generally believed 30 years ago[51], at least three factors indicate that anatomically isolated aortic valve disease (actually either stenosis or pure regurgitation) is nonrheumatic in origin: (1) the low frequency (about 10 percent) of a positive history of acute rheumatic fever, (2) the absence of Aschoff bodies, and, most

416

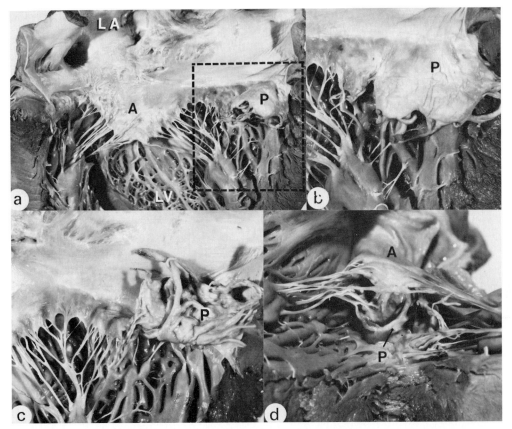

Figure 10. *Floppy mitral valve* in a 38-year-old man who had been well until three years before death, when he experienced a fairly abrupt onset of congestive heart failure. Cardiac catheterization at that time confirmed the presence of pure mitral regurgitation. His blood urea nitrogen at that time was 41 mg./dl. During the next three years he developed severe systemic hypertension (240/140 mm. Hg), severe anemia, severe azotemia (blood urea nitrogen = 230 mg./dl.), and finally, fatal hemorrhagic cardiac tamponade. Necropsy revealed a large segment of posterior mitral leaflet, elongated and prolapsed into the left atrium. Most of the chordae tendineae from this prolapsed segment were ruptured. (The patient never had evidence of infective endocarditis.) The heart weighed 620 gm.

a, Opened left atrium (LA), mitral valve, left ventricle (LV), and prolapsed segment (P). The portion outside the boxed area of mitral leaflets and chordae are normal or near normal (A = anterior mitral leaflet). *b,* Closeup of atrial aspect of the prolapsed segment. *c,* Same view showing the prolapsed segment flipped back into left atrium, exposing its ventricular aspect. *d,* View of mitral valve from left ventricle. In this case mitral prolapse may have been worsened by systemic hypertension; increased closing pressure on the mitral leaflets is created by the elevated systolic pressure.

importantly, (3) the frequency of an underlying congenital malformation of the aortic valve.

The structure of the aortic valve in AS can be correlated to some extent with the age of the patient (Table 2).[43] In patients younger than 15 years, the aortic valve most commonly (60 percent) is congenitally unicuspid and unicommissural;[45,50] in patients 15 to 65 years of age, the valve is most commonly (60 percent) congenitally bicuspid;[46,48] and in patients age older than 65 years, the valve is most commonly (90 percent) tricuspid.[49] The stenosis is either caused by or superimposed on the congenitally malformed aortic valve in virtually all the patients under 15 and in at least 70 percent—possibly as high as 85 percent—of patients between 15 and 65.[43] A congenitally mal-

417

Table 2. Configuration of aortic valve in isolated aortic stenosis in relation to age

	No. valve cusps	<age 15 years	Age 16-65	>age 65 years
1	1	60%	10%	0
2	2	20%	60%	10%
3	3	15%	25%	90%
4	Uncertain	5%	5%	0

formed (in this case congenitally bicuspid) valve appears to be the underlying condition in only about 10 percent of the patients over 65 with AS.[49]

The unicommissural valve, the only type of unicuspid valve observed in the aortic valve position, was described initially by Edwards in 1958[52] (Figs. 11 and 12). This valve, like all other congenitally malformed aortic valves, tends to become more stenotic with time,[50] in contrast to the congenitally bicuspid aortic valve. But the unicuspid aortic valve is almost certainly stenotic from the time of birth, and the fewer the number of aortic valve cusps and commissures, the greater is the likelihood that the valve is stenotic from birth.[43]

Next to the floppy mitral valve, the congenitally bicuspid aortic valve is the most frequent major congenital malformation of the heart or great vessels (Figs. 13 to 19). It is possible that the frequency of this malformation is as high as 2 percent of all human births.[48] In 1800 hearts studied personally, none of which had cardiac valvular, septal, or great vessel abnormalities causing dysfunction, 17 had normally functioning congenitally bicuspid aortic valves. This frequency of nearly 1 percent is similar to that reported by others who examined hearts for the specific purpose of determining presence or absence of congenitally bicuspid aortic valves. Osler[53] found 10 apparently normally functioning congenitally bicuspid aortic valves in 800 autopsies (750 of which were performed by him), an incidence of 1 percent. Eight additional patients had infective endocarditis involving congenitally bicuspid aortic valves. Thus, 18 of 800 (2 percent) had either normally functioning or infected congenitally bicuspid aortic valves. Grant, Wood, and Jones[54] found apparently normally functioning congenitally bicuspid aortic valves in 12 of 1350 (1 percent) necropsy patients. Osler,[53] Lewis and Grant,[55] and Grant and coworkers[54] appear not to have recognized that the bicuspid condition of this valve may underlie severe stenosis or calcification at this site. Thus, if congenitally bicuspid aortic valves that develop complications (stenosis or incompetency with or without infection) are added to those which function normally during the entire lifetime, the frequency of congenitally bicuspid aortic valves may approach 2 percent of the population.

Among the complications of the bicuspid condition of the aortic valve, stenosis is by far the most frequent; pure regurgitation is next, and the latter lesion is most frequently

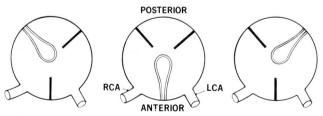

Figure 11. Location of the true commissure in congenitally unicommissural aortic valve stenosis. RCA, LCA = right and left coronary arteries, respectively.

418

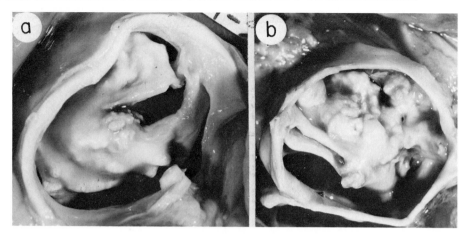

Figure 12. *Congenitally unicommissural stenotic aortic valve* in two men aged 28 *(a)* and 48 years *(b)*.

the result of its being the site of infective endocarditis.[37,38] Why one congenitally bicuspid aortic valve becomes stenotic, another incompetent, and another the site of infective endocarditis is unknown. However, it is clear that stenosis, regurgitation, and infection are complications of the bicuspid condition of the aortic valve and none of them are present at birth. It appears likely that a congenitally bicuspid aortic valve becomes stenotic only as its cusps become fibrotic and calcified; neither cusp of a congenitally bicuspid aortic valve is fibrotic or calcified at the time of birth.

The frequency of development of stenosis or incompetency at the site of a congeni-

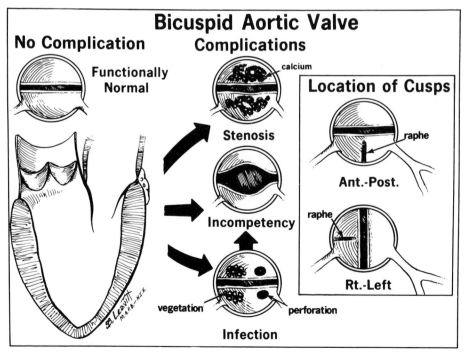

Figure 13. The congenitally bicuspid aortic valve. The location of the cusps and raphes and the acquired complications of the congenital malformation are depicted.

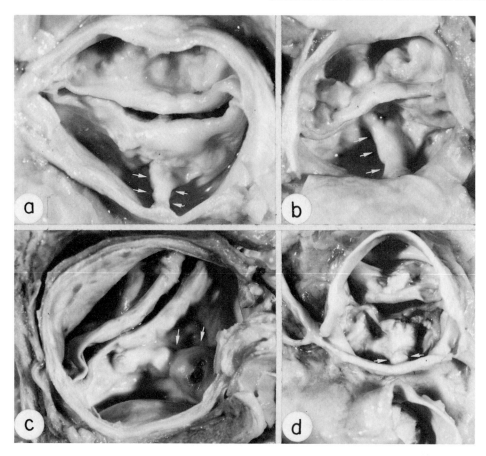

Figure 14. *Calcified, stenotic, congenitally bicuspid aortic valves* in four patients. The cusps are situated anteriorly and posteriorly and the commissures right and left, respectively. Each of the valves has a raphe (white arrows) in the anterior cusp. *a,* Valve of a 61-year-old man. At catheterization two years before his death, the peak systolic gradient (PSG) across the valve was 45 mm. Hg when the cardiac index was 2.6 l./min./m.². He had complete heart block secondary to destruction of the atrioventricular bundle by calcium. *b,* Valve of a 60-year-old man who suddenly collapsed on the street. Electrocardiogram recorded in the emergency room showed left bundle branch block. His only previous symptom of cardiac dysfunction was mild exertional dyspnea. *c,* Valve of a 75-year-old man who died after resection of an asymptomatic abdominal aortic aneurysm which had been discovered during a routine physical examination. A grade 3/6 murmur consistent with aortic stenosis had been heard, but he had no symptoms of cardiac dysfunction. *d,* Valve of a 51-year-old man. The PSG across this valve was only 18 mm. Hg but it was severely incompetent.

tally bicuspid aortic valve also is unknown. Lewis and Grant[55] concluded that vegetations develop at these sites in about 23 percent of adults (16 of 69) with congenitally bicuspid aortic valves. More information is available regarding the incidence of congenitally bicuspid valves in patients with infective endocarditis involving the aortic valve. Of 31 patients with "subacute infective endocarditis" studied at necropsy by Lewis and Grant,[55] 8 had congenitally bicuspid aortic valves. Such valves were found in 4 of 13 patients with infective endocarditis involving aortic valves studied at necropsy by Starling[56] and in 2 of 22 patients studied at necropsy by Fulton and Levine.[57] These investigators apparently were not aware of the fact that congenitally bicuspid aortic valves could become stenotic.

Of the 157 necropsy patients older than 15 years in whom I found congenitally bicuspid stenotic aortic valves, 99 percent had grossly visible extensive calcific deposits in

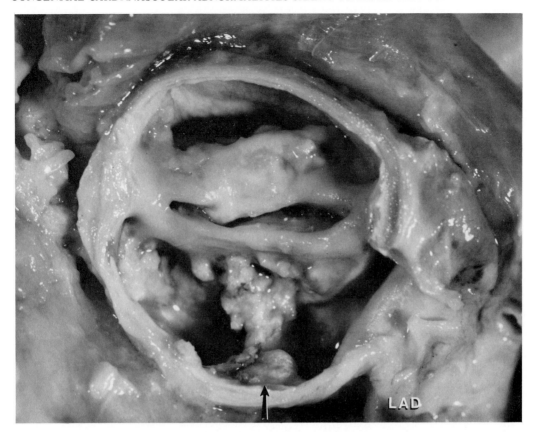

Figure 15. *Congenitally bicuspid, stenotic aortic valve* in an 87-year-old man who developed angina pectoris one year before his sudden death at home. He never had congestive heart failure or syncope. The two cusps are located anteriorly and posteriorly with a raphe (arrow), which is calcified, in the anterior cusp. In addition to the heavy deposits of calcium in the aortic valve, large calcific deposits also were present in the mitral anulus. Aortic stenosis had been diagnosed by physical examination 10 years before he died. LAD = left anterior descending coronary artery.

both cusps. The two patients without calcific deposits were under 30. In contrast, only 5 of the 22 patients with purely incompetent congenitally bicuspid aortic valves had calcific deposits which were focal and small. Calcific deposits are to be expected in adults with stenotic congenitally bicuspid aortic valves. Furthermore, heavy deposits of calcium do not occur in purely incompetent congenitally bicuspid aortic valves; valvular stenosis appears to be a prerequisite for the development of heavy deposits of calcium at this site. Development of infective endocarditis on a heavily calcified valve also is rare.[58] Infective endocarditis was found in only 13 (8 percent) of the 157 patients I studied with stenotic congenitally bicuspid aortic valves; infection was superimposed on a heavily calcified valve in only 4 of them. Of the 22 patients with purely incompetent congenitally bicuspid aortic valves, the valve was the site of vegetative endocarditis in 19 (86 percent), and this infection was the principal cause of incompetency.

The mechanism by which a congenitally bicuspid aortic valve becomes stenotic or incompetent is uncertain. There is no evidence that the valve is stenotic or incompetent at birth. Likewise, there is no evidence that superimposed rheumatic fever or rheumatic heart disease is the cause of the stenosis or incompetency. The explanation advanced by Edwards[59] is attractive. He proposed that it is not mechanically possible for a

421

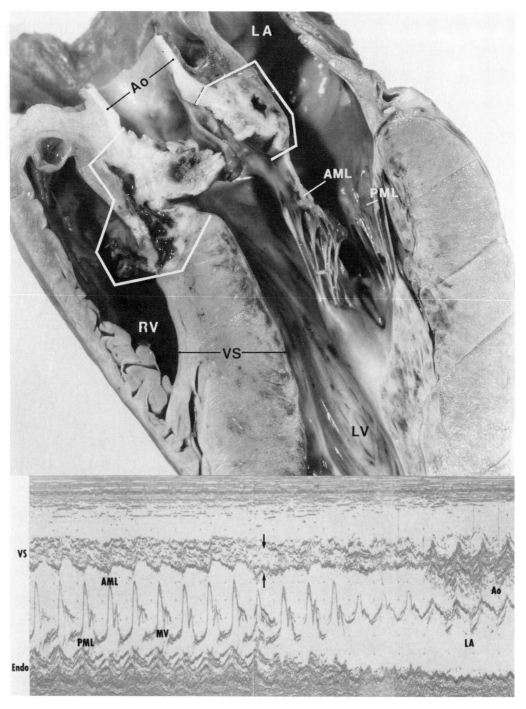

Figure 16. *Congenitally bicuspid aortic valve* with superimposed *Staphylococcus aureus endocarditis* in a 30-year-old man. Before the onset of the infective endocarditis the patient was asymptomatic but before the infection the valve was already mildly stenotic and mildly calcified. Nail biting, to the point of bleeding, apparently was the source of the infection. At necropsy the heart weighed 560 gm. The infection of the aortic valve burrowed into the adjacent soft tissues (brackets) producing large "ring abscesses." Ring abscess caused complete right bundle branch block. There was extensive subendocardial and papillary muscle necrosis of the left ventricle, presumably the result of severely diminished cardiac output. The echocardiogram was recorded several days before death. The arrows in the ventricular septum of the echocardium designate the probable ring abscess. Ao = aorta; LA = left atrium; RV = right ventricle; LV = left ventricle; AML and PML = anterior and posterior mitral leaflets; VS = ventricular septum; MV = mitral valve; Endo = endocardium.

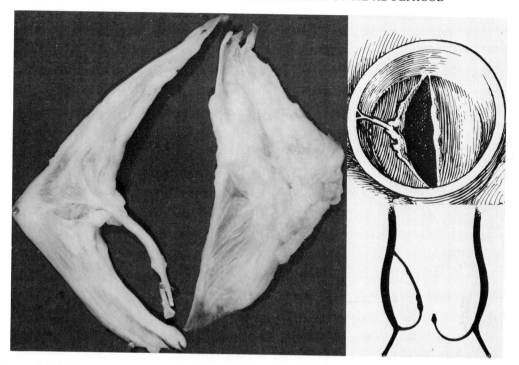

Figure 17. *Purely incompetent congenitally bicuspid aortic valve* in a 27-year-old man who was found to have aortic regurgitation at age 17; he developed exertional dyspnea at age 25. Just before valve replacement, simultaneous left ventricular and brachial arterial pressures were 125/25 and 126/54 mm. Hg, respectively, when the cardiac index was 2.2 l./min./m.². He died suddenly 13 months after valve replacement. The heart weighed 800 gm. Excised aortic valve is pictured at left. The drawing shows the supporting fibrous band that stretched from the margin in the midportion of one cusp to the aortic wall above one sinus of Valsalva (right). This patient is an example of pure severe aortic regurgitation of a congenitally bicuspid valve which was never the site of infective endocarditis.

congenitally bicuspid aortic valve to open and close properly. The distances between lateral attachments of normal aortic valvular cusps along their free margins are curved lines. The extra length allows the cusps to move freely during opening and closing of the valves. In contrast, the distances between lateral attachments of congenitally bicuspid aortic valves along their free margins are almost straight lines. (If the distances were

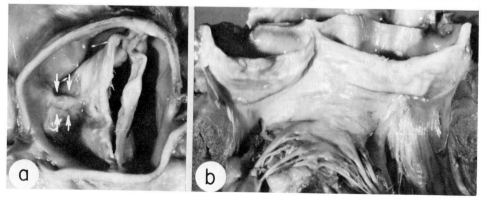

Figure 18. *Functionally normal congenitally bicuspid aortic valve. a,* The right cusp contains the raphe (arrows) and is the larger of the two cusps. *b,* Opened valve.

exactly straight, the valves could not open during ventricular systole.) Consequently, at least one cusp is larger than the other. The excessive length of one or both cusps of a congenitally bicuspid aortic valve produces abnormal contact between the cusps. This abnormal contact, in turn, causes focal fibrous thickening that becomes diffuse with time, eventually causing dystrophic calcification. Thus, stenosis of a congenitally bicuspid aortic valve may be the result of trauma to these cusps produced by their abnormal contact with each other. Although this explanation is appealing, it does not explain why one congenitally bicuspid aortic valve becomes stenotic, another becomes entirely incompetent, and another remains free of complications.

Criteria for differentiating a bicuspid valve of congenital origin from a bicuspid valve of acquired origin have been debated (Fig. 19). There is no controversy over the distinction between a congenitally bicuspid aortic valve devoid of a raphe (false commissure or ridge) and complications (stenosis, incompetency, or infection) and a tricuspid aortic valve devoid of similar complications. There was controversy about the means of differentiating a congenitally bicuspid aortic valve with a raphe from an acquired bicuspid aortic valve resulting from fusion of two cusps at one true commissure.* Osler,[53] from his study of 18 hearts (15 adults), deduced the following characteristics of a congenitally bicuspid aortic valve, all recognizable by gross observation: (1) The raphe is located where the true commissure normally would be, i.e., between the right and left anterior aortic valve cusps; (2) The length of the free margin of the cusp without a raphe is slightly shorter (by an average of 12 percent in his measurements on 7 hearts) than the length of the margin of the cusp containing a raphe, the "conjoint" cusp; (3) The free border of the conjoint cusp is straight or curled and free of nodular thickenings which would indicate bodies of Arantius; (4) The border of attachment of the conjoint cusp, as viewed from the ventricular aspect, presents either the contour of a single semilunar cusp or a shallow groove, indicative of the junction of two cusps; (5) The raphe may be located on the aortic wall alone or may extend onto the cusp for variable distances, but in either case it usually divides the sinus of Valsalva into units of equal size.

In 1923 Lewis and Grant[54] clarified several gross features of "unequivocally" congenital bicuspid aortic valves and presented histologic criteria for differentiating bicuspid valves of "congenital" origin from those of "inflammatory" origin. In contrast to Osler's findings these authors found that fusion could occur not only between right and left anterior cusps but also between right anterior and posterior cusps. A raphe, dividing one of the two cusps, was observed "in about half the cases." The two cusps could be the same size, but usually the conjoined cusp was larger, though less than twice the size of the undivided cusp; or else, "the subdivided cusp is larger than one normal cusp but smaller than two normal cusps." However, Lewis and Grant considered gross distinction between congenital and acquired bicuspid aortic valves unreliable. Elastic tissue stains of transverse sections of congenital raphes showed them to consist mainly of elastic fibers; thus, histologically the raphe was similar to the media of the aorta. In contrast, transverse sections of two fused cusps at a true commissure disclosed that the fused commissure was devoid of elastic fibers and consisted of fibrous valvular tissue. Other investigators[60,61] confirmed these histologic criteria. Koletsky[61] also pointed out that congenital raphes were devoid of vascular channels and inflammatory cells, whereas both were seen in acquired, fused commissures. Since Lewis and Grant de-

---

*The definition of a *commissure* differs depending on whether a semilunar or an atrioventricular (A-V) cardiac valve is under consideration. The aortic valve commissure is the space between two lateral attachments on the aortic wall. Normally each aortic valve cusp is an independent similar sized unit and adherence of one cusp to another at the narrow space (commissure) between the two cusps is abnormal. In contrast to a semilunar valve, the leaflets of an atrioventricular valve are continuous one with another. Thus, the commissures of the A-V valves are the sites of connection between the unequal sized leaflets, not the spaces between the cusps as in the case of the semilunar valves.

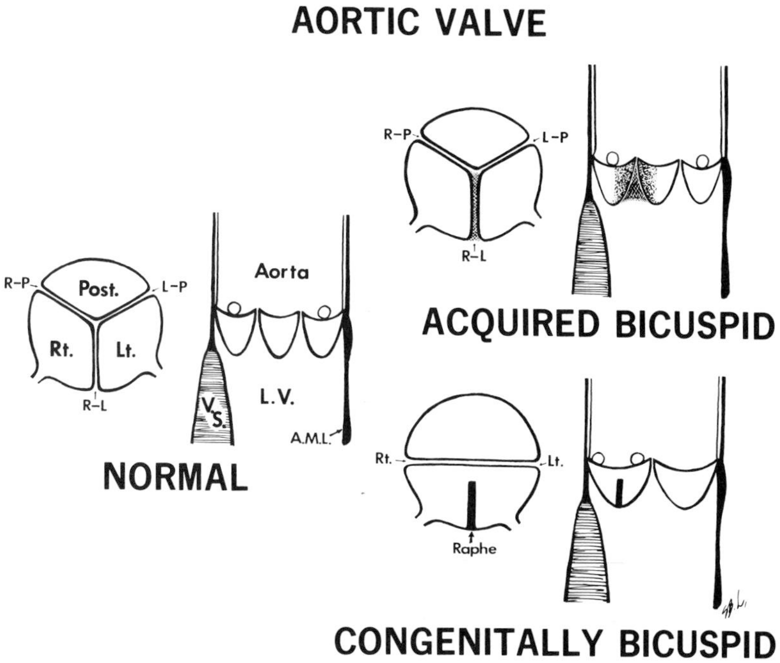

Figure 19. Diagram illustrating differences between *bicuspid aortic valves* of congenital origin as compared to the normal valve. The circumferential distances between each of the three commissures in a normally formed valve are similar. L-P = left-posterior; R-L = right-left, and R-P = right-posterior commissures; Rt., Lt., Post., = right, left, and posterior cusps, respectively; V.S. = ventricular septum; L.V. = left ventricular outflow tract; and A.M.L. = anterior mitral leaflet. In the *acquired bicuspid valve* the circumferential distance between the commissures remains equal, as in a normal valve. The fused commissure is wide, the distal margins of each of the two fused cusps are still usually visible, and the most cephalad margin of the fused commissure is on the same horizontal level as the most cephalad margins of the two nonfused commissures. In the *congenitally bicuspid valve,* the raphe is generally narrow and rarely extends to the free margin of the conjoined cusp or to the cephalad level reached by the two true commissures. The circumferential distances between the two true commissures are greater than this distance between either true commissure and the raphe. The circumferential distance between the true commissures around the conjoined cusp, i.e., the cusp with the raphe, is equal to or slightly greater than the circumferential distance between the true commissures around the cusp devoid of the raphe.

scribed these histologic features, many pathologists have been reluctant to distinguish between congenital and acquired bicuspid aortic valves without microscopic examination of raphes. But however helpful these histologic criteria may be, they are not specific. In some patients certain sections of a raphe show a structure like that of the aortic media, while other sections of the same raphe show only fibrous tissue. Also, the congenital raphe may lose its elastic fibers as the valvular cusps become fibrotic and calcified. The raphe may be the first portion of a congenitally bicuspid aortic valve to calcify, and these deposits destroy existing elastic fibers. Interestingly, Lewis and Grant and others who emphasized the importance of histologic distinction between congenital raphes and fused true commissures were unaware that calcific stenosis was a consequence of a congenitally bicuspid aortic valve. Once the valve is extensively scarred and calcified, histologic examination of the raphe is often fruitless. Furthermore, as Edwards[62] pointed out, in the patient with a bicuspid aortic valve that must be assumed to be congenital—as in infants with aortic coarctation—the raphe may not only be fibrous, but may grossly display features suggesting fusion of two distinguishable, separate cusps.

It appears that tricuspid aortic valves are rarely stenotic at birth. If stenosis is

425

present at birth and the aortic valve has three cusps, the stenosis is usually the result of a very small aortic "anulus" rather than the result of fusion of the cusps; whereas acquired stenosis of a three-cusp aortic valve is common. Of the patients studied personally with clinically isolated AS (with or without regurgitation), aged 16 to 65 years (Table 2), 25 percent had tricuspid valves, and among those over 65, 90 percent had tricuspid valves. In the younger group, about one half of the patients with clinically isolated AS had diffuse fibrous thickening of the mitral leaflets as well. The associated diffuse mitral leaflet thickening is strong evidence that the etiology of AS in this group is rheumatic.[44] Also, nearly 75 percent of this group had positive histories of acute rheumatic fever, whereas 10 percent of the other group, i.e., those with anatomically normal mitral valves and AS, had positive histories.[42,44] The etiology of AS in the patients with anatomically normal mitral valves is unknown. Possibly, as mentioned earlier, minor abnormalities in the sizes of the aortic valve cusps from birth set the stage for abnormal contact of the leaflets with one another, resulting in fibrosis and, finally, stenosis[47] (Fig. 20).

DISCRETE SUBAORTIC STENOSIS

Like valvular AS, discrete subaortic stenosis (DSS), when isolated, usually does not produce symptoms of cardiac dysfunction until adulthood, and it is compatible with a relatively long survival. The average age of death is 35,[63] Unlike valvular AS, however, DSS is rare. In this condition the discrete obstruction is located about 1 cm. caudal to the bases of the aortic valve cusps.[43] The obstruction is on a line corresponding to the site where the atrial septum inserts into the anterior mitral leaflet. The obstruction, at

The Three-cuspid Aortic Valve

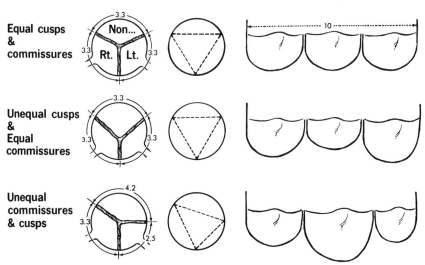

Figure 20. Diagrammatic portrayal of aortic valve cusps equal and unequal in size. *Top row,* The cusps of the aortic valve are equal in size and the circumferential distances between the commissures are equal. The straight-line distances between the commissures (as indicated by the dashed lines in the center circle) also are equal. On the right the aortic valve is opened. *Middle row,* Here the cusps are of unequal size, and they are made unequal by differing cephalocaudal lengths of the individual cusps. The distances between the commissures circumferentially around the aorta and the straight-line distances within the lumen of the aorta are similar to the normal shown in the top panel. *Bottom row,* Here the cephalocaudal lengths of the individual cusps differ and the circumferential distances around the aorta and the straight-line distances within the lumen of the aorta between the commissures (lateral attachments) are different as well.

least in adults, is produced by <u>dense fibrous tissue—not really a "membrane"—which encircles the entire left ventricular outflow tract.</u> The dense fibrous tissue may spread slightly cephalad, approaching the bases of the aortic valve cusps, and caudally for about a centimeter. Because in DSS the obstruction is usually severe and located just below (1 cm.) the aortic valve, the aortic valve cusps are the site of the impact of the blood ejected through the discrete obstruction. As a consequence, <u>the aortic valve cusps become thickened and thus are ideal sites for vegetations.</u> The consequence of cuspal thickening, with or without superimposed infective endocarditis, is development of mild aortic regurgitation. As a result, nearly all adults with DSS have precordial diastolic murmurs of aortic regurgitation in addition to the systolic murmurs of left ventricular outflow obstruction.[64,65] The absence of aortic valve calcific deposits and the absence of dilatation of the ascending aorta in adults, however, helps, before cardiac catheterization, to separate these patients from patients with valvular AS.

Although adequate data is not yet available, it is likely that DSS, on a percentage basis, is the cardiac condition <u>most frequently complicated by infective endocarditis,</u> being more common than that infection's association with congenitally bicuspid or unicuspid aortic valve, prolapsed aortic valve associated with ventricular septal defect, or floppy mitral valve.[58,66] The narrow jet of blood contacting one or more aortic valve cusps under high pressure and velocity provides the ideal circumstance for infective endocarditis to develop. Of five Newfoundland dogs with DSS that were dying naturally, four had active infective endocarditis, which was the cause of death, at necropsy.[66] Among seven patients with DSS whom I studied at necropsy, four had died from active infective endocarditis (Figs. 21 and 22).

Infective endocarditis complicating DSS may be difficult to diagnose clinically, at least before embolic events occur, and early diagnosis in this circumstance is essential to prevent severe damage to the aortic valve cusps. The high pressure jet ejected through the subaortic stenosis damages these cusps naturally, as already mentioned, but when infection is present this damage by the jet is markedly accelerated and the cusps are rapidly destroyed. In patients with destroyed aortic valve cusps and no subaortic stenosis, the consequence is severe aortic regurgitation with progressive left ventricular dilatation and failure. But in patients with destroyed aortic valve cusps associated with DSS, severe aortic regurgitation is prevented by the subaortic obstruc-

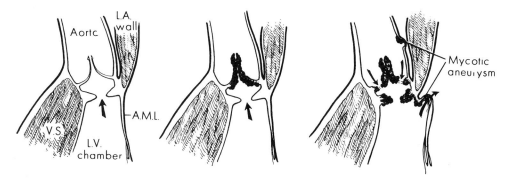

Figure 21. Diagram of aortic-valve region of the patient described in detail in Figure 22. Here the course of the pathologic process suggested by the necropsy findings is illustrated. The left diagram shows the *discrete subvalvular obstruction* before the development of *bacterial endocarditis* when the valve was traumatized by the jet of blood from below. The central diagram depicts the initial formation of bacterial vegetations, exclusively on the aortic valve cusps. As vegetations proliferated, the cusps ruptured (right diagram); the infection then extended to the discrete subvalvular fibrous band and anterior mitral leaflet (A.M.L.) where a mycotic aneurysm formed immediately below the "membrane" where systolic pressure was highest. A second aneurysm in the wall of the ascending aorta resulted from the effects of a systolic jet through the valve. L.A. = left atrium; V.S. = ventricular septum; L.V. = left ventricle.

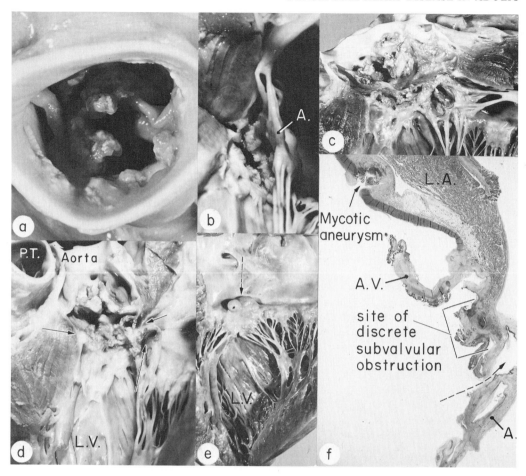

Figure 22. Alpha hemolytic streptococcus endocarditis complicating congenitally *discrete subaortic stenosis* in a 28-year-old man. The infection, which appeared about nine months before death, produced valvular aortic regurgitation. *a,* Aortic valve from above. *b,* Left ventricular outflow tract from below, showing vegetative material on the subvalvular "membrane" and adjacent anterior mitral leaflet (A.). *c,* Opened left ventricular outflow tract showing vegetations on each aortic cusp, on the subvalvular "membrane," and on the ventricular surface of anterior mitral leaflet. *d,* Longitudinal section showing the left ventricular outflow tract. The area of subaortic stenosis is apparent (between the *solid arrows*) and a mycotic aneurysm *(dashed arrow)* is seen in the anterior mitral leaflet. The mitral aneurysm is in the high-pressure portion of the left ventricle (L.V.), i.e., below the discrete subvalvular obstruction. P.T. = pulmonary trunk. *e,* Opened mitral valve showing atrial aspect of the mycotic aneurysm *(dashed arrow)* on the anterior leaflet. *f,* Photomicrograph of section through aorta, left atrium (L.A.), aortic valve (A.V.) cusp, subvalvular "membrane," and anterior mitral leaflet (A.). A mycotic aneurysm is present in the ascending aorta *(solid arrow)* as well as in the anterior mitral leaflet *(dashed arrow)*. Vegetations are present on the aortic valve cusp and on the subvalvular membrane. (Hematoxylin and eosin stain; x 2, reduced 15%)

tion; therefore, the aortic or systemic arterial diastolic pressure does not fall significantly despite an anatomically destroyed aortic valve. As a consequence, the left ventricle does not dilate and congestive cardiac failure may be absent. Because the aortic valve cusps in these patients are previously traumatized by the jet of blood traversing the subaortic stenosis, the infection is superimposed on a previously abnormal valve. In this situation the most common infecting organisms are alpha streptococci, organisms of a relatively low virulence that are compatible with active infective endocarditis over a long period (many months) without antibiotic treatment.[58]

One of the essential reasons for diagnosing DSS before adulthood is to allow operative resection of the "membrane" so that cuspal damage is prevented. When operative treatment is delayed until adulthood, aortic valve replacement is often required in addition to resection of the subaortic "membrane." Then survival becomes dependent on the "survival" of the valvular prosthesis, and anticoagulants usually are required with all of their inherent complications.

A recent anatomic observation in necropsy patients with DSS is severe thickening and luminal narrowing of the intramural coronary arteries located in the ventricular septum.[66] A similar finding has been observed in patients with hypertrophic cardiomyopathy (see next section) and in patients with tunnel subaortic stenosis.[67]

HYPERTROPHIC CARDIOMYOPATHY

In his original description,[68] Teare applied the term *asymmetrical hypertrophy of the heart* to this condition. Subsequently, terms such as *functional subaortic stenosis, diffuse muscular subaortic stenosis, idiopathic hypertrophic subaortic stenosis, hypertrophic obstructive cardiomyopathy,* and *asymmetric septal hypertrophy (ASH)* have been applied. The terms which include the words "stenosis" and "obstruction" appear inappropriate because obstruction is more often absent than present.[69] The terms which emphasize asymmetry of the walls bordering the left ventricular cavity have served a useful purpose in emphasizing a characteristic morphologic feature of this condition,[43] but the ventricular septum may be thicker than the left ventricular free wall in conditions other than hypertrophic cardiomyopathy (HC).[70-77] A few patients (about 5 percent) with HC do not have ASH (i.e., septum thicker than free wall[78,79]) and in rare cases the free wall is not thickened in HC.[78]

Study at necropsy of patients with HC[78] has demonstrated the following morphologic features: (1) greater thickening of the ventricular septum than of the left ventricular free wall (95 percent); (2) small or normal-sized left and right ventricular cavities (95 percent); (3) mural endocardial plaque, left ventricular outflow tract (75 percent, adults only); (4) thickened mitral valve (75 percent, adults only); (5) dilated atria (100 percent, adults only); (6) abnormal intramural coronary arteries (50 percent);[80] and (7) disorganization of myocardial fibers in the ventricular septum (95 percent) (Figs. 23–31; Table 3).

The chief morphologic abnormality in HC resides in the *ventricular septum.* As pointed out by Teare in 1958, the ventricular septum nearly always is thicker than the left ventricular free wall. Among our adult necropsy patients, the maximal thickness of ventricular septum averaged 3.0 cm and the maximal thickness of left ventricular free wall, 1.8 cm. The thickest portion of the septum is that part located about midway between aortic valve and left ventricular apex. This level corresponds approximately to the apex of right ventricle. Although in all our necropsy patients the ventricular septum was thicker than normal, the left ventricular free wall was usually, though not always, thicker than normal.

Although *ventricular asymmetry* (i.e., a significant difference in maximal thickness of ventricular septum and left ventricular free wall) is a characteristic morphologic feature of HC, about 5 percent of our patients with this condition showed *ventricular symmetry* at necropsy (i.e., equal maximal thickness of the ventricular septum and left ventricular free wall). Thus, although asymmetric septal hypertrophy (ASH) is a highly sensitive marker for HC,[69] it is not specific for this condition. Ventricular septa thicker than left ventricular free walls have been reported in conditions causing thinning of the left ventricular free wall relative to the septum and in conditions causing thickening of the septum relative to the free wall. The most common cause of preferential free wall

429

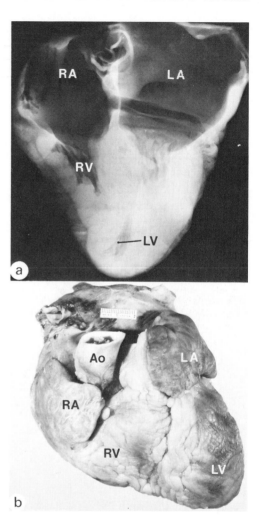

Figure 23. *a,* Radiograph of heart specimen and *b,* the heart itself in a 43-year-old woman with *hypertrophic cardiomyopathy.* Eleven years before she died the peak systolic pressure gradient between left ventricle and aorta was 54 mm. Hg at rest. She had periodic atrial fibrillation, chronic congestive cardiac failure, and an event compatible with cerebral embolus. The radiograph shows very dilated right (RA) and left (LA) atria, small-sized right (RV) and left (LV) ventricular cavities and a ventricular septum thicker than the left ventricular free wall. The exterior view of the specimen also shows very prominent atria. Ao = aorta.

Table 3. Idiopathic dilated (DC) and hypertrophic (HC) cardiomyopathies: morphologic differences

	DC	HC
1. Dilated ventricular cavities	+	0
2. Intracardiac thrombi	+	0
3. Asymmetric septal hypertrophy	0	+
4. Myocardial fiber disorientation	0	+
5. Endocardial plaque, LV outflow tract	0	+
6. Thickened mitral valve	0	+
7. Abnormal intramural coronary arteries	0	+
8. Ventricular scarring (gross)	0 − +	+
9. Thickened ventricular walls	0 − +	+
10. Increased cardiac weight	+	+
11. Dilated atrial cavities	+	+

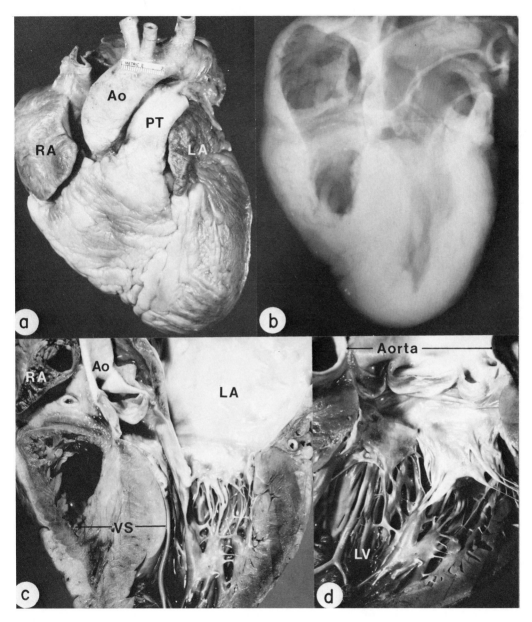

Figure 24. Heart of a 26-year-old man with *hypertrophic cardiomyopathy.* At catheterization three years before his death, a peak systolic pressure gradient of 30 mm. Hg was present between left ventricle and brachial artery and the gradient increased to 85 mm. Hg with provocation (ouabain). The cardiac index was 2.1 l./min./m.². At another catheterization done only six days before his sudden death, the gradient at rest was zero and it rose to only 33 mm. Hg when provoked (isoproterenol). The cardiac index was 2.0 l./min./m.². The anatomic features of hypertrophic cardiomyopathy are demonstrated in these photographs. *a,* Exterior view; both right (RA) and left (LA) atria are dilated. Ao = aorta; PT = pulmonary trunk. *b,* Radiograph of specimen showing the ventricular septum to be thicker than left ventricular free wall. *c,* Coronal section; the septum (VS) is clearly thicker than the left ventricular free wall, and an endocardial mural plaque is present in the left ventricular outflow tract in apposition to the anterior mitral leaflet. *d,* A closer view of the plaque and the thickened anterior mitral leaflet.

431

thinning is myocardial infarction; the most common cause of preferential septal thickening is right ventricular systolic hypertension from any of a variety of conditions.

Among patients with HC, the thickness of the ventricular septum is not dependent on the presence of left ventricular outflow tract obstruction at rest, and, indeed, the thickness of the septum is similar in patients with outflow obstruction at rest and in those without outflow obstruction at rest. Although examination of the septum in patients with HC is not helpful in separating the patients *with* from those *without* left ventricular outflow obstruction at rest, examination of the basal portion of the left ventricular free wall (posterior or posterolateral portion) does permit delineation between these two groups of patients.[81,82] In the patients with the obstructive type of HC, this posterobasal portion of left ventricular free wall represents the thickest portion of free wall, whereas in the patients with the nonobstructive type of HC, this posterobasal portion is thinner than normal and often pointed like a bird's bill (Fig. 25). In the patients with obstruction at rest, the thickest portion of the left ventricular free wall is about midway between the base of posterior mitral leaflet and apex of left ventricle.

Another abnormality in the ventricular septum in patients with HC is focal *myocardial fiber disarray* or disorganization[68,78,81-83] (Fig. 30). This abnormality also was described by Teare in 1958, and occurs in 90 to 100 percent of these patients depending on how "septal disorganization" is defined.[83] Small foci of myocardial fibers not parallel to one another in the ventricular septum are common in normal hearts. When, however, the definition of "septal disorganization" is rigid and quantitation of the amount of disorganization is introduced, about 90 percent of the patients with HC can be clearly delineated from persons with normal hearts or from patients with cardiac conditions other than HC.[83] Studies by Maron and associates[83] have shown that among patients

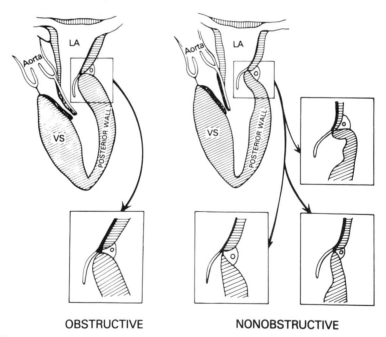

OBSTRUCTIVE   NONOBSTRUCTIVE

Figure 25. Diagram depicting the configuration and thickness of the posterolateral left ventricular free wall just behind the posterior mitral leaflet in the obstructive and nonobstructive types of *hypertrophic cardiomyopathy.* In the obstructive form, the most basal portion of free wall is rounded and thick. In the nonobstructive form, the most basal portion of left ventricular free wall is pointed and thin. In each type the ventricular septum is much thicker than the left ventricular free wall. The mural endocardium in the left ventricular outflow tract and the anterior mitral leaflet in apposition to it is thickened.

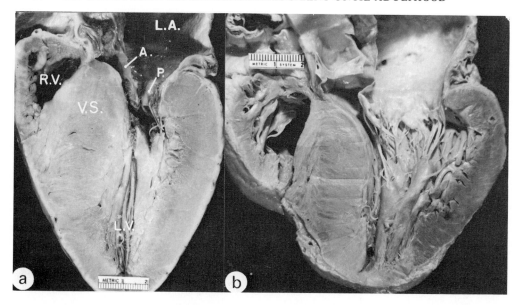

Figure 26. *Hypertrophic cardiomyopathy* in two patients. *a,* Left ventricular outflow obstruction in patient whose gradient at rest was 77 mm. Hg. *b,* Patient with no gradient at rest. The posterobasal portion of left ventricular (L.V.) free wall in the first patient is rounded and thick; this portion of free wall in the second patient is more pointed and thin. The result is a larger left ventricular cavity in the basal portion in *b* than in *a* and, consequently, more room for the mitral valve. The ventricular septum (V.S.) in both patients, however, is severely thickened. A., P. = anterior and posterior mitral leaflets, respectively; R.V. = right ventricle.

with HC nearly 90 percent had 5 percent or more of the area of the ventricular septum showing myocardial fiber disorganization. In contrast, among persons with normal hearts or heart conditions other than HC, less than 5 percent of the area of the ventricular septum showed such disorganization.

Although "septal disorganization" of greater than 5 percent of the area of the ventricular septum occurs in about 90 percent of the patients with HC, about 10 percent of these patients have less than 5 percent of the area of the septum showing disarray and of them a few patients have absolutely no disarray at all.[83] Thus, like ventricular asymmetry, "septal disorganization" of greater than 5 percent of the area of the septum occurs in most patients with HC, but this abnormality may involve a smaller area of the septum, or, rarely, may be entirely absent.

Not only does disorganization of *myocardial fibers* occur; ultrastructural studies have shown disarray of *myofibrils* and *myofilaments* within individual cells.[84] Again, the abnormalities of myofibrils and myofilaments are not absolutely specific for HC, but when disorganization of these subcellular components is found in other cardiac conditions, the abnormal cells are in small numbers. The individual septal myocardial cells in HC also frequently show increased amounts of Z-band material and nonspecific changes of cellular hypertrophy and degeneration.[84]

Myocardial fiber disarray in the left and right ventricular free walls is more difficult to determine by light microscopy than that in the ventricular septum. Ultrastructural examination of the left and right ventricular free walls, however, has disclosed many bizarrely shaped, disorganized cells in the ventricular free walls of patients *without* obstruction whereas the bizarrely shaped and disorganized myocardial fibers are virtually entirely absent from the ventricular free walls in the patients *with* obstruction.[81,82] Thus, the disorientation of groups of myocardial cells and the disarray of myofibrils and myofilaments within individual myocardial cells is not the result of left ventricular outflow obstruction or high intraventricular systolic pressures.

433

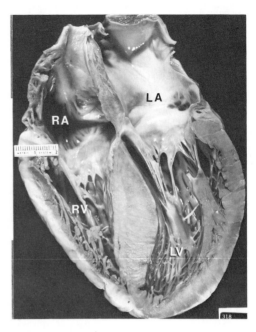

Figure 27. *Hypertrophic cardiomyopathy* (HC) in a 16-year-old girl who was always asymptomatic and died suddenly while jogging. Her mother had HC and three of her four siblings died suddenly. HC had been demonstrated clinically in each of them. The present patient by echocardiograms had systolic anterior motion of the anterior mitral leaflet, an ejection fraction of 87 percent, and no evidence of left ventricular outflow obstruction. She had no precordial murmur. The electrocardiogram had shown narrow Q waves in II, III, and AVF. The heart weighed 310 gm. and the ventricular septum was twice as thick as the left ventricular free wall (19 to 9 mm.). The left ventricular free wall was actually of normal thickness. RA = right atrium; RV = right ventricle; LA = left atrium; LV = left ventricle.

The functional or clinical significance of "septal disorganization" among patients with HC is not entirely clear. Among the patients studied at necropsy by Maron and associates,[83] those with high percentages of disorganization in the septal area were younger, had a higher frequency of premature deaths involving more than one member of the same family,[85,86] and thicker ventricular septa than those with lower percentages. A comparison of the presence or degree of left ventricular outflow obstruction, length of symptoms of cardiac dysfunction, mode of death, arrhythmias, etc., revealed no significant difference between the patients with high percentages and those with low percentages of septal area disorganization.[83]

Another abnormality of ventricular septum with HC is the presence of *abnormal intramural coronary arteries,* found in about one half of the patients[80] (Fig. 31). The abnormalities observed in the intramural coronary arteries in these patients are striking and consist of increased number and size of arteries with thickened walls and narrowed lumens. The thickening results from proliferation of smooth-muscle cells and collagen in both the media and the intima. Also, mucoid deposits (acid mucopolysaccaride material) are more numerous. Like disproportionate septal thickening (causing ventricular asymmetry) and septal disorganization, however, abnormality of the intramural coronary arteries is not specific for HC, though it is certainly more striking in HC than in most other conditions. Similar abnormality of the intramural coronary arteries may be observed in patients and in Newfoundland dogs with discrete subaortic stenosis,[66] in patients with tunnel subaortic stenosis,[67] and in newborns with aortic-valve atresia.[87]

The significance of the changes in the intramural coronary arteries in patients with HC is unknown. Their presence or absence does not correlate with any analyzed clinical parameter including age, sex, presence or degree of left ventricular outflow tract obstruction, presence of cardiac dysfunction including chest pain, or length of symptoms of cardiac dysfunction.

The cause of the striking abnormalities of the intramural coronary arteries also is uncertain. In each of the four conditions in which this degree of abnormality have been observed, namely, HC, discrete and tunnel subaortic stenosis and aortic-valve atresia, the septum is extremely thick and movement of the septum during life as shown by

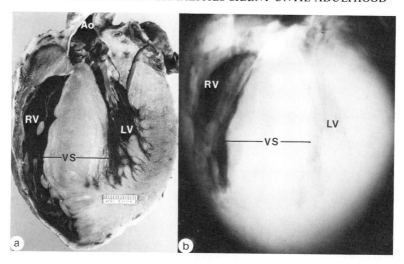

Figure 28. *Hypertrophic asymmetric obstructive* (right-sided) *cardiomyopathy.* This 18-year-old boy described in detail in the text was first studied when he was asymptomatic at age eight; his brother had died suddenly at age nine from idiopathic hypertrophic subaortic stenosis (left-sided obstruction). At catheterization no systolic pressure gradient was observed between the left ventricle and the systemic artery, but a systolic pressure gradient of 35 mm. Hg was recorded between the right ventricle (56/5) and the pulmonary artery (21/9). An electrocardiogram showed right axis deviation, right ventricular hypertrophy, and a right ventricular conduction delay. The child remained asymptomatic until age 12, when he developed chest pain while playing football. Precordial pain recurred frequently thereafter and was precipitated by exertion of decreasing intensity so that he was forced to limit his activities to a sedentary level. When he was restudied at age 13, a grade 1/6 systolic ejection-type precordial murmur was heard which was loudest along the left sternal border. Electrocardiography now showed more severe right ventricular hypertrophy. Cardiac catheterization showed a peak systolic pressure gradient of 118 mm. Hg between the right ventricle (135/7) and pulmonary artery (17/7) and there was no systolic gradient between the left ventricle (108/4) and the brachial artery (108/63 mm. Hg). Resection of the right ventricular outflow myocardium with insertion of a patch at the right ventriculuotomy was performed, and catheterization seven months postoperatively showed virtually no systolic pressure gradient between the right ventricle (30/4 mm. Hg) and the pulmonary artery (28/12). He was asymptomatic. Electrocardiograms now showed a right bundle branch block. This boy apparently remained asymptomatic until the day of death, when he felt faint while driving a car. He pulled over to the side of the road and collapsed. No anatomic explanation for death was revealed at necropsy. His heart weighed 660 gm. The right ventricular (RV) outflow tract was wide open. The ventricular septum (VS) was much thicker than the left ventricular (LV) free wall (1.0 compared to 1.9 cm.), and the right ventricular wall was of normal thickness. The endocardium of the left ventricular outflow tract was not thickened and the mitral valve was normal. Mild interstitial fibrosis involved the ventricular septum. *a,* A longitudinal section of the ventricles shows the disproportionate ventricular septal hypertrophy. The right ventricular cavity is larger than the left. Ao = Aorta. *b,* The radiograph of the heart was taken before it was opened.

echocardiogram is extremely limited. It is possible that the severe septal thickening prevents adequate expansion of these vessels during ventricular diastole and thus reduces flow. The fibrous-smooth muscle cell response, in turn, may serve to obliterate the unused lumen. However, this explanation does not explain the large size of these arteries. It is possible that the proliferation of the smooth-muscle cells in the walls of these arteries represents a response to the same stimulus which is causing severe hypertrophy and abnormal configuration of many striated myocardial cells.

A fourth abnormality of the ventricular septum in adults with HC is the occurrence of a fibrous plaque on the mural endocardium of the outflow portion of the septum[77] (Fig. 24). This fibrous thickening is located in direct apposition to the ventricular aspect of the anterior mitral leaflet and is the result of contact between the valvular and mural endocardium. The mural plaque, in other words, is the anatomic equivalent of the "systolic anterior motion" (SAM) of the anterior mitral leaflet observed on echocar-

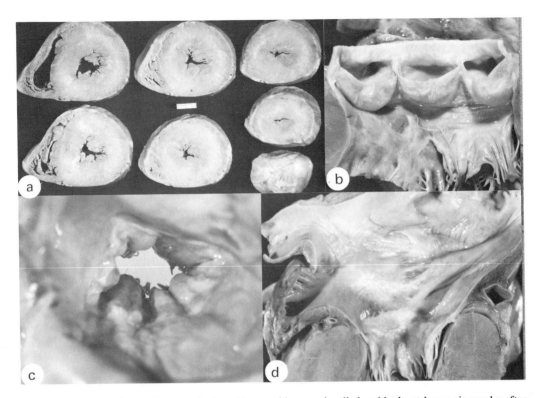

Figure 29. *Hypertrophic cardiomyopathy* in a 53-year-old man who died suddenly at home six weeks after onset of atrial fibrillation. Catheterization when he was asymptomatic (but had cardiomegaly) at age 46 disclosed a left ventricular to systemic arterial peak systolic gradient of 8 mm. Hg at rest, and a gradient of 69 mm. Hg with provocation (isoproterenol). Thereafter, he developed exertional dyspnea, dizziness, and angina. *a,* "Bread loaf" slices of cardiac ventricles. Although the echocardiogram had shown the ventricular septum to be thicker than left ventricular free wall during ventricular diastole, both were of similar thickness at necropsy (25 mm.). *b,* Opened aortic valve showing thickening of the mural endocardium in apposition to the thickened anterior mitral leaflet. *c,* View of mitral valve from left atrium. Thickening of its leaflets is typical of hypertrophic cardiomyopathy. *d,* Opened left atrium and thickened mitral valve. The basal portion of left ventricular wall is rounded and thick.

diogram in patients with HC and occasionally in other conditions.[76] When present in HC, the obstruction almost certainly begins at a level corresponding to the distal margin of the anterior mitral leaflet and with the caudal margin of the septal endocardial plaque. The mural endocardial septal plaque is present more frequently and is thicker in the patients with obstruction at rest compared to those without obstruction at rest.

It appears that HC is primarily a disease of the ventricular septum and that the morphologic abnormalities in it are apparent at the gross, microscopic, and ultrastructural levels. Other portions of the heart, however, are affected in HC but it seems likely that these other abnormalities are secondary to the abnormalities of the ventricular septum. These other abnormalities include *decreased ventricular cavity size* or, at least, lack of ventricular cavity dilatation, *increased atrial cavity size,* varying degrees of interstitial and replacement *myocardial fibrosis* (particularly in the ventricular septum), thickening of the posterior as well as the anterior mitral leaflet and, in elderly patients, calcification of the mitral anulus.[77,88,89]

The cause of the relatively small size of ventricular cavities in HC is unclear. The septum, being on the average about twice normal thickness, surely occupies space normally represented by cavity. The ventricular free walls are, on the average, about a

436

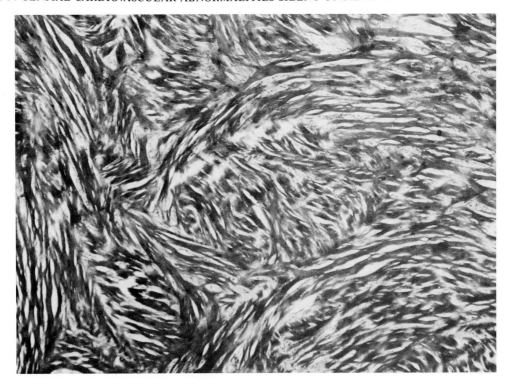

Figure 30. Photomicrograph of portion of ventricular septum in a 19-year-old man with *hypertrophic cardiomyopathy* showing the myocardial fiber disarray typical of this condition. (Masson stain; x 60 magnification)

third thicker than normal; this probably compromises slightly the intracavitary space even further. The greater thickness of the septum makes it relatively noncompliant (as demonstrated by its absent or minimal movement on echocardiogram). Although the left ventricular free wall in HC (by echocardiogram) usually contracts vigorously (in contrast to the septum), it appears to have little capacity to distend outwardly. Whatever the explanation, ventricular cavity size is rarely enlarged in these patients. The patients I have studied with dilated ventricular cavities at necropsy (4 of 65 with HC) have either nonscarred left and/or right ventricular free walls of normal thickness or scarred ventricular free walls of less than normal thickness. Dilatation may occur after operative septotomy-septectomy in HC.[90]

The impression of ventricular cavity size as observed at necropsy in patients with HC may be somewhat misleading because the cavity at necropsy in patients with HC represents the size at the end of ventricular systole.[91] This information was derived by comparing the left ventricular free wall thickness at necropsy to that measured by echocardiogram during life.[91] The thickness at necropsy corresponds to the thickness during ventricular systole, not diastole, which is observed by echocardiogram.

In contrast to the ventricular cavities, the atrial cavities in HC, at least in adults, are always dilated. The dilatation appears to be a response to difficulty in filling the relatively small ventricular caivities.

Not only is the anterior mitral leaflet thickened, but often (more frequently in the patients with obstruction) the posterior mitral leaflet too is thickened. The thickening of both leaflets is probably the consequence of the small left ventricular cavity. It is important to recall that the mitral valve resides in the left ventricle, which because of its

437

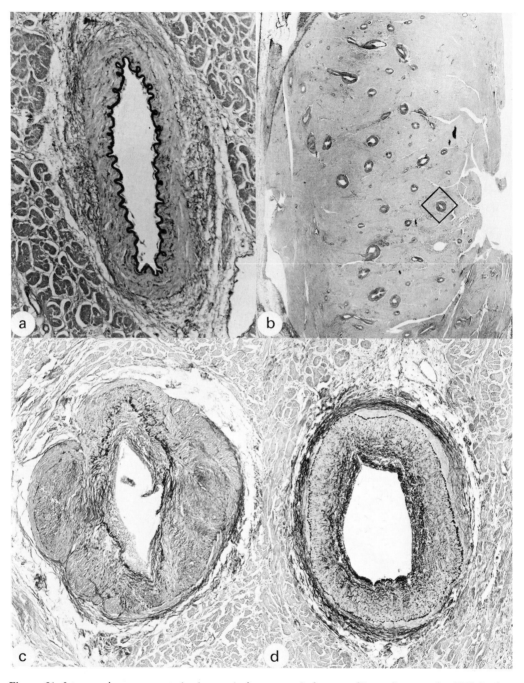

Figure 31. *Intramural coronary arteries in ventricular septum in hypertrophic cardiomyopathy* (HC) *in three different patients. a,* A normal artery (in a patient with HC) x 140. *b,* Low-power (x 4) photomicrograph of portion of ventricular septum showing marked prominence of the intramural coronary arteries in another patient. The arteries appear to be increased in number, size, and wall thickness. *c,* The artery enclosed by the box in *b* is shown here x 90. *d,* This artery, from another patient, has marked intimal thickening by fibroelastic proliferation, in contrast to the artery shown in *c,* which shows no delineation between intima and media. (Elastic van Gieson stains.) (Reduced 18%.)

438

small size, causes abnormal contact of the leaflets with themselves and also causes the anterior one to contact the septum. In the patients without obstruction, the basal portion of the left ventricular cavity is larger than in the patients with obstruction because of the thinning of the basal portion of free wall posteriorly and laterally. The focal fibrous thickening of the posterior mitral leaflet probably results from abnormal contact during ventricular systole since there is not enough room in the ventricular cavity to easily accommodate the leaflets and chordae. In this respect the ventricle and mitral leaflets mimic the movement of an accordion. The mitral leaflet thickening in HC is somewhat analogous to that which occurs normally as a consequence of aging. With aging, the left ventricular cavity becomes smaller, presumably in response to the lowered cardiac output; the mitral leaflets thicken; the left ventricular muscle becomes less compliant; and the left atrium dilates in response to increased work required to fill the small left ventricle. The same mechanisms appear to be accelerated in HC.

Most patients with HC have some degree of mitral regurgitation. It is not related to anular dilatation because the mitral anulus in this condition is not dilated.[78] Furthermore, the leaflet thickening in and of itself is not extensive enough to cause valvular regurgitation. The most likely explanation appears to be abnormal bending of the papillary muscles, particularly the anterolateral one.[69] These structures may be bent abnormally by the bulging ventricular septum with resulting excessive tension on the chordae tendineae preventing closure of the mitral orifice. Although they are usually present in the papillary muscles in HC, focal scars cannot account for the regurgitation. Although it is usually mild in HC, mitral regurgitation may be the predominant clinical feature of this condition. Despite advocacy by some investigators,[92,93] mitral valve replacement in HC is hazardous and unwarranted for a number of reasons.[94] The small left ventricular cavity is rarely capable of freely accommodating a prosthesis, and the mitral regurgitation in patients with HC nearly always either disappears or is strikingly lessened by adequate partial septectomy-septotomy.

SINUS OF VALSALVA ANEURYSM

Dilatation of each of the three sinuses of Valsalva is a normal consequence of aging and this "senile-type dilatation" appears to be more common in hypertensive than in normotensive persons.[21] In addition to aging, there are at least three other causes of dilatation of each of the three sinuses of Valsalva; these are the Marfan and Marfan-like syndromes,[14] syphilis,[95] and ankylosing spondylitis.[96,97] A congenital type of dilatation of all three aortic sinuses unassociated with other congenital anomalies of the heart or great vessels also has been recorded,[98] but its occurrence, if indeed of congenital origin, must be unique.

In contrast to the common occurrence of dilatation of all three aortic sinuses, aneurysmal dilatation of only one or two of the three sinuses is quite unusual (Figs. 32 to 34). The most common cause is probably infective endocarditis with spread of the infective process into adjacent structures and formation of one or more ring abscesses.[99] Aneurysmal dilatation of only one aortic sinus unassociated with infective endocarditis is extremely rare. In this circumstance the localized aneurysmal dilatation is generally attributed to a congenital absence of media in the wall of the aorta behind the sinus of Valsalva[100] (Fig. 35). The wall of aorta behind the sinus may rupture, and when this occurs, aortic regurgitation into either right ventricle or right atrium is the usual consequence (Fig. 33). Less commonly, the sinus aneurysm may obstruct right ventricular outflow or cause a conduction disturbance.[101]

The basic defect in patients with aneurysms involving only one or two of the three aortic valve sinuses is an absence of a portion or all of the media in the wall of aorta behind the sinus. Just because the media is deficient, however, does not assure the

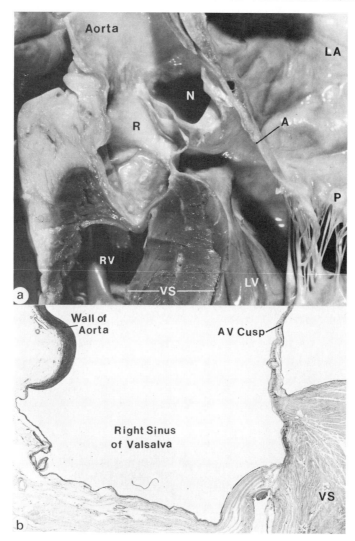

Figure 32. *Unruptured sinus of Valsalva aneurysm* in an 82-year-old man who died of cancer. An unexpected finding at necropsy was aneurysmal dilatation of the right sinus of Valsalva. The right sinus was 2.5 cm. deep and held 15 ml. of fluid, while the left and noncoronary sinuses of Valsalva were only 1.5 cm. deep and held only 5 ml. of fluid.

a, Longitudinal section of heart showing the aneurysmal dilatation of the right (R) sinus of Valsalva. N = noncoronary sinus of Valsalva; A, P = anterior and posterior mitral leaflets, respectively; LA = left atrium; LV = left ventricle; VS = ventricular septum. *b*, Histologic section of wall of right sinus of Valsalva showing the absence of aortic media in the caudal portion of the aneurysm. AV = aortic valve.

appearance of an aortic sinus aneurysm. When a deficiency of aortic media occurs, the wall involved most commonly is that behind the right anterior cusp (about 70 percent of patients); occasionally it is the portion behind the noncoronary (posterior) cusp (about 29 percent); it rarely (< 1%) involves that portion behind the left anterior cusp.[102] The explanation for these differences is uncertain.

Whether or not a sinus of Valsalva aneurysm is ever present from birth is uncertain; most likely the aneurysm is acquired, presumably the result of the aortic pressure. The higher the aortic pressure (for example, in patients with coarctation of the aortic

440

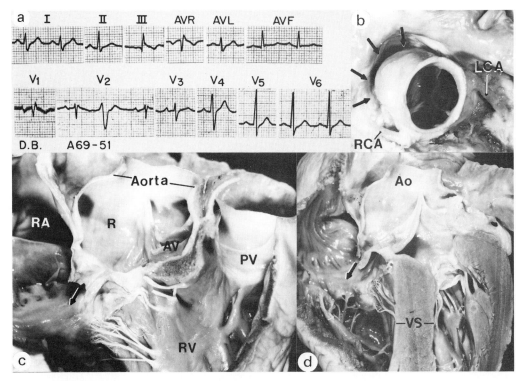

Figure 33. *Rupture of right (R) sinus of Valsalva aneurysm into right ventricle* (RV) in a 31-year-old woman who had been well until about 60 days before death when exertional dyspnea appeared. Eighteen days before death, she developed acute pulmonary edema and a murmur of aortic regurgitation. She died of progressive congestive cardiac failure. *a,* An electrocardiogram taken several days before her death. At necropsy the heart weighed only 300 gm. *b,* An aneurysm of the right sinus of Valsalva was present and bulged to the right (arrows). LCA, RCA = left and right coronary arteries, respectively. *c,* Opened right ventricle (RV) and wall of aorta behind right (R) sinus of Valsalva showing the aneurysm which had ruptured (arrow) into the right atrium (RA) anatomically and into right ventricle functionally. AV = aortic valve; PV = pulmonic valve. *d,* In this view the anterior half of the heart has been removed; the ruptured (arrow) aneurysm's relation to the right side of the heart and to the ventricular septum (VS) is apparent. Ao = aorta.

isthmus), the more likely is the possibility that an aortic sinus aneurysm will develop. The youngest child described with isolated sinus of Valsalva aneurysm was four years old.[103] Although the aneurysm itself may or may not be congenital, the deficiency in aortic media behind the sinus must be congenital.[101]

Both the natural history and the frequency of media-deficient aortic sinus wall are uncertain. The number of persons with a media-deficient aortic sinus wall in whom a sinus aneurysm developed is uncertain, as is the frequency of rupture of a developed sinus aneurysm. Among 78 cases of sinus of Valsalva aneurysm collected from previous publications by Kieffer and Winchell,[104] 59 (76 percent) had ruptured and 19 (24 percent) had not. In some of these cases, however, the aneurysms involved all three sinuses and were therefore probably associated with the Marfan syndrome. Among seven hearts with aneurysm of one aortic sinus studied at necropsy by Edwards and Burchell,[100] four aneurysms had ruptured and three had not. Of six single (one of three sinuses involved) aortic sinus aneurysms which I studied at necropsy, five had ruptured and only one[101] was unruptured. The latter patient was 82 years old; the five patients with ruptured aneurysms ranged in age from 31 to 49 years (average, 38). These figures indicate that among reported cases of aortic sinus aneurysm, rupture is more common than nonrupture. These data are probably considerably biased in favor of ruptured aneurysms;

441

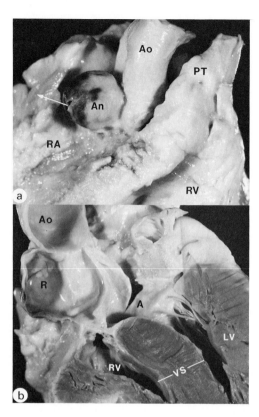

Figure 34. *Rupture of right sinus of Valsalva aneurysm into pericardial sac* in a 33-year-old woman who had been well until she died suddenly while house cleaning. At necropsy the pericardial sac was filled with blood. *a,* The right sinus of Valsalva is exteriorly round and a rupture (arrow) is visible in its right lateral wall. Extravasation was into the pericardial space only and not into a cardiac chamber. An = aneurysm; Ao = aorta; PT = pulmonary trunk; RA = right atrium; RV = right ventricle. *b,* The anterior portion of the heart has been removed again showing the right (R) sinus of Valsalva aneurysm. A = anterior mitral leaflet; LV = left ventricle; VS = ventricular septum.

nonruptured sinus aneurysm may be missed at necropsy, while the nonruptured aneurysm, with few exceptions, produces no evidence of cardiac dysfunction. Therefore, at necropsy there may be no clinical sign or symptom to alert the pathologist to the presence of an aortic sinus aneurysm. Furthermore, incidental necropsy findings, which an aortic sinus aneurysm usually represents, are infrequently reported. Thus, it

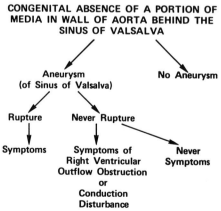

Figure 35. Diagram showing possible outcome in patients with *congenital absence of a portion of media in aortic wall behind sinus of Valsalva.* If no aneurysm occurs, the congenital defect will go unrecognized. If an aneurysm does occur it may or may not rupture. Rupture will virtually always produce clinical symptoms and signs of cardiac dysfunction. If rupture does not occur, symptoms will usually be present only if there is right ventricular outflow obstruction or conduction disturbances.

442

is likely that the frequency of unruptured aortic sinus aneurysm is considerably greater than has been reported.

On rare occasion an unruptured single aortic sinus aneurysm may produce evidence of cardiac dysfunction. Kerber and associates[105] described clinical and operative findings in a 62-year-old man who had evidence of right ventricular outflow obstruction as the result of an aortic sinus aneurysm's bulging into the crista supraventricularis. Complete heart block has also been described in a patient with unruptured aortic sinus aneurysm.[106] The latter patient, however, also had calcific aortic stenosis, and thus it is not certain that the sinus aneurysm was responsible for the conduction defect.

Rupture of the sinus of Valsalva aneurysm is clearly the most frequent complication of aneurysm involving only one of the three aortic sinuses. Rupture rarely occurs before adulthood. Like all conditions affecting the aorta and the aortic valve, it is more common in males than females (about 4 to 1). Death occurs suddenly if the rupture is into the pericardial space rather than into a cardiac cavity (Fig. 34). Death usually occurs, however, within a year after rupture with regurgitation into a cardiac chamber. Death most commonly is the result of congestive cardiac failure.

THE MARFAN SYNDROME

This inheritable disorder may involve the bones, joints, eyes, heart, and blood vessels. The extremities are long and thin (dolichostenomelia), the ligaments and joint capsules are redundant, the lenses may be dislocated (ectopia lentis), the ascending aorta often is dilated, and one or both left-sided cardiac valves usually are incompetent. Cardiovascular disease is by far the most common cause of death in patients with the Marfan syndrome. Of 18 patients that I studied at necropsy, all fulfilled McKusick's rigid criteria for this syndrome,[107] and all died prematurely from cardiovascular disease (average age, 34; range, 15 to 52). Of 56 decreased patients with this syndrome studied by Murdoch and associates,[108] cardiovascular disease was the cause of death in 52 (93 percent) and the average age at death was 32 years.

A variety of cardiovascular lesions have been observed in the aorta and heart of patients with the Marfan syndrome.[107] The 18 necropsy patients with this syndrome just

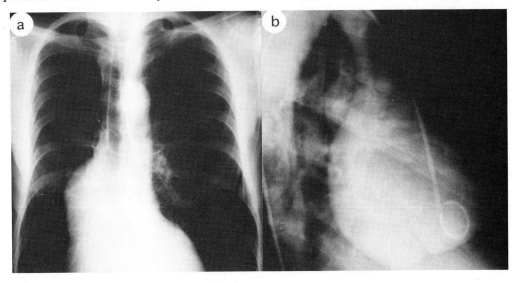

Figure 36. Chest radiograph *(a)* and aortogram *(b)* in a 38-year-old man with *Marfan syndrome.* A large aortic "root" aneurysm is present. (see Figure 37 for additional findings in this patient)

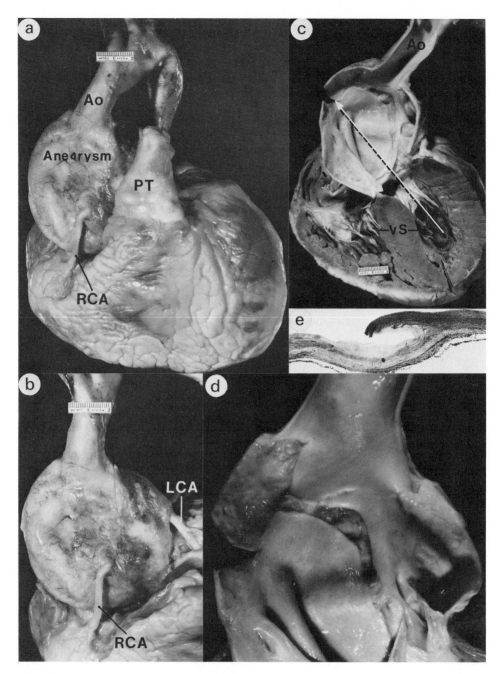

Figure 37. *The Marfan syndrome with rupture of ascending aortic aneurysm* in a 38-year-old black man. The patient was known to have a murmur of aortic regurgitation (aortic pressure 115/55 mm. Hg) but there was no evidence of congestive heart failure. He died suddenly at home and at necropsy the pericardial space was filled with blood and a tear was present in a large aneurysm involving all three sinuses of Valsalva and the proximal tubular portion of ascending aorta. *a,* View of heart shows the size of the aneurysm in comparison to the sizes of other structures. Ao = aorta; PT = pulmonary trunk; RCA = right coronary artery. *b,* A closer view of the large aneurysm with the coronary arteries arising from it. LCA = left coronary artery. *c,* The anterior half of the heart and aorta have now been removed. The dashed line depicts the direction of the blood ejected from the left ventricle. The arrow points to the rupture site in the wall of the aneurysm. The right lateral wall is the site of the rupture. VS = ventricular septum. *d,* Closeup of interior lining of aortic aneurysm at site of rupture. Several healed incomplete tears are present in the wall of the aneurysm and these have been confused with aortic dissections. *e,* Photomicrograph through one of the aortic tears showing massive degeneration of elastic fibers.

mentioned were readily separated into three distinct groups on the basis of their cardiovascular lesions. Group 1 included 12 patients with *saccular aneurysms of ascending aorta* (Figs. 36 to 38). All 12 patients had aortic regurgitation and 6 of them also had associated mitral regurgitation. Their aneurysms involved the sinus portion and the proximal tubular portion of ascending aorta, and two also had saccular aneurysms in the descending thoracic aorta. Histologic study of the wall of the ascending aorta disclosed the typical lesion of this syndrome, i.e., massive degeneration of elastic fibers and increase in mucoid material in the media (Fig. 38).

Group 2 included three patients with *dissection of the entire aorta* (Fig. 39). Before dissection, the aorta was of normal size in all three patients, and histologic study of the aortic wall disclosed that the typical lesion of this syndrome was absent; in fact, except for the dissection itself, the wall of aorta was histologically normal save for some aging changes.[109,110] Only one of the three patients had aortic regurgitation and then only after the dissection; one had mitral regurgitation and two had systemic hypertension before the aortic dissection.

Group 3 included two patients *without aortic saccular aneurysm or aortic disease* but with *pure mitral regurgitation* with floppy mitral leaflets and markedly dilated mitral anuli (Fig. 6). The aorta was of normal size and its wall was histologically normal in both.

Thus, the major lesions in the aorta in patients with this syndrome are saccular root aneurysms and dissection. In contrast to that described clinically by others,[111] our study of 18 necropsy patients suggests that the two rarely go together, since none of these patients had both a saccular aortic aneurysm and aortic dissection. These two aortic lesions may be mutually exclusive. None of the 12 patients with saccular aortic root aneurysms had evidence of dissection, although 9 of the 12 had focal intimal and medial tears in the wall of the saccular aneurysms (Figs. 37 and 38). These aortic tears have been mistakenly called "dissections" in a number of reports. None of the three with aortic dissection had saccular aneurysms of the aorta which was of normal size before the dissection. Histologically, the wall of the aorta varies with the type of lesion. In all 12 patients with aortic root saccular aneurysms, there was massive degeneration of the elastic fibers associated with increased amounts of collagen and mucoid material in the media of the aneurysmal wall. The increased amount of collagen in the aortic wall in these patients may actually prevent longitudinal dissection. In each of the three patients with aortic dissection, the wall of the aorta appeared histologically "normal," i.e., as it does in patients with aortic dissection who do not have the Marfan syndrome,[112] with no changes other than aging. Interestingly, two of the three patients with aortic dissection had evidence of diastolic systemic hypertension, whereas none of the other 16 patients had diastolic hypertension.

The term applied to the characteristic histologic lesion in the aorta in patients with the Marfan syndrome has been "cystic medial necrosis," a term first used by Erdheim in 1929[113] and an outgrowth of the term "medionecrosis" coined by Gsell[114] a year earlier. This term, however, is not ideal because "cysts" as such are infrequent and "necrosis," to my knowledge, has never been observed in the aortic media in this condition. Gsell used the term "medionecrosis" to designate areas in the aortic media with a diminished number of nuclei. Becker[109] recently showed that these areas devoid of nuclei actually consisted of large amounts of fibrous tissue and were a regular feature of the normal, aging aorta. Furthermore, the striking histologic aortic lesion in the Marfan syndrome is *massive degeneration of elastic fibers* in the media and this feature is ignored by the term "cystic medial necrosis." When Erdheim coined this term, stains for elastic fibers were poor or rarely used, and loss or degeneration of elastic fibers are difficult to appreciate on hematoxylin-eosin stained sections. Thus, he apparently could not appreciate this histologic feature of this condition.

445

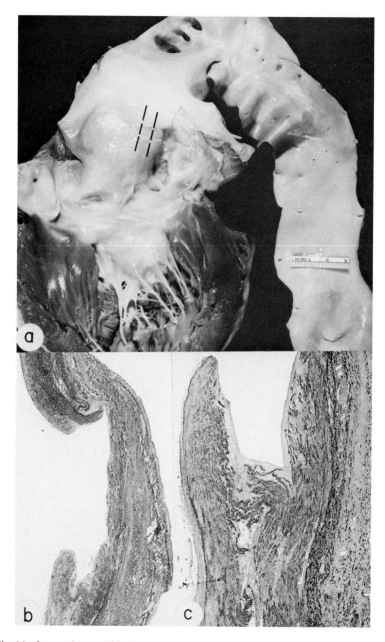

Figure 38. *The Marfan syndrome.* This 21-year-old man had the typical skeletal and optic features of this syndrome but had always been asymptomatic. He was found dead in his parked car after playing in a band for several hours. At necropsy the pericardial sac was filled with blood. *a,* Evidence of a through-and-through rupture is visible in the ascending aorta just above the aortic valve. In addition, several partial ruptures or tears are also present in the ascending aorta. *b,* A histologic section of one tear (shown between dashed lines in *a*). *c,* A closeup of an adjacent section of *b* reveals severe degeneration of elastic fibers of the media. (Elastic tissue stains; *b,* x 7 and *c,* x 18 magnification)

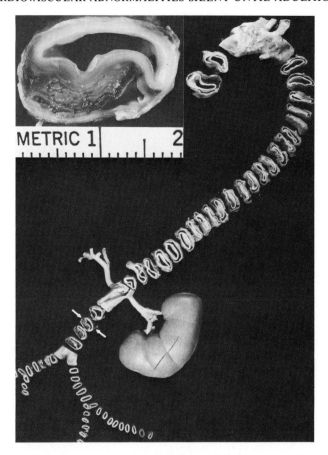

Figure 39. *Aorta* in a 43-year-old man known to have *Marfan syndrome*. He died 15 days after the sudden onset of typical clinical features of *aortic dissection*. Before the aortic dissection there was no precordial murmur. At necropsy, except for the acute dissection, there was no enlargement of the aorta, and except at the site of the entrance into the false channel, there were no tears in the aorta. Shown here is the complete aorta with both true and false channels and a hematoma in the false channel of the abdominal portion. A closeup of the transverse section indicated by the arrows is shown in the upper left. Histologically, there was no evidence of elastic fiber degeneration in the media of aorta. The heart weighed 500 gm. and neither ventricle was dilated. Thus, although this patient had both aortic dissection and Marfan syndrome, the typical histologic aortic medial lesion of this syndrome was absent. Therefore, it is more likely that the systemic hypertension was a more important contributing factor to the aortic dissection.

When elastic fibers disappear from the aortic wall in this condition, the space previously occupied by them appears to be replaced by collagen fibrils and mucoid material. Although the increased acid mucopolysaccharide material has been considered an inherent defect in this condition, it is just as reasonable to believe that this material serves simply as "a filler" for the lost elastic fibers and even smooth muscle cells. It is not clear whether or not the numbers of the elastic lamellae are normal or decreased at the time of birth in patients with the Marfan syndrome; however, aortic root aneurysm, with or without tears, has not been described in newborns with this syndrome. Thus, it appears that although the composition of the aortic media may be defective at birth, the aneurysms form later, presumably as a consequence of intra-aortic pressure on an inherently weak wall. The possible consequences of the inherently or congenitally weakened aortic media is shown diagrammatically in Figure 40.

Aortic regurgitation in patients with the Marfan syndrome is usually the result of

447

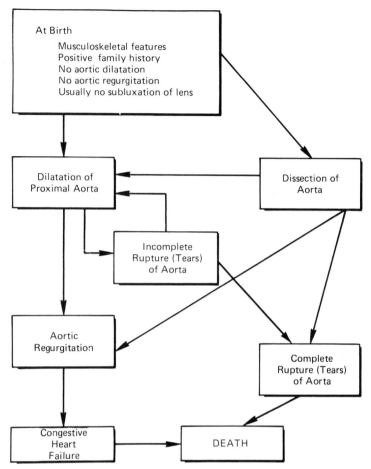

Figure 40. *The Marfan syndrome.* Schema of development of the aortic complications.

severe dilatation of the aortic "root" by the saccular aneurysm. The amount of regurgitation may not, however, correlate directly with the size of the aortic root aneurysm.[111] The aortic regurgitation is the consequence of aortic dissection even less commonly. The aortic valve cusps in patients with the Marfan syndrome appear to have an increased amount of mucoid material (acid mucopolysaccharide), irrespective of the presence of aortic regurgitation.

Mitral regurgitation also is frequent. At least five factors may be important in causing mitral regurgitation in patients with this syndrome. These are (1) floppiness of the mitral leaflets and/or chordae tendineae, (2) dilatation of the mitral anuli, (3) calcification of the mitral anuli, (4) rupture of mitral chordae tendineae, and (5) papillary muscle dysfunction. Of these factors, the first three appear to cause the most severe mitral regurgitation. Of the necropsy patients mentioned, 9 had mitral regurgitation: it was isolated in two and combined with aortic regurgitation in seven. Six of the nine with mitral regurgitation had floppy mitral valves and none of the nine without mitral regurgitation had floppy valves. The "floppiness" involved the posterior mitral leaflet in all six patients. Furthermore, of the nine patients with mitral regurgitation, the circumference of the mitral anulus ranged from 10 to 17 cm. (average, 15 cm.; normal, 9 cm.); of the nine patients without mitral regurgitation this circumference ranged from 9 to 12.5 cm. (average, 11 cm.). In the six patients with floppy mitral valves, the mitral circumference ranged from 14 to 17 cm. (average, 16 cm.). Thus, the average circumference of the mitral anulus in the nine patients with mitral regurgitation (15 cm.) was dilated 67 percent over normal (9 cm.) and in the nine patients without mitral regurgitation it was only 22 percent over normal (12 cm.). It therefore seems reasonable to conclude that both mitral leaflet floppiness and anular dilatation play significant roles in causing mitral regurgitation in these patients. Calcification of the mitral anulus is known to cause or at least be associated with mitral regurgitation.[21] The degree of regurgitation produced by this mechanism alone, however, is nearly always mild or minimal, and the mitral anuli in non-Marfan patients with mitral anular calcification is nearly always of normal or near-normal circumference. Of the 18 patients seen, four had mitral anular calcific deposits with associated mitral regurgitation; three also had floppy mitral leaflets. All four showed a mitral anulus which was quite dilated (range, 13 to 17 cm.; average, 15 cm.). Evidence for rupture of mitral chordae tendineae was found in four of the nine patients with mitral regurgitation. Two of these four patients had histories of infective endocarditis which had healed.[38] All four patients with evidence of mitral chordae rupture had floppy mitral leaflets and dilated mitral anuli (range, 15 to 17 cm.; average, 16 cm.).

The role played by "papillary muscle dysfunction" in causing mitral regurgitation in these patients is less clear.[115] All our 18 patients had dilated left ventricles and all had increased left ventricular masses. The hearts of the 18 patients ranged in weight from 375 to 850 gm. (average, 654 gm.). In 13 of the 18 patients the mitral leaflets were elongated from their basal attachments to their distal margins. This "stretching" probably was the result of the elongation (apex to base) of the left ventricular cavities, resulting primarily from the associated aortic regurgitation. The resulting left ventricular dilatation may have altered the normal angulation between the papillary muscles and the mitral leaflets. Whether or not mitral regurgitation was increased by this mechanism is uncertain.

Although the foregoing discussion concerns only patients with typical features of the Marfan syndrome, the cardiovascular features described in them also occur in patients without the skeletal or ocular manifestations of this syndrome or with histories of this syndrome in other family members. In addition, the characteristic histologic features in the wall of ascending aorta also have been observed in the aorta of patients with congenitally malformed aortic valves, particularly the bicuspid condition, and in patients with aortic stenosis when superimposed on congenitally malformed valves.[116,117] In individuals with the characteristic ascending aortic root aneurysms and histologic evidence of massive elastic-fiber degeneration of aortic media, features of the Marfan syndrome are more often absent than present.

REFERENCES

1. BARLOW, J. B., POCOCK, W. A., MARCHAND, P., ET AL.: *The significance of late systolic murmurs.* Am. Heart J. 66:443,1963.

2. BARLOW, J. B., AND BOSMAN, C. K.: *Aneurysmal protrusion of the posterior leaflet of the mitral valve: an auscultatory-electrocardiographic syndrome.* Am. Heart J. 71:166,1965.

3. CRILEY, J. M., LEWIS, K. B., HUMPHRIES, J. O., ET AL.: *Prolapse of the mitral valve: clinical and cine-angiocardiographic findings.* Br. Heart J. 28:488,1966.

4. STANNARD, M., SLOMAN, J. G., HARE, W. S., ET AL.: *Prolapse of the posterior leaflet of the mitral valve. A clinical, familial and cineangiographic study.* Br. Med. J. 3:71,1967.

5. BARLOW, J. B., BOSMAN, C. K., POCOCK, W. A., ET AL.: *Late systolic murmurs and non-ejection ('mid-late') systolic clicks: An analysis of 90 patients.* Br. Heart J. 30:203,1968.

6. MARKIEWICZ, W., STONER, J., LONDON, E., ET AL.: *Mitral valve prolapse in one hundred presumably healthy young females.* Circulation 53:464,1976.

7. PROCACCI, P. M., SAVRAN, S. V., SCHREITER, S. L., ET AL.: *Prevalence of clinical mitral-valve prolapse in 1169 young women.* N. Engl. J. Med. 294:1086,1976.

8. PROMERANCE, A.: *Ballooning deformity (mucoid degeneration) of atrioventricular valves.* Br. Heart J. 31:343,1969.

9. SHERMAN, E. B., CHAR, F., DUNGAN, W. T., ET AL.: *Myxomatous transformation of the mitral valve producing mitral insufficiency. Floppy valve syndrome.* Am. J. Dis. Child. 119:171,1970.

10. MCCARTHY, L. J., AND WOLF, P. L.: *Mucoid degeneration of heart valves: Blue valve syndrome.* Am. J. Clin. Pathol. 54:582,1970.

11. DAVIS, R. H., SCHUSTER, B., KNOEBEL, S. B., ET AL.: *Myxomatous degeneration of the mitral valve.* Am. J. Cardiol. 28:449,1971.

12. EDWARDS, J. E.: *Mitral insufficiency resulting from "overshooting" of leaflets.* Circulation 43:606,1971.

13. KERN, W. H., AND TUCKER, B. L.: *Myxoid changes in cardiac valves: pathologic, clinical, and ultrastructural studies.* Am. Heart J. 84:294,1972.

14. ROBERTS, W. C., DANGEL, J. C., AND BULKLEY, B. H.: *Non-rheumatic valvular cardiac disease: a clinicopathologic survey of 27 different conditions causing valvular dysfunction.* Cardiovasc. Clin. 5(2):333,1973.

15. RANGANATHAN, N., SILVER, M. D., ROBINSON, T. I., ET AL.: *Angiographic-morphologic correlation in patients with severe mitral regurgitation due to prolapse of the posterior mitral valve leaflet.* Circulation 48:514,1973.

16. MARSHALL, C. E., AND SHAPPELL, S. D.: *Sudden death and the ballooning posterior leaflet syndrome: detailed anatomic and histochemical investigation.* Arch. Pathol. 98:134,1974.

17. GUTHRIE, R. B., AND EDWARDS, J. E.: *Pathology of the myxomatous mitral valve: nature, secondary changes and complications.* Minn. Med. 59:637,1976.

18. SHRIVASTAVA, S., GUTHRIE, R. B., AND EDWARDS, J. E.: *Prolapse of the mitral valve.* Mod. Concepts Cardiovasc. Dis. 46:57,1977.

19. BULKLEY, B. H., AND ROBERTS, W. C.: *Dilatation of the mitral anulus. A rare cause of mitral regurgitation.* Am. J. Med. 59:457,1975.

20. RENTERIA, V. G., FERRANS, V. J., JONES, M., ET AL.: *Intracellular collagen fibrils in prolapsed ("floppy") human atrioventricular valves.* Lab. Invest. (in press).

21. ROBERTS, W. C., AND PERLOFF, J. K.: *Mitral valvular disease. A clinicopathologic survey of the conditions causing the mitral valve to function abnormally.* Ann. Intern. Med. 77:939,1972.

22. JERESATY, R. M.: *Etiology of the mitral valve prolapse-click syndrome.* Am. J. Cardiol. 36:110,1974.

23. MCDONALD, A., HARRIS, A., JETTERSON, K., ET AL.: *Association of prolapse of posterior cusp of mitral valve and atrial septal defect.* Br. Heart J. 33:383,1971.

24. POCOCK, W. A., AND BARLOW, J. B.: *An association between billowing posterior mitral leaflet syndrome and congenital heart disease, particularly atrial septal defect.* Am. Heart J. 81:720,1971.

25. BETRIU, A., WIGLE, E. D., FELDERHOF, C. H., ET AL.: *Prolapse of the posterior leaflet of the mitral valve associated with secundum atrial septal defect.* Am. J. Cardiol. 35:363,1975.

26. LEACHMAN, R. D., COKKINOS, D. V., AND COOLEY, D. A.: *Association of ostium secundum atrial septal defects with mitral valve prolapse.* Am. J. Cardiol. 38:167,1976.

27. EDYNAK, G. M., AND RAWSON, A. J.: *Ruptured aneurysm of the mitral valve in a Marfan-like syndrome.* Am. J. Cardiol. 11:674,1963.

28. RAGIB, G., JUE, K. L., ANDERSON, R. C., ET AL.: *Marfan's syndrome with mitral insufficiency.* Am. J. Cardiol. 16:127,1965.

29. READ, R. C., THAL, A. P., AND VERNON, E. W.: *Symptomatic valvular myxomatous transformation (the floppy valve syndrome); a possible forme fruste of the Marfan syndrome.* Circulation 32:897,1965.

30. SHANKAR, K. R., HULTGREN, M. K., LAVER, R. M., ET AL.: *Lethal tricuspid and mitral regurgitation in Marfan's syndrome.* Am. J. Cardiol. 20:122,1967.

31. DIETZMAN, R. H., PETER, E. T., WANG, Y., ET AL.: *Mitral insufficiency in Marfan's syndrome. A case report of surgical correction.* Dis. Chest 51:650,1967.

32. CROCKER, D. W.: *Marfan's syndrome confined to the mitral valve region: two cases in siblings.* Am. Heart J. 76:538,1968.

33. GROSSMAN, M., KNOTT, A. P., JR., AND JACOBY, W. J., JR.: *Calcified annulus fibrosis with mitral insufficiency with Marfan's syndrome.* Arch. Intern. Med. 121:561,1968.

34. JORTNER, R., SHAHIN, W., ESHKOL, D., ET AL.: *Cardiovascular manifestations and surgery for Marfan's syndrome.* Dis. Chest 56:24,1969.

35. GOODMAN, D., KIMBIRIS, D., AND LINHART, J. W.: *Chordae tendineae rupture complicating the systolic click-late systolic murmur syndrome.* Am. J. Cardiol. 33:681,1974.

36. LACHMAN, A. S., BRAMWELL-JONES, D. M., LAKIER, J. B., ET AL.: *Infective endocarditis in the billowing mitral leaflet syndrome.* Br. Heart J. 37:326,1975.

450

37. ARNETT, E. N., AND ROBERTS, W. C.: *Active infective endocarditis: a clinicopathologic analysis of 137 necropsy patients.* Curr. Probl. Cardiol. 1(7):1,1976.

38. ROBERTS, W. C., AND BUCHBINDER, N. A.: *Healed left-sided infective endocarditis. A clinicopathologic study of 59 patients.* Am. J. Cardiol. 40:876,1977.

39. DEMARIA, A. N., AMSTERDAM, E. A., VISMARA, L. A., ET AL.: *Arrhythmias in the mitral valve prolapse syndrome. Prevalence, nature and frequency.* Ann. Intern. Med. 84:656,1976.

40. BARNETT, H. J., JONES, M. W., BOUGHNER, D. R., ET AL.: *Cerebral ischemic events associated with prolapsing mitral valve.* Arch. Neurol. 33:777,1976.

41. ROBERTS, W. C.: *Coronary embolism. A review of causes, consequences and diagnostic considerations.* Cardiovasc. Med. 3:699,1978.

42. ROBERTS, W. C.: *Anatomically isolated aortic valvular disease. The case against its being of rheumatic etiology.* Am. J. Med. 49:151,1970.

43. ROBERTS, W. C.: *Valvular, subvalvular, and supravalvular aortic stenosis: morphologic features.* Cardiovasc. Clin. 5(1):97,1973.

44. ROBERTS, W. C., AND VIRMANI, R.: *Aschoff bodies at necropsy in valvular heart disease. Evidence from an analysis of 543 patients over 14 years of age that rheumatic heart disease, at least anatomically, is a disease of the mitral valve.* Circulation 57:803,1978.

45. ROBERTS, W. C., AND MORROW, A. G.: *Congential aortic stenosis produced by a unicommissural valve.* Br. Heart J. 27:505,1965.

46. ROBERTS, W. C., AND ELLIOTT, L. P.: *Lesions complicating the congenitally bicuspid aortic valve. Anatomic and radiographic features.* Radiol. Clin. North Am. 6:409,1968.

47. ROBERTS, W. C.: *The structure of the aortic valve in clinically-isolated aortic stenosis. An autopsy study of 162 patients over 15 years of age.* Circulation 42:91,1970.

48. ROBERTS, W. C.: *The congenitally bicuspid aortic valve. A study of 85 autopsy cases.* Am. J. Cardiol. 26:72,1970.

49. ROBERTS, W. C., PERLOFF, J. K., AND COSTANTINO, T.: *Severe valvular aortic stenosis in patients over 65 years of age. A clinicopathologic study.* Am. J. Cardiol. 27:497,1971.

50. FALCONE, M. W., ROBERTS, W. C., MORROW, A. G., ET AL.: *Congenital aortic stenosis resulting from unicommissural valve. Clinical and anatomic features in twenty-one adult patients.* Circulation 44:272,1971.

51. KARSNER, H. T., AND KOLETSKY, S.: *Calcific Disease of the Aortic Valve.* J. B. Lippincott, Philadelphia, 1947.

52. EDWARDS, J. E.: *Pathologic aspects of cardiac valvular insufficiencies.* Arch. Surg. 77:634,1958.

53. OSLER, W.: *The bicuspid condition of the aortic valves.* Trans. Assoc. Am. Physicians 2:185,1886.

54. GRANT, R. T., WOOD, J. E., AND JONES, T. D.: *Heart valve irregularities in relation to subacute bacterial endocarditis.* Heart 14:247,1928.

55. LEWIS, T., AND GRANT, R. T.: *Observations relating to subacute infective endocarditis. Part 1. Notes on the normal structure of the aortic valve. Part 2. Bicuspid aortic valves of congenital origin. Part 3. Bicuspid aortic valves in subacute infective endocarditis.* Heart 10:21,1923.

56. STARLING, H. J.: *Endocarditis lenta.* Q. J. Med. 16:263,1923.

57. FULTON, M. N., AND LEVINE, S. A.: *Subacute bacterial endocarditis, with special reference to the valvular lesions and previous history.* Am. J. Med. Sci. 183:60,1932.

58. ROBERTS, W. C.: *Characteristics and consequences of infective endocarditis (active or healed or both) learned from morphologic studies.* In Rahimtoola, S. H. (ed.): *Infective Endocarditis,* Grune & Stratton, New York, 1978, pp. 55–123.

59. EDWARDS, J. E.: *The congenital bicuspid aortic valve.* Circulation 23:485,1961.

60. BISHOP, L. F., JR., AND TRUBEK, M.: *Bicuspid aortic valve. A differential study between inflammatory and congenital origin.* J. Tech. Meth. 15:111,1936.

61. KOLETSKY, S.: *Congenital bicuspid aortic valves.* Arch. Intern. Med. 67:129,1941.

62. EDWARDS, J. E.: *Congenital malformations of the heart and great vessels: C. Malformations of the valves.* In Gould, S. E. (ed.): *Pathology of the Heart and Blood Vessels,* ed. 3. Charles C Thomas, Springfield, Ill., 1968, p. 341.

63. FONTANA, R. S., AND EDWARDS, J. E.: *Congenital Cardiac Disease. A Review of 357 Cases Studied Pathologically.* W. B. Saunders, Philadelphia, 1962.

64. MORROW, A. G., FORT, L., III, ROBERTS, W. C., ET AL.: *Discrete subaortic stenosis complicated by aortic valvular regurgitation. Clinical, hemodynamic, and pathologic studies and the results of operative treatment.* Circulation 20:1003,1959.

65. REIS, R. L., PETERSON, L. M., MASON, D. T., ET AL.: *Congenital fixed subvalvular aortic stenosis. An anatomical classification and correlations with operative results.* Circulation 43,44(Suppl. I):11,1971.

66. MUNA, W. F. T., FERRANS, V. J., PIERCE, J. E., ET AL.: *Discrete subaortic stenosis in Newfoundland dogs: association of infective endocarditis.* Am. J. Cardiol. 41:746,1978.

67. MARON, B. J., REDWOOD, D. R., ROBERTS, W. C., ET AL.: *Tunnel subaortic stenosis. Left ventricular outflow tract obstruction produced by fibromuscular tubular narrowing.* Circulation 54:404,1976.

68. TEARE, D.: *Asymmetrical hypertrophy of the heart in young adults.* Br. Heart J. 20:1,1958.

69. EPSTEIN, S. E., HENRY, W. L., CLARK, C. E., ET AL.: *Asymmetric septal hypertrophy.* Ann. Intern. Med. 81:650,1974.

70. MARON, B. J., EDWARDS, J. E., FERRANS, V. J., ET AL.: *Congenital heart malformations associated with disproportionate ventricular septal thickening.* Circulation 52:926,1975.

71. MARON, B. J., CLARK, C. E., HENRY, W. L., ET AL.: *Prevalence and characteristics of disproportionate ventricular septal thickening in patients with acquired or congenital heart disease: echocardiographic and morphologic findings.* Circulation 55:489,1977.

72. MARON, B. J., SAVAGE, D. D., CLARK, C. E., ET AL.: *Prevalence and characteristics of disproportionate ventricular septal thickening in patients with coronary artery disease.* Circulation 57:250,1978.

73. MARON, B. J., VERTER, J., AND KAPUR, S.: *Disproportionate ventricular septal thickening in the developing normal human heart.* Circulation 57:520,1978.

74. MARON, B. J., EDWARDS, J. E., AND EPSTEIN, S. E.: *Disproportionate ventricular septal thickening in patients with systemic hypertension.* Chest 73:466,1978.

75. SPRAY, T. L., MARON, B. J., MORROW, A. G., ET AL.: *A discussion on hypertrophic cardiomyopathy.* Am. Heart J. 95:511,1978.

76. MARON, B. J., GOTTDIENER, J. S., ROBERTS, W. C., ET AL.: *Disproportionate ventricular septal thickening (ASH) with systolic anterior motion of the anterior mitral leaflet secondary to valvular heart disease.* Br. Heart J. (in press).

77. ISNER, J. M., FALCONE, M. W., VIRMANI, R., ET AL.: *Cardiac sarcoma causing "ASH" and simulating coronary heart disease.* Am. J. Med. (in press).

78. ROBERTS, W. C., AND FERRANS, V. J.: *Pathologic anatomy of the cardiomyopathies. Idiopathic dilated and hypertrophic types, infiltrative types, and endomyocardial disease with and without eosinophilia.* Hum. Pathol. 6:287,1975.

79. MARON, B. J., GOTTDIENER, J. S., ROBERTS, W. C., ET AL.: *Left ventricular outflow tract obstruction due to systolic anterior motion of the anterior mitral leaflet in patients with concentric left ventricular hypertrophy.* Circulation 57:527,1978.

80. MCREYNOLDS, R. A., AND ROBERTS, W. C.: *The intramural coronary arteries in hypertrophic cardiomyopathy.* Am. J. Cardiol. 35:120,1975.

81. MARON, B. J., FERRANS, V. J., HENRY, W. L., ET AL.: *Differences in distribution of myocardial abnormalities in patients with obstructive and nonobstructive asymmetric septal hypertrophy (ASH). Light and electron microscopic findings.* Circulation 50:436,1974.

82. HENRY, W. L., CLARK, C. E., ROBERTS, W. C., ET AL.: *Differences in distribution of myocardial abnormalities in patients with obstructive and non-obstructive asymmetric septal hypertrophy (ASH). Echocardiographic and gross anatomic findings.* Circulation 50:447,1974.

83. MARON, B. J., EPSTEIN, S. E., AND ROBERTS, W. C.: *Cardiac muscle cell disorganization in the ventricular septum: evidence from quantitative histology that it is a highly sensitive marker of hypertrophic cardiomyopathy.* Am. J. Cardiol. 41:435,1978.

84. FERRANS, V. J., MORROW, A. G., AND ROBERTS, W. C.: *Myocardial ultrastructure in idiopathic hypertrophic subaortic stenosis. A study of operatively excised left ventricular outflow tract muscle in 14 patients.* Circulation 45:769,1972.

85. MARON, B. J., ROBERTS, W. C., EDWARDS, J. E., ET AL.: *Sudden death in patients with hypertrophic cardiomyopathy. Characterization of 26 patients without functional limitation.* Am. J. Cardiol. 41:803,1978.

86. MARON, B. J., LIPSON, L. C., ROBERTS, W. C., ET AL.: *"Malignant" hypertrophic cardiomyopathy. Identification of a subgroup of families with unusually frequent premature deaths.* Am. J. Cardiol. 41:1133,1978.

87. ROBERTS, W. C., PERRY, L. W., CHANDRA, R. S., ET AL.: *Aortic valve atresia: a new classification based on necropsy study of 73 cases.* Am. J. Cardiol. 37:753,1976.

88. EWY, G. A., MARCUS, F. I., BOHJALIAN, O., ET AL.: *Muscular subaortic stenosis. Clinical and pathologic observations in an elderly patient.* Am. J. Cardiol. 22:126,1968.

89. ROBERTS, W. C.: *Cardiomyopathy and myocarditis: morphologic features.* Adv. Cardiol. 22:184,1978.

90. MERRILL, W. H., HENRY, W. L., MARON, B. J., ET AL.: *Echocardiographic assessment of the left ventricle following myotomy and myectomy for idiopathic hypertrophic subaortic stenosis (IHSS).* Am. J. Cardiol. 41:435,1978.

91. MARON, B. J., HENRY, W. L., ROBERTS, W. C., ET AL.: *Comparison of echocardiographic and necropsy measurements of ventricular wall thicknesses in patients with and without disproportionate septal thickening.* Circulation 55:341,1977.

92. COOLEY, D. A., LEACHMAN, R. D., AND WUKASCH, D. C.: *Diffuse muscular subaortic stenosis: surgical treatment.* Am. J. Cardiol. 31:1,1973.

93. COOLEY, D. A., GRACE, R. R., WUKASCH, D. C., ET AL.: *Replacement and/or repair of the mitral valve as treatment of idiopathic hypertrophic subaortic stenosis.* Cardiovasc. Dis. Bull. Texas Heart Inst. 3:381,1976.

94. ROBERTS, W. C.: *Operative treatment of hypertrophic obstructive cardiomyopathy. The case against mitral valve replacement.* Am. J. Cardiol. 32:377,1973.

95. ROBERTS, W. C.: *Left ventricular outflow tract obstruction and aortic regurgitations.* In Edwards, J. E., LEV, M., and Abell, M. R. (eds.): *The Heart,* Williams & Wilkins, Baltimore, 1974, pp. 110–175.

96. BULKLEY, B. H., AND ROBERTS, W. C.: *Ankylosing spondylitis and aortic regurgitation. Description of the characteristic cardiovascular lesion from study of eight necropsy patients.* Circulation 48:1014,1973.

97. ROBERTS, W. C., HOLLINGSWORTH, J. F., BULKLEY, B. H., ET AL.: *Combined mitral and aortic regurgitation in ankylosing spondylitis. Angiographic and anatomic features.* Am. J. Med. 56:237,1974.

98. POMERANCE, A., AND DAVIES, M. J.: *Congenital aneurysms of all three sinuses of Valsalva.* J. Pathol. Bacteriol. 89:607,1965.

99. ARNETT, E. N., AND ROBERTS, W. C.: *Valve ring abscess in active infective endocarditis. Frequency, location, and clues to clinical diagnosis from the study of 95 necropsy patients.* Circulation 54:140,1976.

100. EDWARDS, J. E., AND BURCHELL, M. B.: *Specimen exhibiting the essential lesion in aneurysm of the aortic sinus.* Mayo Clin. Proc. 31:407,1956.

101. FISHBEIN, M. C., OBMA, R., AND ROBERTS, W. C.: *Unruptured sinus of Valsalva aneurysm.* Am. J. Cardiol. 35:918,1975.

102. SAKAKIBARA, S., AND KONNO, S.: *Congenital aneurysm of the sinus of Valsalva. Anatomy and classification.* Am. Heart J. 63:405,1962.

103. FOWLER, R. E. L., AND BEVEL, H. H.: *Aneurysms of the sinus of Valsalva.* Pediatrics 8:340,1951.

104. KIEFFER, S. A., AND WINCHELL, P.: *Congenital aneurysms of the aortic sinuses with cardioaortic fistula.* Dis. Chest 38:79,1960.

105. KERBER, R. W., RIDGES, J. D., KRISS, J. P., ET AL.: *Unruptured aneurysm of the sinus of Valsalva producing right ventricular outflow obstruction.* Am. J. Med. 53:775,1972.

106. DURAS, P. F.: *Heart block with aneurysm of the aortic sinus.* Br. Heart J. 6:61,1944.

107. MCKUSICK, V. A.: *Heritable Disorders of Connective Tissue.* C. V. Mosby Co., St. Louis, 1972, pp. 61–223.

108. MURDOCH, J. L., WLAKER, B. A., HALPERN, B. L., ET AL.: *Life expectancy and causes of death in the Marfan syndrome.* N. Engl. J. Med. 286:804,1972.

109. BECKER, A. E.: *Medionecrosis aortae.* Pathol. Microbiol. (Basel) 43:124,1975.

110. SCHLATMANN, T. J. M., AND BECKER, A. E.: *Histologic changes in the normal aging aorta: implications for dissecting aortic aneurysm.* Am. J. Cardiol. 39:13,1977.

111. LEMON, D. K., AND WHITE, C. W.: *Anuloaortic ectasia: angiographic, hemodynamic and clinical comparison with aortic valve insufficiency.* Am. J. Cardiol. 41:482,1978.

112. SCHLATMANN, T. J. M., AND BECKER, A. E.: *Pathogenesis of dissecting aneurysm of aorta. Comparative histopathologic study of significance of medial changes.* Am. J. Cardiol. 39:21,1977.

113. ERDHEIM, J.: *Medionecrosis aortae idiopathica.* Virchows Arch. (Pathol. Anat.) 273:454,1929.

114. GSELL, O.: *Wandnekrosen der Aorta als selbstandige Erkrankung und ihre Beziehung zur Spontanruptur.* Virchows Arch. (path. Anat.) 270:1,1928.

115. ROBERTS, W. C., AND COHEN, L. S.: *Left ventricular papillary muscles. Description of the normal and a survey of conditions causing them to be abnormal.* Circulation 46:138,1972.

116. MCKUSICK, V. A., LOGUE, R. B., AND BAHNSON, H. T.: *Association of aortic valvular disease and cystic medial necrosis of the ascending aorta. Report of four instances.* Circulation 16:188,1957.

117. FUKUDA, T., TADAVARTHY, S. M., AND EDWARDS, J. E.: *Dissecting aneurysm of aorta complicating aortic valvular stenosis.* Circulation 53:169,1976.

453

Pulmonary Arteries in Congenital Heart Disease: A Structure-Function Analysis

Renu Virmani, M.D. and William C. Roberts, M.D.

For many years students of congenital heart disease were unable to explain the lack of survival patterns in patients with similar-sized, isolated communications between systemic and pulmonary circulations. Although in 1927 Moschcowitz[1] suggested that the explanation may be the result of pulmonary hypertension, hemodynamic and histologic studies during the past 30 years of the pulmonary vessels have helped enormously in explaining these differences. In 1935 Oscar Brenner in Birmingham, England, described histologic features of the normal pulmonary arteries and veins.[2] A year later Parker and Weiss,[3] at Boston City Hospital, described changes in the lungs and blood vessels in patients with mitral stenosis. Jesse Edwards, who also trained at Boston City Hospital in the late 1930s, began describing anatomic changes in the pulmonary vasculature in patients with congenital heart disease in the late 1940s; he too attributed the changes to the effects of pulmonary hypertension. Edwards, his colleagues, and many others described changes in a variety of congenital cardiac diseases,[4-45] and by 1958 a classification of the hypertensive pulmonary changes was formulated.[13] The recognition of the intimate association between the lung and the heart has been a major contribution to the understanding of congenital heart disease. Today it is well known that the state of the lung is the primary determinant of operability in a patient with a shunt. This chapter describes changes observed in the pulmonary vessels of adults with certain congenital cardiovascular malformations.

ANATOMIC CLASSIFICATION OF PULMONARY ARTERIAL HYPERTENSIVE CHANGES IN CONGENITAL HEART DISEASE

The anatomic classification of pulmonary hypertensive changes by Heath and Edwards[13] was based primarily on observations of patients with large ventricular septal defects, but it also was based on studies of a few patients with large patent ductus arteriosus and other defects associated with a free communication between the systemic and pulmonary circulations which causes *pulmonary hypertension from birth.** Their study also included a few patients with primary pulmonary hypertension.

The classification of Heath and Edwards is reproduced in Table 1. Although their classification of histologic changes observed in the pulmonary arteries in patients with

---

*This classic paper by Heath and Edwards included 27 photomicrographs of lung from 22 patients, only 5 of whom had ventricular septal defect. Of particular interest is that 17 of the 22 patients were over 20 years of age.

Table 1. Classification of hypertensive pulmonary vascular changes by Heath and Edwards in 1958.[13] (Reproduced with permission.)

	Grade of hypertensive pulmonary vascular disease					
	1	2	3	4	5	6
Type of intimal reaction	←——None——→					
				——— Cellular ———		→
			←——— Fibrous and fibroelastic ———→			
				←———Plexiform lesion———→		
State of media of arteries and arterioles	←——————————— Hypertrophied ——					→
				←——— Some generalized dilatation ———→		
				←——— Local "dilatation lesions"* ———→		
					←——— Pulmonary hemosiderosis† ———→	
						←—Necrotizing—→ arteritis

*Vein-like branches of hypertrophied muscular pulmonary arteries, angiomatoid lesion, and cavernous lesion

†Associated with distended, thin-walled, arterial vessels throughout the lung

pulmonary hypertension brought organization to a complex, previously unorganized subject, on re-evaluation, it is now apparent, 20 years later, that their classification has certain deficiencies. Considerable overlap exists between their grades 2 and 3, and between their grades 4 and 5. *Alveolar hemosiderosis* (grade 5) does not concern a pulmonary artery and is common in patients without pulmonary arterial hypertension. In our view, a classification of pulmonary arterial changes should not include changes in alveolar spaces (hemosiderosis). The grade 6 category implies that grades 1 through 5 are prerequisites, when, in actuality, necrotizing vasculitis may occur in the absence of grades 1 to 5. It seems to us that a classification of hypertensive changes in the pulmonary arteries should be applicable to all patients with pulmonary hypertension irrespective of cause and irrespective of whether the hypertension is congenital or acquired.

The classification of pulmonary arterial changes used herein is based entirely on the histologic alterations observed independent of etiology, time of appearance, and hemodynamic documentation of the pulmonary arterial pressure (Fig. 1). The major changes in the pulmonary arteries include: (1) *medial thickening* (MT), (2) *intimal thickening* (IT), and (3) *plexiform lesions* (PL). Only MT is grade I; MT and IT are grade II; and MT and IT with PL are grade III. We do not include arteritis (vasculitis), either necrotizing or non-necrotizing, in the grading system since pulmonary arteritis may occur in the absence of pulmonary hypertension.

Histologic Features of Normal Pulmonary Vessels

Much has been written on this subject.[1,9,13,25,45,-47] Table 2 summarizes some of the features of normal adult pulmonary vessels. The extrapulmonary arteries, i.e., the pulmonary trunk and right and left main pulmonary arteries, are *elastic* arteries. At birth the media of the pulmonary trunk consists of parallel elastic lamellae which are identical in number and configuration to those in the media of ascending aorta (Fig. 2). If the pulmonary arterial pressure falls to its normal level in the first few weeks of life, the thickness of the wall of the pulmonary trunk and its branches diminishes, and the number of elastic lamellae decrease; those which remain are disrupted (Fig. 2). In between the elastic fibers are smooth muscle cells and collagen fibrils. The integrity of the elastic pulmonary arteries in adults is dependent not on the disrupted elastic fibers

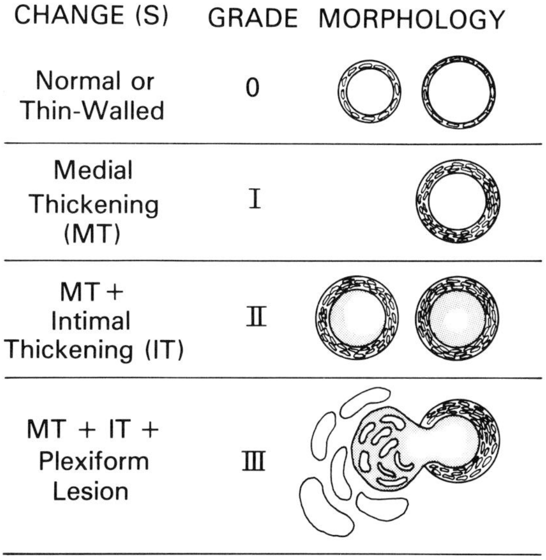

Figure 1. Types and grading of the morphologic pulmonary arterial changes in the patients studied (see text).

but on the integrity of the smooth muscle cells and collagen. The elastic pulmonary arteries extend into the lungs to the levels of the intrapulmonary cartilaginous bronchi.

The *muscular* pulmonary arteries begin, obviously, where the elastic arteries end. Although it contains occasional elastic and collagenous fibrils, the media consists predominantly of smooth muscle cells bordered by internal and external elastic membranes. The muscular arteries are adjacent to or associated with the terminal bronchioles, respiratory bronchioles, and alveolar ducts.

The pulmonary *arterioles* are branches of the muscular arteries. Except at their origin from the muscular arteries—where they have a thin muscular media between internal and external elastic membranes—the media is absent. An easily discernible elastic membrane covered by a single layer of endothelial cells borders the lumen. The arteriole divides into *capillaries* which course directly into the alveolar septa. The walls of the capillaries consist primarily of a single layer of endothelial cells covered by basement membrane. The capillary has a spiraling course within the alveolar septum rather than running parallel to the lining of the adjacent alveolus, as was originally believed.[3]

The capillaries drain into the pulmonary *venules* which are larger than, but virtually identical in structure to the capillaries: they consist of an endothelial layer covered by an elastic membrane. The *veins* have a thicker internal elastic membrane and are bordered by several irregularly arranged bundles of smooth muscle cells interspersed with collagenous fibrils and elastic fibrils.

The *bronchial arteries* are located within the walls of the bronchi, but otherwise are similar to the muscular pulmonary arteries. The *bronchial veins* also are in the bronchial walls and have thinner walls and larger lumens than the bronchial arteries. *Lymphatics* are present adjacent to pulmonary arteries and bronchi and in the interlobular septa and subpleural areas.

Histologic Features and Proposed Causes of Abnormal Pulmonary Arteries

Medial Thickening

This applies to an increase in the thickness of the media, either in the wall of the pulmonary artery or in the proximal portion of the pulmonary arteriole. Whether this

Table 2. Histologic features of normal pulmonary vessels in adults

| | External Diameter | Media | | | Lumen Diameter ÷ Wall Thickness | Internal Elastic Membrane | External Elastic Membrane | Adventitia (0–4) |
		Elastic Fibers (0–4)	SM Cells (0–4)	Collagen (0–4)				
Extrapulmonary Arteries								
Pulmonary trunk	1.6 cm.	+ + + +	+ +	+		+	+	+
Right main PA	1.3 cm.	+ + + +	+ +	+		+	+	+
Left main PA	1.3 cm.	+ + + +	+ +	+		+	+	+
Intrapulmonary Vessels								
Elastic arteries	>1000μ	+ + +	+ +	+	10	+	+	+
Muscular arteries	100–1000μ	+	+ + + +	+	4	+	+	+
Arterioles	<100μ	0	0*	0	6	+	0	+ +
Capillaries	<10μ	0	0	0		0**	0	0
Venules	10–100μ	0	0	0		+	0	+ +
Veins	>100μ	+ +	+	+ +	4	+	0	+ + +
Bronchial arteries	100–300μ	+	+ + + +	+	4	+	±	+
Bronchial veins		0	+	+	2	+	0	+
Lymphatic channels		0	0	0		0***	0	0

*A thin muscular media is present in its most proximal portion
**Endothelial layer plus basement membranes
***Actually an endothelial lining rather than an internal elastic membrane
SM = smooth muscle

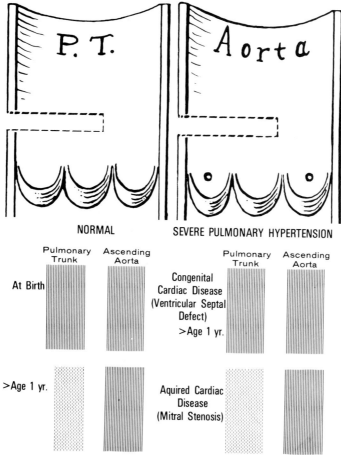

Figure 2. Configuration of elastic fibers in the pulmonary trunk at birth, after 1 year of age, with pulmonary hypertension from birth (VSD), and with an acquired condition (mitral stenosis). The sketch (top) shows the sites in the pulmonary trunk (P.T.) and aorta at which the sections for histologic examination were taken. At birth the configuration of the elastic fibers in both the pulmonary trunk and ascending aorta are identical and wall thicknesses are similar. Normally, after a year of age the number of elastic fibers in the pulmonary trunk diminishes considerably to reach an "adult configuration," and the thickness of the wall also diminishes. If a large VSD or aorticopulmonary defect is present from birth, both the configuration of the elastic fibers and wall thickness of the pulmonary trunk remains similar to that of the ascending aorta ("fetal configuration"). If pulmonary hypertension is acquired later in life, however, as in mitral stenosis, the configuration of the elastic fibers of the pulmonary trunk remains like that of the normal adult but wall thickness increases. The information on the configuration of elastic fibers in the pulmonary trunk is based on original work by Heath and associates.[69]

occurs entirely from hypertrophy of smooth muscle cells or whether both hypertrophy and hyperplasia cause the thickening is unclear.

Intimal Thickening

There are two types of intimal thickening—cellular and acellular. In the cellular variety the proliferated intima consists primarily of strap cells with collagen in between. The strap cells appear to be primarily smooth muscle cells. The acellular variety consists mostly of dense fibrous tissue (collagen) with minimal smooth muscle cells or none at all.

Plexiform Lesion

This is an aneurysmal or glomus-like structure which emerges at a right angle from a muscular pulmonary artery. The beginning of the right-angle branch is usually apparent; from there it rapidly dilates into a plexus of channels, the walls of which consist primarily of fibrous tissue covered by endothelial cells. The plexiform structure ends by giving off thin-walled channels, which probably are dilated arterioles; these branch quickly into alveolar septal capillaries. When these thin-walled channels are considerably dilated they are sometimes called *dilatation lesions*.

Proposed Causes

Medial thickening is a response of the arterial wall to increased pressure and therefore occurs only in patients with pulmonary arterial hypertension. As mentioned earlier, whether the thickening of the media is a consequence of hypertrophy alone, of hypertrophy and hyperplasia, or of hyperplasia alone, is unclear. Medial thickening is never simply a normal consequence of aging.

Intimal thickening, be it cellular or acellular, is not necessarily the consequence of pulmonary arterial hypertension, but it is accelerated by elevation of pulmonary arterial pressure. Cellular and acellular intimal proliferation is observed commonly in older persons, most of whom have normal pulmonary arterial pressures.[47] The occurrence of intimal thickening combined with medial thickening, however, is indicative of pulmonary hypertension.

Plexiform lesions occur only in patients with severe pulmonary hypertension, although some patients with severe pulmonary hypertension do not have them. These lesions can occur in patients with large left-to-right shunts or primary pulmonary hypertension, but do not occur in patients with severe pulmonary hypertension secondary only to left-sided cardiac disease (i.e., mitral stenosis). Plexiform lesions do not occur if the cause of the pulmonary hypertension is located distal to the pulmonary capillary level, or, stated differently, if the pulmonary arterial hypertension is the consequence of pulmonary venous hypertension. For plexiform lesions to occur the cause of the hypertension must orginate at the capillary or precapillary level.[48]

The exact cause of plexiform lesions is unknown. Serial sections of lung at sites of plexiform lesions generally show extreme narrowing or almost total obstruction of the lumen of the muscular pulmonary artery distal to the origin of the small muscular pulmonary artery or arteriole which is the site of the lesions.[25] Kanjuh and colleagues[30] have speculated that the plexiform lesion is a consequence of a *jet lesion* caused by blood rapidly changing its course because of the distal obstruction of the relatively large muscular pulmonary artery distal to the site of the plexiform lesion. Thus, the plexiform lesion might act as a dissipater of the extremely high pulmonary arterial pressure.

Other proposed causes of plexiform lesions are that they represent *sites of anastomoses of pulmonary arteries and veins*[49–52] or that they are a *congenital malformation.*[53,54] The latter theory appears particularly unlikely because plexiform lesions have never been observed in the lungs at birth. The earliest these pulmonary lesions have been observed is 2 months of age;[24,30,55,56] they are rare, however, under the age of 5 years. Another proposal is that the plexiform lesions represent *sites of thrombosis which have subsequently recanalized.*[57,58] Recently, Wagenvoort[45] proposed that plexiform lesions represent sites of necrotizing arteritis and, therefore, *represent healing of a necrotizing inflammatory process.* The arteritis weakens the arterial wall which becomes focally aneurysmal. Fibrin and platelets are deposited in the aneurysm and organization of the resulting thrombus produces multiluminal channels lined by endothelial cells.

460

We believe that plexiform lesions may represent aneurysms formed at sites of *congenitally underdeveloped or weak media* (analagous to the formation of intracerebral berry aneurysms in systemic hypertension) and that the aneurysm is filled by thrombus which organizes into multiple minute vascular channels. Distal to the weak or thin media, the lumen of the muscular artery is obliterated.

NECROPSY OBSERVATIONS OF PATIENTS OVER AGE 15 YEARS WITH CONGENITAL HEART DISEASE

To secure information on the lungs of adults with congenital cardiovascular anomalies, we reviewed clinical records accessioned in the Pathology Branch of the National Heart, Lung, and Blood Institute of the National Institutes of Health, often re-examining the heart itself and histologic sections of lung. All patients over age 15 with major anomalies of the heart and great vessels associated with a communication between pulmonary and systemic circulations were examined. A few cases were eliminated because histologic sections of lung were not available; a total of 87 patients were analyzed. At least five blocks of lung portions (all larger than 2 by 2 cm.) had been processed in alcohol and xylene and embedded in paraffin from each patient. At least one section of lung from these paraffin blocks was stained by hematoxylin and eosin, and at least one additional section from each paraffin block was stained for elastic fibers by either the Van Gieson or the Movat method. The status of the intrapulmonary pulmonary arteries was determined by histologic examination of each of the stained sections of lung, and the presence or absence of medial thickening, intimal thickening, plexiform lesions, and luminal thrombus was recorded. The presence and frequency of cholesterol-ester granulomas were also recorded.

Operated and Unoperated Patients

Certain clinical and morphologic observations in the 87 study patients are summarized in Tables 3–14. The 87 patients ranged in age from 16 to 83 (mean 34); 47 (54 percent) were women and 40 (46 percent) were men. One or more cardiovascular operations had been performed in 65 patients (75 percent), and observations in this group are summarized in Table 3. The other 22 patients (25 percent) never had a cardiovascular operation, and observations in this group are summarized in Table 4. The 22 unoperated patients ranged in age from 16 to 33 (mean 36), and the 65 operated patients were between 16 and 64 years old (mean 33). In Tables 3 and 4 the patients are grouped by the type of congenital cardiovascular malformation present. Patients with multiple nonobligatory anomalies—those who presumably represent more than a single embryologic defect—are grouped together under the term "complex anomaly;" observations in them are summarized in Table 5.

Patients with Abnormal Pulmonary Arteries

Medial thickening with or without intimal thickening or plexiform lesions was observed in the intrapulmonary pulmonary arteries by examination of lung sections of 44 (50 percent) of the 87 patients. The abnormalities consisted entirely of medial thickening in 6 patients (14 percent), medial and intimal thickening in 25 patients (57 percent), and medial and intimal thickening with plexiform lesions in 13 patients (29 percent). In addition, fibrin or fibrin-platelet thrombi were observed in the lumen of one or more small pulmonary arteries in 31 patients: 12 (39 percent) had neither medial nor intimal thickening, nor plexiform lesions; one or more of these three lesions were present in 19 (61 percent).

461

Table 3. Observations in 65 necropsy patients with various congenital cardiovascular malformations and one or more cardiovascular operations

Malformation: Sex of Patients/Age Range/Mean Age	PA Systolic Pressure, mm. Hg					Shunts			Pulmonary Arterial Changes				
	<30	30-60	61-90	>90	U	L→R	R→L	Both	None	MT only	MT + IT	PL	T
ASD													
Fossa ovale: 8F/43-64/61	1	4	2	1	0	8	0	0	4	1	3	0	4
Partial AV canal: 5F/21-54/38	1	3	0	0	1	4	0	1	2	1	2	0	2
Sinus venosus: 1M/37	1	0	0	0	0	1	0	0	1	0	0	0	0
VSD: 4F, 2M/16-54/29	0	1	4	1	0	4	1	1	1	2	2	1	2
Patent ductus arteriosus: 2F, 5M/16-44/30	0	0	1	6	0	5	2	0	0	0	1	6	1
VSD + PS (TOF): 5F, 10M/16-53/29	9	0	0	0	6	1	11	3	14	0	0	1	5
VSD + PV atresia: 1F/22	0	0	0	0	1	0	0	1	1	0	0	0	1
Complete transposition + VSD													
With PS: 3F/21-59/32	1	0	0	0	2	0	2	1	3	0	0	0	0
Without PS: 0													
Corrected transposition + VSD: 1M/38	0	0	1	0	0	0	0	1	0	0	1	0	1
Double outlet right ventricle: 1F/24	0	1	0	0	0	1	0	0	0	0	1	0	0
Ebstein's anomaly + ASD: 1F, 1M/20-31/25	1	0	0	0	1	0	1	1	0	0	2	0	1
PS with intact VS + ASD: 3F/28-43/36	2	0	0	0	1	0	3	0	3	0	0	0	1
Tricuspid atresia: 1M/27	0	0	0	0	1	0	1	0	1	0	0	0	0
Parachute MV syndrome: 1F/24	0	0	1	1	0	1	0	0	0	0	1	0	0
Complex anomaly: 5F, 5M/16-39/27*	4	0	0	1	4	2	3	5	7	0	2	1	2
TOTALS: 39F, 26M/16-64/33	20	9	9	10	17	27	24	14	37	4	15	9	20

*See Table 5 for additional information on these cases.

ASD = atrial septal defect; AV = atrioventricular; F = female; IT = intimal thickening; L = left; M = male; MT = medial thickening; MV = mitral valve; PA = pulmonary artery; PL = plexiform lesions + MT + IT; PS = pulmonic stenosis; PV = pulmonic valve; R = right; T = thrombi; TOF = tetralogy of Fallot; U = unknown; VS = ventricular septum; VSD = ventricular septal defect.

Table 4. Observations in 22 unoperated necropsy patients with various congenital cardiovascular malformations*

Malformation: Sex of Patients/ Age Range/Mean Age	PA Systolic Pressure, mm. Hg					Shunts			Pulmonary Arterial Changes				
	<30	30–60	61–90	>90	U	L→R	R→L	Both	None	MT only	MT + IT	PL	T
ASD													
Fossa ovale: 5F, 2M/29–83/55	0	1	1	1	4	6	0	1	3	1	2	1	4
Partial AV canal: 0													
Sinus venosus: 1M/58	0	0	0	1†	0	1	0	0	0	0	1	0	1
VSD: 2M/16–37/27	1	0	0	0	1	2	0	0	1	0	1	0	0
PDA: 3F/17–34/21	0	0	0	2	1	0	1	2	0	1	0	2	1
VSD + PS (TOF): 1M/22	0	0	0	0	1	0	1	0	1	0	0	0	1
VSD + PV atresia: 1M/28	0	0	0	0	1	0	0	1	1	0	0	0	0
Complete transposition + VSD													
With PS: 0													
Without PS: 1F, 1M/21–39/30	0	0	0	0	2	1	0	1	0	0	2	0	1
Complex anomaly: 5M, /20–41/26**	0	1	0	1	3	2	2	1	0	0	4	1	3
TOTALS: 9F, 13M/16–83/36	1	2	1	5	13	12	4	6	6	2	10	4	11

* Abbreviations listed in Table 3.
** See Table 5 for additional information on these cases.
† This patient died of carcinoma of the lung; some of this elevation probably is the result of the severe pulmonary cancer.

Table 5. Observations in 15 necropsy patients with complex anomalies*

| Patient Age (years)/Sex | Malformation | | | | PA Pressure mm. Hg (s/d) | SA Pressure mm. Hg (s/d) | Shunt | | SA O₂ Sat., % | OP | Pulmonary Arterial Changes | | | | |
	PS	VSD	ASD	Other			L→R	R→L			None	MT only	MT+IT	PL	T
WITHOUT RIGHT VENTRICULAR OUTFLOW OBSTRUCTION															
31/F	0	+	0	CS→LA	75/25	130/75	+	0	81	+	0	0	+	0	+
39/M	0	+	0	COA	105/54	152/64	+	+	87	0	0	0	0	+	0
41/M	0	+	0	PDA+CT+IAA		120/70	0	+		0	0	0	0	+	0
21/M	0	+	0	DORV+CT	92/48	104/64	+	0	90	0	0	0	+	0	0
21/M	0	+	0	DORV+CT		102/64	+	0	90	0	0	0	+	0	0
WITH RIGHT VENTRICULAR OUTFLOW OBSTRUCTION															
33/M	+	0	+	AS		80/62	+	+	81	+	+	0	0	0	0
19/M	+	0	+	RPV→RA	18/9	144/78	+	+	97	+	+	0	0	0	0
20/M	+	0	+	AV canal		180/100	0	+		0	0	0	+	0	+
25/F	+	+	+	AS		100/65	0	+	61	+	+	0	0	0	+
38/F	+	+	0	CT		125/48	0	+	62	+	+	0	+	0	0
17/M	+**	+	+	DORV, CT	20/12	90/60	+	0	93	+	+	0	0	0	0
22/F	+**	+	0	SV	15/6	100/65	+	+	81	+	+	0	0	0	0
16/M	+**	+	0	SV+CT		100/75	+	+	51	+	+	0	0	0	0
25/M	+	0	+	TAPVC	55/20	110/50	+	+	72	0	0	0	+	0	0
17/M	+**	0	+	TAPVC	20/8	95/60	0	+	92	+	+	0	0	0	+

*Last category in Tables 3 and 4.

**Subvalvular

AS = aortic stenosis; ASD = atrial septal defect; AV = atrioventricular; COA = coarctation of aorta; CS = coronary sinus; CT = corrected transposition; DORV = double outlet right ventricle; F = female; IT = intimal thickening; L = left; LA = left atrium; M = male; MT = medial thickening; OP = cardiovascular operation; PA = pulmonary artery; PDA = patent ductus arteriosus; PL = plexiform lesion + MT + IT; PS = pulmonic stenosis; R = right; RA = right atrium; RPV = right pulmonic vein; RV = right ventricle; SA = systemic artery; Sat. = saturation; s/d = systolic/diastolic; SV = single ventricle; T = thrombi; TAPVC = total anomalous pulmonary venous connection; VSD = ventricular septal defect.

Pulmonary Arterial Systolic Pressure and Shunt Direction

Of the 57 patients in whom pulmonary arterial pressures were recorded, the systolic pressure was ≤ 30 mm. Hg in 21 (37 percent); 30 to 60 mm. Hg in 11 (19 percent); 61 to 90 mm. Hg in 10 (18 percent); and > 90 mm. Hg in 15 (26 percent). All 87 patients had one or more communications between systemic and pulmonary circulations and were comprised as follows: (1) 39 patients with left-to-right shunt only (Tables 6 through 8); (2) 28 patients with right-to-left shunt only (Tables 6, 7, and 9); and (3) 20 patients with both left-to-right and right-to-left shunts (Tables 6, 7, and 9). Right ventricular outflow obstruction occurred in 36 (41 percent) of the 87 patients, including 18 of the 57 patients in whom pulmonary arterial systolic pressures were recorded. Pulmonary arterial systolic pressures were ≤ 30 mm. Hg in 5 (13 percent) of the 39 patients without right ventricular outflow obstruction, and in 16 (89 percent) of the 18 patients with obstruction. Conversely, the pulmonary arterial systolic pressure was elevated (>30 mm. Hg) in 34 (87 percent) of 39 patients without right ventricular outflow obstruction and in 2 (11 percent) of the 18 patients with obstruction (Tables 6, 8, and 9).

Anatomic Features of the Pulmonary Vessels

Figures 3 to 13 illustrate some of the anatomic features observed in the pulmonary vessels of the study patients.

Left-to-Right Shunts

Of these 39 patients, the pulmonary arterial pressure had been recorded in 31: 4 patients (13 percent) had only medial thickening; 13 patients (42 percent) had medial and intimal thickening; 3 patients (10 percent) had medial and intimal thickening with plexiform lesions; and 11 patients (35 percent) had none of these changes. The pulmonary arterial systolic pressures in the 11 patients ranged from 20 to 63 mm. Hg (mean 36 mm. Hg): in 5 it was ≤ 30 mm. Hg. In the 4 patients with medial thickening only, this pressure ranged from 58 to 80 mm. Hg (mean 70 mm. Hg). In the 13 patients with medial and intimal thickening, pressures ranged from 37 to 118 mm. Hg (mean 81 mm. Hg). In the 3 patients with plexiform lesions, pulmonary arterial systolic pressure was 120 mm. Hg in 2 and 136 mm. Hg in the other.

Right-to-Left Shunts

Of these 13 patients, 9 had pulmonary arterial systolic pressures ≤ 30 mm. Hg (mean 15 mm. Hg) from right ventricular outflow obstruction, and none of them had morphologic changes in the pulmonary arteries. The 4 other patients who had no right ventricular outflow obstruction had pulmonary arterial systolic pressures ranging from 98 to 132 mm. Hg (mean 114 mm. Hg) and all had plexiform lesions in the pulmonary arteries.

Both Left-to-Right and Right-to-Left Shunts

Of these 13 patients, 6 had right ventricular outflow obstruction and 7 did not. There were no morphologic changes in the pulmonary arteries in 6 patients whose pressures ranged from 15 to 20 mm. Hg (mean 15 mm. Hg); 4 had medial and intimal thickening and their pressures ranged from 22 to 83 mm. Hg (mean 55 mm. Hg). The 3 patients with plexiform lesions had pressures of 108, 110 and 138 mm. Hg.

Table 6. Observations in 87 necropsy patients over age 15 with congenital cardiovascular malformations

								Pulmonary Arterial Changes				
Direction of Shunt	*Totals*	*L→R*	*R→L*	*Both*	*L→R*	*R→L*	*Both*	*None*	*MT only*	*MT + IT*	*PL*	*T*
No. Patients	87	3	22	11	36	6	9	43	6	25	13	31
RV Outflow Obst.		3	22	11	0	0	0					
PA systolic Pressure (mm. Hg.)												
≤30	21	2	9	5	3	0	2	20	0	1	0	5
31-60	11	0	0	1	9	0	1	5	1	5	0	2
61-90	10	1	0	0	8	0	1	1	3	6	0	5
>90	15	0	0	0	8	4	3	0	0	5	10	7
Unknown (U)	30	0	13	5	8	2	2	17	2	8	3	12
Morphologic changes in PAs												
None	43	3	19	10	10	0	1					
MI alone	6	0	0	0	6	0	0					
MT + IT	25	0	2	1	17	1	4					
PL	13	0	1	0	3	5	4					
Thrombi	31	1	8	2	13	2	5					

IT = intimal thickening; L = left; MT = medical thickening; obst = obstruction; PA = pulmonary artery; PL = plexiform lesions + MT + IT; R = right; RV = right ventricle; T = thrombi

Table 7. Observations in 36 necropsy patients over age 15 with right ventricular outflow or inflow obstruction

Malformation: Sex of Patients/ Age Range/Mean Age	PA Systolic Pressures (mm. Hg)						SA O₂ Sat. (%)	Pulmonary Arterial Changes						
	<30	31-60	61-90	>90	U	OP		None	H	IT only	MT only	MT + IT	ARL	T
LEFT-TO-RIGHT SHUNT ONLY														
VSD+PS(TOF):1M/22	1	0	0	0	0		92	1	0	0	0	0	0	1
VSD+RVOTO:1F/25	0	0	1	0	0	1	91	1	0	0	0	0	0	0
Complex anomaly:1M/17	1	0	0	0	0	1	93	0	1	0	0	0	0	0
RIGHT-TO-LEFT SHUNT ONLY														
VSD+PS(TOF):5F, 7M/17–36/27	5	0	0	0	7	11	9(82)	2	7	6	0	1(PL)	5	5
CT+PS+VSD+DORV:1F/55	1	0	0	0	0	1		0	1	1	0	0	0	0
CT+PS+VSD+ASD:1M/21	0	0	0	0	1	1		0	1	1	0	0	0	0
TVA+ASD:1M/27	0	0	0	0	1	1	83	0	0	1	0	0	0	0
PS+IVS+ASD:3F/28–43/36	2	0	0	0	1	3	2(75)	1	3	1	0	0	0	1
Complex anomaly:2F, 2M/17–38/34	1	0	0	0	3	3	3(72)	1	1	2	0	2	0	3
BOTH LEFT-TO-RIGHT AND RIGHT-TO-LEFT SHUNTS														
VSD+PS(TOF):3M/16–53/37	3	0	0	0	0	3	3(81)	0	1	2	0	0	2	0
VSD+PVA:1F, 1M/22–28/25	0	0	0	0	2	1	2(67)	0	0	2	0	0	1	1
CT+VSD+PS:1M/21	0	0	0	0	1	1	71	0	0	1	1	0	0	1
Complex anomaly:1F, 4M/16–33/23	2	1	0	0	2	4	4(83)	1	1	2	0	1	0	0

ARL = Arnold Rich lesions; ASD = atrial septal defect; CT = corrected transposition; DORV = double outlet right ventricle; F = female; H = hypoplastic; IT = intimal thickening; M = male; MT = medial thickening; OP = cardiovascular operation; PA = pulmonary artery; PL = plexiform lesions + MT and IT; PS = pulmonic stenosis; PVA = pulmonary valve atresia; RVTO = right ventricular outflow tract obstruction; SA = systemic artery; Sat. = saturation; T = thrombus; TOF = tetralogy of Fallot; TVA = tricuspid valve atresia; U = unknown; IVS = intact ventricular septum; VSD = ventricular septal defect.

Table 8. Clinical and morphologic observations in 36 necropsy patients over age 15 with CHD, L-R shunts, and no right ventricular outflow or inflow obstruction

Malformation / Sex of Patients / Age Range/Mean Age	PA Systolic Pressure (mm. Hg)						Pulmonary Arterial Changes				
	<30	31–60	61–90	>90	U	OP	None	MT only	MT + IT	PL	T
ASD											
Fossa ovale: 13F, 1M/43–83/57	1	5	3	1	4	8	7	2	5	0	7
Partial AV canal: 4M/21–54/39	0	3	0	0	1	4	1	1	2	0	2
Sinus venosus: 2M/37–58/48	1	0	0	1	0	1	1	0	1	0	1
VSD: 2F, 3M/16–54/28	1	0	3	0	1	4	1	2	2	0	1
PDA: 1F, 4M/16–44/28	0	0	1	4	0	5	0	1	1	3	0
Complete transposition with VSD: 1F/39	0	0	0	0	1	0	0	0	1	0	0
DORV: 1F/24	0	1	0	0	0	1	0	0	1	0	0
Parachute MV syndromes: 1F/24	0	0	0	1	0	1	0	0	1	0	0
Complex anomaly: 1F, 2M/21–31/26	0	0	1	1	1	1	0	0	3	0	2
TOTALS: 20F, 16M/16–83/42	3	9	8	8	8	27	10	6	17	3	13

Abbreviations as in Tables 3, 5, and 6.

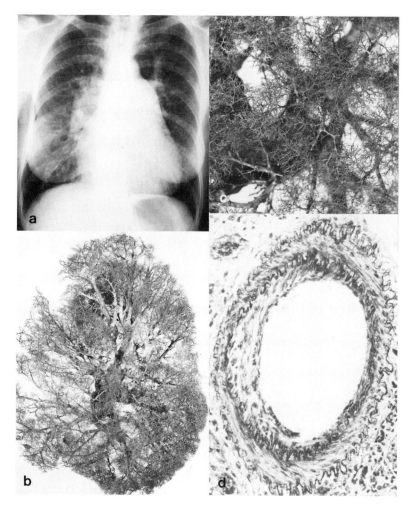

Figure 3. Atrial septal defect in a 45-year-old woman who died 11 days after operative closure. Preoperative pulmonary arterial pressure was 40/14 mm. Hg; left-to-right shunt was 2.8 to 1; and pulmonary to systemic resistance was 0.17 to 1. *a,* Radiograph immediately before operation. *b,* Mold of pulmonary arteries in one lung. *c,* Close-up of wide-open arteries. *d,* Typical muscular pulmonary artery showing mild medial and intimal thickening. (Movat stain, x 252; reduced 30%.)

Table 9. Clinical and morphologic observations in 15 necropsy patients over age 15 with CHD and R-L shunts only or both R-L and L-R shunts, without right ventricular outflow or inflow obstruction

	F	M	ASD	VSD	PDA	Other	PA Systolic Pressure mm. Hg	OP	PA Lesions
						RIGHT-TO-LEFT SHUNT ONLY			
17	+	0	0	0	+	0	120	0	PL,T
20	+	0	+	0	0	Ebstein's + LSVC	U	+	MT +IT
25	+	0	0	+	0	0	98	+	PL
33	0	+	0	+	+	0	106	+	PL,T
40	+	0	0	0	+	0	132	+	PL
41	0	+	0	+	+	IAA + CT	U	0	PL
						BOTH RIGHT-TO-LEFT AND LEFT-TO-RIGHT SHUNTS			
16	+	0	0	+	0	0	60	+	MT +IT,T
21	+	0	0	+	+	0	138	0	PL,T
21	0	+	+	+	0	Comp T	U	0	MT +IT
24	+	0	0	0	+	0	U	0	PL
29	+	0	+	0	0	0	110	0	PL,T
31	0	+	+	0	0	Ebstein's	22	+	MT +IT,T
38	0	+	0	+	0	CT	83	+	MT +IT,T
39	0	+	0	+	0	COA	108	+	PL
40	+	0	+	0	0	TAPVC	20	+	O

Abbreviations as in Table 5 and 6; EA = Ebstein's anomaly.

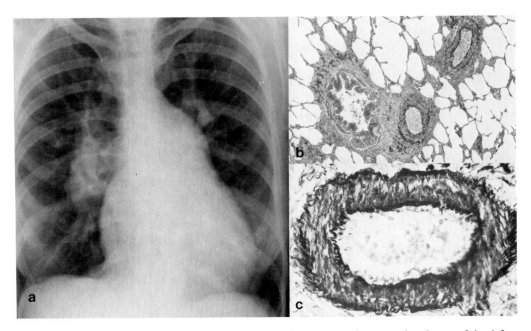

Figure 4. Atrial septal defect in a 50-year-old woman who died 11 days after operative closure of the defect. Preoperative pulmonary arterial pressure was 95/30 mm. Hg; the shunt was entirely left-to-right. *a,* Radiograph immediately before operation. *b,* Two muscular pulmonary arteries with thickened media (x 60). *c,* Close-up (x 330) of one of the two muscular pulmonary arteries shown in *b.* (Movat stains; reduced 30%.)

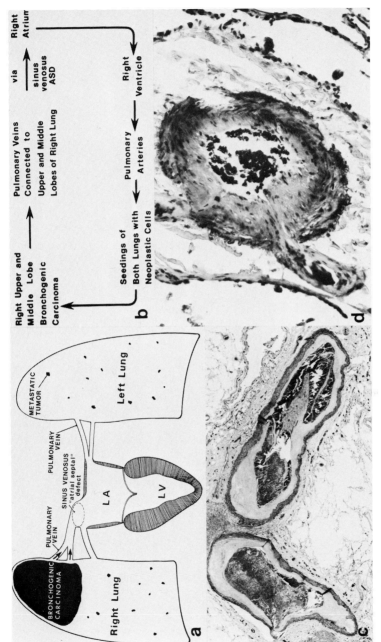

Figure 5. Sinus venosus type ASD with anomalous pulmonary venous return from the right lung associated with bronchogenic carcinoma in a 58-year-old man. Three years before he died his pulmonary arterial pressure was 100/22 mm. Hg and left-to-right shunt was 1.5 to 1. *a*, Diagram of the heart and lungs. LA = left atrium; LV = left ventricle. *b*, Path of metastatic spread of the tumor in both lungs. *c*, Large pulmonary arteries with thickened intima and antemortem blood clot (x 85). *d*, Typical muscular artery and branching arteriole with thickened media and intima (x 220). (Movat stains; reduced 12%.)

471

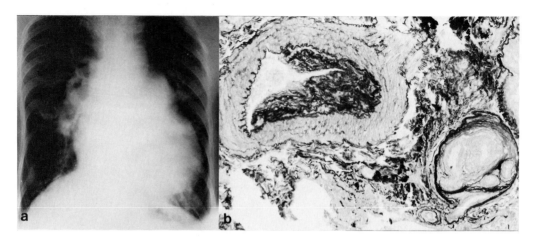

Figure 6. Patent ductus arterosus in a 36-year-old man who died during attempted closure of the calcified ductus. Preoperative pulmonary arterial pressure was equal to systemic arterial pressure (136/96 mm. Hg). The shunt was entirely left to right. *a,* Radiograph immediately before operation. *b,* Muscular pulmonary artery showing marked medial and intimal thickening and a plexiform lesion. (Elastic van Gieson stain; x 220; reduced 30%.)

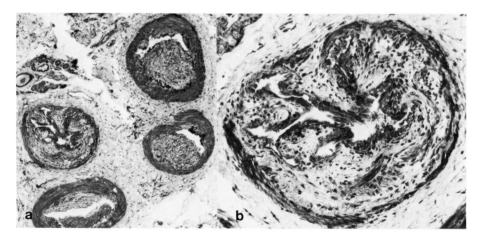

Figure 7. Patent ductus arteriosus in a 40-year-old woman who died during attempted operative closure. Simultaneous pulmonary arterial and femoral arterial pressures were 110/58 (mean 80) and 128/46 mm. Hg (mean 80), respectively. The shunt was right-to-left, femoral arterial oxygen saturation was 70 percent, and blood hematocrit was 46 percent. *a,* Muscular pulmonary arteries with thickened media and intima and narrowed lumens (x 80). *b,* Plexiform lesions (x 240). (Movat stains; reduced 30%.)

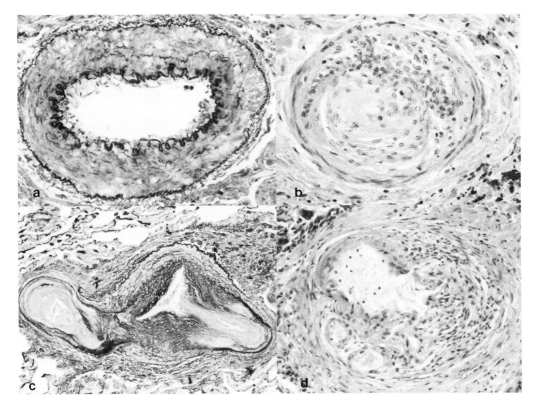

Figure 8. Combined PDA and discrete subaortic stenosis in a 17-year-old boy. Peak systolic pressure gradient between left ventricle and brachial artery was 78 mm. Hg. Pulmonary arterial pressure was 128/70 mm. Hg and the shunt was entirely left-to-right. Muscular pulmonary arteries (*a* through *d*) shows severe medial hypertrophy and luminal narrowing by intimal thickening. *c, d,* Plexiform lesions. (Elastic Van Gieson stains: x 255 (*a*) and x 65 (*c*); hematoxylin and eosin stains: x375 (*b*) and x 240 (*d*); reduced 34%.)

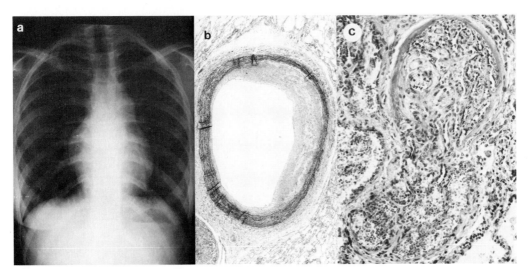

Figure 9. Combined PDA and VSD in a 21-year-old woman who died soon after catheterization. The pulmonary and systemic arterial pressures were both 138/86 mm. Hg (mean 107). The shunt through the ductus was mainly right-to-left and the shunt through the VSD was minute. Oxygen saturation was 89 percent in the brachial artery and 75 percent in the femoral artery; blood hematocrit was 66 percent. *a,* Chest radiograph. *b,* Intrapulmonary elastic artery (x 27). *c,* Plexiform lesion (x 225). (Hematoxylin and cosin stains; reduced 40%.)

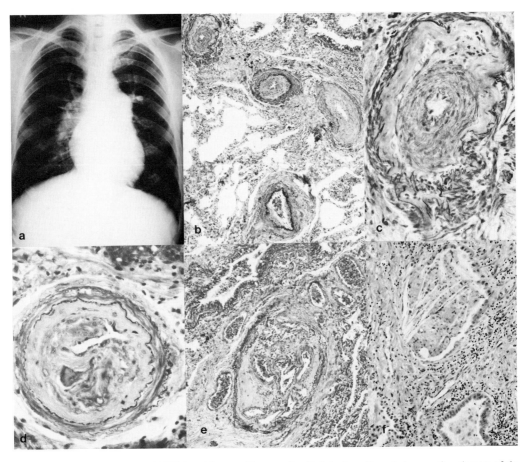

Figure 10. Combined PDA and VSD in a 33-year-old man who died during attempted operative closure of the ductus. Simultaneous pulmonary and femoral arterial pressures were 106/64 and 132/52 mm. Hg, respectively. The femoral and brachial arterial oxygen saturations were 69 and 80 percent, respectively. Blood hematocrit was 54 percent but severe iron deficiency anemia was present. The shunt at the ductus was primarily right-to-left and no shunt was detected at the ventricular level. *a,* Chest radiograph immediately before operation. *b, c, d,* Severe medial and intimal thickening with luminal narrowing (x 95, x 380, x 385, respectively). *e,* Plexiform lesions (x 130). *f,* Cholesterol-ester granuloma (x 160). (Movat stains: *b, c, d, e;* hematoxylin and eosin stain: *f;* reduced 42%.)

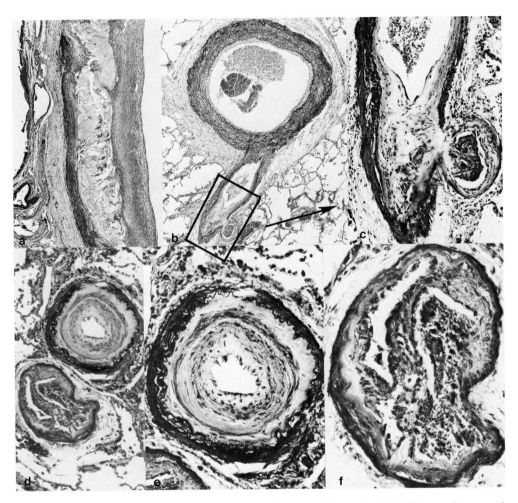

Figure 11. Combined VSD and coarctation of aorta in a 39-year-old man who died 24 hours after operative closure of the defect. Simultaneous pulmonary arterial and aortic pressures were 131/76 (mean 93) and 144/84 (mean 100) mm. Hg, respectively. Left brachial arterial oxygen saturation was 87 percent, blood hematocrit was 54 percent, and the shunt was bidirectional, but predominantly left-to-right. The pulmonary arteries had thick media, thick intima, narrowed lumens, and plexiform lesions. *a,* Intrapulmonary elastic artery (media stains black) with a huge atherosclerotic plaque (x 40). *b,* Large pulmonary artery with a muscular branch which has an obliterated lumen (x 60). *c,* Close-up of the area in brackets shown in *b* (x 155). This is a plexiform lesion. *d,* Muscular pulmonary artery (x 130). *e,* Close-up of artery shown in *d* (x 248). *f,* Close-up of plexiform lesion shown in *d* (x 330). (Movat stains; reduced 40%.)

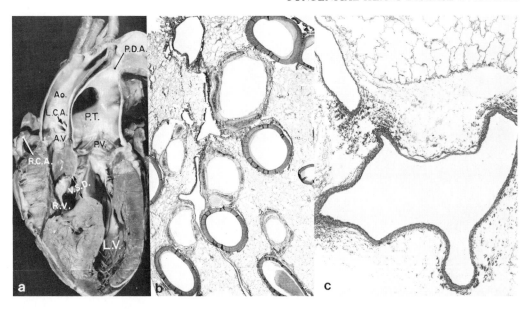

Figure 12. Ventricular septal defect and PDA associated with the Taussig-Bing malformation in a 39-year-old woman described in detail elsewhere.[70] Pulmonary arterial pressure was 91/58 mm. Hg; brachial arterial pressure, 93/56 mm. Hg. Blood hematocrit was 75 percent; systemic arterial oxygen saturation, 47 percent. *a,* Longitudinal view of heart showing the pulmonary trunk (P.T.) and pulmonic valve (P.V.) overriding a large ventricular septal defect (V.S.D.). The aorta (A.) arises anteriorly and from the right ventricle (R.V.). The patent ductus arteriosus (P.D.A.) is large. L.V. = left ventricle; L.C.A. = ostium of left coronary artery; R.C.A. = right coronary artery. *b,* Greatly dilated pulmonary arteries near hilum of one lung (x 5). Media is thickened but intima is normal or only minimally thickened. The pulmonary arteries in this patient were everywhere wide open and dilated. *c,* Dilated pulmonary veins (x 40). Despite the balanced pulmonary and systemic arterial pressures maintained over many years the anatomic pulmonary arterial changes were mild. (Elastic Van Gieson and Movat stains; reduced 33%.)

MORPHOLOGIC CHANGES IN THE PULMONARY ARTERIES: THE EFFECTS OF PULMONARY ARTERIAL SYSTOLIC PRESSURE, DIRECTION AND LOCATION OF SHUNT, AND PATIENT AGE

The observations described above and presented in detail in Tables 3 through 14 indicate that the crucial determinant of anatomic change in the muscular pulmonary arteries of patients over age 15 with congenital cardiac disease is the *level of the pulmonary arterial pressure*. These observations in our 57 necropsy patients in whom pulmonary arterial pressures were recorded are summarized in Fig. 14. Of the 26 patients without morphologic pulmonary arterial changes, the average pulmonary arterial systolic pressure was 25 mm. Hg (range 9 to 63 mm. Hg) and only 6 patients had pressures > 30 mm. Hg. In contrast, of the 10 patients with plexiform lesions, the average pulmonary arterial systolic pressure was 119 mm. Hg (range 98 to 138 mm. Hg; p < .01). The 21 patients with medial thickening only or medial and intimal thickening had similar average pulmonary arterial systolic pressures (70 and 75 mm. Hg, respectively). The average pulmonary arterial systolic pressure in the patients with medial thickening with or without intimal thickening was significantly (p < .01) different than the pressures of patients without morphologic pulmonary arterial changes and patients with plexiform lesions (Fig. 14).

The *direction of the intravascular shunt* appeared to have only indirect effect on the pulmonary arteries. As shown in Figures 14 through 16, 15 of the 26 patients without structural pulmonary arterial abnormalities (average pulmonary arterial systolic pres-

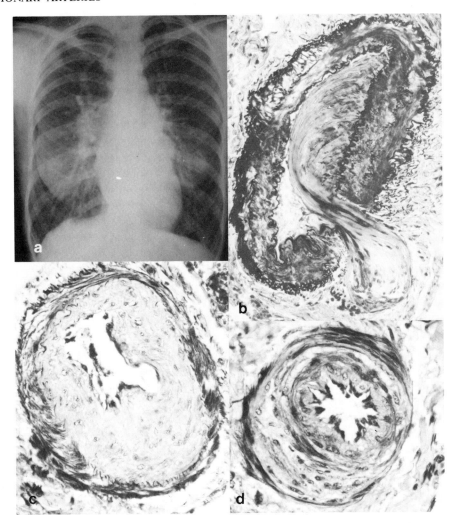

Figure 13. Congenital mitral stenosis, VSD, PDA, and coarctation of aorta in a 25-year-old asymptomatic woman.[71] Pulmonary arterial pressure was 104/60 mm. Hg (mean 82); left ventricular pressure, 122/4 mm. Hg. Left atrial to left ventricular end-diastolic gradient was 20 mm. Hg and cardiac output was normal. *a,* Preoperative chest radiograph. A mitral commissurotomy was performed but considerable mitral regurgitation resulted; the VSD was closed by direct suture, and an unsuspected ductus was ligated. The patient died 20 hours after operation. *b* (x 220), *c* (x 330), *d* (x 435), Pulmonary arteries show severe intimal and medial thickening with luminal narrowing, and pulmonary venous and alveolar septal and space lesions are typical of mitral stenosis.[72-75] (Movat stains; reduced 25%.)

sure = 15 mm. Hg) had right-to-left or bidirectional shunts and 7 of the 10 patients with plexiform lesions (average pulmonary arterial systolic pressure = 116 mm. Hg) (Fig. 15) also had right-to-left or bidirectional shunts. Thus, the pressure and not the direction of the shunt determines anatomic pulmonary arterial changes in these patients. As shown in Figure 16, patients with left-to-right shunts only, also had all degrees of anatomic change in the muscular pulmonary arteries, again demonstrating that structural changes in these patients depend on the pulmonary arterial pressure.

The anatomic changes in the muscular pulmonary arteries were only secondarily dependent on the *location of the shunt* in the heart or great arteries. Among our 40 patients with isolated atrial septal defect (ASD) or ventricular septal defect (VSD) or

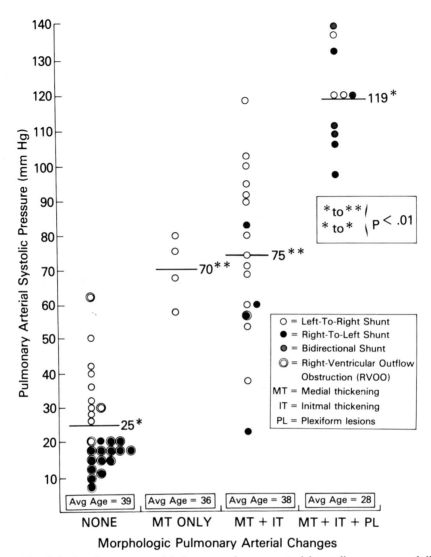

Figure 14. Morphologic pulmonary arterial changes, pulmonary arterial systolic pressure, and direction of shunt in 57 necropsy patients over age 15 with congenital heart disease. In 26 patients the media of the pulmonary arterial wall was normal or thinner than normal, in 4 there was medial thickening only, in 17 there was both medial and intimal thickening, and in 10 there was medial and intimal thickening with plexiform lesions. The average pulmonary arterial systolic pressure in the patients with medial thickening with or without intimal thickening was significantly (p < .01) different from the average pressure in patients without any morphologic changes and from the average pressure in those with plexiform lesions.

patent ductus arteriosus (PDA) (Tables 3 and 4), 33 had pulmonary arterial pressures recorded at catheterization. As shown in Figures 17 and 18, the anatomic changes in the muscular pulmonary arteries in these 33 patients depended not on the location of the shunt but on the pressure in the pulmonary artery. Of course, the location of the communication played a major role in determining the pulmonary arterial pressure. Generally, the closer the shunt is to the pulmonary circulation the greater the pulmonary arterial pressure. Thus, the average pulmonary arterial systolic pressure in our patients was highest (118 mm. Hg) (Fig. 17) in the 9 patients with PDA, lowest (58 mm.

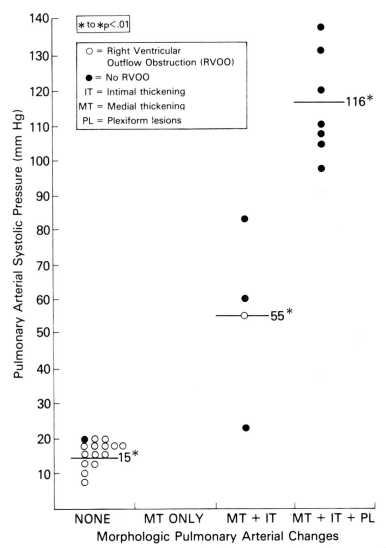

Figure 15. Morphologic pulmonary arterial changes and pulmonary arterial systolic pressure in 26 necropsy patients over age 15 with right-to-left or bidirectional shunts. In 15 patients the media of the pulmonary arteries was normal or thinner than normal; 4 patients had both medial and intimal thickening; 7 patients had both medial and intimal thickening with plexiform lesions. The average pulmonary arterial systolic pressure increased significantly as morphologic pulmonary arterial changes worsened.

Hg) in the 17 patients with ASD, and intermediate (68 mm. Hg) in the 7 patients with isolated VSD. Surprisingly, no significant difference in average pulmonary arterial systolic pressure was observed between the 17 patients with isolated ASD and the 7 patients with isolated VSD (Fig. 17). The average pulmonary arterial systolic pressure in the 9 patients with isolated PDA was nearly twice that of the patients with either ASD or VSD, and this difference was highly significant (p < .001).

Plexiform lesions were observed in 1 of the 17 patients with ASD, in 1 of the 7 with VSD, and in 7 of the 9 with PDA. All 9 patients with plexiform lesions had pulmonary arterial systolic pressures > 90 mm. Hg.

Age was not an important determinant of anatomic changes in the muscular pulmo-

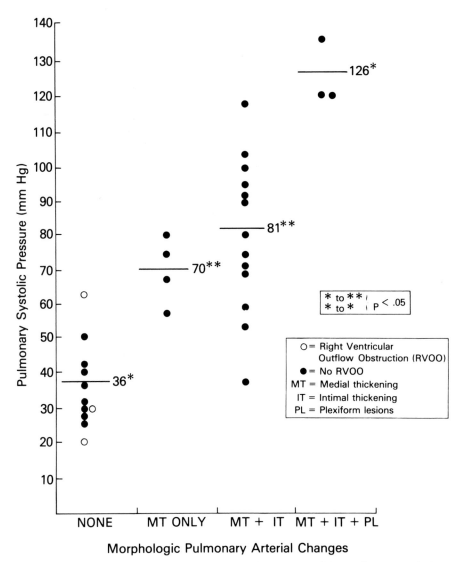

Figure 16. Morphologic pulmonary arterial changes and pulmonary arterial systolic pressure in 31 necropsy patients over age 15 with only left-to-right shunts. In 11 patients the media of the pulmonary arteries was normal or thinner than normal; 4 patients had only medial thickening; 13 patients had both medial and intimal thickening; 3 patients had both medial and intimal thickening with plexiform lesions. The average pulmonary arterial systolic pressure in the patients with medial thickening with or without intimal thickening was significantly (p < .05) different from the average pressure in patients without morphologic changes and from the average pressure in those with plexiform changes.

nary arteries (Fig. 19). Among the 40 patients with isolated ASD or VSD or PDA, the group with ASD was oldest (mean 51 years) and yet they had the least severe pulmonary arterial anatomic changes. Furthermore, the patients with VSD and PDA were younger and had the same mean age (28 years); yet, the anatomic pulmonary arterial changes were far worse among the patients with PDA (p < .001). The lack of severe morphologic pulmonary arterial changes in the patients with ASD appears to explain the much longer survival among these patients than among those with either isolated VSD or PDA (Fig. 19).

Observations of Other Investigators

Although several investigators have described previously the effect of pressure, direction and location of shunt, and age on the anatomic changes in the pulmonary arteries, the only previous study which allows direct comparison to ours is the one by Heath and associates.[14] Among their 40 patients with isolated ASD or VSD or PDA, 23 were over 15 years of age (range 17 to 55; mean 32) and pulmonary arterial systolic pressures were available in all patients. Figures 20 to 22 show our plotting of their observations in 23 patients in the same way we plotted our own observations (Figs. 17

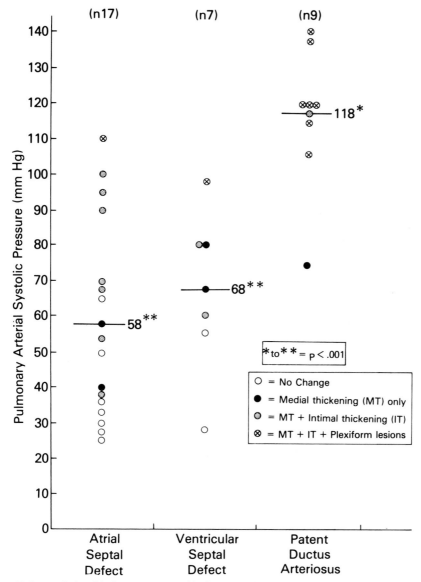

Figure 17. Interrelationship between type of isolated cardiovascular malformation, pulmonary arterial systolic pressure, and morphologic pulmonary arterial changes in 33 necropsy patients over age 15. There was no significant difference in the average systolic pressures in patients with ASD and VSD, but both these averages were significantly (p < .001) different from the average pressure in patients with PDA.

481

through 19). As shown in Figure 21, the pulmonary arterial systolic pressures were significantly (p < .01) lower in the patients in whom the morphologic pulmonary arterial changes consisted only of medial thickening. Surprisingly, in contrast to our patients, no significant differences in these average pressures were observed between the patients with medial and intimal thickening and the patients with plexiform lesions. Furthermore, the average systolic pressure in their patients with isolated ASD was only slightly lower—although significantly (p < 0.01)—than the average pressures in their patients with either VSD or PDA (Fig. 20).

As in our patients, their patients with ASD were significantly older than their patients with either VSD or PDA, even though their pulmonary arterial systolic pressures were significantly lower. As pointed out by Heath and associates,[14] however, in patients with

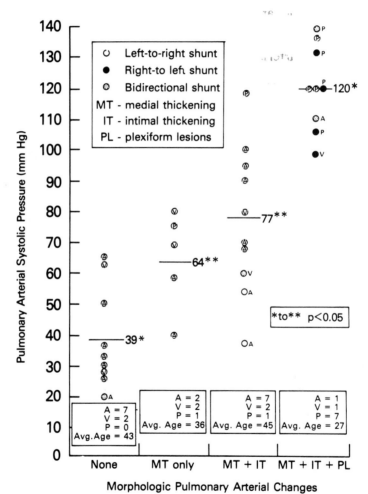

Figure 18. Morphologic pulmonary arterial changes, pulmonary arterial systolic pressure, and shunt direction in 33 necropsy patients over age 15 with isolated ASD or VSD or PDA. The pulmonary arteries were normal in 9 patients; 5 had medial thickening only; 10 had both medial and intimal thickening; 9 had both medial and intimal thickening with plexiform lesions. The average pulmonary arterial systolic pressures in the patients with medial thickening with or without intimal thickening was significantly (p<.05) different from average pressure in patients without morphologic changes and from the average pressure in those with plexiform changes.

large VSD or PDA the systemic pressure is freely propagated into the pulmonary circulation from birth. Hence, the age of the patient is synonymous with the duration of the pulmonary arterial hypertension. As seen in Figure 22, there was an inverse correlation with the morphologic pulmonary arterial changes and the average age of their patients. In patients with medial thickening only, the average age was 37; in the group with medial and intimal thickening, the average age was 34; and in their patients with plexiform lesions the average age was 29. A similar trend occurred in our patients (Fig. 18).

The direction of the shunt, as shown in Figure 21, played a role in causing the morphologic pulmonary arterial changes in that their patients with bidirectional or only right-to-left shunts had higher pulmonary arterial systolic pressures than those with only left-to-right shunts.

Thus, the study by Heath and associates[14] showed no significant pulmonary arterial systolic pressure differences between patients with plexiform lesions and those with both medial and intimal thickening (Fig. 21). Our study, in contrast, showed a significant difference in pulmonary arterial systolic pressure between these two anatomic groups (Fig. 18). Their study showed a clear difference in pulmonary arterial systolic pressure in the patients with only medial thickening compared to those with both medial and intimal thickening and those with plexiform lesions (Fig. 21). Our study (Fig. 18), in contrast, showed no significant difference in the patients with medial thickening only as compared to those with both medial and intimal thickening.

When comparing pulmonary arterial systolic pressures to the location of the shunt, there was no significant difference in pulmonary pressures in their patients with VSD and PDA; there was a significant difference between the pressures of these two groups and pressures of patients with ASD (Fig. 20). In contrast, our study showed a highly significant difference between average pulmonary systolic pressure in patients with PDA and in those with VSD, but no significant difference between patients with ASD and in those with VSD (Fig. 17).

The results of our study were similar to that of Heath and associates[14] in regard to age (Figs. 19 and 22) and direction of the shunt.

How might the differences in the results of the two studies be explained? First, the patients were different. We studied only necropsy patients and many histologic sections from each patient. How many, if any, of their patients were studied at necropsy is not stated. It appears likely that the lung tissue in most of their patients was obtained at biopsy at the time of cardiac operation. Second, the investigators were different and judgments of morphologic changes possibly were different. Third, the numbers of patients in each study were relatively small so that differences may have been magnified. Fourth, their study excluded patients without anatomic changes in the pulmonary arteries whereas ours did not. Nevertheless, when we exclude our patients without anatomic pulmonary arterial changes, the differences between the two studies persist.

Wagenvoort and associates[33,40,41] studied lung tissue biopsied at the time of thoracotomy in patients with various congenital cardiovascular malformations. They also have shown that the primary cause of anatomic pulmonary arterial changes is elevation of the pulmonary arterial pressure, and that the magnitude of pulmonary flow is not, in itself, a determinant of these anatomic changes. This group did find, however, that the location of the shunt was an important factor in determining the extent of the anatomic pulmonary arterial changes. Of 77 lung samples studied from patients with isolated ASD (mean age, 22 years), medial thickening occurred in only 22 (29 percent), intimal thickening occurred in only 14 (18 percent), and none had plexiform lesions. In contrast, of 44 patients with isolated VSD (mean age, 9 years) and of 74 with isolated PDA (mean age, 9 years), 44 (34 percent) had medial thickening, 36 (28 percent) had intimal thickening, and only 2 (2 percent) had plexiform lesions. Severe intimal thicken-

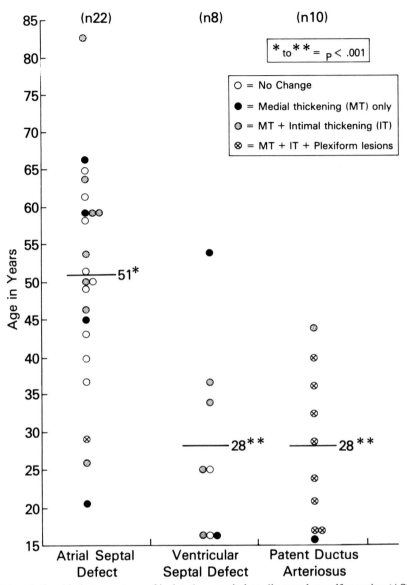

Figure 19. Interrelationship between type of isolated congenital cardiovascular malformation (ASD, n = 22; VSD, n = 8; PDA, n = 10) and morphologic pulmonary arterial changes in 40 necropsy patients over age 15. The average ages of patients with VSD and PDA are significantly (p < .001) different than the average age of patients with ASD.

ing was not observed in any patient with ASD or PDA but it occurred in 12 (27 percent) of the 44 patients with VSD.

The Wagenvoort study emphasized that the pulmonary vessels of their patients with ASD (much younger than ours and Heath's) did not differ significantly from those of his "control subjects." Among Wagenvoort's 105 patients with left-to-right shunts and pulmonary atrial systolic pressures greater than 60 mm. Hg, all had medial thickening and 74 (70 percent) had intimal thickening. In contrast, of his 45 patients with only right-to-left or bidirectional shunts, all had medial thickening and 44 (98 percent) had

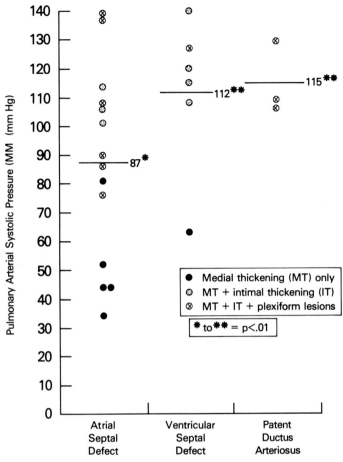

Figure 20. Data from Heath and associates[14] showing interrelationship between type of isolated congenital cardiovascular malformation (ASD, n = 14; VSD, n = 6; PDA, n = 3), pulmonary artery systolic pressure, and morphologic pulmonary arterial changes in 23 patients over age 15. There was no significant difference between the average pulmonary arterial systolic pressures in patients with VSD and in patients with PDA, but pressures in these two groups were significantly (p < .01) different from those in the patients with ASD.

intimal thickening. Plexiform lesions were not described in any of these 150 patients but, again, they were much younger than our patients.

SIGNIFICANCE OF PLEXIFORM LESIONS IN PATIENTS WITH PRIMARY PULMONARY HYPERTENSION

Plexiform lesions in the lung are indicative of severe pulmonary arterial hypertension which is almost always irreversible. Of our 87 patients, 13 (15 percent) had plexiform lesions: they occurred in 12 (23 percent) of the 51 patients without and in 1 (3 percent) of the 36 patients with right ventricular outflow or inflow obstruction (Table 10). The latter patient, however, developed plexiform lesions after operative creation of a large end-to-side communication between aorta and right main pulmonary artery. The pulmonary arterial systolic pressures were known in 11 of our 13 patients with plexiform lesions and in each this pressure was greater than 90 mm. Hg (mean 118 mm. Hg). Of the 13 patients with lesions, 12 had either VSD or PDA and only one had isolated ASD; they were between 17 and 41 years old (mean 28).

Table 10. Observations in 18 necropsy patients over age 15 with CHD, pulmonary arterial systolic pressures >90 mm. Hg, and no right ventricular outflow or inflow obstruction

Patient Age, Sex Malformation	PA Pressure (mm. Hg, s/d)	SA Pressure (mm. Hg, s/d)	Shunt	SA O$_2$ Sat. (%)	Cardiac Operation	Interval (days) OP to Death
WITH PLEXIFORM LESIONS						
29 F/ASD, RPV→SVC	110/60	110/60	both		none	
25 F/VSD	98/62	104/66	R-L	88	VSD closed	1
33 M/VSD, PDA	106/64	136/68	R-L	61	PDA closed	0
21 F/VSD, PDA	138/86	140/88	both	89	none	
39 M/VSD, COA	108/54	152/64	both	87	VSD closed	1
41 M/VSD, PDA, IAA +CT		120/70	none	*	none	
40 F/PDA	132/64	128/68	R-L	70	PDA closed	0
24 F/PDA		128/70	none	*	none	
28 M/PDA	120/60	120/60	L-R	96	PDA closed	1
17 F/PDA	120/65	110/60	R-L	*	none	
36 M/PDA	136/96	136/96	L-R	95	PDA closed	0
17 M/PDA, SS	120/65	122/65	L-R	97	PDA closed; SS resectioned	1
19 F/TOF	105/—	108/78	R-L	70	right PA-DA anastomosis	14 yrs.
WITHOUT PLEXIFORM LESIONS						
50 F/ASD	95/30	105/80	L-R	96	ASD closed	11
58 M/ASD	100/22	140/90	L-R		none	
44 F/PDA	118/52	150/70	L-R	92**	PDA closed	7
24 F/VSD, PDA, MS +COA	104/60	118/70	L-R		PDA and VSD closed; MVC	1
21 M/VSD, DORV +CT	92/48	102/64	L-R	90	none	0

*Central cyanosis present.
**Right brachial artery; 89 percent in femoral artery.
  Abbreviations as in Tables 5 and 6; DA = descending aorta; IAA = interrupted aortic arch; MVC = mitral valve commissurotomy; MS = mitral stenosis; SS = subaortic stenosis; SVC = superior vena cava.

Heath and associates[14] described plexiform lesions in 10 (43 percent) of their 23 patients over 15 years of age with isolated ASD or VSD or PDA (Fig. 21). In their 10 patients with plexiform lesions the pulmonary arterial systolic pressures ranged from 76 to 139 mm. Hg (mean 111 mm. Hg), and in 8 of the 10 this pressure was 90 mm. Hg or greater. These lesions were observed in 6 (43 percent) of their 14 patients with ASD, in 1 (17 percent) of 6 with VSD, and all of the 3 with PDA. Among our patients, in contrast, plexiform lesions were seen in 1 (6 percent) of 17 with ASD, in 1 (14 percent) of 7 with VSD, and in 7 (78 percent) of 9 with PDA. Except for the patients with ASD, the frequency of plexiform lesions in our patients was similar to that observed in the patients studied by Heath and associates.[14]

Plexiform lesions are observed in highest frequency not in patients with congenital cardiovascular malformations but in patients with primary or idiopathic pulmonary hypertension. Observations in 16 necropsy patients with this condition are summarized in Table 11. Fourteen (87 percent) of these 16 patients had plexiform lesions in the lungs; in 13, pulmonary arterial systolic pressures ranged from 60 to 192 mm. Hg (mean 117 mm. Hg). In 11 of these 13 patients this pressure was greater than 90 mm. Hg. In the 2 patients without plexiform lesions, pulmonary arterial systolic pressures were 49 and 101 mm. Hg.

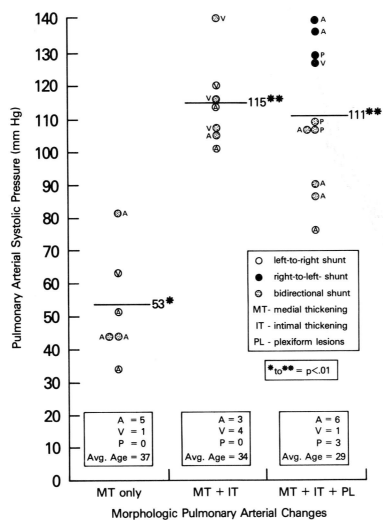

Figure 21. Data from Health and associates[14] showing interrelationship between morphologic pulmonary arterial changes, pulmonary arterial systolic pressure, and direction of shunt in 23 patients over age 15 with isolated ASD or VSD or PDA. Medial thickening only occurred in 6 patients; 7 had medial and intimal thickening; 10 had both medial and intimal thickening with plexiform lesions. The average pulmonary arterial systolic pressures in the patients with medial and intimal thickening were not significantly different from those of patients who had medial and intimal thickening with plexiform lesions. Pressures in both of these groups were significantly (p < .01) different from pressures in patients with only medial thickening.

Of the 10 patients with primary pulmonary hypertension with plexiform lesions and known pulmonary arterial pressures reported by Walcott and associates,[59] the pulmonary arterial systolic pressures ranged from 76 to 168 mm. Hg (mean 99 mm. Hg) and in only 2 patients was this pressure less than 90 mm. Hg.

Wagenvoort and Wagenvoort[60] summarized pulmonary morphologic observations in 110 patients (age range, infancy to 69 years; mean 23) with primary pulmonary hypertension, and 77 (70 percent) had plexiform lesions. Of their 110 patients, however, only 70 were 16 years of age or older and of the remaining 39 patients, many were infants and young children. Had these authors included only patients over age 15 their frequency of plexiform lesions almost certainly would have been higher.

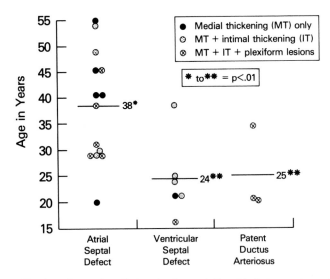

Figure 22. Data from Heath and associates[14] showing interrelationship between type of isolated congenital cardiovascular malformation (ASD, n = 14; VSD, n = 6; PDA, n = 3), age, and morphologic pulmonary arterial changes in 23 patients over age 15. The patients with VSD and PDA were significantly (p < .01) younger than those with ASD.

Table 11. Observations in 16 necropsy patients with primary pulmonary hypertension

Patient Age, Sex	Duration of Symptoms (months)	Pressures (mm. Hg)		CI (ml./min./m.²)	SA O₂ Sat. (%)	Heart Weight (gm.)	PL	CEF-PT
		PA (s/d)	SA (s/d)					
8 F*	24	190/100	90/55			160	+	A + F
17 F*	24	192/5	138/90	2.1	91	340	+	F
18 M	1	135/90	92/68	1.9	66	440	+	A
22 M**	36	88/54	100/60	1.5	86		+	A
25 F	30	92/39	130/78	2.0	98	460	+	A
25 F	54	122/49	122/80	2.7		360	+	A
25 F**	24	91/41	104/67	2.0	95		+	A
25 F	48	112/41	109/70	2.5			+	
28 M	24	108/58	127/80	3.2	92	630	+	A
29 F*	60	120/40	110/80	1.5	91	320	+	A
35 F*	84	101/38	108/72		86	400	0	A
38 M	144	138/88	138/88		↓†	880	+	F
39 F*	30	49/30	96/73		81†	390	0	A
39 F*	6	60/45	112/85			360	+	A
43 M	4	70/30	115/72	2.5		500	+	
56 M**	24		110/80				+	

*Death during or shortly after cardiac catheterization.
**Father-son-daughter relationship reported in detail elsewhere.[76]
†Right-to-left shunt via patent foramen ovale.
CEF-PT = configuration of elastic fibers of pulmonary trunk (A = adult; F = fetal); CI = cardiac index; PA = pulmonary artery; PL = plexiform lesion; SA = systemic artery; Sat. = saturation; s/d = systole diastole.

SIGNIFICANCE OF PULMONARY PARENCHYMAL
CHOLESTEROL-ESTER GRANULOMAS

Among our 87 necropsy patients with various congenital cardiovascular malformations, 8 (11 percent) had pulmonary parenchymal cholesterol-ester granulomas (Table 12, Fig. 23). The cause of these granulomas is uncertain, but most patients who have them also have pulmonary hypertension.[61] We observed 13 necropsy patients with cholesterol-ester pulmonary granulomas (Table 12); 11 had pulmonary arterial systolic pressures recorded and these ranged from 50 to 138 mm. Hg (mean 108 mm. Hg). The other 2 patients had pulmonic stenosis and probably normal or only mildly elevated pulmonary arterial pressures.

PULMONARY ARTERIAL *HYPO*TENSION

To this point we have discussed changes in pulmonary arteries primarily in patients with pulmonary *hyper*tension. Now we focus on patients with pulmonary arterial *hypo*tension. The media of the pulmonary arteries in patients with chronic pulmonary hypertension is usually thicker than normal; the reverse is true in patients with chronic pulmonary hypotension in whom the media is thinner than normal. In addition, the lumens of these arteries, as well as those of the capillaries and pulmonary veins, are dilated.[45] The medial thinning and the luminal widening appears to be a consequence of the decreased pulmonary arterial pressure and not a consequence of decreased pulmonary arterial flow because these findings are present both in patients with isolated pulmonic stenosis (normal pulmonary flow) and in patients with pulmonic stenosis associated with VSD and right-to-left shunt (diminished pulmonary flow) (Figs. 24 and 25).

Table 12. Observations in 13 necropsy patients over age 15 with cholesterol-ester granulomas

| Patient Age, Sex | Diagnosis | Pressure (mm. Hg) | | Shunt | Anatomic Grade of PA Changes |
		PA (s/d)	SA (s/d)		
29 F	ASD	110/60	110/60	both	III
33 M	VSD + PDA	106/60	136/68	R-L	III
21 F	VSD + PDA	138/86	140/88	both	III
38 M	VSD + CT	83/20	102/65	both	II
24 F	VSD + DORV	60/12	80/48	L-R	II
38 F	ASD + PS			R-L	0
24 F	VSD + PDA + MS + COA	104/60	118/70	L-R	II
25 F*	VSD + PS + AS		100/65	R-L	0
25 F	PPH	122/49	122/80	0	III
25 F	PPH	91/41	104/67	0	III
17 F	PPH	192/5**	138/90	0	III
38 M	PPH	138/88	138/88	0	III
39 F	PPH	50/30	96/73	L-R	II

*Patient also had pulmonary tuberculosis.
**Right ventricular pressure; pulmonary artery not entered.
AS = aortic stenosis; ASD = atrial septal defect; COA = coarctation of aorta; CT = corrected transposition; DORV = double outlet right ventricle; MS = mitral stenosis; PDA = patent ductus arteriosus; PPH = primary pulmonary hypertension; PS = pulmonic stenosis; PA = pulmonary artery; SA = systemic artery; s/d = systole/diastole; VSD = ventricular septal defect.

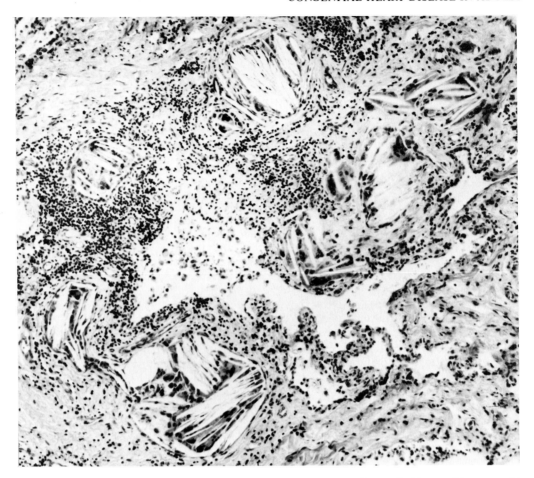

Figure 23. Multiple cholesterol-ester granulomas in the pulmonary parenchyma of a 38-year-old woman with VSD and corrected transposition. She had severe pulmonary hypertension (83/20 mm. Hg). Brachial arterial pressure was 102/65 mm. Hg and the left-to-right shunt was 2.1:1. (Hematoxylin and eosin stain, x 82; reduced 30%.)

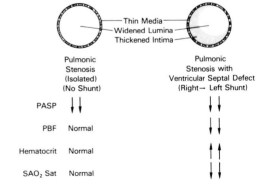

Figure 24. Diagram showing appearance of the pulmonary arteries in patients with pulmonary *hypo*tension. Patients with pulmonic stenosis have thinned media and wide lumina. If isolated, there is usually no thickening of the intima, but if pulmonic stenosis is combined with VSD the intima is usually thickened.

	Thin Media — Widened Lumina — Thickened Intima	
	Pulmonic Stenosis (Isolated) (No Shunt)	Pulmonic Stenosis with Ventricular Septal Defect (Right→ Left Shunt)
PASP	↓ ↓	↓ ↓
PBF	Normal	↓ ↓
Hematocrit	Normal	↑ ↑
SAO₂ Sat	Normal	↓ ↓

Abbreviations: PASP= Pulmonary Arterial Systolic Pressure; PBF = Pulmonary Blood Flow; SA = Systemic Artery; Sat = Saturation

490

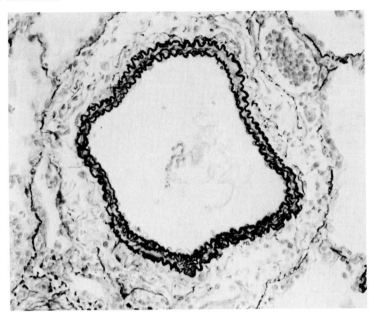

Figure 25. Pulmonic stenosis with ASD and anomalous drainage of the right pulmonary veins into the right atrium in a 19-year-old man who died three days after closure of the defect, pulmonic valvulotomy, and rerouting of the anomalous pulmonary veins. Preoperatively, pulmonary arterial pressure was 18/9 mm. Hg (mean 15), right ventricular pressure was 78/6 mm. Hg, brachial arterial pressure was 144/84 mm. Hg (mean 100), pulmonary to systemic flow ratio was 1.6 to 1, and systemic arterial oxygen saturation was 97 percent. Pulmonary arteries in this patient had thin medial walls and no intimal thickening, changes typical of pulmonary *hypo*tension. (Elastic van Gieson stain, x 272)

Another finding in some patients with pulmonary hypotension caused by congenital cardiovascular malformations is intimal fibrinous and fibrous changes. These intimal lesions were described intially by Arnold Rich[4] and are illustrated in Figure 26. Although pulmonary hypotension accompanies these lesions, it does not appear to be their cause. Evidence for this conclusion is provided by the fact that these lesions are rare in patients with pulmonic stenosis unassociated with communications between systemic and pulmonary circulations, but they are common in patients with pulmonic stenosis associated with VSD and right-to-left shunts (Table 13). The cause for the intimal lesions, therefore, must be related to the decreased pulmonary blood flow and associated polycythemia. It is also possible that "sludging" of blood flowing through the pulmonary vascular bed plays a role. Our observations in necropsy patients over age 15 with pulmonic stenosis are summarized in Table 13.

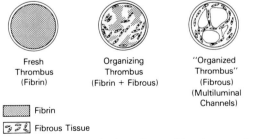

Figure 26. Diagram of Arnold Rich lesions occurring in patients with pulmonary hypotension and inadequate pulmonary blood flow.

Table 13. Observations in 9 necropsy patients over age 15 with pulmonic stenosis associated with either patent foramen ovale or ventricular septal defect

Patient Age, Sex Associated Defect	Pressures (mm. Hg, s/d)			SA O₂ Sat. (%)	Blood Hct. (%)	OP	Interval (days) OP to Death	PAs		
	PA	RV	SA					M	I	AR
28 F/PFO	9/4	170/4	123/70	67	61	PV	4	↓	nl	0
38 F/PFO						PV	60	↓	nl	0
43 F/PFO	13/8	172/12	130/70	83	65	PV	0	↓	↑	+
35 F/VSD	20/10	88/6		87	54	BT	21	↓	nl	0
22 M/VSD		145/9	148/105	88	71	0		↓	nl	0
53 M/VSD	17/8	95/8	110/65	77	69	TC	1	nl	↑	+
30 M/VSD	20/10	124/11	116/73	72	76	TC	45	↓	↑	+
23/M/VSD	12/4	112/4	131/85	68	72	TC	0	↓	↑	0
55 M/VSD	15/7	135/7	125/71	71	65	BT	6	↓	↑	0

AR = Arnold Rich lesions; Art = arterial; BT = Blalock-Taussig; Hct. = hematocrit; I = intima; nl = normal; M = media; OP = Cardiovascular operation; PA = pulmonary artery; PFO = patent foramen ovale; PV = pulmonic valvulotomy; RV = right ventricle; SA = systemic artery; Sat. = saturation; TC = total correction; ↓ = thinner than normal; ↑ = thickened; VSD = ventricular septal defect

Operative Creation of Systemic-to-Pulmonary Arterial Communications in Patients with Pulmonary Hypotension

Although development of pulmonary arterial hypertension is a recognized complication of operative creation of pulmonary-to-systemic arterial anastomoses,[62–66] the actual occurrence of pulmonary hypertension is uncommon. Therefore, anatomic pulmonary arterial changes indicative of pulmonary hypertension are also uncommon (Figs. 27 through 30).

Table 14 summarizes our observations in 10 necropsy patients over 15 years of age in whom pulmonary-to-systemic shunts had been created operatively between 3 and 23 years (mean 14) before death because of inadequate pulmonary blood flow. Nine patients had tetralogy of Fallot and one combined pulmonic stenosis and ASD. Surprisingly, 9 of the 10 patients showed neither pulmonary arterial medial or intimal thickening; 5 showed media of normal thickness and 4 had media thinner than normal. The one patient (Table 14) who did have medial and intimal thickening also had plexiform lesions. This patient, reported elsewhere,[65] was the only one of the 10 patients who had a Potts[67] operation rather than a Blalock-Taussig[68] anastomosis. The anastomosis in her was an end-to-side connection between right pulmonary artery and aorta. The right lung consequently developed systemic pressures and plexiform lesions (Fig. 29).

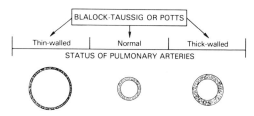

Figure 27. Diagram illustrating the effect of operative creation of systemic to pulmonary arterial communications on pulmonary arteries of patients with pulmonary *hypo*tension. The media of the pulmonary arteries may remain thin-walled and dilated (left), may increase to normal thickness (center), or may develop abnormally thickened media.

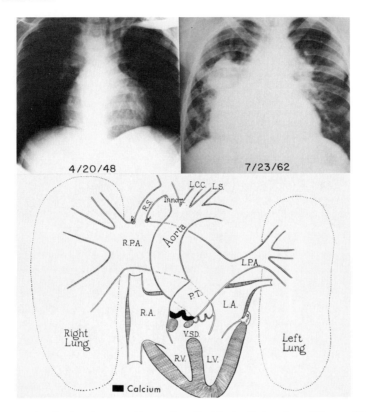

Figure 28. Tetralogy of Fallot in a 35-year-old man described in detail elsewhere.[65] By age 16 he was severely cyanotic and clubbed. Hemoglobin was 19.5 gm./100 ml. Chest radiograph (4/20/48) disclosed decreased pulmonary vascularity, and a subclavian-to-pulmonary arterial anastomosis was performed. Postoperatively, exercise tolerance improved and cyanosis had disappeared. At age 26 he had the first of many episodes of rapid heart action; three years later a chest radiograph (7/23/62) showed aneurysmal dilatation of the right pulmonary artery; systemic blood pressure was 150/25 mm. Hg. The patient died at age 35 of progressive right- and-left-sided congestive heart failure. Shortly before death the hematocrit was 44 percent.

The diagram of the heart and lungs at necropsy shows total obstruction of the pulmonic valve, ventricular septal defect (VSD), severely dilated pulmonary trunk (PT) and right main pulmonary artery (RPA), and widely patent right subclavian (RS) artery and anastomosis. LCC = left common carotid artery; LS = left subclavian artery; LPA = left pulmonary artery; LA = left atrium; LV = left ventricle; RA = right atrium; RV = right ventricle. Histologically, there was neither medial nor intimal thickening of the pulmonary arteries of either lung.

It is now well appreciated that pulmonary hypertension and anatomic pulmonary arterial changes of pulmonary hypertension are far more likely to develop after Potts than after Blalock-Taussig anastomoses. The various changes which may develop after creation of pulmonary to systemic anastomoses in patients with previous pulmonary hypotension are shown diagrammatically in Figure 30.

SUMMARY

Our three-grade anatomic classification of pulmonary arterial changes for patients with pulmonary arterial hypertension is a modification of the classification of Heath and Edwards. Our new classification consists of medial thickening only, grade I; medial and intimal thickening, grade II; and both medial and intimal thickening plus plexiform lesions, grade III. These anatomic changes in the pulmonary arteries result entirely

493

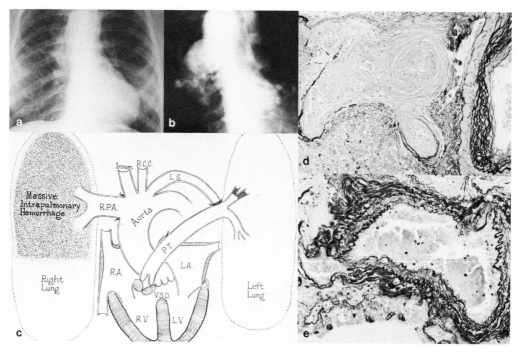

Figure 29. Tetralogy of Fallot in a 19-year-old woman described in detail elsewhere.[65] A left subclavian to left pulmonary arterial anastomosis was performed at age 3. There was little improvement, however, and an end-to-side anastomosis between aorta and right main pulmonary artery was performed two years later. She was nearly asymptomatic thereafter until age 11, when exercise tolerance diminished and cyanosis returned. At age 18 hematocrit was 80 percent. *a,* Chest radiograph shows right-aortic arch, decreased vascularity in the left lung, and increased vascular markings in the central portions of the right lung. The pulmonary trunk could not be entered by catheter from the right ventricle. Simultaneous right ventricular, femoral arterial, and right main pulmonary arterial systolic pressures were equal (108 mm. Hg). Oxygen saturation in the femoral artery was 70 percent. *b,* At right ventricular angiography all contrast material was ejected into the aorta and the lumens of the intrapulmonary branches of the right main pulmonary artery were severely narrowed. The left subclavian artery was occluded just proximal to its connection to the left main pulmonary artery. No contrast material entered the pulmonary trunk, left main pulmonary artery, or left lung. Because of systemic pressure in the right pulmonary arteries and absent blood flow to the left lung, the patient was considered inoperable. At age 19 she died suddenly of massive intrapulmonary hemorrhage. *c,* Diagram of findings in heart and lungs at necropsy (abbreviations in Figure 28). *d,* A portion of wall of a right pulmonary artery. Arising from it (but not connected in this section) is a plexiform lesion. *e,* Left pulmonary artery is normal. (Elastic van Gieson stain, x 160; reduced 41%.)

from pulmonary hypertension. Intimal thickening without medial thickening, however, is observed in older persons, and, in itself, is not a consequence of pulmonary hypertension.

Observations in our 87 necropsy patients over age 15 with major congenital cardiovascular malformations indicate that the changes in the pulmonary arteries are directly related to the level of pulmonary arterial pressure. Direction of the shunt, location of the shunt, and age of the patient were important only by their effect on the pulmonary arterial pressure. The patients with patent ductus arteriosus had the most severe changes in the pulmonary arteries and the highest average pulmonary arterial pressures.

Although not *all* patients with pulmonary arterial systolic pressures >90 mm. Hg had them, plexiform lesions were only observed in patients in whom the pulmonary arterial systemic pressure was >90 mm. Hg. Plexiform lesions indicate the irreversible nature

COMPLICATIONS OF PULMONARY-SYSTEMIC ANASTOMOSIS IN TETRALOGY OF FALLOT

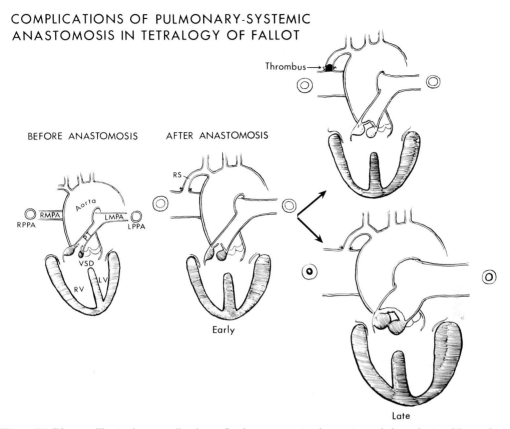

Figure 30. Diagram illustrating complications of pulmonary-systemic anastomosis in patients with tetralogy of Fallot. After anastomosis the early changes are related to the beneficial effects of increased blood flow to the lungs. With the shunt wide open, blood flow through the right ventricular outflow tract decreases and the amount of blood shunted from the right ventricular body to the left ventricle in diastole increases. As a result of the increased blood flow and pressure, the major pulmonary arteries widen and their wall thicknesses increase. Late complications include occlusion of the shunt and of the pulmonic valve or right ventricular infundibulum. LV = left ventricle; LPPA and RPPA = left and right peripheral pulmonary arteries; LMPA and RMPA = left and right main pulmonary arteries; RS = right subclavian artery; RV = right ventricle; VSD = ventricular septal defect.

of pulmonary hypertension and are more frequent in patients with primary pulmonary hypertension than in patients with congenital cardiovascular malformations.

The cause of plexiform lesions is unknown. We believe they are aneurysmal dilatations at sites of congenitally weak and/or thin walls of muscular pulmonary arteries. Distal to the weak or thin media the lumen of the muscular artery is obliterated. The aneurysmal protrusion is filled with thrombus which organizes into multiluminal channels.

Cholesterol-ester granulomas in the lungs usually indicate the presence of pulmonary hypertension; their cause is also uncertain.

In patients with pulmonary *hypo*tension (isolated pulmonic stenosis) and in patients with pulmonic stenosis and ventricular septal defect (tetralogy of Fallot), the media of the pulmonary arteries is thinner than normal and the lumens are larger than normal. Intimal thickening is usually seen in patients with tetralogy of Fallot even though the media is not thickened.

Surgical creation of systemic-to-pulmonary arterial anastomoses may cause the pul-

Table 14. Observations in 10 necropsy patients over age 15 with cyanotic CHD: Pulmonary vascular changes in patients having operatively created systemic to pulmonary arterial shunts for inadequate pulmonary blood flow (or severe systemic arterial desaturation)

Patient Age, Sex	Anomalies	SA* O₂ Sat. (%)	RV Pressure (mm. Hg. s/d) PRE–PO	PA Pressure (mm. Hg. s/d) PRE–PO	SA Pressure (mm. Hg. s/d) PRE–PO	Type Operative Shunt Created	Direction of PO Shunt R→L	L→R	Interval (yrs) OP-Shunt to Death	Cause of Death/ Status of Operative Shunt	Morphologic Pulmonic Arterial Changes
19 F	PS, VSD	70	NA–105/6	NA–108/78**	NA–108/78	(1)LSA→LPA (2)Ao→RPA	+ +	+	16 14	bleeding, lung/(1)C; (2)O	(1)H, (2)PL
35 M	PS, VSD		172/18–NA	20/10–NA	108/85–150/25	RSA→RPA	+	+	19	CHF/O	H, T
36 M	PS, VSD		NA	NA	NA–104/63	Ao→LPA	+		20	reoperation	H, T
24 F	PS, VSD	89	NA–40/0	NA–14/4	NA–90/70	(1)RSA→RPA (2)RSA→RPA	+	0	18 23	reoperation/O↓↓	H
27 M	PS, VSD		NA	NA	NA	LSA→LPA	+	0	9	CHF/(1) + (2)O↓↓↓	H
21 M	PS, VSD, ASD, CT		NA	NA	NA–120/80	LSA→LPA	+	0	11	polycythemia/O↓↓↓	none
21 M	PS, VSD, CT	71	125/0–NA	NA	NA–125/80	(1)LSA→LPA (2)RSA→RPA	+	+	6 3	reoperation/(1)C, (2)O↓	(1)T, (2)none
33 M	PS, ASD	81	NA–130/10	NA	NA–80/55†	LSA→LPA	+	+	20	reoperation/O	none
27 M	PS,VSD,ASD, TA	88	NA	NA	NA–112/66	LSA→LPA	+	+	20	reoperation/O	none
22 F	PS,VSD	72	145/0–154/13	15/0–NA	120/65–196/75	LSA→LPA	+	0	8	reoperation C	none

* Last year of life

** Right pulmonary artery

† Left brachial artery: right femoral artery = 98/58

ASD = atrial septal defect; C = closed; CHF = congestive heart failure; CT = complete transposition; H = hypoplastic; LPA = left main pulmonary artery; LSA = left subclavian artery; NA = data not available; O = open; PA = pulmonary artery; PL = plexiform lesion + medial hypertrophy + intimal proliferation; PO = postoperative; PRE = preoperative; PS = pulmonic or subpulmonic stenosis; RPA = right pulmonary artery; RSA = right subclavian artery; RV = right ventricle; T = thrombi containing fibrin; TA = tricuspid atresia; SA = systemic artery; Sat. = saturation; s/d = systolic/diastolic; VSD = ventricular septal defect.

monary arterial media to thicken to normal widths or even to widths thicker than normal, but the development of pulmonary hypertension after such operations is infrequent.

REFERENCES

1. Moschcowitz, E.: *Hypertension of the pulmonary circulation; its causes, dynamics and relation to other circulatory states.* Am. J. Med. Sci. 174:388,1927.
2. Brenner, O.: *Pathology of the vessels of the pulmonary circulation.* Arch. Intern. Med. 56:211,1935.
3. Parker, F., and Weiss, S.: *The nature and significance of the structural changes in the lungs in mitral stenosis.* Am. J. Pathol. 12:573,1936.
4. Rich, A. R.: *A hitherto unrecognized tendency to the development of widespread pulmonary vascular obstruction in patients with congenital pulmonary stenosis (tetralogy of Fallot).* Bull. Johns Hopkins Hosp. 82:389,1948.
5. Edwards, J. E., Douglas, J. M., Burchell, H. B., et al.: *Pathology of the intrapulmonary arteries and arterioles in coarctation of the aorta associated with patent ductus arteriosus.* Am. Heart J. 38:208,1949.
6. Civin, W. H., and Edwards, J. E.: *Pathology of the pulmonary vascular tree. I. A comparison of the intrapulmonary arteries in the Eisenmenger complex and in stenosis of ostium infundibuli associated with biventricular origin of the aorta.* Circulation 21:545,1950.
7. Heath, D., and Witaker, W.: *The pulmonary vessels in patent ductus arteriosus.* J. Pathol. Bacteriol. 70:285,1955.
8. Brewer, D. B.: *Fibrous occlusion and anastomosis of the pulmonary vessels in a case of pulmonary hypertension associated with patent ductus arteriosus.* J. Pathol. Bacteriol. 70:299,1955.
9. Dammann, J. F., and Ferencz, C.: *The significance of the pulmonary vascular bed in congenital heart disease. I. Normal lungs, 11. Malformations of the heart in which there is pulmonary stenosis.* Am. Heart J. 52:7,1956.
10. Dammann, J. F., Jr., and Ferencz, C.: *The significance of the pulmonary vascular bed in congenital heart disease. III. Defects between the ventricles or great vessels in which both increased pressure and blood flow may act upon the lungs and in which there is a common ejectile force.* Am. Heart J. 52:210,1956.
11. Edwards, J. E.: *Functional pathology of the pulmonary vascular tree in congenital cardiac disease.* Circulation 15:164,1957.
12. Heath, D., Dushane, J. W., Wood, E. H., et al.: *The etiology of pulmonary thrombosis in cyanotic congenital heart disease with pulmonary stenosis.* Thorax 13:213,1958.
13. Heath, D., and Edwards, J. E.: *The pathology of hypertensive pulmonary vascular disease. A description of six grades of structural changes in the pulmonary arteries with special reference to congenital cardiac defects.* Circulation 18:533,1958.
14. Heath, D., Helmholz, H. F., Burchell, H. B., et al.: *Graded pulmonary vascular changes and hemodynamic findings in cases of atrial and ventricular septal defect and patent ductus arteriosus.* Circulation 18:1155,1958.
15. Heath, D., Helmholz, H. F., Burchell, H. B., et al.: *Relation between structural changes in the small pulmonary arteries and the immediate reversibility of pulmonary hypertension following closure of ventricular and atrial septal defects.* Circulation 18:1167,1958.
16. Wagenvoort, C. A.: *The morphology of certain vascular lesions in pulmonary hypertension.* J. Pathol. Bacteriol. 78:503,1959.
17. Ferencz, C.: *The pulmonary vascular bed in tetralogy of Fallot. I. Changes associated with pulmonic stenosis.* Bull. Johns Hopkins Hosp. 106:81,1960.
18. Ferencz, C.: *The pulmonary vascular bed in tetralogy of Fallot. II. Changes following a systemic-pulmonary arterial anastomosis.* Bull. Johns Hopkins Hosp. 106:100,1960.
19. Heath, D.: *Pathology of the pulmonary vessels.* Br. J. Dis. Chest 54:182,1960.
20. Wagenvoort, C. A., Dushane, J. W., and Edwards, J. E.: *Hypertensive pulmonary arterial lesions as a result of anastomosis of systemic and pulmonary circulations.* Mayo Clin. Proc. 35:186,1960.
21. Naeye, R. L.: *Perinatal changes in the pulmonary vascular bed with stenosis and atresia of the pulmonic valve.* Am. Heart J. 61:586,1961.
22. Wagenvoort, C. A., Neufeld, H. N., Dushane, J. W., et al.: *The pulmonary arterial tree in ventricular septal defect. A quantitative study of anatomic features in fetuses, infants, and children.* Circulation 23:740,1961.
23. Wagenvoort, C. A., and Edwards, J. E.: *The pulmonary arterial tree in pulmonic atresia.* Arch. Pathol. 71:646,1961.

24. WAGENVOORT, C. A.: *Pulmonary arteries in infants with ventricular septal defect.* Med. Thorac. 19:354,1962.

25. HARRIS, P., AND HEATH, D.: *The Human Pulmonary Circulation. Its Forms and Function in Health and Disease.* E & S Livingstone, Ltd., Edinburgh and London, 1962.

26. THOMAS, M. A.: *Pulmonary vascular changes in pulmonary stenosis with and without ventricular septal defect.* Br. Heart J. 26:655,1964.

27. FERENCZ, C.: *Pulmonary vascular changes in tetralogy of Fallot.* Dis. Chest 46:664,1964.

28. WAGENVOORT, C. A., HEATH, D., AND EDWARDS, J. E.: *The Pathology of the Pulmonary Vasculature.* Charles C Thomas, Springfield, Ill., 1964.

29. THOMAS, M. A.: *Pulmonary vascular changes in pulmonary stenosis with and without ventricular septal defect.* Br. Heart J. 26:655,1964.

30. KANJUH, V. I., SELLERS, R. D., AND EDWARDS, J. E.: *Pulmonary vascular plexiform lesion.* Arch. Pathol. 78:513,1964.

31. FERENCZ, C.: *Transposition of the great vessels; pathophysiologic consideration based upon a study of the lungs.* Circulation 33:232,1966.

32. ANDERSON, R. A., LEVY, A. M., NAEYE, R. L., ET AL.: *Rapidly progressive pulmonary vascular obstructive disease. Association with ventricular septal defects during early childhood.* Am. J. Cardiol. 19:854,1967.

33. WAGENVOORT, C. A., NAUTA, J., VAN DER SCHAAR, P. J., ET AL.: *Effect of flow and pressure on pulmonary vessels. A semiquantitative study based on lung biopsies.* Circulation 35:1028,1967.

34. WAGENVOORT, C. A., NAUTA, J., VAN DER SCHAAR, P. J., ET AL.: *Vascular changes in pulmonic stenosis and tetralogy of Fallot studied in lung biopsies.* Circulation 36:924,1967.

35. WAGENVOORT, C. A., NAUTA, J., VAN DER SCHAAR, P. J., ET AL.: *The pulmonary vasculature in complete transposition of the great vessels judged from lung biopsies.* Circulation 38:746,1968.

36. VILES, P. H., ONGLEY, P. A., AND TITUS, J. L.: *The spectrum of pulmonary vascular disease in transposition of the great arteries.* Circulation 40:31,1969.

37. WAGENVOORT, C. A.: *Hypertensive pulmonary vascular disease complicating congenital heart disease: A review.* Cardiovasc. Clin. 5:43,1973.

38. HISLOP, A., AND REID, L.: *Stuctural changes in the pulmonary arteries and veins in tetralogy of Fallot.* Br. Heart J. 35:1178,1973.

39. NEWFELD, E. A., PAUL, M. H., MUSTER, A. J., ET AL.: *Pulmonary vascular disease in complete transposition of the great arteries: A study of 200 patients.* Am. J. Cardiol. 34:75,1974.

40. WAGENVOORT, C. A.: *Classification of pulmonary vascular lesions in congenital and acquired heart disease.* Adv. Cardiol. 11:48,1974.

41. WAGENVOORT, C. A., AND WAGENVOORT, N.: *Pathology of the Eisenmenger syndrome and primary pulmonary hypertension.* Adv. Cardiol. 11:123,1974.

42. HOFFMEISTER, H. -E., APITZ, J., AND BACKMANN, R.: *The correlation between pulmonary hypertension and histological findings of the pulmonary vessels in congenital heart disease.* Thoraxchir. Vask. Chir. 23:436,1975.

43. BESSINGER, F. B., BLIEDEN, L. C., AND EDWARDS, J. E.: *Hypertensive pulmonary vascular disease associated with patent ductus arteriosus. Primary or secondary?* Circulation 52:157,1975.

44. NEWFELD, E. A., SHER, M., PAUL, M. H., ET AL.: *Pulmonary vascular disease in complete atrioventricular canal defect.* Am. J. Cardiol. 39:721,1977.

45. WAGENVOORT, C. A., AND WAGENVOORT, N.: *Pathology of Pulmonary Hypertension.* John Wiley & Sons, New York, 1977.

46. CIVIN, W. H., AND EDWARDS, J. E.: *The postnatal structural changes in the intrapulmonary arteries and arterioles.* Arch. Pathol. 51:192,1951.

47. WAGENVOORT, C. A., AND WAGENVOORT, N.: *Age changes in muscular pulmonary arteries.* Arch. Pathol. 79:524,1965.

48. ROBERTS, W. C., AND FREDRICKSON, D. S.: *Gaucher's disease of the lung causing severe pulmonary hypertension with associated acute recurrent pericarditis.* Circulation 35:783,1967.

49. SPENCER, H.: *Primary pulmonary hypertension and related vascular changes in the lungs.* J. Pathol. Bacteriol. 62:75,1950.

50. GORDON, A. J., DONOSO, E., KUHN, C. L. A., ET AL.: *Patent ductus arteriosus with reversal of flow.* N. Engl. J. Med. 251:923,1954.

51. HUFNER, R. F., AND MCNICOL, C. A.: *The pathologic physiology of microscopic pulmonary vascular shunts.* AMA Arch. Pathol. 65:554,1958.

52. ROSSALL, R. E., AND THOMPSON, H.: *Formation of new vascular channels in the lungs of a patient with secondary pulmonary hypertension.* J. Pathol. Bacteriol. 76:593,1958.

53. PLANT, A.: *Hemangioendothelioma of the lung. Report of two cases.* Arch. Pathol. 29:517,1940.

54. MOSCHCOWITZ, E., RUBIN, E., AND STRAUSS, L.: *Hypertension of the pulmonary circulation due to congenital glomoid obstruction of the pulmonary arteries.* Am. J. Pathol. 39:75,1961.

55. CROSS, K. R., AND KOBAYASHI, C. K.: *Primary pulmonary vascular sclerosis: Report of case.* Am. J. Clin. Pathol. 17:155,1947.

56. HRUBAN, Z., AND HUMPHREYS, E. M.: *Congenital anomalies associated with pulmonary hypertension in an infant.* Arch. Pathol. 70:766,1960.

57. NAEYE, R. L., AND VENNART, G. P.: *Structure and significance of pulmonary plexiform structures.* Am. J. Pathol. 36:593,1960.

58. KAPANCI, Y.: *Hypertensive pulmonary vascular disease. Endothelial hyperplasia and its relations to intravascular fibrin precipitation.* Am. J. Pathol. 48:665,1965.

59. WALCOTT, G., BURCHELL, H. B., AND BROWN, A. L.: *Primary pulmonary hypertension.* Am. J. Med. 49:70,1970.

60. WAGENVOORT, C. A., AND WAGENVOORT, N.: *Primary pulmonary hypertension. A patholytic study of the lung vessels in 156 clinically diagnosed cases.* Circulation 42:1163,1970.

61. GLANCY, D. L., FRAZIER, P. D., AND ROBERTS, W. C.: *Pulmonary parenchymal cholesterol-ester granulomas in patients with pulmonary hypertension.* Am. J. Med. 45:198,1968.

62. ROSS, R. S., TAUSSIG, H. B., AND EVANS, M. H.: *Late hemodynamic complications of anastomotic surgery for the treatment of the tetralogy of Fallot.* Circulation 18:553,1958.

63. PAUL, M. H., MILLER, R. A., AND POTTS, W. J.: *Long-term results of aortic-pulmonary anastomosis for tetralogy of Fallot: An analysis of the first 100 cases eleven to thirteen years after operation.* Circulation 23:525,1961.

64. MCCAGG, C. J., ROSS, R. S., AND BRAUNWALD, E.: *The development of elevated pulmonary vascular resistance in man following increased pulmonary blood flow from systemic pulmonary anastomoses.* Am. J. Med. 33:201,1962.

65. ROBERTS, W. C., FRIESINGER, G. C., COHEN, L. S., ET AL.: *Acquired pulmonic atresia. Total obstruction to right ventricular outflow after systemic to pulmonary arterial anastomoses for cyanotic congenital cardiac disease.* Am. J. Cardiol. 24:335,1969.

66. NEWFELD, E. A., WALDMAN, J. D., PAUL, M. H., ET AL.: *Pulmonary vascular disease after systemic-pulmonary arterial shunt operations.* Am. J. Cardiol. 39:715,1977.

67. POTTS, W. J., SMITH, S., AND GIBSON, S.: *Anastomosis of the aorta to a pulmonary artery. Certain types in congenital heart disease.* JAMA 132:627,1946.

68. BLALOCK, A., AND TAUSSIG, H. B.: *Surgical treatment of malformations of the heart in which there is a pulmonary stenosis or pulmonary atresia.* JAMA 128:189,1945.

69. HEATH, D., DUSHANE, J. W., WOOD, E. H., ET AL.: *The structure of the pulmonary trunk at different ages and in cases of pulmonary hypertension and pulmonary stenosis.* J. Pathol. Bacteriol. 77:443,1959.

70. PERLOFF, J. K., URSCHELL, C. W., ROBERTS, W. C., ET AL.: *Aneurysmal dilatation of the coronary arteries in cyanotic congenital cardiac disease.* Am. J. Med. 45:802,1968.

71. GLANCY, D. L., AND ROBERTS, W. C.: *Congenital obstructive lesions involving the major pulmonary veins, left atrium, or mitral valve: A clinical, laboratory, and morphologic survey.* Cathet. Cardiovasc. Diagn. 2:215,1976.

72. PARKER, F., JR., AND WEISS, S.: *The nature and significance of the structural changes in the lungs in mitral stenosis.* Am. J. Pathol. 12:573,1936.

73. HEATH, D., AND WHITAKER, W.: *The pulmonary vessels in mitral stenosis.* J. Pathol. Bacteriol. 70:291,1955.

74. ABER, C. P., CAMPBELL, J. A., AND MEECHAM, J.: *Arterial patterns in mitral stenosis.* Br. Heart J. 25:109,1963.

75. TANDON, H. D., AND KASTURI, J.: *Pulmonary vascular changes associated with isolated mitral stenosis in India.* Br. Heart J. 37:26,1975.

76. KINGDON, H. S., COHEN, L. S., ROBERTS, W. C., ET AL.: *Familial occurrence of primary pulmonary hypertension.* Arch. Intern. Med. 118:422,1966.

Myocardial Ultrastructure in Children and Adults with Congenital Heart Disease

Michael Jones, M.D., and
Victor J. Ferrans, M.D., Ph. D.

Clinical studies in patients with valvular heart disease[1-8] and congenital heart disease[9-18] have suggested that a "myocardial factor" related to dysfunction of the heart muscle may be responsible for unsatisfactory postoperative clinical courses in certain patients who undergo complete, successful correction of their anatomic lesions. From such studies it is evident that myocardial dysfunction may develop as a consequence of longstanding hemodynamic abnormalities, chronic hypoxia, and cardiac hypertrophy associated with congenital heart disease. This dysfunction may not be reversible following surgical correction of the anatomic lesions. Little information is available concerning the course of morphological changes in patients with right ventricular hypertrophy due to congenital heart disease. It is known, however, that exceptional patients with tetralogy of Fallot may survive to middle age without surgical treatment.[19] The average age at death of untreated patients with this disease is 12 years.[20,21] Even patients who have received subclavian to pulmonary arterial anastomoses may have a 50 percent mortality rate in 20 to 28 years after these palliative operations.[22-24] Although successful total correction of tetralogy of Fallot can be accomplished in patients over the age of 30, the perioperative and late mortality rates of such patients are high, in the range of 10 to 20 percent.[25-31] Because of the importance of the problem of myocardial dysfunction in congenital heart disease and because of the paucity of information on cardiac ultrastructure in congenital heart disease, we have made a comparative light and electron microscopic study of operatively resected right ventricular muscle from 75 patients with congenital heart anomalies associated with markedly elevated right ventricular pressures (equal to or greater than systemic systolic pressures). The elevated right ventricular pressures were caused by either obstruction to right ventricular outflow, with or without an intracardiac shunt (70 patients), or by large left-to-right shunts associated with elevated pulmonary arterial pressures (5 patients). Based on these observations, we have identified morphological characteristics of myocardial degeneration which bear relationships to the patients' ages and clinical courses. Before presenting our observations on the incidence of morphological changes of cellular degeneration in the various age groups of patients, it is appropriate to review the ultrastructural features of myocardium as seen in the normal state and in hypertrophy with and without degeneration of the muscle cells.

MATERIALS AND METHODS

Patients Studied

Clinical and hemodynamic data from each group of patients are summarized in Table 1. The 75 patients with right ventricular pressure overload were divided into four

501

Table 1. Clinical and hemodynamic findings in 75 patients with congenital heart disease and right ventricular hypertrophy

Age Group (years)	Number of Patients	Average Age (years)	Hct (%)	PAO$_2$ (%)	RA (mm.Hg)	RV$_s$ (mm.Hg)	RVEDP (mm.Hg)	PSG (mm.Hg)	Preoperative Failure	Postoperative Low Output State	Arrhythmia	Late Postoperative Failure	Death
0.9–10	36	6	45	86	4	94	7	67	0(0%)	4(11%)	0(0%)	0(0%)	3(8%)
11–20	22	14	58	86	5	106	7	81	0(0%)	2(9%)	1(5%)	0(0%)	2(9%)
21–29	8	25	51	90	3	107	8	82	2(25%)	2(25%)	1(12%)	2(25%)	2(25%)
30–53	9	40	51	86	4	117	9	97	4(44%)	5(55%)	3(33%)	1(11%)	3(33%)

HCT = hematocrit; PAO$_2$ = peripheral arterial oxygen saturation; PSG = peak systolic pressure gradient between right ventricle and pulmonary trunk; RA = right atrial mean pressure; RV$_s$ = right ventricular systolic pressure; RVEDP = right ventricular end diastolic pressure.
The values for HCT, PAO$_2$, RA, RV$_s$, RVEDP, and PSG are average values for each age group.

groups: Group I (36 patients), aged 10 months to 10 years; Group II (22 patients), aged 11 to 20 years; Group III (8 patients), aged 21 to 29 years; and Group IV (9 patients), aged 30 to 53 years. The average patient age in Group I was 6 years; in Group II, 14 years; in Group III, 25 years; and in Group IV, 40 years. Average hematocrits were 45, 58, 51, and 51 percent; peripheral arterial oxygen saturations were 86, 86, 90, and 86 percent, respectively. Right atrial mean pressures averaged 4, 5, 3, and 4 mm. Hg; right ventricular end diastolic pressures averaged 7, 7, 8, and 9 mm. Hg, respectively. Right ventricular systolic pressures were equal to or greater than systemic systolic arterial pressures in all patients.

None of the patients in Group I or II had signs or symptoms of cardiac failure preoperatively; however, one fourth of the patients in Group III and 44 percent (four) of the patients in Group IV had clinical evidence of cardiac failure. Four (11 percent) Group I patients, two (9 percent) Group II patients, two (25 percent) Group III patients, and five (55 percent) Group IV patients had the low cardiac output syndrome postoperatively and required inotropic support for over 24 hours. Eight percent of the Group I patients, 9 percent of the Group II patients, 25 percent of the Group III patients, and 33 percent of the Group IV patients died either early or late in their postoperative courses. No patient in Group I, one patient (5 percent) in Group II, two patients (22 percent) in Group III, and three patients (33 percent) in Group IV had clinically significant arrhythmias early or late postoperatively. Only two patients (22 percent) in Group IV had no functional abnormalities at all early or late postoperatively.

Preparation of Tissues

Portions of crista supraventricularis muscle were obtained from each patient at the time of correction of the anomaly. Operations were performed between 1971 and 1975 at the National Heart, Lung, and Blood Institute and The Johns Hopkins Hospital. All operations were performed with cardiopulmonary bypass and core hypothermia of 20 to 30°C. Tissue from the parietal band of the crista supraventricularis was immediately minced into 1- to 2-mm. pieces in cold, buffered glutaraldehyde and fixed in this solution for 12 hours. Postfixation processing included 2 hours in a cold solution of 1 percent osmium tetroxide in Millonig's prosphate buffer; dehydration in ethanol and propylene oxide; and embedding in Maraglas.[32] Five to twenty blocks of tissue from each patient were sectioned at a thickness of 1 μ and stained with alkaline toluidine blue. Light microscopic evaluation of these sections was used to estimate transverse cell diameters and to select specimens for ultrathin sectioning for electron microscopy. Other portions of the tissue were fixed in formalin, embedded in paraffin, and stained with hematoxylin-eosin and Masson's trichrome stain for estimation of the extent of interstitial fibrosis. Ultrathin sections were stained with lead citrate and uranyl acetate and examined with an RCA EMU-3G or a JEOL 100B electron microscope.

RESULTS

Ultrastructure of Normal Myocardium

Our knowledge of normal human myocardial ultrastructure has been derived primarily from observations on normal-sized cardiac muscle cells in tissues obtained at open heart operations, and from comparisons of these observations with those made on myocardium of various normal animals. Normal myocardium consists of cardiac muscle cells and interstitial tissue components. Normal human cardiac muscle cells (Figs. 1 through 3) are elongated, measure from 10 to 15 μ in diameter, are arranged in parallel, and are connected end-to-end by intercellular junctions known as intercalated discs.

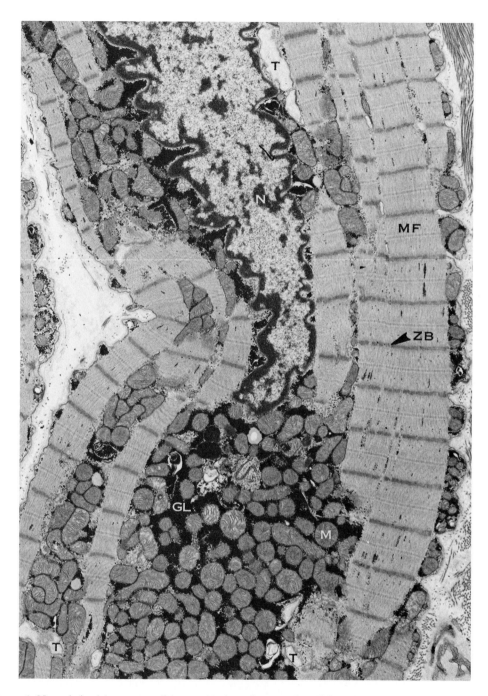

Figure 1. Normal-sized (transverse diameter, 11 μ) cardiac muscle cell from 7-year-old girl with ventricular septal defect and aortic regurgitation. Note the myofibrils (MF) with prominent Z bands (ZB), glycogen particles (GL), and T-tubules (T) of various sizes. The mitochondria (M) form a large cluster at the pole of the nucleus (N). ($\times$ 8600)

504

Side-to-side junctions (lateral junctions) are less frequently present. Cellular organelles include: nuclei, myofibrils, mitochondria, T-tubules, sarcoplasmic reticulum, ribosomes (both free and bound to the membranes of the reticulum), cytoskeletal filaments (100 Å in diameter), glycogen particles of the β- or monoparticulate type, Golgi complexes, lysosomes, and residual bodies (Fig. 1). The plasma membrane and a finely fibrillar external lamina or basement membrane constitute the sarcolemma (Fig. 2).

The myofibrils (Figs. 1 through 3) are composed of sarcomeres; these are the contractile units that contain two types of myofilaments arranged into a characteristic pattern of repeating bands or striations. The thick filaments form the A bands, measure from 120 to 160 Å in diameter and contain myosin. The thin filaments form the I bands, measure from 50 to 80 Å in diameter and contain actin and other proteins. The thin filaments terminate at the Z bands; how they are attached has not been fully elucidated. The thick filaments are not attached to other myofibrillar structures at their terminations. The thick and thin filaments interdigitate so that each thick filament is surrounded by six thin filaments (Figs. 2 and 3), thus providing the basis for the sliding filament mechanism of muscle contraction.

The intercellular junctions (Fig. 3) in cardiac muscle cells have four distinct structural components: (1) undifferentiated regions, in which the apposed plasma membranes have no specialized components and are separated by a space of 200 Å; (2) desmosomes, which are similar to those of other cell types and serve as points of reinforcement of intercellular adhesion; (3) myofibrillar insertion sites, in which the thin myofilaments of the terminal sarcomeres insert into a mass of material that resembles that in Z bands and is adherent to the inner (cytoplasmic) aspect of the plasma membrane; and (4) nexuses, which serve as points of low resistance for transmission of the electrical impulse from one cell to another, and are characterized by narrowing of the space between the apposed plasma membranes to a width between 30 and 40 Å.

The nucleus (Fig. 1) is composed of the inner and the outer nuclear membranes, the nuclear chromatin, and the nucleolus. Nuclear pore complexes, which provide direct routes for nucleocytoplasmic interaction, are present throughout the nuclear membranes. The transverse tubules, or T-tubules (Fig. 2), are cylindrical invaginations of the plasma membranes. These invaginations course at the levels of the Z bands, extend deep into the interior of the cell, and provide a means for rapid activation of the contractile elements located away from the cell surfaces. The mitochondria are located in the interfibrillary spaces and usually form clusters in the myofibril-free areas at the nuclear poles, where the Golgi complexes and numerous glycogen particles are also present.

The sarcoplasmic reticulum (SR) forms a network of intracellular tubules that do not communicate with the extracellular space. This network has at least three morphologically distinct components: free SR, junctional SR, and extended junctional SR. The free SR forms a network of branching and anastomosing tubules that surround the myofibrils. The junctional SR consists of specialized saccular dilatations known as terminal cisterns. These cisterns have an electron-dense content (junctional granules) and are closely approximated to the sarcolemma, either at the free surface of the cell or at the level of the T-tubules (Fig. 2). The structures resulting from the apposition of one or two terminal cisterns of SR to a T-tubule are known as dyads and triads, respectively. The terminal cisterns participate in the excitation-contraction coupling by providing sites for the sequential release and binding of calcium during activation and relaxation. The extended junctional SR is composed of cisterns that resemble those of junctional SR but do not become closely apposed to the sarcolemma. Extended junctional SR is relatively abundant in atrial myocardium, in which T-tubules are absent in some cells and poorly developed in others; it is very scarce in ventricular myocardium, in which T-tubules are well developed.

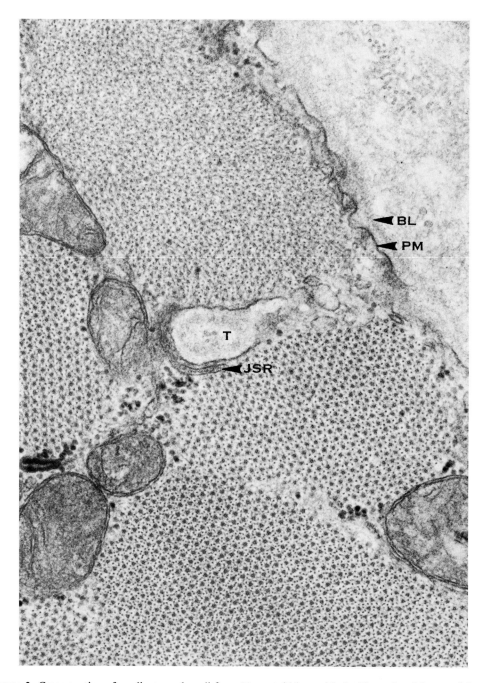

Figure 2. Cross section of cardiac muscle cell from 11-year-old boy with double outlet right ventricle and infundibular pulmonic stenosis shows: hexagonal array of thick and thin myofilaments; a dyad, composed of a T-tubule (T) and closely apposed cistern of junctional sarcoplasmic reticulum (JSR); the sarcolemma, composed of the plasma membrane (PM) and the basal lamina (BL) or basement membrane; and a cluster of connective tissue microfibrils (upper right). ($\times$ 57,500)

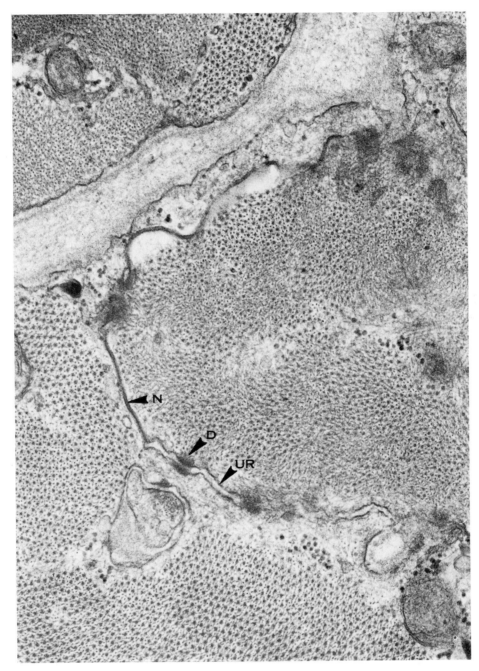

Figure 3. Part of intercellular junction in same tissue shown in Figure 2, showing a long, convoluted nexus (N), a desmosome (D) and several undifferentiated regions (UR). (× 43,500)

Interstitial components consist of vascular and neural elements and cellular (fibroblasts, primitive mesenchymal cells, occasional macrophages and mast cells) and extracellular (collagen fibrils, elastic fibers, connective tissue microfibrils, acid mucopolysaccharide-rich ground substance) components of connective tissue.

General Ultrastructural Features of Hypertrophied Myocardium

This section summarizes morphologic aspects of cardiac hypertrophy as evidenced in the present study and as described in other studies.[33] Data concerning the incidence of ultrastructural changes in the four groups of patients in the study are presented in the next section of this chapter.

Hypertrophying cardiac muscle cells increase in size but not in number, except under very special circumstances. The mechanisms by which cell size increases are complex and result in an increase in the number and/or size of the organelles of the individual myocardial cells. Most of the increment in cardiac muscle cell constituents involves increases in mitochondria and in contractile elements. It has been shown that the dimensions of the sarcomeres and myofilaments are not altered in hypertrophy.[34] Ideally, the synthesis of certain cellular components should be synchronous; however, the synthesis of different cellular components may exceed that of others, producing an imbalance in the relative amounts of different organelles, particularly mitochondria and myofibrils. Increased synthesis of collagen occurs very early in hypertrophy.[35] At certain periods during the hypertrophy process, usually in the late stages, the deposition of collagen and other interstitial structures may appear more prominent morphologically than the formation of organelles of cardiac muscle cells.

Based on biochemical and morphologic studies of experimental animals, Meerson delineated three stages of cardiac hypertrophy.[36-38] The first of these, the stage of developing hypertrophy, is followed by a stage of stable hyperfunction or compensated hypertrophy. The third stage of hypertrophy, that of cellular exhaustion, may develop eventually, in association with deterioration of the function of the heart and the appearance of morphological changes of fibrosis and cellular degeneration. Previous studies from this laboratory[33,39-43] have indicated that the concept of Meerson is applicable not only to animals with experimentally induced hypertrophy but also to humans with hypertrophy secondary to various types of clinical heart disease. The three stages of hypertrophy sometimes are not as clearly defined morphologically as might be implied by the definitions given above. The myocardium of an individual patient may show either hypertrophied, nondegenerated cells or a continuum of morphological changes ranging from hypertrophied, nondegenerated cells to hypertrophied, severely degenerated cells.

Hypertrophy Without Degeneration

Hypertrophied, nondegenerated muscle cells may be qualitatively normal in every respect except for their size (20 to 60 μ in transverse diameter). Considerable variability in muscle cell size may exist in myocardium of a given patient (Fig. 4), and even among immediately adjacent muscle cells in a tissue block. Normal-sized cells may be found next to severely enlarged ones. Variability in the size of mitochondria also occurs, and it may be related to the fact that mitochondrial replication involves a poorly understood interaction between nuclear and mitochondrial DNA. Other alterations in myocardial hypertrophy include enlargement of Golgi complexes and of nuclei (Fig. 5); the latter often show an increase in the degree of convolution of the nuclear membranes. Intranuclear tubules may develop as the most extreme form of alteration in nuclear membranes.[44] Ribosomes are increased in number, and T-tubules become di-

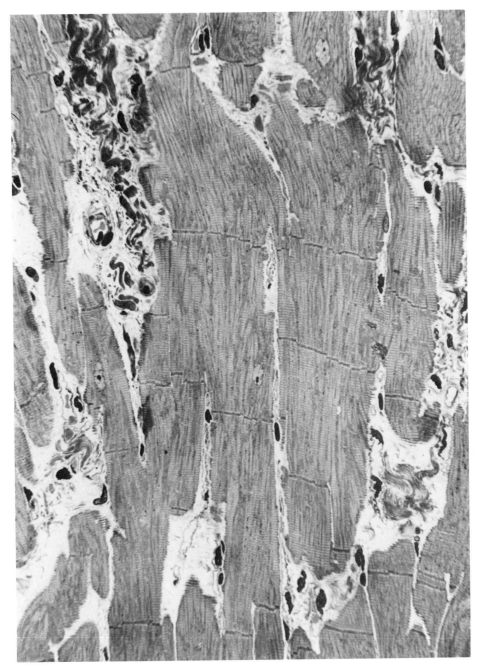

Figure 4. Light micrograph of severely hypertrophied muscle cells from 25-year-old woman with atrial septal defect and combined infundibular and valvular pulmonic stenosis. Focal accumulations of fibrous tissue are present between the myocytes. (Toluidine blue stain, × 550)

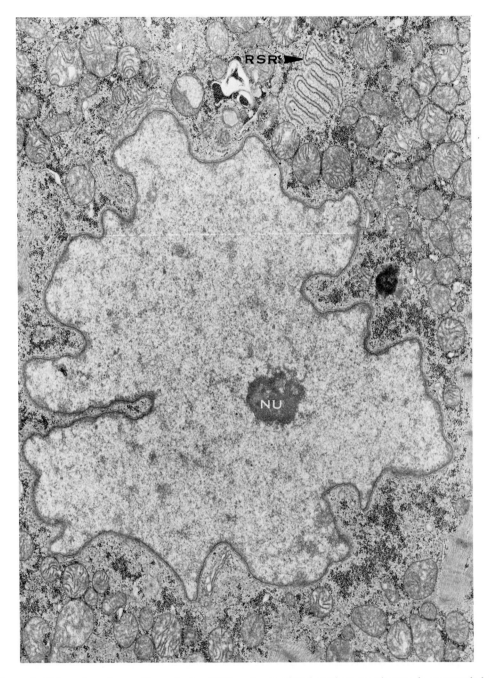

Figure 5. Enlarged nucleus with nucleolus (NU) and convoluted nuclear membranes is surrounded by mitochondria and a group of cisterns of rough-surfaced endoplasmic reticulum (RSR). From myocardium of 33-year-old man with tetralogy of Fallot. (× 12,000)

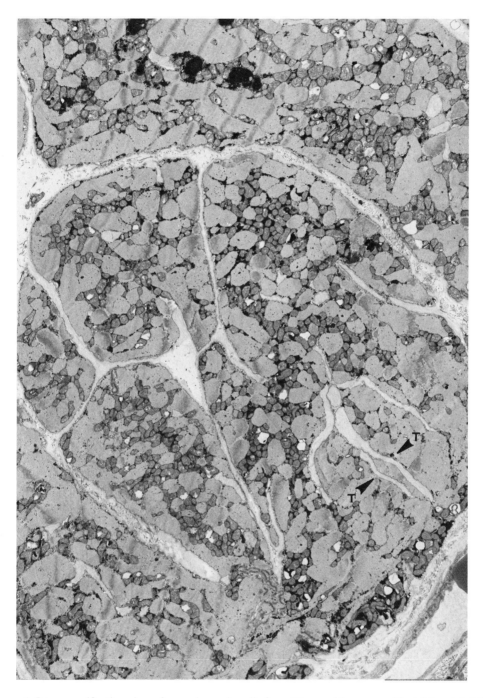

Figure 6. Low magnification view of several muscle cells from 36-year-old woman with atrial septal defect and combined infundibular and valvular pulmonic stenosis, showing marked irregularities in the shapes of whole cells and of T-tubules (T) which course in various directions. ($\times$ 5100)

lated and tortuous (Fig. 6). The extent of folding of intercellular junctions exceeds that present in normal myocardium. Cell shapes become more irregular and multiple inter-calated discs are found more frequently than in normal hearts. These structures have been defined as consisting of two or more parallel segments of intercalated discs sepa-rated by ten or less sarcomeres. Multiple intercalated discs are the junctions of cyto-plasmic processes interlocking along the sides of the muscle cells.[45] Focal accumula-tions of Z-band material and increased lipofuscin granules also occur. The accumula-tions of Z-band material may serve as the loci of new sarcomere formation. In addition to the changes just described, quantitative abnormalities may occur with respect to the relative amounts of cytoplasm (cytoplasmic volume fraction) occupied by mitochon-dria, myofibrils, and other organelles.

Hypertrophy With Degeneration

Chronic degenerative myocardial changes in hypertrophy include: interstitial fibrosis (Fig. 7); cellular atrophy (Fig. 8); cellular and myofibrillar disorganization (Fig. 9); Z-band abnormalities (Figs. 10 and 11); myofibrillar lysis (Figs. 11 and 12); myelin figures (Fig. 13); proliferation of sarcoplasmic reticulum (Figs. 14 and 15); lipid accumulation (Fig. 14); spherical microparticles associated with the plasma membranes (Figs. 16 through 18); intramitochondrial glycogen (Figs. 14 and 15); thickened basal laminae (Fig. 17); intracytoplasmic junctions (Fig. 16); and cellular isolation with partial dis-sociation or complete loss of intercellular connections (Figs. 16 through 18).

Several studies by our group and by other investigators[33-39] have documented the fact that these degenerative alterations are not specific for any one given type of heart disease. Such alterations occur in chronic mitral and aortic valvular disease, congestive cardiomyopathy, and congenital heart diseases. In the present study of patients with congenital heart disease, we found a clear relationship between the patients' ages and the incidence of degenerative changes. The ultrastructural features of these degenera-tive changes are outlined below, and the incidence of such changes in the four groups of patients in the study is given in Table 2.

Foci of interstitial fibrosis usually are present in proximity to atrophied, disorganized, or degenerated cells. Deposits of mature collagen, microfibrils, small elastic fibers, and ground substance (Fig. 7) separate adjacent cardiac muscle cells, indicating either: (1) interstitial tissue replacement of areas vacated by lysed myocardial cells, or (2) in-creased amounts of interstitial tissue in areas where lysis of cells has not occurred.

Certain cardiac muscle cells, which appear pale by light microscopy, show disruption and loss of the normal structure of sarcomeres. These cells may be isolated from other cardiac muscle cells and located in or adjacent to areas of interstitial fibrosis. Cellular atrophy, as defined by transverse cell diameters less than five microns, often accom-panies myofibrillar degenerative changes (Fig. 8). Atrophic cells are identified as car-diac muscle cells only with difficulty using light microscopy.

Sarcomeric disruption, perhaps the most important alteration in degenerated cells, is apparent by lysis of both thick and thin myofilaments, but usually with preferential loss of the thick filaments (Figs. 11 and 12). Because of this preferential loss, large areas of cells affected by this change appear devoid of myofibrils and contain disorganized tangles of actin filaments and 100 Å filaments. Lysis of myofibrils is often accompanied by the formation of masses of Z-band material arranged in clumps or in streaming patterns. Some of these masses of Z-band material have a complex, paracrystalline structure (Fig. 10). Cells with loss of contractile elements are distinguishable from necrotic cardiac muscle cells by the preservation of other cellular organelles (mitochondria, glycogen, nuclei, and sarcolemma) which are disrupted in cellular nec-rosis.

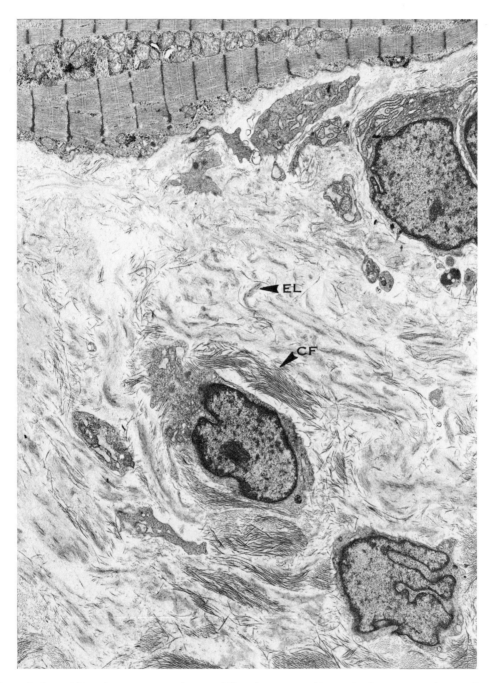

Figure 7. Several fibroblasts are present in area of fibrosis (center and bottom) adjacent to cardiac muscle cell (top). The fibrotic tissue contains accumulations of microfibrils and small elastic fibers (EL) as well as collagen fibrils (CF). Same patient tissue shown in Fig. 5. (× 6700)

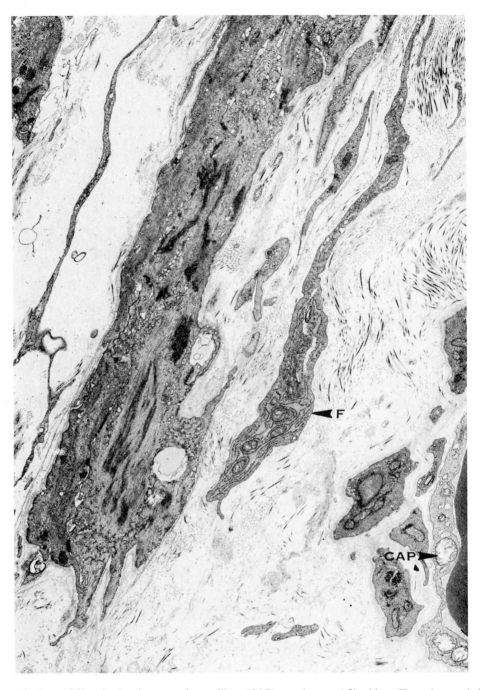

Figure 8. Area of fibrosis showing part of a capillary (CAP), an elongated fibroblast (F), and several thin, atrophic muscle cells that have partially lysed myofibrils and are connected by extensive areas of intercellular junction. Same patient tissue shown in Figures 5 and 7. (× 9000)

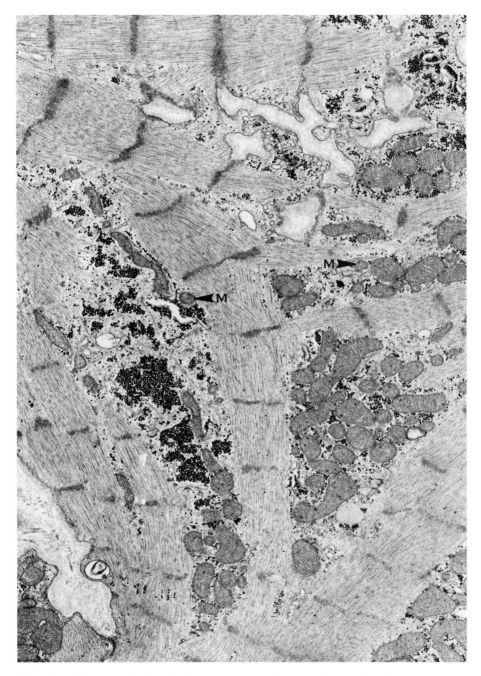

Figure 9. Marked divergence in the orientation of contractile elements is evident in muscle cell from 30-year-old woman with tetralogy of Fallot. Mitochondria (M), some of which are extremely small, show great variation in size. (× 18,500)

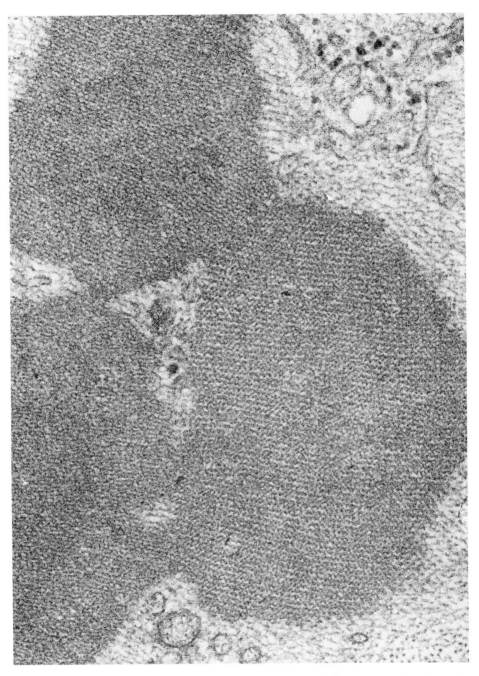

Figure 10. Large masses of Z-band material in degenerated muscle cell (from same patient tissue shown in Figure 2) exhibit highly organized substructure with a complex tetragonal array. (× 97,000)

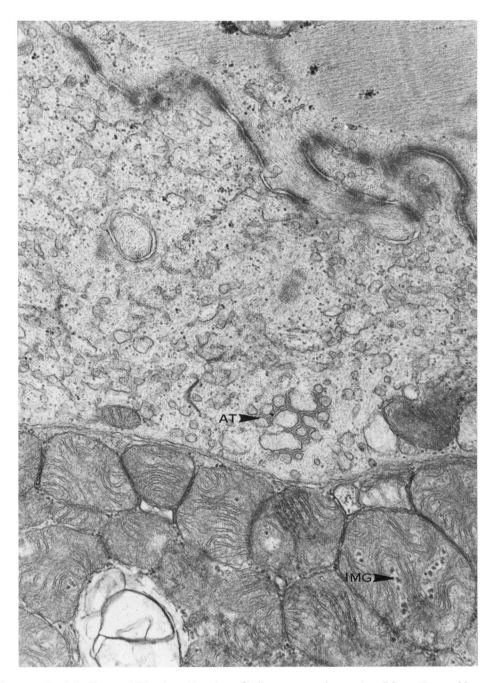

Figure 11. Partially disrupted Z bands and lysed myofibrils are present in muscle cell from 45-year-old woman with tetralogy of Fallot. ($\times$ 52,500)

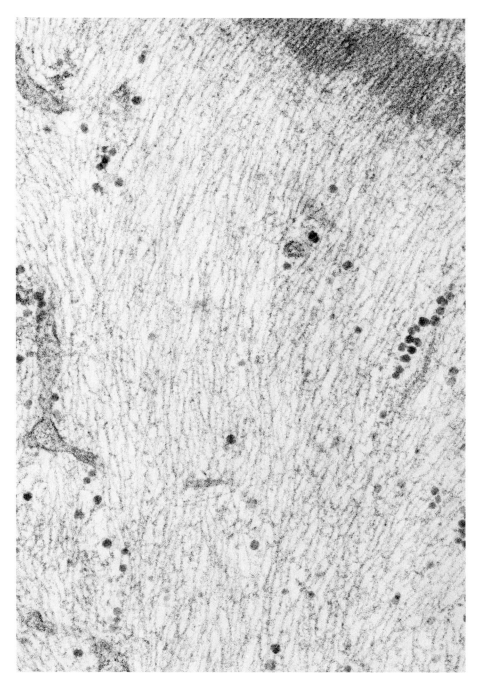

Figure 12. Part of myofibril (from same patient tissue shown in Figure 2) that has lost its thick (myosin) filaments and consists of a widened Z band (top right) and thin (actin) filaments that do not interdigitate with thick filaments. (× 82,000)

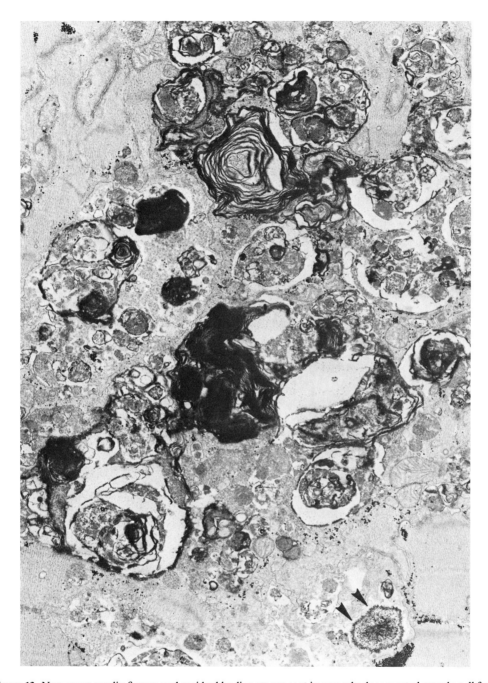

Figure 13. Numerous myelin figures and residual bodies are present in severely degenerated muscle cell from 53-year-old man with ventricular septal defect and combined infundibular and valvular pulmonic stenosis. Structure at lower right (arrowheads) probably is a calcific deposit. (× 14,500)

519

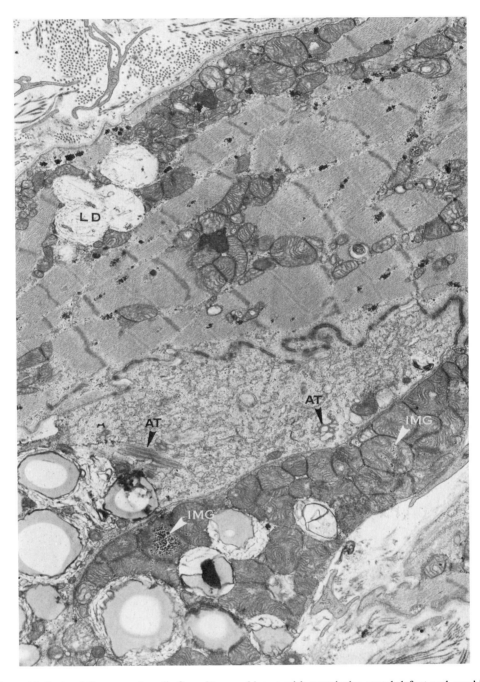

Figure 14. Parts of three muscle cells from 21-year-old man with ventricular septal defect and combined infundibular and valvular pulmonic stenosis. All three cells contain lipid droplets (LD). Cell at center is connected to cell at top by long area of intercellular junction, although closely apposed cells at center and bottom are not connected by specialized junctions. Cell at center is devoid of myofibrils and contains numerous elements of sarcoplasmic reticulum, including two aggregates of tubules (AT). Intramitochondrial glycogen deposits (IMG) are present in the cell at the bottom. (× 11,200)

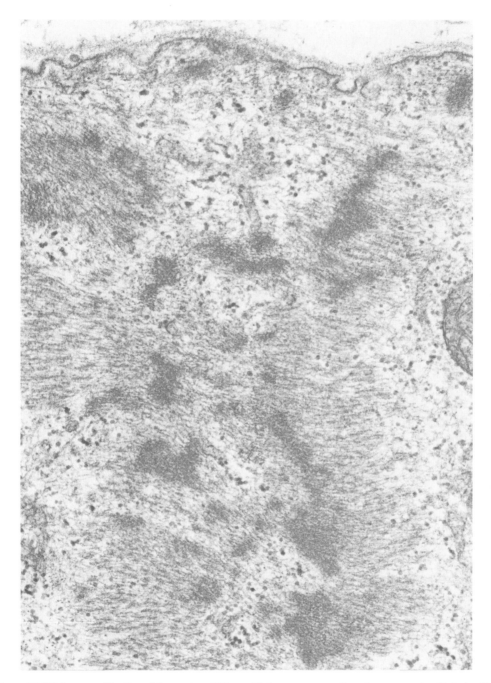

Figure 15. Higher magnification of the center of Figure 14 shows cross section of an aggregate of tubules (AT) of sarcoplasmic reticulum and intramitochondrial glycogen deposits (IMG). ($\times$ 33,200)

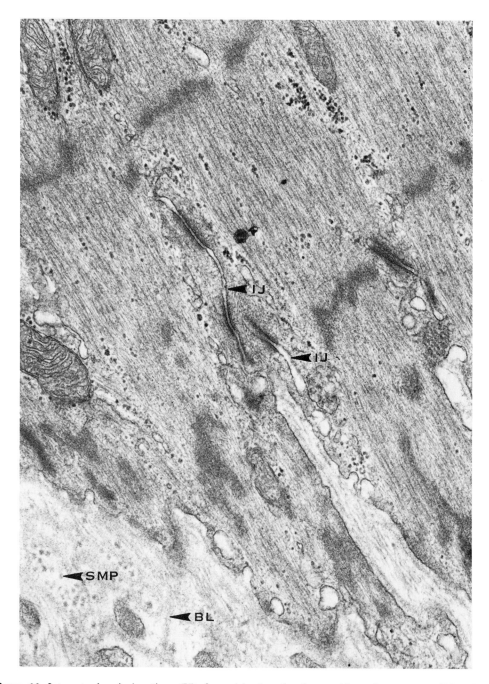

Figure 16. Intracytoplasmic junctions (IJ), formed by junctional apposition of two areas of the plasma membrane of the same cell, are present at the free end of muscle cell that terminates at edge of area of fibrosis. Spherical microparticles (SMP) are associated with areas of thickening of the basal lamina of the muscle cell. Myocardium from patient tissue shown in Figure 5. ($\times$ 37,500)

522

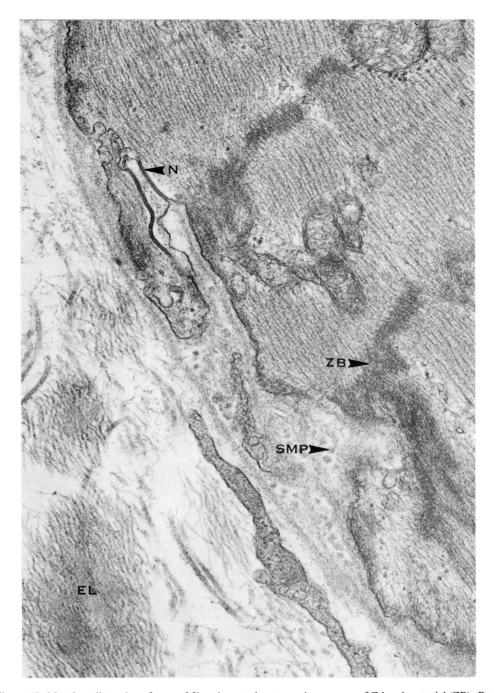

Figure 17. Muscle cell at edge of area of fibrosis contains streaming masses of Z-band material (ZB). Basal lamina is reduplicated and associated with spherical microparticles (SMP). A convoluted nexus (N) forms an intercellular junction with small process of another cardiac muscle cell (area enclosed by nexus). Numerous microfibrils, a few collagen fibrils and an elastic fiber (EL) are present in the interstitium. Myocardium from patient tissue shown in Figure 5. (× 44,500)

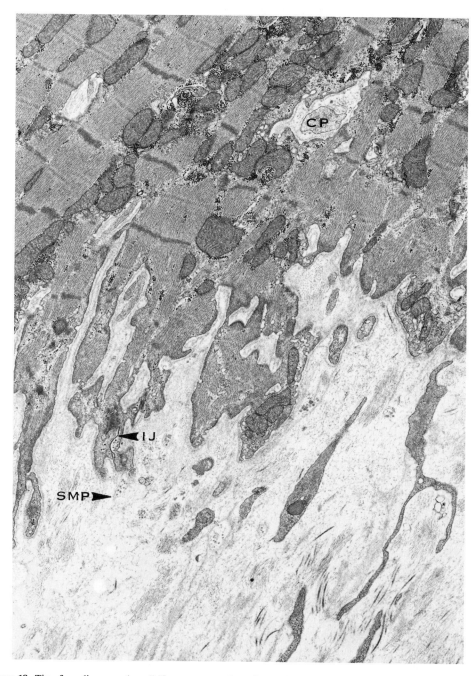

Figure 18. Tip of cardiac muscle cell (from same patient tissue shown in Figure 5) that terminates in area of fibrosis shows marked surface convolutions. Basal lamina is thickened, reduplicated, and associated with spherical microparticles (SMP). Small area of intercellular junction (IJ), similar to that shown in Figure 17, is present at the free end of cell. Pale cytoplasmic process (CP) at top right may represent site of previous intercellular junction that has undergone complete dissociation. ($\times$ 13,000)

524

Foci of cellular and myofibrillar disorganization are manifested by cells which are randomly arranged, stellate in shape, and irregularly connected to each other. These cells, which usually are located in areas of interstitial fibrosis, have myofibrils coursing in several directions rather than in parallel directions (Fig. 9). This disorganization is qualitatively similar to but much less extensive than that present[46] in myocardium of patients with hypertrophic cardiomyopathy.

Some cardiac muscle cells contain large, spherical lipid droplets (Fig. 14). These cells usually show other morphologic signs of degeneration, such as myofibrillar lysis or proliferation of SR. Cardiac muscle cells from similar areas contain large numbers of myelin figures composed of electron-dense, concentrically arranged lamellae (Fig. 13). These lamellae may form by the aggregation of phospholipid material derived from the breakdown of mitochondria.

Other cardiac muscle cells, which appear pale and nonstriated by light microscopy, contain networks of tubules of free SR which almost entirely fill the sarcoplasm (Figs. 14 and 15). Tubular and vesicular proliferation of free SR may completely replace other cardiac muscle organelles. The proliferation of SR may be associated with the formation of complex aggregates of tubules.[42,47] Proliferation of junctional or extended junctional SR can be extensive in hypertrophied human atria,[42] but it has not been described in human ventricles. In certain degenerated cardiac muscle cells the myofibril-free areas may be completely occupied by large numbers of mitochondria or glycogen granules. A small percentage (< 1 percent) of the mitochondrial population may contain glycogen deposits located in the outer mitochondrial compartment; these deposits may be related to hypoxia.[48]

The ends of isolated cardiac muscle cells have finger-like projections that extend into the interstitium, suggesting that intercellular connections have been lost from previously adjacent cardiac muscle cells (Figs. 8, 17, and 18). Isolated cells often contain intracytoplasmic junctions,[49] which are formed by the junctional apposition of two areas of the plasma membrane of the same cell (Fig. 16). Spherical microparticles[50] composed of central, dense cores surrounded by single, trilaminar membranes are found in close relationship to the basement membranes and outer surfaces of the plasma membranes of cardiac muscle cells in areas of cellular dissociation and/or interstitial fibrosis (Figs. 16 through 18). These particles are thought to be the result of budding from the plasma membranes. Such a process mediates the shedding of certain areas of plasma membranes, particularly those of junctions, where remodeling of cardiac muscle cell surfaces occurs.[50]

Relationship Between Patient Age and Incidence of Degenerative Myocardial Changes

Morphological findings in the four groups of patients are summarized in Table 2. Cellular hypertrophy was present in all patients, but larger cells were more prominent in the older patients. Changes associated with myocardial hypertrophy (cells over 20 μ in diameter, lobulated nuclei, multiple intercalated discs, dilated T-tubules, and increased numbers of ribosomes) were present in all patients, but were more common in the patients 20 years old or older. Myocardial interstitial fibrosis was observed in Groups I, II, III, and IV at frequencies of 19, 23, 25, and 100 percent, respectively. Myofibrillar lysis, myelin figures, sarcoplasmic reticulum proliferation, and spherical microparticles associated with cell membranes were present infrequently in Groups I, II, and III (0 to 25 percent) but commonly in Group IV (67 to 100 percent). Cellular atrophy, disorganization of cells and myofibrils, lipid accumulation, intramitochondrial glycogen, intracytoplasmic junctions, and thickened basal laminae were frequent also in cardiac muscle from patients over 30 years old. Certain alterations (myelin figures,

Table 2. Incidence of degenerative changes (expressed as percentages of the total number of patients in each group) in myocardium of four groups of patients with congenital heart disease

Type of Change	Group I 0.9–10 years (36 patients)	Group II 11–20 years (22 patients)	Group III 21–29 years (8 patients)	Group IV 30–53 years (9 patients)
Interstitial fibrosis	19	23	25	100
Myofibrillar lysis	0	0	25	100
Z-band abnormalities	22	59	25	100
Myelin figures	0	4	12	78
Proliferation of SR	0	0	12	67
Spherical microparticles	0	0	0	78
Cell/myofibrillar disorganization	3	27	25	44
Lipid accumulation	0	0	25	22
Intramitochondrial glycogen	22	18	38	44
Intracytoplasmic junctions	3	0	0	22
Thickened basal laminae	0	0	0	22

myofibrillar lysis, smooth endoplasmic reticulum proliferation, lipid vacuoles) were absent in Groups I and II (patients less than 20 years old), were present in Group III and were common in Group IV. Thus, morphological evidence of chronic myocardial degeneration was unusual in the patients less than six years old, but was present in all patients over 30. In general, patients between the ages of 6 and 30 had intermediate frequencies of degenerative myocardial changes.

DISCUSSION

The "myocardial factor" in patients with surgically correctable heart disease has been of considerable interest in recent years.[1–17] Only too commonly, patients undergo successful operative correction of their anatomic lesions but fail to obtain functionally satisfactory results because of poor myocardial function, arrhythmias, or inadequately explained sudden death. Although this problem has been well recognized in patients with valvular heart disease,[1–8] it also occurs in patients with congenital heart disease.[9–18,20]

Higgins and Mulder[20] found congestive heart failure in more than one third of the patients with tetralogy of Fallot surviving without operative correction to the third decade of life. McIntosh and Cohen[10] found low right ventricular outflow gradients and decreased cardiac output at rest, as well as abnormal hemodynamic responses to exercise, in 10 patients who were asymptomatic after total correction of tetralogy of Fallot. Pouleur and coworkers[12] also noted depression of right ventricular function in patients who had undergone total correction of tetralogy of Fallot. Jarmakani and coworkers[17] studied right ventricular end-diastolic volume, ejection fraction, and cardiac output in patients with tetralogy of Fallot, and found evidence indicative of impaired right ventricular function and abnormal right ventricular compliance.

James and coworkers[18] evaluated heart rate, blood pressure, physical working capacity, and electrocardiographic changes during exercise in 43 asymptomatic patients (ages 7 to 41 years) 1 to 14 years after total correction of tetralogy of Fallot; 109 normal subjects (ages 5 to 42 years) served as controls. When comparing males to males and females to females with body surface area equal to or greater than 1.2 m², maximal heart rates and working capacities were lower in the patient groups than in the control groups. An inverse relationship was observed between maximal working capacity and

Table 3. Morphologic alterations that may result in decreased myocardial contractility

1. Interstitial fibrosis
2. Cellular and myofibrillar disorganization
3. Abnormalities of Z-band material
4. Myofibrillar lysis
5. Proliferation of sarcoplasmic reticulum
6. Increased thickness of basal laminae
7. Cellular atrophy
8. Loss of intercellular connections

age at the time of surgery in both male and female patient groups. In contrast to this, the maximal heart rates and working capacities in the males with body surface areas less than 1.2 m² (average age at operation, 6.5 years) did not differ significantly in the patient and control groups. Premature atrial or ventricular contractions were recorded after exercise in 23 percent of the patients with tetralogy and in none of the patients in the control group.

It is evident from the studies just reviewed that myocardial dysfunction eventually develops in certain patients with congenital heart disease, and that such dysfunction may not be reversible upon operative correction of the lesion. Poor myocardial function in patients who have had complete operative correction of congenital heart disease may be the result of irreversible damage or degeneration suffered by hypertrophied myocardium as a consequence of the longstanding hemodynamic burden. These anatomic changes correspond to those observed in animal hearts in the third stage of hypertrophy or stage of cellular exhaustion as defined by Meerson.[36-38] No systematic morphologic assessment has been made previously of the cardiac cellular damage and degeneration that occur in patients with congenital heart disease, although several limited descriptions of these changes have appeared.[39] The present study, comparing the characteristics of myocardium from patients subjected to similar hemodynamic stresses for different periods of time, allows certain generalizations to be made with respect to structural and functional changes associated with the late stages of hypertrophy in cyanotic congenital heart disease. Our present state of knowledge makes it impossible to relate directly an unsatisfactory clinical postoperative course (i.e., development of low cardiac output state, chronic right ventricular failure, and arrhythmias) to specific cardiac morphologic alterations. Nevertheless, such a relationship is suggested by the age-related increase in myocardial dysfunction and myocardial degenerative changes in patients with tetralogy.

Many of the myocardial alterations observed in our older patients could affect cardiac function adversely and cause right ventricular failure and a low cardiac output state postoperatively (Table 3). Deterioration of cardiac function would be an expected result of acute ischemic injury, caused by the elective cardiac arrest at operation, superimposed upon pre-existing long-term degenerative alterations. Another factor contributing to myocardial degeneration may be inadequacy of blood supply producing a chronic state of relative ischemia in severely hypertrophied myocardium. This latter problem may be further complicated by the arterial oxygen desaturation in cyanotic congenital heart disease.

The most important structural changes observed in this study involved the loss of myocardial contractile elements and of normal myocardial intercellular relationships. These changes were consistently associated with interstitial fibrosis. Cellular dissociation and isolation are produced by separation from, or loss of, adjacent cells; these changes are commonly associated with proliferation of fibrous tissue. These anatomic changes promote asynergistic contraction and focally delayed activation because of the interruption of cell-to-cell transmission of mechanical and electrical forces. Decreased myocardial contractility also would be expected to result from: (1) derangements of the contractile apparatus, such as disorganization of sarcomeres and myofibrillar lysis; (2) dilatation and proliferation of sarcoplasmic reticulum; and (3) loss of T-tubules. The ultimate replacement of degenerated cells by noncontracting, noncompliant interstitial tissue components would contribute further to mechanical dysfunction of the heart. Irritability and increased automaticity, with a tendency to produce ectopic mechanisms, may be clinically important consequences of the cellular dedifferentiation and isolation that occur in myocardial degeneration.

CONCLUSION

Our findings on the presence of cardiac muscle cell degeneration in patients with longstanding right ventricular hypertrophy indicate that operative correction of the anatomic defects should be undertaken as early in life as is technically feasible. These observations also emphasize the need for providing the best possible degree of intraoperative myocardial protection, particularly in older patients who are likely to have myocardial degeneration. Morphological evaluation of operatively resected myocardium may have predictive value for immediate and long-term myocardial function.

REFERENCES

1. HARVEY, R. M., FERRER, M. I., AND SAMET, P.: *Mechanical and myocardial factors in rheumatic heart disease with mitral stenosis.* Circulation 11:531,1955.

2. FLEMING, H. A., AND WOOD, P.: *Myocardial factor in mitral valve disease.* Br. Heart J. 21:117,1959.

3. PETERSON, C. R., HERR, R., AND CRISERA, V. R.: *The failure of hemodynamic improvement after valve replacement surgery.* Ann. Intern. Med. 66:1,1967.

4. HILDNER, F. J., JAVIER, R. P., COHEN, L. S., ET AL.: *Myocardial dysfunction associated with valvular heart disease.* Am. J. Cardiol. 30:319,1972.

5. SCHEUER, J.: *Ventricular dysfunction associated with valvular heart disease.* Am. J. Cardiol. 30:445,1972.

6. BRISTOW, J. D., AND KREMKAU, E. L.: *Hemodynamic changes after valve replacement with Starr-Edwards prostheses.* Am J. Cardiol. 35:716,1975 .

7. BOLOOKI, H., AND KAISER, G.: *Significance of cardiac function in surgical management of patients with valvular heart disease.* Am. J. Cardiol. 37:319,1976.

8. SELZER, A.: *Cardiac valve replacement: an unanswered question.* Am. J. Cardiol. 37:322,1976.

9. QUATTELBAUM, T. D., VARGHESE, P. J., NEILL, C. A., ET AL.: *Sudden death among postoperative patients with tetralogy of Fallot: A follow-up study of 251 patients for an average of twelve years.* Am. J. Cardiol. 35:164,1975.

10. MCINTOSH, H. D., AND COHEN, A. I.: *Pulmonary stenosis: the importance of myocardial factor in determining the clinical course and surgical results.* Am. Heart J. 65:715,1963.

11. EPSTEIN, S. E., BEISER, G. D., GOLDSTEIN, R. E., ET AL.: *Hemodynamic abnormalities in response to mild and intense upright exercise following operative correction of an atrial septal defect or tetralogy of Fallot.* Circulation 47:1065,1973.

12. POULEUR, H., GOENEN, M., JAUMIN, P. M., ET AT.: *Cardiac function early after repair of tetralogy of Fallot.* J. Thorac. Cardiovasc. Surg. 70:24,1975.

13. GRAHAM, T. P., JR.: *Myocardial performance after anatomic or physiologic corrective surgery.* Prog. Cardiovasc. Dis 17:439,1975.

14. JARMAKANI, J. M., GRAHAM, T. P., JR., AND CANENT, R. V., JR.: *Left ventricular contractile state in children with successfully corrected ventricular septal defect.* Circulation 45 (Suppl. I): 102,1972.

15. PERLOFF, J. K.: *Pediatric congenital cardiac becomes a postoperative adult. The changing population of congenital heart disease.* Circulation 47:606,1973.

16. PARR, G. V. S., BLACKSTONE, E. H., AND KIRKLIN, J. W.: *Cardiac performance and mortality early after intracardiac surgery in infants and young children.* Circulation 51:867,1975.

17. JARMAKANI, J. M., NAKAZAWA, M., ISABEL-JONES, J., ET AL.: *Right ventricular function in children with tetralogy of Fallot before and after aortic-to-pulmonary shunt.* Circulation 53:555,1976.

18. JAMES, F. W., KAPLAN, S., SCHWARTZ, D. C., ET AL.: *Response to exercise in patients after total surgical correction of tetralogy of Fallot.* Circulation 54:671,1976.

19. MARQUIS, R. M.: *Longevity and the early history of the tetralogy of Fallot.* Br. Med. J. 1:819,1956.

20. HIGGINS, C. B., AND MULDER, D. G.: *Tetralogy of Fallot in the adult.* Am. J. Cardiol. 29:837,1972.

21. HOLLADAY, W. E., AND WITHAM, A. C.: *The tetralogy of Fallot.* Arch. Intern. Med. 100:400,1957.

22. TAUSSIG, H. B., CROCETTI, A., ESHAGHPOUR, E., ET AL.: *Long-term observations of the Blalock-Taussig operation. I. Results of first operations.* Johns Hopkins Med. J. 129:243,1971.

23. TAUSSIG, H. B., JOSEPHS, H., SCHAFFER, A. J., ET AL.: *Long-time observations on the Blalock-Taussig operation. VIII. 20 to 28 year follow-up on patients with tetralogy of Fallot.* Johns Hopkins Med. J. 137:13,1975.

24. DEUCHAR, D., BESCOS, L. L., AND CHAKORN, S.: *Fallot's tetralogy: a 20 year surgical follow-up.* Br. Heart J. 34:12,1972.

25. SISEL, R. J., WELDON, C. S., AND OLIVER, G. C.: *Successful operative repair of acyanotic tetralogy of Fallot in a 61-year-old man.* Ann. Thorac. Surg. 11:598,1971.

26. FREISINGER, G. C., AND BAHNSON, H. T.: *Tetralogy of Fallot. Report of a case with total correction at 54 years of age.* Am. Heart J. 71:107,1966.

27. BJERNULF, A., AND CULLHED, I.: *Open correction of Fallot's anomaly in three patients over forty years of age.* Acta Med. Scand. 183:515,1968.

28. ROSS, C. D., BAXLEY, W. A., KARP, R. B., ET AL: *Tetralogy of Fallot over age 30: clinical and surgical aspects.* Circulation 51, 52(II):234,1975.

29. BENDER, H. W., HALLER, J. A., BRAWLEY, R. K., ET AL.: *Experience in repair of tetralogy of Fallot malformation in adults.* Ann. Thorac. Surg. 11:508,1971.

30. WOLF, M. D., LANDTMAN, B., AND NEILL, C. A.: *Total correction of tetralogy of Fallot. Follow-up study of 104 cases.* Circulation 31:385,1965.

31. CHIARIELLO, L., MEYER, J., WUKASCH, D. C., ET AL.: *Intracardiac repair of tetralogy of Fallot. Five-year review of 403 patients.* J. Thorac. Cardiovasc. Surg. 70:529,1975.

32. FREEMAN, J., AND SPURLOCK, B.: *A new epoxy embedment for electron microscopy.* J. Cell Biol. 13:437,1962.

33. MARON, B. J., FERRANS, V. J., AND ROBERTS, W. C.: *Ultrastructural features of degenerated cardiac muscle cells in patients with cardiac hypertrophy.* Am. J. Pathol. 79:387,1975.

34. RICHTER, G. W., AND KELLNER, A.: *Hypertrophy of the human heart at the level of fine structure: an analysis and two postulates.* J. Cell Biol. 18:195,1963.

35. CUTILLETTA, A. F., DOWELL, R. T., RUDNIK, M., ET AL.: *Regression of myocardial hypertrophy. I. Experimental model, changes in heart weight, nucleic acids and collagen.* J. Mol. Cell. Cardiol. 7:767,1975.

36. MEERSON, F. Z.: *Compensatory hyperfunction of the heart and cardiac insufficiency.* Circ. Res. 10:250,1962.

37. MEERSON, F. Z., ZALETAGEVA, T. A., AND LAGUTIHEV, S. S.: *Structure and mass of mitochondria in the process of compensatory hyperfunction and hypertrophy of the heart.* Exp. Cell Res. 36:568,1964.

38. MEERSON, F. Z.: *The myocardium in hyperfunction, hypertrophy and heart failure.* Circ. Res. 25 (Suppl. II):1,1969.

39. JONES, M., FERRANS, V. J., MORROW, A. G., ET AL.: *Ultrastructure of crista supraventricularis muscle in patients with congenital heart diseases associated with right ventricular outflow tract obstruction.* Circulation 51:39,1975.

40. MARON, B. J., FERRANS, V. J., AND ROBERTS, W. C.: *Myocardial ultrastructure in patients with chronic aortic valve disease.* Am. J. Cardiol. 35:725,1975.

41. MARON, B. J., FERRANS, V. J., AND JONES, M.: *The spectrum of degenerative changes in hypertrophied human cardiac muscle cells: an ultrastructural study.* In Roy, P.-E., and Harris, P. (eds.): *Recent Advances in Studies on Cardiac Structure and Metabolism, Vol. VIII. The Cardiac Sarcoplasm.* University Park Press, Baltimore, 1975, p. 447.

42. THIEDEMANN, K.-U., AND FERRANS, V. J.: *Ultrastructure of sarcoplasmic reticulum in atrial myocardium of patients with mitral valvular disease.* Am J. Pathol. 83:1,1976.

43. JONES, M., AND FERRANS, V. J.: *Myocardial degeneration in congenital heart disease: a comparison of morphologic findings in young and old patients with congenital heart diseases associated with muscular obstruction to right ventricular outflow.* Am. J. Cardiol. 39:1051,1977.

44. FERRANS, V. J., JONES, M., MARON, B. J., ET AL.: *The nuclear membranes in hypertrophied human cardiac muscle cells.* Am. J. Pathol. 78:427,1975.

45. MARON, B. J., AND FERRANS, V. J.: *Significance of multiple intercalated discs in hypertrophied human myocardium.* Am. J. Pathol. 73:81,1973.

529

46. FERRANS, V. J., MORROW, A. G., AND ROBERTS, W. C.: *Myocardial ultrastructure in idiopathic hypertrophic subaortic stenosis.* Circulation 45:769,1972.
47. MARON, B. J., AND FERRANS, V. J.: *Aggregates of tubules in human cardiac muscle cells.* J. Mol. Cell. Cardiol. 6:249,1974.
48. MARON, B. J., AND FERRANS, V. J.: *Intramitochondrial glycogen deposits in hypertrophied human myocardium.* J. Mol. Cell. Cardiol. 7:697,1975.
49. BUJA, L. M., FERRANS, V. J., AND MARON, B. J.: *Intracytoplasmic junctions in cardiac muscle cells.* Am. J. Pathol. 74:613,1974.
50. FERRANS, V. J., THIEDEMANN, K.-U., MARON, B. J., ET AL.: *Spherical microparticles in human myocardium. An ultrastructural study.* Lab. Invest. 35:349,1976.

The Eisenmenger Reaction and Its Management

Thomas P. Graham, Jr., M.D.

HISTORICAL PERSPECTIVE

In 1897 Victor Eisenmenger described the clinical and pathological findings of a 32-year-old man who had a large ventricular septal defect (VSD) and a history of cyanosis and moderate shortness of breath since infancy.[1] The patient was able to lead an active life until he was 29 years old; then dyspnea increased and manifestations of heart failure began. Physical examination revealed cyanosis, clubbing, and signs of right heart failure. The right heart was enlarged and a loud systolic murmur of tricuspid regurgitation was maximal at the lower left sternal border. There was also a diastolic murmur of pulmonary regurgitation. The patient improved with rest and anticongestive therapy but collapsed and died suddenly several months later following a large hemoptysis. At necropsy a large VSD was located in the membranous septum measuring 2 by 2.5 cm. in diameter. The left and right ventricles were of equal thickness. The right ventricle was considerably dilated and the tricuspid valve ring was widely stretched. There was considerable atherosclerosis of the pulmonary trunk and its branches, and pulmonary infarction was present secondary to multiple thrombosis. Following Eisenmenger's report, little insight into the pathophysiology of this disease process was gained until the classic work of Paul Wood was published in 1958.[2] Wood studied 127 patients with the Eisenmenger syndrome over a period of 11 years and lucidly described the syndrome in a series of publications.

The term "Eisenmenger's complex" is commonly used to apply to the condition of a large ventricular septal defect associated with marked elevation of pulmonary vascular resistance and a predominant right-to-left shunt. The more general term, "Eisenmenger's syndrome," is used to indicate any large defect allowing free communication between the pulmonary and systemic circuits at the aortic, ventricular, or atrial level with a balanced or predominant right-to-left shunt secondary to marked elevation of pulmonary vascular resistance. This chapter deals with the latter, more general definition. From the foregoing description it is obvious that a large number of different pathological entities can present with elevated pulmonary vascular resistance and be classified in the Eisenmenger's syndrome category. A list of these disorders is provided in Table 1.

The incidence of this complicating feature in patients with VSD is not certain. It is clear that this complication does not occur in patients with small ventricular defect or with associated severe pulmonary stenosis. It does occur with defects that allow equalization of pressure between the right and left ventricles and are approximately the size of the aortic valve ring or larger. In infants born with a defect of this size, the usual

Table 1. Congenital cardiac lesions which can be complicated by the Eisenmenger reaction

A. Aortic Shunts
 1. Patent ductus arteriosus
 2. Aorticopulmonary septal defect (window)
 3. Truncus arteriosus
 4. Pulmonary atresia, VSD, and large "bronchial" collateral vessels
B. Ventricular Shunts
 1. VSD
 2. Single ventricle
 3. Transposition of the great arteries with VSD
 4. Double outlet right ventricle
 5. Tricuspid atresia, VSD, and no pulmonary stenosis
 6. Mitral atresia and VSD or single ventricle
 7. Atrioventricular canal
C. Atrial Shunts
 1. Atrial septal defect: secundum, primum, sinus venosus
 2. Common atrium
 3. Total anomalous pulmonary venous return
 4. Partial anomalous pulmonary venous return
 5. Transposition with atrial septal defect

course is the development of symptoms of severe congestive heart failure during the first several months of life. Most of these patients now are treated medically and improve or undergo reparative operation when medical therapy is unsuccessful. Because of the small but definite incidence of elevated pulmonary vascular resistance developing during the first year or certainly the first two years of life in patients with large shunts, it has now been recommended that infants with large defects and systemic pulmonary artery pressure have their defects repaired by one year of age. A large majority of the patients who are allowed to continue with their pulmonary hypertension will develop increasing pulmonary vascular resistance during late childhood and early adolescence.

Patients who have elevated pulmonary vascular resistance from an early age and do not exhibit a period of severe congestive heart failure in infancy comprise a smaller group. It appears that these patients do not have the normal fall in pulmonary vascular resistance following birth and, therefore, do not show signs of congestive heart failure in the first 6 months of life. These patients may be extremely difficult to identify and may present to physicians dealing with adolescents and young adults with no history of a precordial murmur or congestive heart failure in infancy. There may be a time in which the pulmonary resistance in these patients is at such a level that repair could be performed in the first year or two of life. However, it is obvious that they will be difficult to identify early in life. This group of patients may account for <5 percent of all patients with large VSD.

Patients with atrial shunts have a much lower overall incidence of the Eisenmenger reaction. It is probable that only 10 to 15 percent of patients with a large atrial defect show elevation of pulmonary vascular resistance as adolescents or young adults.[2] This figure probably increases slowly with increasing age, a possible consequence of pulmonary thromboembolic disease in some patients.

CLINICAL FEATURES

History

The majority of patients with the Eisenmenger reaction will give a history of symptoms suggesting congestive heart failure in infancy. These patients usually have amelioration of the symptoms after the first year of life as the result of a gradual increase in pulmonary vascular resistance and decreasing left-to-right shunting. Patients with an atrial septal defect generally do not have symptoms suggestive of heart failure early in life unless they have a common atrium or an ostium primum atrial defect; if present, congestive heart failure may not be a prominent feature. As already indicated, a number of patients may give no history of congestive failure during infancy and have, by inference, elevated resistance from an early age. Symptoms are generally related to shortness of breath with exertion and are usually more prominent in patients with ventricular shunting rather than aortic shunting. This suggests that the breathlessness may be related to decreased oxygen saturation of the arterial supply to the brain, since patients with right-to-left ductal shunting will not have central nervous system desaturation.

Right-sided congestive heart failure is a late manifestation and usually is brought on by the development of tricuspid regurgitation or an atrial arrhythmia. The length of time the tricuspid valve remains competent in patients with elevated right ventricular pressure is variable, but it is unusual for these symptoms to occur before age 30 years. Atrial arrhythmias appear to be more common in the patients with atrial level shunting. Syncope and hemoptysis are rare before age 20 years.[2]

Anginal-like pain, which probably results from right ventricular hypoxia secondary to an imbalance between myocardial oxygen demands and supply, is rare before late adolescence or early adulthood; it occurred in 14 percent of Wood's patients with VSD, in 20 percent of his patients with patent ductus arteriosus, and in 15 percent of his patients with atrial shunting. A history of squatting is uncommon but was found in 15 percent of patients with VSD, 5 percent of patients with atrial septal defect, and 3 percent of patients with patent ductus arteriosus.[2]

Physical Examination

The physical examination is usually quite revealing and generally allows a presumptive but reasonably accurate diagnosis. Obvious central cyanosis with clubbing is present in the most severe cases, and redness of the nail beds is present in mild cases. Cyanosis of the toes with pink nail beds on the right hand indicates the diagnosis of a reversed shunting ductus arteriosus. When the right hand is blue and the toes are pink, transposition of the great arteries with a reversed ductus is the diagnosis.

The venous pulse usually reveals mild to moderate elevation of the systemic venous pressure. A prominent A wave may be present. Palpation is most helpful and a right ventricular parasternal life is present in virtually all patients. The left ventricular apical impulse usually is absent because of right ventricular hypertrophy which results in a posterior displacement of the left ventricle. The upper left sternal border generally reveals a prominent main pulmonary artery impulse and a palpable pulmonary closure. Auscultation discloses a loud second heart sound with the aortic and pulmonary components fused into a single sound in most patients with ventricular, atrial, or aortic communications. However, patients with atrial communications can have the persistent fixed splitting heard in patients without severe elevation of pulmonary resistance, and patients with a reversed ductus arteriosus can have a variably split second heart sound.[2] A pulmonary ejection click is present in a large number of patients, as is an early decrescendo murmur of pulmonary regurgitation. The murmur of tricuspid regurgitation is present in a varying number of patients, and increases in frequency with increasing age. An inspiratory increase in the intensity of this murmur usually allows correct identification of the source.

Chest X-ray

The chest roentgenogram usually does not show prominent cardiomegaly. The left atrium and left ventricle are normal in size. The right atrium and ventricle are only mildly to moderately enlarged, but significant tricuspid regurgitation can produce severe right heart enlargement. The main pulmonary artery segment and the hilar vessels usually are quite prominent. A definite cutoff or decrease in the size of the peripheral arteries is present in many patients. Chest films which appear to be virtually normal except for a prominent pulmonary trunk can be seen in patients with the full-blown Eisenmenger syndrome.

Electrocardiogram

The electrocardiogram usually shows right atrial enlargement, right axis deviation, and right ventricular hypertrophy. The left ventricular complexes generally are normal or decreased in magnitude.

Echocardiogram

The echocardiogram can frequently be helpful in identifying a large pulmonary artery located anteriorly in patients without transposition but with abnormal systolic time intervals characteristic of elevated pulmonary vascular resistance.[3] Overriding of the aorta may be present in patients with large VSD or truncus arteriosus. Other characteristic features of various congenital defects, including atrioventricular canal, single ventricle, or transposition of the great arteries, can be extremely useful in identifying the intracardiac anatomy.

Catheterization Studies

Catheterization studies are indicated in any patient in whom the history, physical examination, and accessory laboratory findings do not definitely indicate the anatomical and physiological diagnosis. These studies do carry with them some increased risk; but if systemic hypertension and arrhythmia can be avoided, complete catheterization studies are possible with only a small increase in risk. Any arrhythmia must be treated rapidly because these patients have very little tolerance for any decrease in cardiac output or fall in coronary perfusion pressure. Simultaneous pressure measurements in the pulmonary artery and aorta as well as left atrial or pulmonary wedge pressures with concomitant shunt measurements are essential for diagnosis. Oxygen determinations and indicator dilution curves are of obvious importance. Alterations in pulmonary flows or pressures with oxygen breathing and tolazoline injection should be evaluated, although these maneuvers usually are of little benefit at or near sea level in the older patient with bidirectional shunting. At high altitude these procedures can be of considerable use. It is important to measure both systemic and pulmonary flows and resistances before and after oxygen breathing because oxygen can raise systemic resistance and decrease right-to-left shunting in the absence of any significant change in pulmonary resistance.[4]

Angiocardiographic studies carry with them a slightly increased risk. This is probably associated with the known fall in systemic vascular resistance which occurs following injection of contrast media. Any fall in systemic resistance will, of course, increase right-to-left shunting and may result in sudden deterioration in the patient. However, careful monitoring of aortic pressure and the use of pressor agents to increase systemic resistance can be utilized to obviate any problem in this regard. In particular, pulmonary artery cineangiocardiography can be the most deleterious. Ventricular injections are usually well tolerated. It is usually necessary to perform these studies to delineate the intracardiac and great vessel anatomy. It is important to rule out potentially correctable causes of elevated pulmonary vascular resistance leading to right-to-left shunting by measuring pulmonary wedge to left ventricular diastolic pressure gradients. These latter conditions include any anatomical cause for pulmonary venous hypertension such as cor triatriatum, pulmonary vein stenosis, supravalvular mitral stenosis, and valvular mitral stenosis.

Natural History

Most patients with the Eisenmenger syndrome do well throughout adolescence and early adult life, but become increasingly symptomatic during their 30s. The average age of death in Wood's series[2] was 33 for aortic and ventricular septal defects and 36 for atrial septal defects. Maximum age reached was 65 for patients with ventricular or atrial septal defect and 55 for patients with patent ductus arteriosus. Hemoptysis is exceedingly rare before age 20. It was not seen in Wood's group before age 24, but thereafter it occurred with increasing frequency and reached 100 percent by age 40. Other authors have reported a much lower incidence of this complication.[5-7] Hemoptysis can be secondary to pulmonary infarction and pulmonary thrombosis or to rupture of pulmonary arterial plexiform lesions. Angina pectoris is uncommon in patients under 20 years of age, and the incidence in older patients varies from 2 to 20 percent.[2,5-7]

Medical Therapy

With the exception of patients with transposition of the great arteries and VSD, who can benefit from an atrial repair by the technique of Mustard without closure of the VSD,[8] patients with the Eisenmenger syndrome are not candidates for intracardiac surgery. Medical therapy is symptomatic and can be addressed within the following categories.

Polycythemia

With increasing polycythemia there is a decrease in cardiac output, related probably both to autoregulation in varying organ beds and increasing blood viscosity. Rosenthal and coworkers[9] have shown the acute beneficial effects of red cell volume reduction and replacement with plasma in patients with cyanotic congenital heart disease and marked polycythemia. With the reduction of hematocrit, the very annoying problem of excessive headache, particularly with exertion, will usually be markedly ameliorated. In addition, the patient's general sense of well being and effort tolerance can be improved. The duration of this symptomatic improvement may last from several weeks to several months. The benefits of a repeated red cell exchange, as described by Rosenthal,[9] will depend on the individual patient. The indications and method for this procedure are outlined in Table 2.

Congestive Heart Failure

Congestive heart failure frequently is associated with tricuspid regurgitation or an atrial arrhythmia. Conversion of the atrial arrhythmia by pharmacological means is certainly indicated, as is treatment of the congestive failure with digoxin and diuretics. The combination of a thiazide diuretic and spironolactone usually is quite useful in this situation. A low-salt diet is also helpful, but unlimited fluid intake is advisable, particularly during the summer months, to avoid hemoconcentration.

Hemoptysis

Heath and Edwards' classic paper[11] provides a ready explanation for hemoptysis in patients with pulmonary vascular obstructive disease. These patients have dilated or

Table 2. Effects, indications, and method of red cell volume reduction in polycythemia of cyanotic congenital heart disease[9]

A. Acute effects of 10% decrease in hematocrit
    1. 38% increase in systemic blood flow (Qs)
    2. 23% decrease in systemic vascular resistance (Rs)
    3. 20% increase in systemic oxygen transport (Qs x arterial O_2 content)
B Indications
    1. For temporary symptomatic relief—weeks to months
       a. Decrease in headaches
       b. Increase in exercise tolerance
    2. Reduces coagulation abnormalities
    3. Rarely indicated if hematocrit $\leq$ 70%, nearly always beneficial if hematocrit $\geq$ 80%
C. Method
    1. Removal of whole blood and replacement by equal amount of fresh frozen plasma or 5% human albumin
    2. Never remove blood without replacement
    3. 30 ml. aliquots
    4. Monitor blood pressure and heart rate
    5. Whole blood volume (WBV) to be removed: WBV = weight (kg.) x 0.11 x (v hematocrit i − v hematocrit d)/v hematocrit i where 0.11 = assumed blood volume as fraction of weight, v hematocrit i = initial hematocrit, v hematocrit d = desired hematocrit.
    6. Attempt only 10% reduction in hematocrit

---

angiomatoid lesions of pulmonary arterioles, which may represent outgrowths of small pulmonary arteries or dilated, degenerating bronchial arteries.[12] These vessels are thin-walled and can rupture even with mild trauma, such as excessive coughing. Another cause for hemoptysis is pulmonary infarction secondary to thromboembolic disease, which can be fatal.[2]

Clarkson and coworkers[5] found no history of hemoptysis in 40 patients under 20 years of age, but 11 of 23 (48 percent) patients 20 years or older had this complication. Of these 11 patients, 7 died within a 7-year followup period. Of the 12 patients without hemoptysis, 5 died within 17 years. Wood[2] found hemoptysis in 33 percent of his patients but never before the age of 24. It occurred in all his patients by age 40 and was a contributing cause of death in 29 percent. Although Wood[2] believed this complication frequently heralded a downhill course, other authors have not agreed.[6,7,12] A difference in etiology for the hemoptysis might explain this discrepancy; pulmonary infarction with thromboembolic disease certainly can be life-threatening, whereas rupture of small angiomatoid lesions need not be.

There is no effective treatment for this complication. If there is evidence for peripheral venous disease, then therapy toward this problem is indicated. Supportive treatment and cough supression are indicated also. However, long term anticoagulation is not beneficial.

Anginal Type Chest Pain

Chest pain, which is rare in young patients, is probably related to an imbalance between right ventricular oxygen demands and oxygen delivery. It is possible that red cell volume reduction[9] might reduce the chest pain, although there are no data indicating that this is true. Nitroglycerin or other agents that lower systemic resistance are potentially harmful because they increase right-to-left shunting. The use of propranolol in this situation has not been reported; it could decrease oxygen demands, particularly at times of stress when tachycardia may be precipitated. If propranolol is used, the patient must be watched carefully for signs of congestive heart failure which might ensue.

Pregnancy

There are a number of reports indicating that Eisenmenger's syndrome is associated with a high maternal mortality rate in late pregnancy and in the postpartum period.[13-15] The changes in late pregnancy may be caused by increased right-to-left shunting due to lowering of the systemic resistance by the placental circulation. There is also a possibility of an increase in pulmonary artery occlusion due to thromboembolic disease during the postpartum period. A recent report indicates that heparin prophylaxis does not improve the maternal morbidity or mortality rate in this situation.[15] Therefore, it is advisable for women with this condition to avoid pregnancy.

Contraception[10]

Oakley and Somerville[16] reported a rapid downhill course in three patients with Eisenmenger's syndrome who were taking oral contraceptives. The risk of thromboembolic disease with oral contraceptives, particularly of the estrogenic type, makes this form of contraception unacceptable. Sterilization is the most effective method of contraception, but the operation to perform sterilization carries with it its own risk. Intrauterine devices may cause excessive bleeding and predispose to endocarditis. Therapeutic abortion is indicated in patients with severe pulmonary vascular disease. It should be performed as early as possible, with careful monitoring, and with prophylaxis for infective endocarditis.

Syncope and Sudden Death

Wood[2] reported a 14 percent incidence of sudden death in 42 autopsied patients. Clarkson and coworkers[5] found that 7 of 17 (41 percent) of their autopsied patients died suddenly of unexplained cause. Young and Marks[6] found that 8 of 17 (47 percent) adult patients with Eisenmenger's syndrome died suddenly at ages ranging from 17 to 47 years. Thus, sudden death presumably from an arrhythmia, is the leading mode of death in these reported patients.

Syncope can occur with effort and can result from a fall in systemic vascular resistance with increased right-to-left shunting and a decrease in central nervous systemic oxygenation. Another possible cause of syncope is arrhythmia, and patients with this disorder should have Holter monitoring to try to detect a treatable rhythm disturbance. Strenuous activity should be avoided, but this is seldom a problem since most of these patients regulate their own activity just below a level that causes dyspnea.

Anemia

Iron and folic acid deficiency anemias can be detrimental to these patients. Symptoms include dizziness, fatigability, and anorexia. Red cell indices and a blood smear usually are sufficient to detect these abnormalities. Treatment of iron deficiency anemia with ferrous sulfate for 6 to 8 weeks is recommended at a dose of 6 mg. elemental iron/kg./day in three divided doses. Indices and smear should be rechecked at this time and if they are not normal, hematological consultation is recommended.

Bleeding Disorders

Cyanotic patients can have a variety of abnormalities of hemostasis.[17] Fortunately, laboratory abnormalities are much more common than clinical bleeding problems. In most cases modest red cell reduction, as described by Rosenthal and coworkers,[9] will correct significant bleeding problems. In acute hemorrhage, platelet transfusion may be necessary in patients with thrombocytopenia.[10]

Hyperuricemia and Gout

Elevated serum uric acid is common in patients with severe polycythemia. The reported incidence of gout is 0.3 percent in the general population and 2 percent in all cyanotic congenital heart disease; in the adult patients with Eisenmenger's syndrome reported by Young and Marks[6] it was 5 percent (2/42). Elevated uric acid levels usually are not treated unless the serum level is $\geq$ 10 mg./100 ml., or unless the patient has renal disease or symptoms of gout.[10] Treatment includes allopurinol with or without other uricosuric agents,[10] and discontinuation of any drugs (such as thiazides) which could contribute to the hyperuricemia.

Scoliosis

This orthopedic abnormality occurs in the general population with an incidence between 0.03 and 6 percent; in patients with congenital heart disease its incidence is 3 to 19 percent.[18] Roth and coworkers[18] found an overall incidence of 12 percent in a pediatric and adolescent population of congenital heart disease patients. The prevalence increased to 36 percent in patients over 13 years of age. Scoliosis was three times more common in cyanotic congenital heart disease. This complication should be watched for and treated early to avoid compromised pulmonary function and exercise tolerance.

Brain Abscess[19]

This complication should be considered in any cyanotic patient with unexplained fever, headache, vomiting, and/or focal or generalized neurological abnormalities. These patients must be monitored closely because they can rapidly develop increasing intracranial pressure with changing neurological signs and become a neurosurgical emergency.

Infective Endocarditis (IE)

These patients must be protected from IE at times of potential infection. These include dental procedures, oral surgery, endotracheal intubation, and genitourinary surgery. Although the risk of IE may be low in patients without large pressure gradients, the Eisenmenger patient is at risk and prophylaxis is indicated.

Cerebrovascular Accident

This complication can occur with a brain abscess, with infective endocarditis as a result of embolus and/or mycotic aneurysm, or with thromboembolic disease. Erythropheresis[9] is indicated if severe polycythemia (hematocrit $\geq$ 70 percent) is present. Systemic anticoagulation has not proved useful. Supportive treatment with hydration, physiotherapy, and therapy of possible seizures is required. Seizures can begin as late as 4 to 8 weeks after the cerebrovascular accident.

Special Considerations[10,20]

Patients with Eisenmenger's syndrome obviously do better at higher atmospheric partial oxygen pressures. At 7500 feet atmospheric pO_2 is 118 mm. Hg versus 159 mm.

Hg at sea level. At 7500 feet alveolar pO_2 is 62.5 mm. Hg and arterial blood pO_2 57.5 mm. Hg in a normal individual. The cabin pressure of many commercial aircrafts corresponds to an altitude of 7500 feet when flying at 40,000 feet. Such variations in inspired O_2 could be dangerous for these patients. Therefore, they should avoid trips at high altitude whenever possible. If a commercial aircraft flight is unavoidable, consultation with the airline prior to the flight is advisable. Cabin altitude is maintained at sea level up to 22,000 feet. Special arrangements can be made for a personal supply of oxygen if higher altitudes are reached.

ILLUSTRATIVE PATIENT PROFILES

Patient A

This 17-year-old male gave no history of congestive heart failure as an infant. At age 2 a heart murmur was detected, and at 3½ cardiac catheterization was performed at another hospital, revealing an ostium primum atrial septal defect with a large left-to-right shunt and mitral regurgitation. The mean pulmonary artery pressure was 32 mm. Hg and Qp/Qs was 2.7/1. At age 4, open heart surgery was performed but the atrial defect was not repaired because the mitral valve appeared too abnormal to repair, and ASD closure in the presence of significant mitral regurgitation was considered unwise. Thereafter he experienced gradually increasing fatigability with moderate exercise. During the 6 months prior to his admission to our center, he noted even greater effort intolerance, a decrease in activity, headaches with mild exercise, and weight loss. Three weeks before admission he had hemoptysis on three occasions without antecedent cough or exercise. Cyanosis had been questionably present since the age of 4½, and it increased during the 6 months prior to our evaluation.

On admission to Vanderbilt he weighed 135 lb. and was 70 in. tall. He had moderate mucous membrane and nailbed cyanosis; fingers and toes were clubbed bilaterally. Blood pressure was 102/70 mm. Hg. Heart rate was 86/min. and cardiac rhythm was regular. The pulses were normal. Palpation revealed a right ventricular parasternal lift, a palpable pulmonary artery impulse, and a palpable S_2 at the upper left sternal border. There was a grade 2/6 blowing systolic murmur at the lower left sternal border, and it radiated to the apex and left axilla. S_2 was split widely with very little respiratory variation and a loud pulmonary component.

The electrocardiogram showed sinus rhythm, right atrial enlargement, a superior QRS axis with a counterclockwise frontal loop, and right ventricular hypertrophy. The hemoglobin was 19.6 mg. percent. The chest film (Fig. 1) showed a normal-sized heart in the frontal view, with a cardiothoracic ratio of 0.48. The main pulmonary artery and the central pulmonary arteries were prominent. In contrast, the more peripheral vessels appeared normal to decreased in size.

Cardiac catheterization revealed pulmonary artery pressure of 95/40 mm. Hg (mean 65) with simultaneous femoral artery pressure of 115/75 mm. Hg (mean 75). There was no left-to-right shunt by O_2 determinations, but a 40 percent atrial right-to-left shunt was demonstrated. The Qp/Qs was 0.68 with an Rp/Rs of 1.26. The Rp was 24 mm. Hg/l./min./M². There was no change in pulmonary artery pressure or degree of shunting following the inhalation of 100 percent oxygen or following the injection of 50 mg. of tolazoline into the pulmonary artery. Angiocardiography revealed an ostium primum type atrial septal defect with mild mitral regurgitation.

This young man's history indicates the progression of an operable, predominant left-to-right shunt atrial defect at age 3½ to an inoperable lesion with severe elevations of pulmonary vascular resistance by age 17. As is the case with most patients with atrial

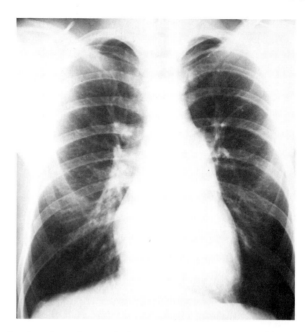

Figure 1. Chest film of patient A, a 17-year-old boy with an ostium primum type atrial septal defect and the Eisenmenger reaction. The pulmonary trunk and the proximal pulmonary arteries are prominent, in contrast to the normal or small peripheral pulmonary arteries.

septal defects, congestive heart failure in infancy or childhood was not a problem. The progression to severe elevation of pulmonary vascular resistance was accompanied by increasing fatigability with exercise, polycythemia, headaches, and hemoptysis. The chest film illustrates the normal heart size and abnormal pulmonary artery size and appearance in this syndrome.

Patient B

This 18-year-old girl was first referred at 14 years of age because of an elevated hemoglobin of 17.1 gm. percent. There was no past history of heart failure or precordial murmur. However, she had experienced increasing fatigability with strenuous exercise accompanied by circumoral cyanosis during the previous year. At age 14 she weighed 113 lb. and was 62 in. tall. Blood pressure was 130/90 mm. Hg. Heart rate was 112/min. The pulses were normal. There was mild cyanosis of her feet but no cyanosis of the hands or lips. There was a prominent right ventricular parasternal lift, a palpable pulmonary artery impulse, and a palpable S_2 at the upper left sternal border. S_1 was normal. S_2 was single or closely split with a loud pulmonary component. There was a grade 1/6 soft, short systolic murmur at the upper left sternal border.

The electrocardiogram showed sinus rhythm, right atrial enlargment, right axis deviation, and right ventricular hypertrophy. The chest film (Fig. 2) showed a normal-sized heart in the frontal plane, with a cardiothoracic ratio of 0.44. The main pulmonary artery segment was prominent, as were the peripheral pulmonary arteries. There was no distinct cutoff or disparity between the proximal and distal pulmonary arteries.

Cardiac catheterization revealed a pulmonary artery pressure of 105/70 mm. Hg (mean 85), aortic pressure of 105/60 mm. Hg (mean 85), and no detectable left-to-right shunt by O_2 determinations. There was a large right-to-left ductal shunt by O_2 and indicator dilution studies. There was no detectable change in pulmonary pressure or

540

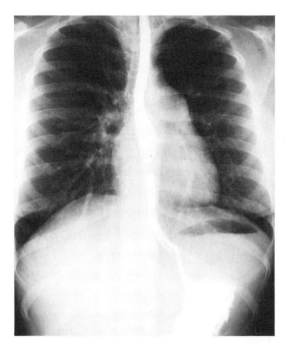

Figure 2. Chest film in patient B, an 18-year-old girl with a reversed shunting patent ductus. The heart size is normal with a prominent pulmonary trunk. Both the proximal and distal pulmonary arteries also appear prominent.

calculated flow with O_2 inhalation or tolazoline injection. Rp was 29 mm. Hg/l./min./M^2. Angiography revealed only a large, reversed shunting patent ductus arteriosus.

This patient illustrates the severe elevation of pulmonary vascular resistance which can occur with no antecedent history indicating a large left-to-right shunt. By inference, this patient had an elevated Rp from an early age since there was no indication of progression from a large left-to-right shunt with symptoms of left heart failure in infancy or childhood to a severe elevation of pulmonary vascular resistance in adolescence. Over the last 4 years her condition has remained stable, with no worsening of her effort intolerance or polycythemia.

CONCLUSION

Eisenmenger's syndrome is a condition of severe elevation of pulmonary vascular resistance occurring in a patient with balanced or predominant right-to-left shunting at the ventricular, aortic, or atrial level. Most of these patients can lead a reasonably active and productive life throughout adolescence and young adulthood by avoiding strenuous exertion. Some continue to do well into their 30s and 40s. These patients do need continuing supportive care for various medical problems from a physician who is interested in and knowledgable about congenital heart disease.

REFERENCES

1. EISENMENGER, V.: *Congenital defects of the ventricular septum.* Z. Klin. Med. Suppl. 32:1,1897.
2. WOOD, P.: *The Eisenmenger syndrome.* Br. Med. J. 2:701,755,1958.
3. HIRSCHFELD, S., MEYER, R., SCHWARTZ, D. C., ET AL.: *The echocardiographic assessment of pulmonary artery pressure and pulmonary vascular resistance.* Circulation 52:642,1975.

4. KRONGRAD, E., HELMHOLZ, H. J., JR., AND RITTER, D. G.: *Effect of breathing oxygen in patients with severe pulmonary vascular obstructive disease.* Circulation 47:94,1973.

5. CLARKSON, P. M., FRYE, R. L., DuSHANE, J. W., ET AL.: *Prognosis for patients with ventricular septal defect and severe pulmonary vascular obstructive disease.* Circulation 38:129,1968.

6. YOUNG, D., AND MARKS, H.: *Fate of the patient with the Eisenmenger syndrome.* Am. J. Cardiol. 28:659,1971.

7. BRAMMELL, H. S., VOGEL, J. H. K., PRYOR, R., ET AL.: *The Eisenmenger syndrome.* 28:679,1971.

8. LINDESMITH, G. G., STILES, Q. R., TUCKER, B. L., ET AL.: *The Mustard operation as a palliative procedure.* J. Thorac. Cardiovasc. Surg. 63:75,1972.

9. ROSENTHAL, A., NATHAN, D. G., MARTY, A. T., ET AL.: *Acute hemodynamic effects of red cell volume reduction in polycythemia of cyanotic congenital heart disease.* Circulation 42:297,1970.

10. ROSENTHAL, A., AND TYLER, D. C.: *General principles in the treatment of congenital heart disease.* In Gellis, S., and Kagan, B. M. (eds.): *Current Pediatric Therapy,* ed. 7. W B. Saunders, Philadelphia, 1976, pp. 137–140.

11. HEATH, D., AND EDWARDS, J. E.: *The pathology of hypertensive pulmonary vascular disease.* Circulation 18:533,1958.

12. HAROUTUNIAN, L. M., AND NEILL, C. A.: *Pulmonary complications of congenital heart disease: hemoptysis.* Am. Heart J. 84:540,1972.

13. JONES, A. M., AND HOWITT, G.: *Eisenmenger syndrome in pregnancy.* Br. Med. J. 1:1627,1965.

14. NEILSON, G., GALEA, E. G., AND BLUNT, A.: *Eisenmenger syndrome in pregnancy.* Med. J. Aust. 1:431,1971.

15. PITTS, J. A., CROSBY, W. M., AND BASTA, L. L.: *Eisenmenger syndrome in pregnancy.* Am. Heart J. 93:321,1977.

16. OAKLEY, C., AND SOMERVILLE, J.: *Oral contraceptives and progressive pulmonary vascular disease.* Lancet 1:890,1968.

17. MAURER, H. M.: *Hematologic effects of cardiac disease.* Pediat. Clin. N. Am. 19:1083,1972.

18. ROTH, A., ROSENTHAL, A., HALL, J. E., ET AL.: *Scoliosis and congenital heart disease.* Clin. Orthop. 93:95,1973.

19. FISCHBEIN, C. A., ROSENTHAL, A., FISCHER, E. G., ET AL.: *Risk factors for brain abscess in patients with congenital heart disease.* Am. J. Cardiol. 34:97,1974.

20. LIEBMAN, J., LUCAS, R., MOSS, A., ET AL.: *Airline travel for children with chronic pulmonary disease.* Pediatrics 57:408,1976.

Surgical Considerations in Treating Adults with Congenital Heart Disease

Gordon K. Danielson, M.D., and
Dwight C. McGoon, M.D.

Many congenital heart lesions are still being diagnosed or treated in adults. In many ways the surgical considerations and techniques of repair are similar to those used for infants and children, but for some lesions there are special features to be considered when surgical treatment is proposed and carried out in adult life.

How many patients with congenital heart disease are seen and treated as adults? A number of our surgical series were reviewed to determine what percentage of patients have undergone treatment of their congenital heart disease in adult life; the data are shown in Table 1. Atrial septal defect was the most common congenital heart defect seen in adults. In an early series of 397 patients undergoing repair of secundum atrial septal defect, 65 percent were between the ages of 20 and 69. Currently, more patients would be diagnosed in the infant and pediatric age group, but we still see many patients whose diagnosis is first made in adult life. Of 101 patients with partial AV canal, 15 percent were over age 20. Untreated complete atrioventricular canal, however, is a more lethal lesion and none of our patients were operated upon as adults. A significant number of patients with total anomalous pulmonary venous connection and anomalous systemic venous connection were adults, and the majority of patients with aortic sinus fistula were age 21 or older. A summary of two large series[1,2] supplies statistics for coarctation of the aorta; 36 percent of this large group were between 20 and 60 years of age.

A small number of patients with corrected transposition are first encountered in adult life. Even a few patients with coronary artery disease are found to have congenital heart defects. In the first 154 patients undergoing saphenous vein bypass grafting on one surgical service, three were found to have congenital defects; one of these patients had a two-chambered right ventricle and ventricular septal defect (VSD), another had VSD, and a third had atrial septal defect. Double outlet right ventricle, Ebstein's anomaly, patent ductus arteriosus, and pulmonary atresia are also encountered in adults.

Although the current incidence of pulmonary stenosis and tetralogy of Fallot in adults is less than the percentages shown in Table 1, which are taken from our earlier series, these conditions are still being encountered in adult patients. Transposition of the great arteries and truncus arteriosus are two severe anomalies which usually result in early death, and patients over the age of 23 were not encountered in the series shown. Two of ten patients who underwent the Fontan procedure for tricuspid atresia were ages 22 and 31.

In a review of 122 patients with univentricular heart (single or common ventricle) examined at our institution, 30 percent were in the adult group. As a number of forms of this anomaly are now correctable, proper diagnosis and evaluation of this condition are assuming increasing importance.

Finally, VSD is another congenital cardiac defect which may be first diagnosed or treated in adult life.[4]

In addition to the statistics for individual anomalies shown in Table 1, a review was made in 1976 of the 1333 operations performed with the aid of extracorporeal circulation at our institution. Of the 394 patients undergoing repair of congenital heart disease, 62 (16 percent) were over 21 years of age.[5]

ATRIAL SEPTAL DEFECT

Figure 1 shows the chest x-ray of a 71-year-old woman who was admitted for cataract surgery. During her workup the diagnosis of *atrial septal defect* was made. She had a known murmur for six years and had been in congestive heart failure with atrial fibrillation for five years. She remained in borderline cardiac compensation while taking digoxin and hydrochlorothiazide. The catheterization data showed normal pulmonary artery pressure (21/6 mm. Hg), low pulmonary resistance (2.6 units m^2), and a pulmonary blood flow twice systemic flow (Qp/Qs = 2). The decision for operation was rather straightforward here, in spite of her age, and she underwent successful patch closure of two atrial septal defects. One might question the decision to operate upon a patient in this age group, or even upon a somewhat younger patient who is less symptomatic. However, these patients do return with significant symptoms at a still older age when their operative risk is much higher.

Figure 2 shows the chest x-ray of a 79-year-old inventor who was known to have an atrial septal defect for many years. He had successfully avoided operation until he had reached "end-stage" cardiac disability. He had giant cardiomegaly, tricuspid regurgita-

Table 1. Incidence of congenital heart disease in adults repaired at the Mayo Clinic

Anomaly	No. of Patients	Adults No.	%	Age Range, years
ASD—secundum	397	259	65	20–69
ASD—primum				
Partial A-V canal	101	15	15	20–48
Complete A-V canal	27	0	0	——
Total anomalous pulmonary venous connection	54	10	19	20–37
Anomalous systemic venous return	100	7	7	20–50
Aortic sinus fistula	21	15	71	21–52
Coarctation*	671	242	36	20–60
Corrected transposition	25	4	16	15–48
Coronary artery disease	154	3	2	37–55
Double outlet right ventricle	40	1	3	33
Ebstein's anomaly	20	8	40	20–51
Patent ductus arteriosus	223	81	36	20–54
Pulmonary atresia	103	22	21	20–38
Pulmonary stenosis	221	49	22	21–66
Tetralogy of Fallot	285	66	23	15–54
Transposition of great arteries	128	—	—	up to 23
Tricuspid atresia	10	2	—	22, 31
Truncus arteriosus	92	—	—	up to 21
Univentricular heart	122	36	30	20–38
Ventricular septal defect*	300	34	11	20–49

* Series taken from the literature

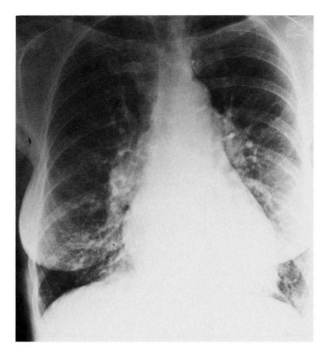

Figure 1. AP chest x-ray of a 71-year-old woman with symptomatic atrial septal defect.

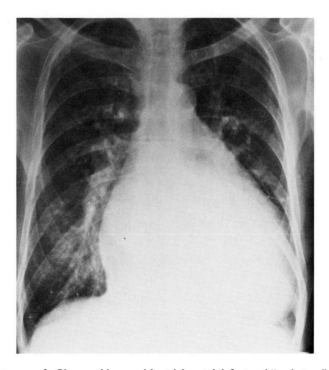

Figure 2. AP chest x-ray of a 79-year-old man with atrial septal defect and "end-stage" cardiac disability.

tion, and massive peripheral edema with associated stasis dermatitis. He was taking furosemide, 200 mg. a day, spironolactone, 75 mg. a day, and digoxin as well as other medications. The cardiac rhythm was chronic atrial fibrillation with multiple ventricular premature beats. The catheterization data on this patient showed moderately severe pulmonary hypertension (55/25 mm. Hg), but the calculated pulmonary resistance (4.2 units m²) was only moderately elevated. He still had a large pulmonary shunt (Qp/Qs = 2.8). The patient and his wife were now very desirous of operation in spite of the risks involved, so we accepted him as an operative candidate. An umbrella closure of atrial septal defect was considered, but the defect was too large to be closed by the largest umbrella available at that time (for defects < 40 mm.). He underwent patch closure of the defect and tricuspid annuloplasty, but could not be weaned from cardiopulmonary bypass after one hour of assisted circulation, so an intra-aortic balloon was inserted. The balloon could be removed 20 hours after operation and he was discharged from the hospital on the thirteenth postoperative day. Clearly it would have been preferable to correct this man's defect at an earlier stage in his disease.

Figure 3A shows the anterior-posterior (AP) chest x-ray taken on a 73-year-old woman who underwent suture closure of atrial septal defect and tricuspid annuloplasty for pulmonary hypertension, chronic atrial fibrillation, and intractable congestive heart failure. She had been seen at our institution five years earlier when she was minimally symptomatic, but she was not considered to be a surgical candidate then because of her age (68 years). We have seen a number of patients who have followed this same clinical course; we now advise closure of all atrial septal defects regardless of age, unless there is some other serious medical contraindication. Figure 3B shows her chest x-ray eight days after operation.

Another reason for closing an atrial septal defect upon diagnosis is illustrated by a 55-year-old engraver-designer whose x-ray is shown in Figure 4. Note the aneurysmal, calcified pulmonary arteries. He had severe pulmonary vascular obstructive disease (Rp = 15.1 units m²), right-to-left shunt, and was clearly inoperable. Although this was explained to him by several physicians, when last seen he was making the rounds of various medical clinics trying to persuade someone to operate upon him.

Between 1965 and 1976, 24 patients between the ages of 60 and 78 underwent surgical

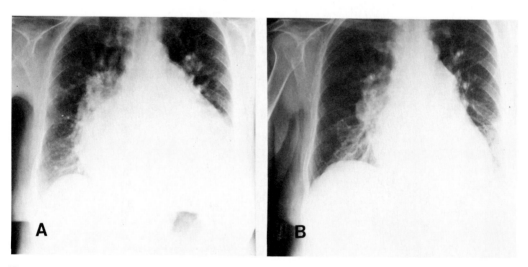

Figure 3. A, AP chest x-ray of a 73-year-old woman with atrial septal defect, pulmonary hypertension, chronic atrial fibrillation, and intractable congestive heart failure. B, AP chest x-ray eight days after suture closure of atrial septal defect and tricuspid annuloplasty. Note the marked reduction in heart size.

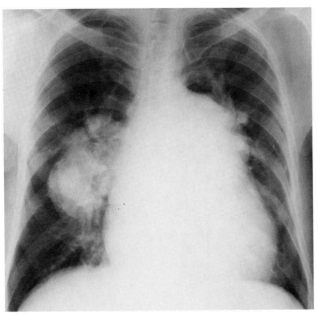

Figure 4. AP chest x-ray of a 55-year-old man with atrial septal defect, severe pulmonary vascular obstructive disease, and aneurysmal, calcified pulmonary arteries.

repair of their atrial septal defect at our institution.[6] Three patients underwent concomitant tricuspid annuloplasty. There was one death (mortality, 4 percent). This deceased patient also had severe three-vessel coronary artery disease. There were no operative deaths in 79 consecutive patients whose ages ranged from 40 to 60 years. If one excludes the operative mortality, survival curves are identical to those of patients matched for age and sex in a general population. By contrast, without operation 90 percent of adults with atrial septal defect have died by age 60; and after age 50, the annual mortality is 6 to 8 percent per year.[6]

Sometimes the decision regarding operability can be difficult, as in the case of a 26-year-old cachectic woman who had undergone attempted closure of a septum primum atrial septal defect at age 12. She now had a large residual atrial septal defect, severe mitral regurgitation, and progressive congestive heart failure (Fig. 5A). The cardiac catheterization data were very worrisome. The total pulmonary resistance was greater than 28 units, and even the pulmonary arteriolar resistance was calculated at 16.5 units. In patients with left-to-right shunts we have generally considered resistance between 8 and 10 units or higher as contraindicating operation on the basis of severe pulmonary vascular obstructive disease. However, this patient did have severe mitral regurgitation, and it was reasoned she might behave more like a patient who had a mitral valve replacement than one who had a shunt closed following operation. Furthermore, she still had a moderate left-to-right shunt (Qp/Qs = 1.4). Operation was performed by patching the atrial septal defect and replacing the mitral valve with a 35-mm. Hancock prosthesis. Cardiac catheterization performed prior to discharge showed that the pulmonary arterial pressure was still at systemic levels. One year later, however, the heart size had decreased considerably and she was asymptomatic (Fig. 5B). She had gained 25 pounds, had developed secondary sexual characteristics, and had taken a job as a key punch operator. Pulmonary pressure had fallen to 33/15 mm. Hg. Thus, in this patient the elevated pulmonary vascular resistance was caused in

547

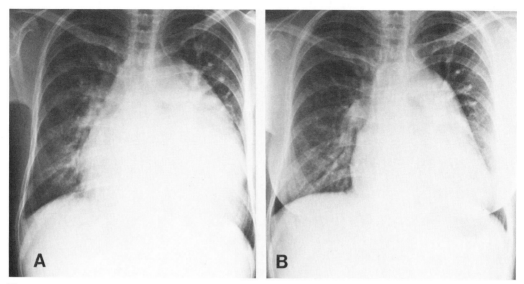

Figure 5. A, AP x-ray of a 26-year-old cachectic woman with septum primum atrial septal defect, severe mitral regurgitation, and advanced congestive heart failure. B, Chest x-ray of the same woman one year after patch closure of atrial septal defect and mitral valve replacement with Hancock prosthesis.

large measure by the severe mitral regurgitation, and her pulmonary hypertension proved to be largely reversible.

TOTAL ANOMALOUS PULMONARY VENOUS CONNECTION

Total anomalous pulmonary venous connection (TAPVC) in adults has hemodynamics similar to those of atrial septal defect. Figure 6 shows the chest x-ray of a 29-year-old salesman who complained of dyspnea on exertion and occasional bouts of tachycardia.

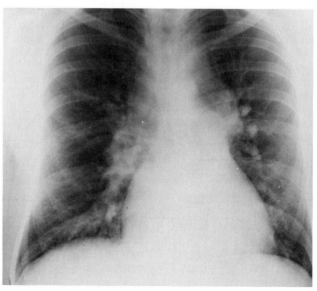

Figure 6. AP chest x-ray of a 29-year-old man with supracardiac total anomalous pulmonary venous connection.

548

He was first evaluated at a medical center where he was believed to have a mediastinal tumor. He was seen four years later at a second medical center where he was correctly diagnosed as having supracardiac TAPVC. There is a widening of the superior mediastinum on both the right and left sides of the midline; this is the result of an anomalous pulmonary venous connection to a left vertical vein together with a large superior vena cava (snowman configuration). He underwent successful repair of his anomaly. The hemodynamic assessment for patients with TAPVC is the same as for patients with atrial septal defect unless there is pulmonary venous obstruction, in which case calculation of the pulmonary vascular (arteriolar) resistance is more difficult and less meaningful. The mortality risk of surgical repair is related to the degree of pulmonary hypertension and currently averages less than 5 percent for adults.[7]

ANOMALOUS SYSTEMIC VENOUS CONNECTION

Anomalous systemic venous connection in the adult can take many forms.[8] Figure 7A shows the chest x-ray of a 37-year-old housewife who had intense cyanosis with digital clubbing, progressive dyspnea on exertion, and fatigue. At cardiac catheterization and at subsequent operation she was found to have isolated dextrocardia; right superior vena cava draining to right atrium; azygos continuation of the left inferior vena cava to the left superior vena cava and from there to the left atrium; hepatic venous and coronary sinus drainage to the left atrium; atrial septal defect; and VSD (Fig. 7B). Repair was accomplished by inserting a prosthetic baffle into the left lateral and cephalad portions of the left atrium so as to direct the hepatic and left superior vena caval blood to the right atrium. The atrial septal defect was closed with the same patch and the VSD was sutured (Fig. 7C). Most patients with anomalous systemic venous connection have associated cardiovascular defects, and the risk of operation is that of the associated defects. When this condition is recognized, either preoperatively or intraoperatively, it need not prevent successful intracardiac repair of associated anomalies or affect operative mortality or postoperative morbidity.

COARCTATION OF THE AORTA

In some reported series over 30 percent of patients with *coarctation of the aorta* have been first diagnosed or treated in adult life (Table 1).[1,2] Surgical treatment is more difficult in adults since the aorta is more sclerotic, aneurysms of the intercostal arteries are common, and there may be associated cardiovascular disease. Repair is facilitated by use of bypass or interposition grafts[2] or patch graft angioplasty.[9] An example is a 36-year-old hypertensive housewife who was admitted with a blood pressure of 190/110 mm. Hg. Systemic hypertension had been diagnosed 14 years earlier; subsequently a heart murmur developed suddenly and significant mitral regurgitation was noted. A thoracic aortogram revealed severe coarctation of the aorta with two poststenotic aneurysms (Fig. 8A). Cardiac catheterization demonstrated associated massive mitral regurgitation with pulmonary hypertension (pulmonary artery pressure 96/47 mm. Hg). Repair of both lesions was undertaken through a left thoracotomy. Figure 8B shows the operative specimen including the involved aorta, coarctation, and two aneurysms. The opened specimen is shown in Figure 8C. The defect was bridged with a graft (Fig. 8D). During the operation cardiopulmonary bypass was instituted and the mitral valve was inspected and found to have ruptured chordae along the anterior leaflet. The mitral regurgitation was alleviated by plication of the anterior leaflet and construction of an eccentric posterior annuloplasty.

In adults with coarctation the inelastic aortic segments may be difficult to bring together following excision of the stenosed segment. Thus, use of a graft or patch-graft

549

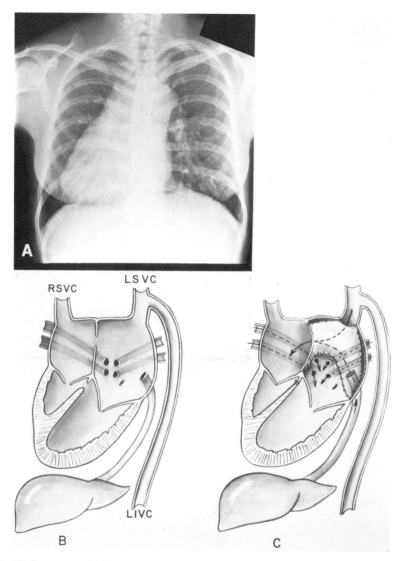

Figure 7. A, AP chest x-ray of a 37-year-old woman who had intense cyanosis with digital clubbing, progressive dyspnea on exertion, and fatigue. B, Diagram of intracardiac anatomy showing isolated dextrocardia, right superior vena cava draining to right atrium; azygos continuation of the left inferior vena cava to the left superior vena cava, and from there to the left atrium; hepatic venous and coronary sinus drainage to the left atrium; atrial septal defect; and VSD. C, Repair was accomplished by inserting a prosthetic baffle into the left lateral and cephalad portions of the left atrium so as to direct the hepatic and left superior vena caval blood to the right atrium. The atrial septal defect was closed with the same patch and the VSD was sutured.

angioplasty facilitates repair in the majority of adults. These techniques also obviate the need for extensive dissection and mobilization of the aorta with ligation of intercostal arteries, and thus decrease the hazards of serious hemorrhage and spinal cord ischemia. The operative risk for repair of coarctation of the aorta in the adult is less than 5 percent,[2,10] but the chances for complete relief of hypertension are not as good as for younger patients. The reasons for this are unknown, although many mechanisms have been suggested.[11,12]

550

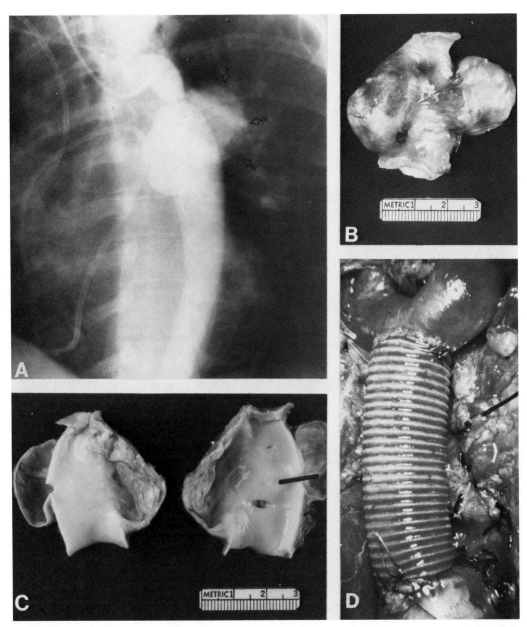

Figure 8. Thoracic aortogram from a 36-year-old hypertensive housewife showing severe coarctation of the aorta with two poststenotic aneurysms. Arrows point to lateral aneurysm. Cardiac catheterization demonstrated associated massive mitral insufficiency with pulmonary hypertension. Repair of both lesions was undertaken through a left thoracotomy. B, Photograph of the operative specimen showing involved aorta, coarctation, and two aneurysms. C, Opened specimen with black marker at ostium of lateral aneurysm. D, The defect was bridged with a prosthetic graft. During the operation cardiopulmonary bypass was instituted, the mitral valve was inspected and found to have ruptured chordae along the anterior leaflet, and repair was carried out by plication of the anterior leaflet and construction of an eccentric posterior annuloplasty.

CORRECTED TRANSPOSITION

Of our 25 patients with *corrected transposition,* 4 (16 percent) ranged in age from 15 to 48 years (Table 1). The oldest patient was asymptomatic until he developed sudden complete heart block and required implantation of a pacemaker (Fig. 9). Repair of anomalies associated with corrected transposition involves many technical considerations and should be undertaken with the aid of intracardiac electrophysiologic mapping. In situs solitus patients with this condition the conduction bundle runs anterior to the pulmonary trunk and anterior to the VSD; this is in contrast to the typical location of the conduction bundle in other congenital cardiac anomalies—posterior and inferior to the VSD. The incidence of surgical heart block has been high in earlier series but has been reduced recently by knowledge of the course of the conduction system, intracardiac mapping of the specialized conduction tissue, use of external conduits to bypass pulmonary valvular and subvalvular stenosis, and proper placement of the ventriculotomy in the pulmonary ventricle.[13,14] Insufficiency of the right or left atrioventricular valve, or both, is common in corrected transposition and adds to the difficulty of repair. The risk for operation, which depends on the type and number of associated anomalies, has been reduced from 50 percent to 12 percent.[13,14]

One special technical problem may be encountered in adult patients who have longstanding right ventricular hypertension, especially in the presence of arterial desaturation (e.g., cyanotic heart disease with pulmonic stenosis and VSD). Typically, the ventricles in these patients are massively hypertrophied and diffusely fibrotic. However, the myocardium is friable and holds sutures poorly in spite of the fibrotic appearance. Sutures must be placed deeply and tied carefully to avoid cutting through the tissues. The problem is compounded if there is residual right ventricular hypertension after the repair, which may result from a number of conditions including hypoplastic distal pulmonary arteries and longstanding shunts which have caused pulmonary vascular obstructive disease. In some patients the septum is also friable, making secure closure of the VSD difficult. Use of mattress sutures passed through pledgets of Teflon felt and reinforcement of suture lines with over-and-over sutures are useful technical adjuncts.

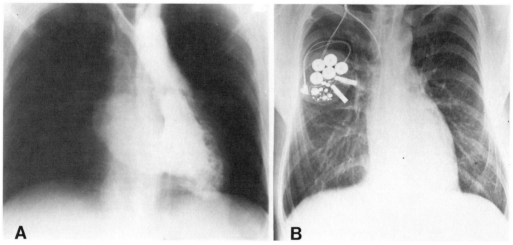

Figure 9. A, Angiogram from systemic ventricle in a 48-year-old man with corrected transposition who developed sudden complete heart block. A morphological right ventricle fills a left-sided (and anterior) aorta. Some reflux into the left atrium through an insufficient left AV (tricuspid) valve is seen. B, Transvenous pacemaker lead could be satisfactorily located in the pulmonary (morphological left) ventricle for treatment of the complete heart block.

EBSTEIN'S ANOMALY

Repair of *Ebstein's anomaly* can be performed well in both childhood and adult life. We prefer a reconstruction in which the atrialized portion of the right ventricle is plicated, the tricuspid valve is narrowed by annuloplasty, and the atrial septal defect is closed. This repair avoids replacement of the tricuspid valve with a prosthesis, reduces the cardiac size, and has given good to excellent results in 14 of 16 patients.[15,16]

TRANSPOSITION OF THE GREAT ARTERIES

Transposition of the great arteries is a rare anomaly in patients over age 20 (Table 1).[17,18] The oldest patient we know of in whom repair was successfully accomplished was a 44-year-old man who had associated VSD, pulmonary stenosis, and juxtaposition of the atrial appendages on the left (Fig. 10A). His parents had expected him to die at any time, so he had not been taught to read or write. He had marked cyanosis and digital clubbing and also had severe osteoarthropathy with thickened periosteum and pain in the extremities (Fig. 10, B and C). Repair was accomplished by the Rastelli technique in which blood is directed from the left ventricle through the VSD to the aorta with an intraventricular patch, and blood is directed from the right ventricle to the pulmonary

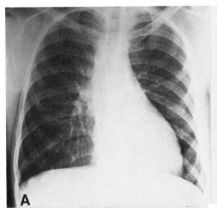

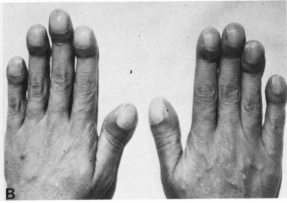

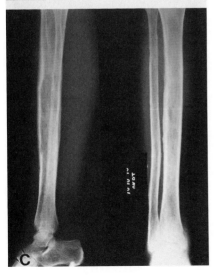

Figure 10. A, AP chest x-ray of a 44-year-old man who had transposition of the great arteries, VSD, pulmonary stenosis, and juxtaposition of the atrial appendages on the left. B, Photograph of hands showing marked digital clubbing. C, X-ray of the legs demonstrated changes of osteoarthropathy with thickened periosteum. Repair was successfully carried out by the Rastelli technique[18] with subsequent regression of the digital clubbing and osteoarthropathy.

553

artery by an external valved conduit.[18] It is interesting that his extremity pain disappeared immediately postoperatively when the arterial saturation was raised to normal levels. The current surgical risk for repair of transposition with VSD and pulmonary stenosis is 8 percent.[18]

PATENT DUCTUS ARTERIOSUS

Repair of *patent ductus arteriosus* is more hazardous in adults than in infants because the majority of adults have calcific deposits in the walls of the ductus and adjoining aorta. Application of a clamp on a calcified ductus or aorta may result in catastrophic hemorrhage. We have encountered patients in whom the calcium has not been seen by fluoroscopy or by laminagrams but who nevertheless had significant calcific deposits present at operation. Thus, any adult with patent ductus arteriosus should be suspected of having significant calcific deposits until proven otherwise. Several operative approaches are available. In one, the left chest is opened and cardiopulmonary bypass is instituted with venous cannulation of the right atrial appendage, right ventricle, or pulmonary trunk and with arterial cannulation of the aorta or its branches both above and below the level of the ductus.[19] The aorta is clamped proximal and distal to the ductus, well away from the calcific deposits in the wall of the aorta. If the ductus near the pulmonary artery is not calcified, a clamp can be placed at that level. Alternatively, the orifice can be temporarily occluded with a balloon catheter, or the proximal pulmonary trunk can be clamped to initiate total cardiopulmonary bypass. The aorta is opened opposite the ductus and the orifice is closed with a large patch sewn inside the aorta beyond the area of calcific deposits. We have used this technique successfully on several occasions but now prefer the following approach, which is simpler and easier.

The patient is placed in a supine position and a standard median sternotomy is performed. Total bypass is instituted by separate caval cannulation. The pulmonary arterial end of the ductus is dissected free. Usually this will be found to be free of calcium and it can then be clamped and excised from the pulmonary artery, taking a small portion of the pulmonary artery wall. The end is then oversewn and the defect in the pulmonary artery closed by direct suture. Alternatively, the pulmonary artery can be opened as for a Potts shunt[20] and oversewn from within. This method is particularly useful for the recanalized or incompletely ligated patent ductus.

As in all patients who have congenital cardiac lesions which allow left-to-right shunts, patients with patent ductus arteriosus must be carefully evaluated preoperatively with regard to the presence and severity of pulmonary vascular obstructive disease. In patent ductus the hemodynamics are similar to those for a Potts anastomosis.[21] Pulmonary resistance between 8 and 10 units or higher is considered indicative of severe pulmonary vascular disease and contraindicates closure of the shunt. Operative mortality in the absence of severe vascular disease is less than 1 percent.

PULMONARY STENOSIS

Of the first 221 patients with *pulmonary stenosis* who underwent repair at the Mayo Clinic, 22 percent were between 21 and 66 years of age.[22] It is generally agreed that patients who have a peak systolic pressure gradient across the pulmonary valve of 80 mm. Hg or more should undergo surgical relief of the obstruction even if they are asymptomatic when first seen, in view of the poor natural history of severe pulmonary stenosis.[23] Patients with a gradient from 50 to 79 mm. Hg fare much better clinically, but their outcome is even more favorable after surgical treatment.[23] Patients with mild gradients of 49 mm. Hg or less can be followed, and they may do well for many years. However, we have seen such patients return in congestive heart failure with cyanosis from right-to-left shunting at the atrial level in later life. The surgical risk for correction of pulmonary stenosis in adults is less than one percent if performed before cyanosis and congestive heart failure appear.[22,23]

PULMONARY ATRESIA

In our series of 103 patients with *pulmonary atresia*, 21 percent were between 20 and 38 years of age.[24] Subsequently, we have had patients as old as 54 years undergo successful operation for repair or palliation. New concepts of management have enlarged the possibilities for surgical improvement of many patients who were previously considered inoperable. The various forms of pulmonary atresia are shown in Figure 11. Figure 12 diagrams the technique for repair when there is no discontinuity between the

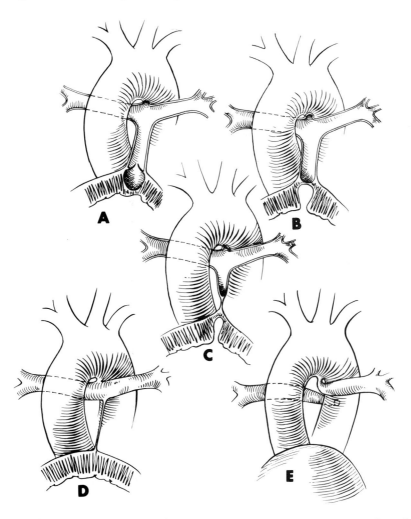

Figure 11. Types of pulmonary atresia classified according to most downstream extent of atretic zone. A, Atresia of right ventricular outflow tract. B, Pulmonary valve atresia. C, Proximal pulmonary arterial atresia. D, Distal pulmonary arterial atresia. E, Proximal branch arterial atresia (nonconfluence). In this example the left pulmonary artery arises from left ductus arteriosus and right pulmonary artery is supplied by a collateral artery arising from descending thoracic aorta.

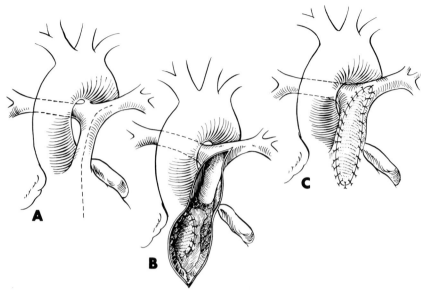

Figure 12. Repair of valvular, infundibular, or localized proximal pulmonary arterial atresia. A, Incision is made across outflow tract, pulmonary valve, and main pulmonary artery into left pulmonary artery, if main pulmonary artery is hypoplastic. B, Pulmonary valve and obstructing infundibular tissue are resected and VSD is closed with a knitted Teflon patch. C, Outflow tract is enlarged with a pericardial patch.

right ventricle and pulmonary artery. Figure 13 shows repair with a Hancock prosthesis when discontinuity is present.

After the ventricular anatomy has been defined in patients with pulmonary atresia, a thoracic aortogram is performed (Fig. 14A). This is followed by selective injection of the systemic-pulmonary collateral arteries with late filming. The patient in Figure 14 has hypoplastic confluent right and left pulmonary arteries (Fig. 14, B and C). Figure 15A shows an operative photograph of reconstruction of the right ventricular outflow tract with a pericardial patch. If a significant gap is present between the right ventricle and confluent pulmonary arteries, the pericardial patch can be closed posteriorly at its midportion to form a tube conduit. Figure 15B shows the postoperative right ventriculogram and demonstrates a direct connection and improved blood flow to the confluent pulmonary arteries. With time the pulmonary arteries increase in size under the high pressure from the right ventricle, and many of these patients are expected to be candidates for total repair when the pulmonary arteries have grown sufficiently. In the absence of complicating problems the risk of palliation is less than five percent; the operative risk for total repair is less than ten percent.

TETRALOGY OF FALLOT

Tetralogy of Fallot in adults can be repaired with a mortality risk similar to that for repair in children (5 percent or less). Figure 16 shows the AP chest x-ray of a 44-year-old executive who had tetralogy of Fallot. He had undergone a previous Brock valvotomy, and subsequently the pulmonary valve calcified. Complete repair was undertaken in the usual manner by resection of the infundibular pulmonary stenosis and pulmonary valve, patch closure of the VSD, and pericardial patch enlargement of the right ventricular outflow tract. For some adults, particularly those who have had previous shunts and

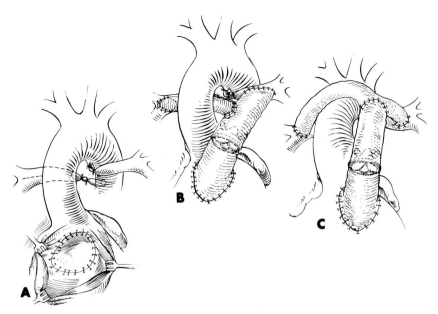

Figure 13. Repair of pulmonary atresia by means of a valved conduit. In this example the left pulmonary artery receives blood from a left patent ductus arteriosus and right pulmonary artery is supplied by a collateral artery. A, After institution of cardiopulmonary bypass, the ductus and collateral artery are doubly ligated. Vertical ventriculotomy is made and VSD is closed with a knitted Teflon patch; cephalad end of patch is attached to cephalad end of ventriculotomy. B, Dacron graft containing a glutaraldehyde-preserved porcine valve is sewn end-to-side to left pulmonary artery. Smaller graft, without valve, is carried behind aorta to join prosthesis to right pulmonary artery. Proximal portion of prosthesis is trimmed and used to close right ventriculotomy. C, Alternatively, a straight-tube graft can be used to connect right and left pulmonary arteries, and distal end of valved conduit can be sewn end-to-side to tube graft. If graft to right pulmonary artery does not lie satisfactorily posterior to ascending aorta, it may be arched cephalad and anterior to ascending aorta, as shown, to prevent compression beneath sternum.

elevated pulmonary arterial pressures, placing a valved conduit in the outflow tract might be considered to improve hemodynamics and decrease right ventricular diastolic pressures. As mentioned previously, a technical aspect which may be troublesome relates to a defective right ventricular muscle which holds sutures poorly.

UNIVENTRICULAR HEART

Univentricular heart (common or single ventricle) is another condition encountered in adult life. In a review of 122 patients seen at our institution, 30 percent were between 20 and 38 years of age.[3] An improved understanding of the anatomy, conduction system, and physiology of univentricular heart with two atrioventricular valves now allows patients with this anomaly to be accepted for operation if they show significant or progressive symptoms. The most favorable types of univentricular heart are those with outlet chambers, especially where the chamber is anterior and to the left; the most favorable subtype of the latter group includes those with natural pulmonary stenosis. For this group surgical repair can now be undertaken with an expected mortality of 20 percent or less. The results of our experience with septation of univentricular heart have been summarized recently.[25,26]

Figure 17A shows univentricular heart with an outlet chamber located anteriorly and to the left, from which the aorta arises. Pulmonary stenosis is present. The conduction

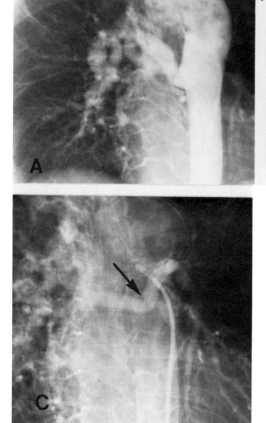
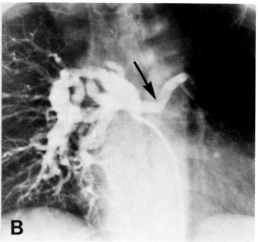

Figure 14. A, Thoracic aortogram of a 54-year-old woman with pulmonary atresia. No pulmonary arteries are identified. B, Selective injection of one systemic-pulmonary collateral artery suggests presence of a confluent right and left pulmonary artery (arrow). C, Late films confirm the presence of confluent right and left pulmonary arteries (arrow).

bundle courses along the cephalad and anterior rim of the bulboventricular foramen. In Figure 17B repair has been carried out by placing the septation patch to the right of both semilunar valves at the cephalad line of attachment. The proximal pulmonary artery has been ligated and a valved conduit (Hancock) has been placed between the "right" ventriculotomy and the distal pulmonary artery.

VARIOUS LEFT-TO-RIGHT SHUNTS

Ventricular septal defect, left ventricular-to-right atrial fistula, aortic sinus fistula, and *other left-to-right shunts* are repaired in a standard fashion. The major concern is to identify those patients who have developed pulmonary vascular obstructive disease and whose risk for operation is thereby increased or made prohibitive. In the absence of significant pulmonary arterial hypertension, the risk for repair in adults is between 1 and 2 percent.

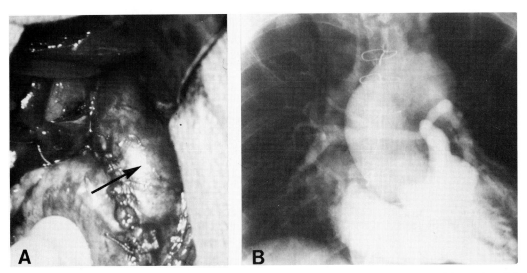

Figure 15. A, Operative photograph of reconstruction of the right ventricular outflow tract with a pericardial patch (arrow). B, Postoperative right ventriculogram demonstrating a direct connection and improved blood flow to the confluent pulmonary arteries.

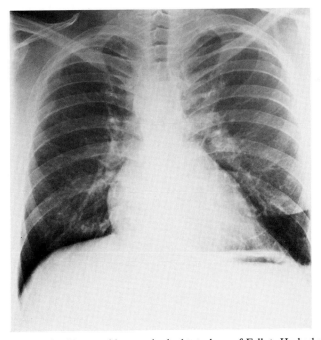

Figure 16. AP chest x-ray of a 44-year-old man who had tetralogy of Fallot. He had previously undergone a Brock valvotomy and now has a calcified pulmonary valve.

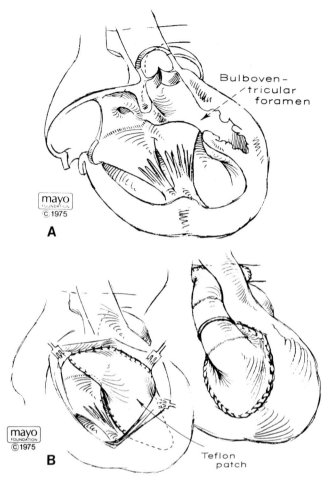

Figure 17. A, Diagram of univentricular heart with an outlet chamber located anteriorly and to the left, from which the aorta arises. Pulmonary stenosis is present. B, Repair is carried out by placing a septation patch to the right of both semilunar valves at the cephalad line of attachment. The proximal pulmonary artery has been ligated and a valved conduit (Hancock) has been placed between the "right" ventriculotomy and the distal pulmonary artery.

In summary, a wide spectrum of congenital cardiac anomalies can be encountered in adults, and most can be corrected with a low risk of surgical mortality and good to excellent clinical results. Special features to be considered when surgical treatment is proposed and carried out in adult life have been reviewed.

REFERENCES

1. SCHUSTER, S. R., AND GROSS, R. E.: *Coarctation of the aorta: a review of 500 surgically corrected cases.* Heart Bulletin 11:105,1962.
2. MORRIS, G. J., JR., COOLEY, D. A., DEBAKEY, M. E., ET AL.: *Coarctation of the aorta with particular emphasis upon improved techniques of surgical repair.* J. Thorac. Cardiovasc. Surg. 40:705,1960.
3. MOODIE, D. S., TAJIK, A. J., AND RITTER, D. G.: *The natural history of common (single) ventricle.* Am. J. Cardiol. 39:311,1977.

4. COOLEY, D. A., GARRETT, H. E., AND HOWARD, H. S.: *The surgical treatment of ventricular septal defect: an analysis of 300 consecutive surgical cases.* Prog. Cardiovasc. Dis. 4:312,1962.

5. RITTER, D. G.: Unpublished data.

6. SUCHOR, R. J., AND TAJIK, A.: Unpublished data.

7. GOMES, M. M. R., FELDT, R. H., McGOON, D. C., ET AL.: *Total anomalous pulmonary venous connection: surgical considerations and results of operation.* J. Thorac. Cardiovasc. Surg. 60:116,1970.

8. DELEVAL, M. R., RITTER, D. G., McGOON, D. C., ET AL.: *Anomalous systemic venous connection: surgical considerations.* Mayo Clin. Proc. 50:599,1975.

9. MOOR, G. F., IONESCU, M. I., AND ROSS, D. N.: *Surgical repair of coarctation of the aorta by patch grafting.* Ann. Thorac. Surg. 14:626,1972.

10. OSTERMILLER, W. E., JR., SOMERNDIKE, J. M., HUNTER, J. A., ET AL.: *Coarctation of the aorta in adult patients.* J. Thorac. Cardiovasc. Surg. 61:125,1971.

11. BAILEY, C. P.: *Surgical treatment of coarctation of the aorta: report of the section on cardiovascular surgery.* Dis. Chest 31:468,1957.

12. MARON, B. J., HUMPHRIES, J. O., ROWE, R. D., ET AL.: *Prognosis of surgically corrected coarctation of the aorta: a 20-year postoperative appraisal.* Circulation 47:119,1973.

13. DANIELSON, G. K., McGOON, D. C., WALLACE, R. B., ET AL.: *Surgery of corrected transposition. Second European Symposium on Paediatric Cardiology. London, June 13–15, 1977. Proceedings of the Paediatric Cardiology Symposium, Churchill Livingstone, in press.*

14. MARCELLETTI, C., MALONEY, J. D., RITTER, D. G., ET AL.: *Corrected transposition and ventricular septal defect: surgical experience.* Unpublished data.

15. McFAUL, R. C., DAVIS, Z., GIULIANI, E. R., ET AL.: *Ebstein's malformation.* J. Thorac. Cardiovasc. Surg. 72:910,1976.

16. DANIELSON, G. K., MALONEY, J. D., and Devloo, R. A. E.: *Surgical repair of Ebstein's anomaly.* Mayo Clin. Proc. In press.

17. DANIELSON, G. K., MAIR, D. D., ONGLEY, P. A., ET AL.: *Repair of transposition of the great arteries by transposition of venous return.* J. Thorac. Cardiovasc. Surg. 61:96,1971.

18. MARCELLETTI, C., MAIR, D. D., McGOON, D. C., ET AL.: *The Rastelli operation for transposition of the great arteries: early and late results.* J. Thorac. Cardiovasc. Surg. 72:427,1976.

19. MORROW, A. G., AND CLARK, W. D.: *Closure of the calcified patent ductus: a new operative method utilizing cardiopulmonary bypass.* J. Thorac. Cardiovasc. Surg. 51:534,1966.

20. KIRKLIN, J. W., AND DEVLOO, R. A.: *Hypothermic perfusion and circulatory arrest for surgical correction of tetralogy of Fallot with previously constructed Potts anastomosis.* Dis. Chest 39:87,1961.

21. VON BERNUTH, G., RITTER, D. G., FRYE, R. L., ET AL.: *Evaluation of patients with tetralogy of Fallot and Potts anastomosis.* Am. J. Cardiol. 27:259,1971.

22. DANIELSON, G. K., EXARHOS, N. D., WEIDMAN, W. H., ET AL.: *Pulmonic stenosis with intact ventricular septum: surgical considerations and results of operation.* J. Thorac. Cardiovasc. Surg. 61:228,1971.

23. NUGENT, E. W., FREEDOM, R. M., NORA, J. J., ET AL.: *Clinical course in pulmonary stenosis. Report from the Joint Study on the Natural History of Congenital Heart Defects.* Circulation 56(Suppl. I):38,1977.

24. OLIN, C. L., RITTER, D. G., McGOON, D. C., ET AL.: *Pulmonary atresia: surgical considerations and results in 103 patients undergoing definitive repair.* Circulation 54(Suppl. II):35,1976.

25. DANIELSON, G. K., McGOON, D. C., MALONEY, J. D., ET AL.: *Surgery of primitive ventricle with outlet chamber. Second European Symposium on Paediatric Cardiology. London, June 13–15, 1977. Proceedings of the Pediatric Cardiology Symposium, Churchill Livingstone, in press.*

26. McGOON, D. C., DANIELSON, G. K., RITTER, D. G., ET AL.: *Correction of the univentricular heart having two atrioventricular valves.* J. Thorac. Cardiovasc. Surg. 74:218,1977.

Index